Skin in Rheumatologic Diseases

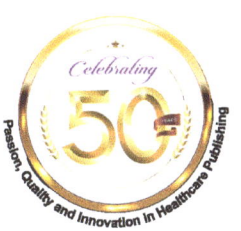

Skin in Rheumatologic Diseases

Editors

Savita Yadav MD
Consultant Dermatologist
Skin Care World Clinic
Dermatology and Dermatosurgery Hospital
Gurugram, Haryana, India

Uma Kumar MD
Professor and Head
Department of Rheumatology
All India Institute of Medical Sciences
New Delhi, India

Somesh Gupta MD
Professor
Department of Dermatology and Venereology
All India Institute of Medical Sciences
New Delhi, India

Foreword
Anurag Agrawal

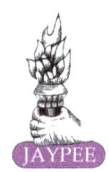

JAYPEE

JAYPEE BROTHERS MEDICAL PUBLISHERS
The Health Sciences Publisher
New Delhi | London

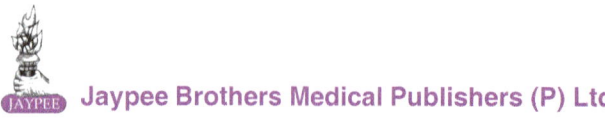 **Jaypee Brothers Medical Publishers (P) Ltd**

Headquarters

Jaypee Brothers Medical Publishers (P) Ltd
4838/24, Ansari Road, Daryaganj
New Delhi 110 002, India
Phone: +91-11-43574357
Fax: +91-11-43574314
Email: jaypee@jaypeebrothers.com

Overseas Offices

J.P. Medical Ltd
83 Victoria Street, London
SW1H 0HW (UK)
Phone: +44 20 3170 8910
Fax: +44 (0)20 3008 6180
Email: info@jpmedpub.com

Website: www.jaypeebrothers.com
Website: www.jaypeedigital.com

© 2020, Jaypee Brothers Medical Publishers

The views and opinions expressed in this book are solely those of the original contributor(s)/author(s) and do not necessarily represent those of editor(s) of the book.

All rights reserved. No part of this publication may be reproduced, stored or transmitted in any form or by any means, electronic, mechanical, photocopying, recording or otherwise, without the prior permission in writing of the publishers.

All brand names and product names used in this book are trade names, service marks, trademarks or registered trademarks of their respective owners. The publisher is not associated with any product or vendor mentioned in this book.

Medical knowledge and practice change constantly. This book is designed to provide accurate, authoritative information about the subject matter in question. However, readers are advised to check the most current information available on procedures included and check information from the manufacturer of each product to be administered, to verify the recommended dose, formula, method and duration of administration, adverse effects and contraindications. It is the responsibility of the practitioner to take all appropriate safety precautions. Neither the publisher nor the author(s)/editor(s) assume any liability for any injury and/or damage to persons or property arising from or related to use of material in this book.

This book is sold on the understanding that the publisher is not engaged in providing professional medical services. If such advice or services are required, the services of a competent medical professional should be sought.

Every effort has been made where necessary to contact holders of copyright to obtain permission to reproduce copyright material. If any have been inadvertently overlooked, the publisher will be pleased to make the necessary arrangements at the first opportunity. The **CD/DVD-ROM** (if any) provided in the sealed envelope with this book is complimentary and free of cost. **Not meant for sale.**

Inquiries for bulk sales may be solicited at: jaypee@jaypeebrothers.com

Skin in Rheumatologic Diseases / Savita Yadav, Uma Kumar, Somesh Gupta

First Edition: **2020**

ISBN: 978-93-5270-505-4

CONTRIBUTORS

Editors

Savita Yadav MD
Consultant Dermatologist
Skin Care World Clinic
Dermatology and Dermatosurgery Hospital
Gurugram, Haryana, India

Uma Kumar MD
Professor and Head
Department of Rheumatology
All India Institute of Medical Sciences
New Delhi, India

Somesh Gupta MD
Professor
Department of Dermatology and Venereology
All India Institute of Medical Sciences
New Delhi, India

Contributing Authors

Abir Saraswat MD
Consultant Dermatologist
Department of Dermatology
Indushree Skin Clinic
Lucknow, Uttar Pradesh, India

Ajaz K Khan MD FACR
Director
Centre for Arthritis and Rheumatism
Shifa Super Speciality Hospital
Srinagar, Jammu and Kashmir, India

Aman Sharma MD FACR FRCP
Professor
Department of Internal Medicine
Post Graduate Institute of Medical Education and Research
Chandigarh, India

Amita Aggarwal MD DM
Professor, Department of Clinical Immunology and Rheumatology
Sanjay Gandhi Postgraduate Institute of Medical Sciences
Lucknow, Uttar Pradesh, India

Ankan Gupta MD
Consultant Dermatologist
SK Hospital
Trivandrum, Kerala, India

Aparna Palit MD
Professor
Department of Dermatology, Venereology and Leprosy
Shri BM Patil Medical College Hospital and Research Center
Vijayapura, Karnataka, India

Skin in Rheumatologic Diseases

Arvind Ganapathi MD
Senior PG Registrar
Department of Clinical
Immunology and Rheumatology
Christian Medical College
Vellore, Tamil Nadu, India

Avinash Jain MD DM
Clinical Immunologist and
Rheumatologist
Department of Immunology and
Rheumatology
Sanjay Gandhi Postgraduate
Institute of Medical Sciences
Lucknow, Uttar Pradesh, India

Biju Vasudevan MD FRGUHS
Professor
Department of Dermatology
Base Hospital
Lucknow, Uttar Pradesh, India

CR Srinivas MD
Professor
Department of Dermatology
PSG Institute of Medical Sciences
and Research
Coimbatore, Tamil Nadu, India

Debashish Danda MD DM FRCP FACR FAMS
Professor and Head
Department of Clinical
Immunology and Rheumatology
Christian Medical College
Vellore, Tamil Nadu, India

Devendra S Dadhwal MD DM
Associate Professor
Department of Pulmonary
Medicine
Dr Rajendra Prasad Government
Medical College
Kangra, Himachal Pradesh, India

Dipankar De MD
Associate Professor
Department of Dermatology
Post Graduate Institute of
Medical Education and Research
Chandigarh, India

Garima MD
Senior Resident
Department of Dermatology,
Venereology and Leprology
Post Graduate Institute of
Medical Education and Research
Chandigarh, India

Gitesh U Sawatkar MD
Senior Resident
Department of Dermatology,
Venereology and Leprology
Post Graduate Institute of
Medical Education and
Research
Chandigarh, India

Gomathy Sethuraman MD FIAD MNAMS
Professor
Department of Dermatology
and Venereology
All India Institute of Medical
Sciences
New Delhi, India

Iffat Hassan MD
Professor
Head of the Department
Postgraduate Department
of Dermatology, Sexually
Transmitted Diseases and
Leprosy (University of Kashmir)
Government Medical College
Srinagar (University of Kashmir)
Jammu and Kashmir, India

Kusum Sharma MD
Professor
Department of Medical
Microbiology
Post Graduate Institute of
Medical Education and Research
Chandigarh, India

Liza Rajasekhar MD
Professor and Head
Department of Rheumatology
Nizam's Institute of Medical
Sciences
Hyderabad, Telangana, India

Neetu Bhari MD DNB MNAMS
Assistant Professor
Department of Dermatology and
Venereology
All India Institute of Medical
Sciences
New Delhi, India

Pradeep Balasubramanian MD
Assistant Professor
Department of Dermatology
Institute of Medical Sciences
Port Blair, Andaman and Nicobar
Islands, India

Prasan D Rath MD FACR Dip Musculoskeletal Ultrasound
Associate Director and Head
Department of Rheumatology
Max Super Speciality Hospital
New Delhi, India

Rahul Mahajan MD MNAMS
Assistant Professor
Department of Dermatology and
Venereology
Postgraduate Institute of
Medical Education and
Research
Chandigarh, India

Rajiv Joshi MD DVD DNB
Consultant
Department of Dermatology
PD Hinduja Hospital and
Medical Research Centre
Mumbai, Maharashtra, India

Ranjan Gupta MD DM
Assistant Professor
Department of Rheumatology
All India Institute of
Medical Sciences
New Delhi, India

Renu George MD DVL
Professor
Department of Dermatology
Christian Medical College
Vellore, Tamil Nadu, India

Contributors

Riti Bhatia MD
Senior Resident
Department of Dermatology
and Venereology
All India Institute of
Medical Sciences
New Delhi, India

Sanat Phatak MD DM
Senior Resident
Department of Clinical
Immunology and Rheumatology
Sanjay Gandhi Postgraduate
Institute of Medical Sciences
Lucknow, Uttar Pradesh, India

Sanjeev Handa MD FAMS FAAD FRCP (Edin.)
Professor and Head
Department of Dermatology,
Venereology and Leprology
Post Graduate Institute of
Medical Education and Research
Chandigarh, India

Sapan C Pandya MD DM
Assistant Professor
Department of Medicine
Smt. NHL Municipal Medical
College, VS Hospital and Vedanta
Institute of Medical Sciences
Ahmedabad, Gujarat, India

Sauvik Dasgupta MD
Senior Resident
Department of Rheumatology
All India Institute of
Medical Sciences
New Delhi, India

Shankar Naidu MD
Senior Resident
Department of Internal Medicine
Post Graduate Institute of
Medical Education and Research
Chandigarh, India

Silas S Nelson MD
Associate Professor
Department of Medicine
Netaji Subhash Chandra Bose
Medical College
Jabalpur, Madhya Pradesh,
India

Sramana Mukhopadyay MD
Assistant Professor
Department of Pathology
Christian Medical College
Vellore, Tamil Nadu, India

Sunil Dogra MD DNB FRCP
Dip Derma
Professor
Department of Dermatology,
Venereology and Leprology
Post Graduate Institute of
Medical Education and
Research
Chandigarh, India

Tanvi Dev MD
Senior Resident
Department of Dermatology
All India Institute of
Medical Sciences
New Delhi, India

Varun Dhir MD DM
Associate Professor
Department of Internal
Medicine
Post Graduate Institute of
Medical Education and
Research
Chandigarh, India

Vikram K Mahajan MD
Professor and Head
Department of Dermatology,
Venereology and Leprosy
Dr Rajendra Prasad Government
Medical College
Kangra, Himachal Pradesh,
India

Vishal Gupta MD
Senior Research Associate
Department of Dermatology
and Venereology
All India Institute of Medical
Sciences
New Delhi, India

Yasmeen Jabeen Bhat MD
Assistant Professor
Department of Dermatology
Government Medical College
Srinagar, Jammu and Kashmir,
India

FOREWORD

Why is "skin-deep" a derogatory word for superficiality, when it takes a lifetime of experience to just scratch the surface of what there is to be known about the skin? I expect that it is because we do not appreciate the hidden intricacy of what lies in plain sight, marveling only at its cosmetic aspects. The skin is a window, revealing much to the astute eye and mind about what lies inside. Despite my personal deficiencies in this area, it has always been a great inspiration to me to see how distinction between confounding diseases is sometimes made by observing a rash. Conversely, the simplest of things, such as loss or gain of pigment, is the termination point of an amazingly rich network of events that have been the focus of researchers at my institute for almost a decade.

In this context, it is my pleasure to write the foreword for this important book, which is expected to bring greater clarity to our understanding of skin in rheumatologic diseases. The editors, Dr Savita Yadav, Dr Uma Kumar and Dr Somesh Gupta must be commended for compiling an extensive body of work that provides descriptive as well as analytic insights from multiple perspectives. Skin lesions may not just be the first sign of deeper rheumatologic disease, but may serve as critical decision-points in differential diagnosis. The wide range of expertise that this book brings—immunology, rheumatology, pathology, dermatology, and good old fashioned clinical acumen—creates a whole that is much more than the sum of its parts. It is a matter of great pride to me that distinguished academicians from my alma mater, All India Institute of Medical Sciences, Delhi, have led and continued to lead, the way forward in professional training and knowledge dissemination.

I look forward to this book becoming a staple reading material for clinicians and researchers working in this area and confidently predict that this will be the first of many editions, bringing to readers, the latest at the intersection of dermatology and rheumatology.

Anurag Agrawal MBBS PhD
Diplomate American Board
Director
CSIR Institute of Genomics and Integrative Biology
New Delhi, India

PREFACE

Skin is the mirror for many internal diseases. This holds even truer for *Skin in Rheumatologic Diseases*. Overwhelming majority of rheumatologic diseases has preceding, simultaneous or subsequent involvement of skin. This intimate association of these two organ systems need closer interaction of two specialties of dermatology and rheumatology. The conception of this book project was an attempt to fill the void of a dedicated book on *Skin in Rheumatologic Diseases* which has inputs from the experts from both the specialties.

Studying skin in rheumatologic diseases is important. These diseases often seriously affect the quality of life of patients and at times make them bedridden. A consistent effort is needed for improvement in diagnosis and management of these patients, as well as understanding the pathophysiology of these diseases. Recent developments have provided more effective therapeutic options in the form of biologic therapies, however, many of these drugs remain beyond the affordable range of the majority of patients. Nevertheless, the new additions in the therapeutic armamentarium are welcome and we hope that as the demand rises the cost would come down. These drugs are discussed in the book.

A picture speaks for a thousand words. This book is full of visuals which will help the readers to understand and learn about the skin manifestations. A good coverage of histopathology, laboratory investigations, and treatment makes this book complete. Each contributor is an expert in his or her field, thus reader can rest assured that the content is authentic and coming from opinion leaders. We hope you enjoy reading the book.

Savita Yadav
Uma Kumar
Somesh Gupta

CONTENTS

1. **Introduction** — 1
   Savita Yadav, Uma Kumar, Somesh Gupta

2. **Basic Skin Lesions Related to Rheumatologic Disorders** — 2
   Abir Saraswat

3. **Dermatopathology of Rheumatologic Diseases** — 11
   Rajiv Joshi

4. **Immunodiagnostics in Rheumatologic Diseases** — 20
   Sanat Phatak, Amita Aggarwal

5. **Chronic Cutaneous and Subacute Cutaneous Lupus Erythematosus** — 26
   Garima, Dipankar De, Sanjeev Handa

6. **Systemic Lupus Erythematosus** — 55
   Ranjan Gupta, Amita Aggarwal

7. **Dermatomyositis** — 68
   Aparna Palit

8. **Systemic Sclerosis** — 89
   Savita Yadav, Neetu Bhari

9. **Morphea and Morpheaform Disorders** — 118
   CR Srinivas, Pradeep Balasubramanian

10. **Mixed Connective Tissue Disease** — 134
    Varun Dhir

11. **Scleredema and Scleromyxedema** — 140
    Biju Vasudevan, Ankan Gupta

12. **Sjögren's Syndrome** — 150
    Sapan C Pandya, Avinash Jain

13. **Sarcoidosis** — 165
    Vikram K Mahajan, Devendra S Dadhwal

14.	Cryoglobulinemic Vasculitis Liza Rajasekhar	188
15.	Psoriatic Arthritis Sunil Dogra, Gitesh U Sawatkar	195
16.	Reactive Arthritis Riti Bhatia, Somesh Gupta	213
17.	Rheumatoid Arthritis Sauvik Dasgupta, Uma Kumar	221
18.	Cutaneous Association of Rheumatological Disorders Neetu Bhari, Rahul Mahajan	233
19.	Approach to a Patient with Livedo Reticularis Prasan D Rath, Silas S Nelson, Ajaz K Khan	249
20.	Dermatological Manifestations of Large and Medium Vessel Vasculitides: Rheumatologists' Perspective Arvind Ganapathi, Sramana Mukhopadyay, Renu George, Debashish Danda	259
21.	Antinuclear Cytoplasmic Antibody-associated Small Vessel Vasculitis Aman Sharma, Shankar Naidu, Kusum Sharma	274
22.	Small Vessel Vasculitis of the Skin Neetu Bhari, Tanvi Dev, Gomathy Sethuraman	292
23.	Behçet's Disease Iffat Hassan, Yasmeen Jabeen Bhat, Debashish Danda	301
24.	Miscellaneous Rheumatological Disorders with Skin Manifestations Savita Yadav, Vishal Gupta	312
	Appendix 1: 6-minute Walk Test Report of a Systemic Sclerosis Patient Presenting with Dyspnea	325
	Index	327

CHAPTER 1

Introduction

Savita Yadav, Uma Kumar, Somesh Gupta

"Rheumatology" is a subspecialty of internal medicine which takes care of the patients with clinical problems involving the joints, soft tissues, vessels, and connective tissue. Majority of the "rheumatologic disorders" are immune-mediated diseases and the main subgroups comprise of inflammatory arthropathies, immune-mediated connective tissue diseases with multisystem involvement, and soft-tissue rheumatism. In a large number of "rheumatological disorders", the skin is also affected and these patients are often referred or present to the "dermatologists". Clear understanding of cutaneous manifestations of these disorders is essential for both the "dermatologists" as well as the "rheumatologists".

The skin manifestations can be the initial presenting symptom in some of these diseases, such as vasculitis, lupus erythematosus, systemic sclerosis, and sarcoidosis. These skin manifestations often help in establishing the diagnosis; therefore, provide a good window to the systemic disease. In addition, the skin lesions are easily amenable to biopsy and histopathological evaluations clinching the diagnosis and invasive systemic investigations for diagnostic purposes can be avoided in some patients. Nail fold capillary examination using dermatoscope serves as a good tool for diagnosing several immune-mediated connective tissue diseases. Often improvement in skin lesions correlate with improvement in systemic features and some of the skin manifestations have prognostic significance as well.

This book will serve as a ready reference for cutaneous manifestations of rheumatologic diseases and an interface between the "dermatologists" and the "rheumatologists". It is a multi-author book written by eminent "dermatologists" and "rheumatologists". It will enhance the understanding of the skin manifestations of rheumatologic diseases among the "rheumatologists" as well as "dermatologists" and thereby will go a long way in contributing to the patient care.

In this book, we have focused on the "rheumatological disorders" which have the cutaneous involvement. In all the chapters, the main emphasis is on the clinical presentation of the diseases. Chapters will provide a detailed description of the classical and the uncommon variants of the skin manifestations of these disorders as well as the comprehensive understanding of the joint and other organ involvement. The diagnostic and prognostic significance of skin manifestations has been elaborated. Besides the clinical manifestations, we have also discussed the etiopathogenesis of diseases in succinct and the latest guidelines and updates on the treatment of these diseases are presented. We have also included chapters on basic skin lesions seen in various "rheumatologic disorders" and approach to diagnostic workup in these patients. "A picture speaks for a thousand words". This book has around 500 images which will help the reader to visualize the skin lesions.

We hope you will enjoy reading this book.

CHAPTER 2

Basic Skin Lesions Related to Rheumatologic Disorders

Abir Saraswat

INTRODUCTION

Rheumatologic disorders often have concomitant cutaneous involvement. Some of the skin lesions are specific to particular disorder, while others are nonspecific but still help in establishing diagnosis and sometimes in prognosticating about the disease. In this chapter, we are going to present and discuss the common and important skin lesions which can occur in various rheumatologic diseases. There understanding is required for suspecting the diagnosis and planning set of investigations to be done in a particular patient.

PURPURA

Purpura is the general term used to describe visible hemorrhage in the skin or mucous membranes (Fig. 1). Clinically, these lesions cannot be blanched fully upon diascopy. Based mainly on the size and depth of lesions, it is classified into the following three clinical types:

1. Petechia: Typically an area of hemorrhage less than 3 mm in diameter. It is usually bright red in color, especially an early lesion.
2. Ecchymosis: A deep reddish-blue (Fig. 2), purplish or black macule at least 0.5–1.5 cm in its greatest dimension. It may arise *de novo* or result from the coalescence of petechiae. In the latter case, there are always some petechiae at the periphery of the ecchymosis.
3. Contusion: A deep, palpable, trauma-induced lesion that is frequently purpuric on the surface.

Purpuric lesions can be macular or palpable. Palpable purpura is a sign of vascular inflammation.

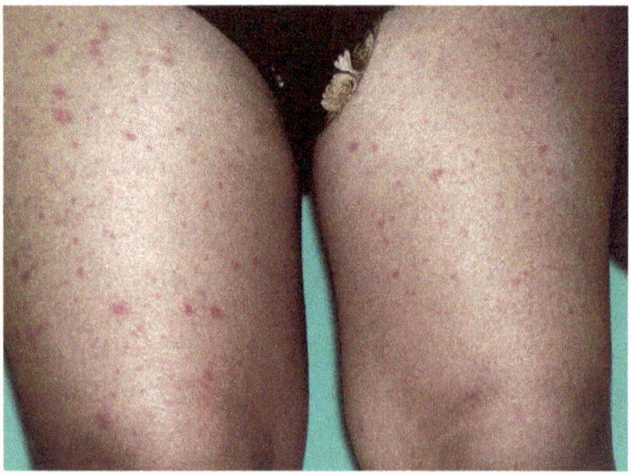

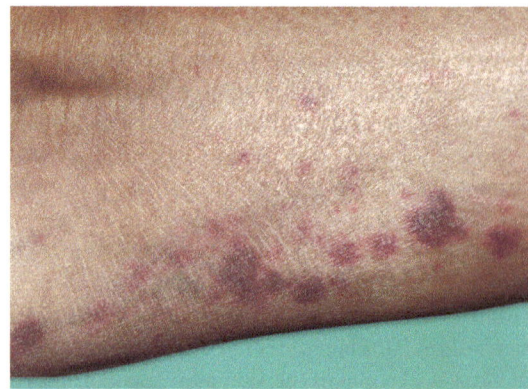

FIGURE 1: Palpable purpura over both thighs in a cutaneous small vessel vasculitis patient.

FIGURE 2: Multiple fresh ecchymotic patches over right lower leg in a patient with inherited coagulopathy.

Pathogenesis

Purpura can be caused by intravascular (Table 1), vascular (Table 2), or extravascular causes (Table 3). Intravascular causes are related to congenital or acquired disorders that lead to problems with the amount/number or function of platelets, procoagulant, or anticoagulant factors. Vascular causes of purpura are mainly

Table 1: Intravascular causes of purpura	
Type	Causes
Platelet count-related (petechiae)	• Thrombocytopenia below 50,000/mm^3 caused by: Idiopathic thrombocytopenic purpura, thrombotic thrombocytopenic purpura, disseminated intravascular coagulation, drug-induced thrombocytopenia and bone marrow defect due to infiltration, fibrosis, or failure
Platelet function-related (petechiae)	• Congenital platelet function defects • Acquired platelet function defects such as: Kidney or liver dysfunction, monoclonal gammopathy • Thrombocytosis above 1,000,000/mm^3 usually due to myeloproliferative disorders
Elevated intravascular pressure (petechiae)	• Valsalva maneuver-like causes, viz. forceful vomiting, violent coughing, straining during childbirth
Coagulation cascade-related (ecchymoses)	• Procoagulant defect caused by: Hemophilia, vitamin K deficiency, anticoagulants, disseminated intravascular coagulation, hepatic failure leading to poor procoagulant synthesis

Table 2: Vascular causes of purpura	
Type	Causes
Inflammatory causes (palpable, usually partially blanchable, early lesions erythematous)	• Small vessel leukocytoclastic vasculitis (Fig. 3) • Pityriasis lichenoides et varioliformis acuta • Erythema multiforme • Chronic pigmented purpura (Fig. 4)
Noninflammatory causes (palpable or nonpalpable, retiform, may be ecchymotic, no early erythema)	• Platelet-plugging disorders: Thrombocytosis, paroxysmal nocturnal hemoglobinuria, heparin necrosis • Pathogen-related vessel invasion: Strongyloidiasis, fungemia e.g., aspergillus, ecthyma gangrenosum • Cholesterol or oxalate emboli • Cryoglubulinemia/cryofibrinogenemia • Coagulation disorders: Inherited or acquired severe protein C/protein S deficiency due to sepsis, antiphospholipid antibody syndromes • Cutaneous calciphylaxis • Degos disease

Table 3: Extravascular causes of purpura	
Type	Causes
Major trauma-related (usually ecchymosis or contusion)	Obvious trauma
Perifollicular petechiae	Scurvy
Minor trauma-related (extensors of arms or shins, dorsa of hands or linearly along excoriations)	• Senile/actinic purpura • Long-term corticosteroid use/endogenous hypercortisolism • Systemic amyloidosis • Ehlers-Danlos syndrome • Pseudoxanthoma elasticum

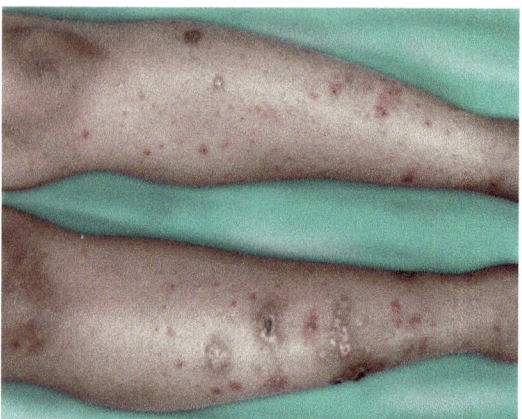

FIGURE 3: Palpable purpura and superficial ulcers over both legs in a cutaneous small vessel vasculitis patient.

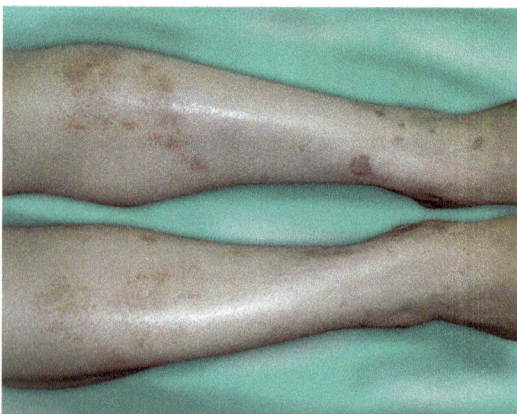

FIGURE 4: Petechial spots seen in pigmented purpuric dermatosis.

Box 1: In purpura, the features that suggest a need of further evaluation
- Systemic symptoms like arthralgias, malaise, or fever
- Large lesions on covered areas
- Lesions occurring in crops
- Tender or palpable lesions
- Hematuria, malena or hematochezia, subconjunctival hemorrhages or upper gastrointestinal bleed
- Reticulate or ulcerated lesions, targetoid lesions, pustules, perifollicular lesions

caused by vessel wall inflammation leading to intracutaneous bleed or intravascular thrombosis. Noninflammatory vascular causes of purpura include several conditions that cause occlusion. Extravascular causes include minor trauma with a background of reduced dermal support for the vessels, or major trauma alone.

Clinical Features of Purpura

Purpura can be a nonsignificant finding, not needing much evaluation or a sinister sign of severe underlying problems.[1-3] The overall clinical context decides the seriousness of this finding. Examples of nonserious purpuric lesions include purpuric lesions occurring on sun-exposed and trauma-prone sites in elderly patients with significant actinic damage, or purpuric linear excoriations in patients suffering from severely itchy dermatoses. In the latter cases, it often helps to see if purpuric lesions are present on areas like the mid-back which are usually not accessible, although patients can use back-scratchers, pencils, and combs to scratch otherwise inaccessible areas. Clinical clues that suggest deeper evaluation of purpura are shown in box 1.

Some typical distributions and patterns of purpura can give a clue to the diagnosis:
- Lesions due to immune-complex deposition disorders like cutaneous leukocytoclastic vasculitis[4] usually occur on dependent areas, i.e., back and buttocks in bed-ridden patients and lower legs and feet of mobile patients
- Clinically identical lesions due to anti-neutrophil-cytoplasmic antibodies (ANCA) are much more likely to occur at random sites like ears in addition to dependent areas
- Lesions on the eyelids are characteristically seen due to violent coughing or vomiting. Relatively mild coughing may produce the "panda sign" in patients with systemic amyloidosis
- Ear lesions are seen in cold-induced purpura syndromes like cryoglobulinemia and drug-induced purpura due to levamisole, and propylthiouracil
- Acral purpura is seen in embolic causes, cryoglobulinemia and rickettsial disease

- Friction sites are affected in purpuric contact dermatitis due to textile dyes/finishes, Henoch-Schönlein purpura and ecchymoses of Ehlers-Danlos syndrome and pseudoxanthoma elasticum
- Oral mucosal purpura is common in thrombocytopenia and amyloidosis.

The color of lesions can be bright red, bluish-purple or black depending on the oxygenation level of the blood and the age of the lesion. Chronic lesions can be brown or golden-hued due to the deposition of hemosiderin. However, this color cannot be clinically distinguished from the color of melanin or other pigments.

Blanchability is assessed by pressing the lesion firmly with a glass slide or hand lens. It is an important finding for two reasons. One, partial or total nonblanchability confirms that a lesion is actually purpuric. Second, the degree of blanchability can give a clue to the intensity of inflammation present in the purpuric lesion as well as the age of the lesion. The inflammatory component can be blanched with pressure whereas the hemorrhagic component does not blanch. However, deeper lesions that occur due to the noninflammatory occlusion of vessels can develop a late erythema. This develops at the periphery of livedo racemosa as a result of ischemic necrosis. That is why diascopy to assess blanchability should always be done on a newly developed lesion. Extensive noninflammatory retiform purpura is seen due to disseminated intravascular coagulation caused by sepsis, malignancy or other serious underlying disorders.

The size of lesions can suggest etiology, although there is a lot of overlap and exceptions to this. Generally, petechial lesions occur due to thrombocytopenia, platelet dysfunction, increased intravascular pressure or in types of capillaritis. In contrast, ecchymoses are seen due to coagulation disorders or poor extravascular support. Variable sized lesions can be seen in scurvy, drug-induced purpura and patients with very low platelet counts.

Investigations

These depend solely on the clinical features and history, which suggests the possible underlying causes of purpura.

Skin Biopsy

It should only be done if vasculitis is suspected, e.g., if palpable and partially blanchable lesions are present. Large and nonblanchable lesions should only be biopsied if platelet number and function is normal and coagulopathy is ruled out. In this scenario, deposition disorders and vessel wall disease may be present which can be seen on histopathology.

Bleeding Time and Clotting Time

These tests are supposed to give a clue to platelet function and coagulation status respectively, but are too nonspecific to give much clinically useful information.

Complete Blood Count

Platelet counts below $50,000/mm^3$ is usually needed for cutaneous hemorrhage to occur; counts below $10,000/mm^3$ can cause large ecchymoses. Thrombocytosis can cause altered platelet function as well. Disorders of platelet function need in vitro testing. Other blood cell counts can give a clue to myeloproliferative disorders or marrow failure. Further testing depends on abnormalities found on complete blood count and the clinical context.

Tests of Other Bleeding Sites

Funduscopy, stool for occult blood and urinalysis should be done since these simple tests can rule out occult bleeding. Hematuria is important to look for as a sign of renal vasculitis.

Coagulation Screen

Partial thromboplastin time and prothrombin time are good screening tests to rule out coagulation cascade defects. In case of noninflammatory retiform purpura, protein C and S testing may be done. Anticardiolipin antibodies and Venereal Disease Research Laboratories (VDRL) testing along with partial thromboplastin time (PTT) are used in antiphospholipid antibody syndromes.

Serological Testing

If collagen vascular disease is suspected, appropriate serological tests should be done, viz. antinuclear antibody (ANA), ANCA, etc.

TELANGIECTASIA

Telangiectasia (telangiectases) represents dilatations of the capillaries or venules that may or may not disappear with the application of pressure. They are usually quite small, but an individual lesion may range from a barely visible pinpoint to a bluish nodule a centimeter or more in size. They may be punctate, linear, arborizing or stellate and can present on the skin or mucous membranes.[5] Their color can range from bright red to dull blue, smaller telangiectases usually being more toward the red side of the spectrum. Some indicative causes of telangiectases are mentioned in box 2.

As it is evident from the table, there are several mechanisms that can lead to the formation of telangiectasia. The cause of the dilatation may be systemic, as seen in hepatic failure, related to the vessel wall itself as in several primary telangiectatic syndromes or extravascular, seen in photodamaged skin. Macular, fine telangiectasia seen in collagen vascular diseases and generalized essential telangiectasia are formed by the dilatation of postcapillary venules and the upper capillary plexus. Nailfold telangiectasia and cherry angiomas are formed from dilated capillary loops in the dermal papillae. In hereditary hemorrhagic telangiectasia (HHT), they are formed by microvascular arteriovenous anastomoses.

Secondary telangiectasia can be caused by a lack/loss of extravascular connective tissue leading to dilatation of the vessels. Topical steroid misuse, actinic damage, and poikiloderma are common examples of this mechanism. Smoking is known to exacerbate actinic damage. Prolonged vasodilatation can also cause telangiectasia, as seen in rosacea and varicose veins. Increased pressure in the vascular bed leads to the weakest parts, viz. the postcapillary venules and capillaries to dilate permanently. On the legs, the presence of telangiectasia can thus be a sign of significant abnormalities in the main leg veins leading to venous hypertension.

Telangiectasias are a common sign in diseases like lupus erythematosus, scleroderma (Fig. 5) and dermatomyositis (Figs 6 and 7), and are commonly seen in patients suffering from Raynaud's phenomenon, with or without underlying collagen vascular disease. When seen under magnification, nailfold capillary architecture and morphology can be very helpful in the diagnosis of scleroderma or dermatomyositis. Telangiectatic loops and capillary dropouts on the nailfolds can be very helpful in establishing the diagnosis, in association with other findings.

Even though telangiectasias represent very superficially located dilated thin-walled blood vessels, significant bleeding from these lesions is quite rare. An exception to this is the autosomal dominant disorder hereditary HHT, also called

Box 2: Causes of telangiectasia

Primary telangiectasia
Vascular nevi, hereditary hemorrhagic telangiectasia, ataxia-telangiectasia, spider telangiectasia, Bloom's syndrome, cutis marmorata telangiectatica, angioma serpiginosum

Secondary telangiectasia
- Collagen vascular disease: Lupus erythematosus, scleroderma, dermatomyositis, morphea
- Environmental causes: Photoaging, prolonged tar exposure

Radiation dermatitis
- Altered estrogen metabolism: Hepatic failure
- Prolonged vasodilation: Rosacea, varicose veins
- Lack of extravascular support: Topical corticosteroid abuse, poikiloderma
- Mastocytosis: Telangiectasia macularis eruptiva perstans

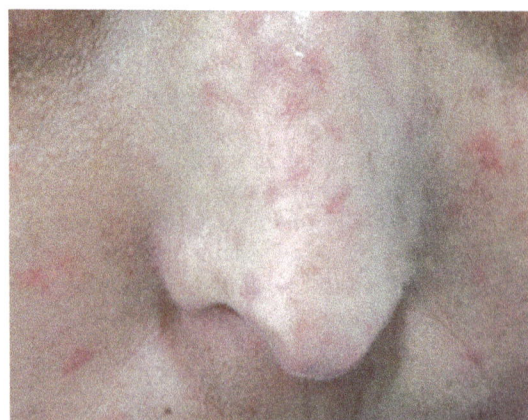

FIGURE 5: Matt like telangiectasia in a systemic sclerosis patient.

Basic Skin Lesions Related to Rheumatologic Disorders

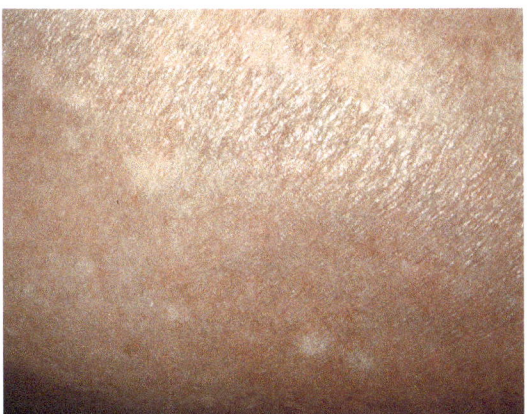

FIGURE 6: Telangiectasia in a poikilodermatous patch seen in dermatomyositis patient.

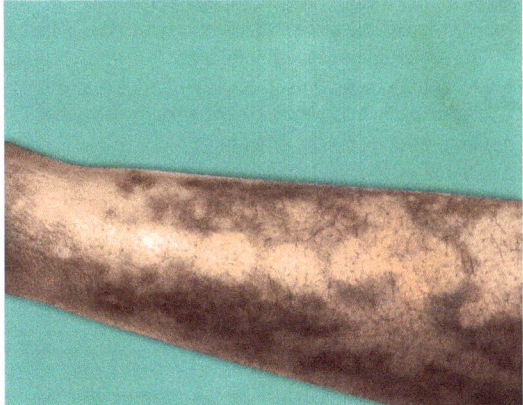

FIGURE 8: Livedo reticularis.

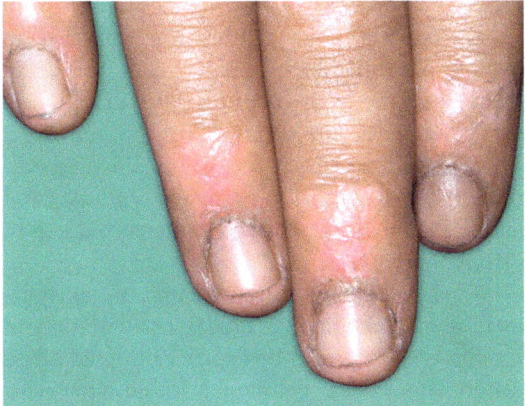

FIGURE 7: Nail fold capillary dilatation in a dermatomyositis patient.

Osler-Rendu-Weber disease, where recurrent epistaxis from nasal mucosal telangiectases is the most common symptom. Lesions in patients with CREST (calcinosis, Raynaud's phenomenon, esophageal dysmotility, sclerodactyly, and telangiectasia)-type of scleroderma can also bleed.

Spider telangiectasias are found in up to 15% of normal people. They are comprised of a central pulsatile vessel, an arteriole, from which multiple spider-like vessels radiate outward. They are usually located on the upper half of the body. They are almost always found if looked for in pregnant women, and increase with gestational age. If found in increasing numbers in any individual, an underlying liver disease must be looked for.

LIVEDO RETICULARIS

Livedo reticularis (Livedo racemosa, cutis marmorata, livedo annularis) refers to a fixed, reddish blue pattern of mottling seen on the skin in a "broken fishnet" pattern (Fig. 8).[6]

The exact cause of this highly characteristic pattern on the skin is not known, but spasm or occlusion of the small vertically oriented arterioles in the dermis that connect the deep and superficial vascular plexuses is probably responsible. Increased sympathetic nerve activity is also associated with livedo reticularis, especially in essential or benign livedo reticularis. The reddish-blue blotches conform to deoxygenated blood pooling in the superficial venous plexus. Raising or warming the affected limb can therefore reverse these changes in many cases. A defect in the thrombolytic system, tissue abnormalities leading to arteriolar thrombosis, decreased protein C/protein S activity and hyperhomocysteinemia have all been reported to play a role in the pathogenesis of livedo. Different causes of livedo reticularis are shown in box 3.

All types of livedo are seen most commonly on the lower extremities of young women under the age of 40 years. Patients with primary idiopathic livedo are asymptomatic, except for cosmetic concerns. Patients of secondary livedo may complain of symptoms of the underlying disease. The affected limb may feel cold and numb to the patient. In livedoid vasculitis, small, painful, and

Skin in Rheumatologic Diseases

> **Box 3: Varieties of livedo reticularis**
> - Primary idiopathic livedo reticularis
> - Livedo reticularis with summer/winter ulceration, also called livedoid vasculitis or atrophie blanche
> - Drug-induced livedo: Amantadine
> - Secondary livedo: vasculitis, atheromatous embolism, collagen vascular disease especially lupus erythematosus, Sneddon's syndrome (livedo with cerebrovascular lesions), hyperviscosity states, obstructive arterial disease, endocrine disorders, antiphospholipid antibody syndrome, Raynaud's phenomenon

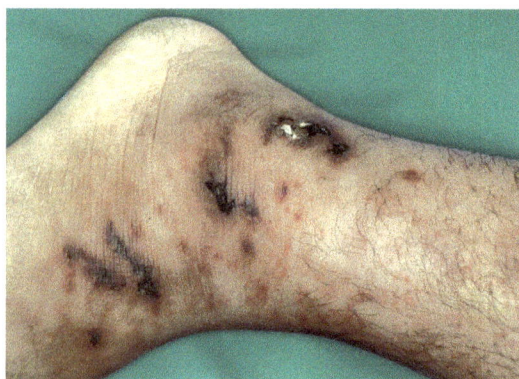

FIGURE 9: Superficial retiform necrotic ulcers in a livedoid vasculopathy patient.

extremely tender ulcers covered with eschar may be seen on the feet or ankles (Fig. 9). Nodules, purpuric macules, and ankle edema may also be present. There may be a seasonal pattern to the ulceration, with exacerbations occurring in the winters or less commonly summers. Subsided ulcers leave behind small white scars surrounded by telangiectatic erythema.

Biopsies show intravascular thrombosis and thickening/hyalinizing changes in mid-dermal vessel walls. Red blood cells extravasation and a perivascular lymphocytic infiltrate are also seen. In primary idiopathic livedo, no specific biopsy findings are seen.

Treatment of livedo reticularis depends on the underlying cause, severity, and symptomatic nature of the disease. Attempts should be made to find out a cause in all symptomatic/ulcer-associated cases. Only if no obvious cause is found, should a diagnosis of livedoid vasculitis be made. Limbs should be kept as warm as possible and underlying abnormalities of coagulation or blood vessels should be corrected or treated. In livedoid vasculitis, the treatment primarily consists of antiplatelet, anticoagulant or fibrinolytic agents.[1,7] Anabolic steroids like danazol or stanozolol are also useful.

RAYNAUD'S PHENOMENON

Raynaud's phenomenon is the occurrence of episodes of sudden blanching or cyanosis of one or more digits, usually on cold exposure (Fig. 10).[8,9] Primary Raynaud's phenomenon occurs with no detectable underlying disease and is usually seen in young women. Men constitute only a quarter or less of all affected individuals.

The exact cause of the episodic vasospasm seen in Raynaud's phenomenon is not known. However, a localized defect of the digital artery which renders them abnormally sensitive to cold is proposed to be responsible. The exact defect may lie with α-2 adrenoceptors or S-2 serotonergic receptors, but it is not conclusively proven. Sympathetic overactivity, cold temperature, platelet-derived vasoactive agents, and endothelial dysfunction have all been blamed in this phenomenon.

Typically, patients complain of episodic attacks of blanching or bluish discoloration of the digits precipitated by exposure to cold air or water. Sometimes, emotional stimuli may also be blamed. Hands are more commonly involved than the feet and thumbs are usually spared in the early stages. Involvement may initially be

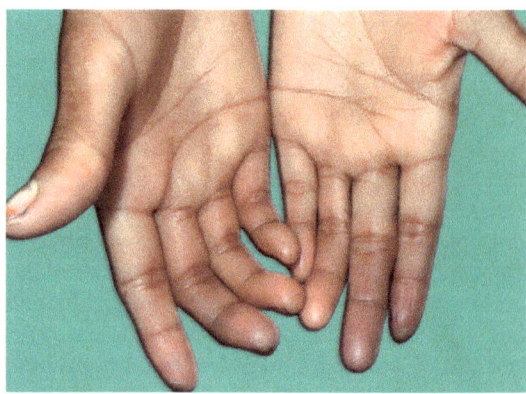

FIGURE 10: Raynaud's phenomenon in a systemic sclerosis patient.

very patchy with only one or a few fingers or toes being affected. In dark-skinned patients, the color changes may be difficult to appreciate and symptomatic features of numbness of fingers followed by painful engorgement on re-warming may be elicited. If the initial ischemic phase is accompanied by pain, a secondary cause of Raynaud's phenomenon should be suspected. More proximal involvement than the fingers and toes also points to a secondary cause. The textbook triphasic response of blanching followed by cyanosis and erythema on re-warming is seldom seen in its entirety. The frequency of attacks is widely variable.

On examination, the digits may look normal, although sometimes they are cool and clammy to the touch. Hyperhidrosis may be associated. Peripheral pulses are normally felt. Nails may show cuticle hypertrophy or pterygium formation. Cutaneous atrophy and deformed anteroposteriorly curved nails are seen in longstanding cases, especially if associated with scleroderma. Fingertip ulcers or scars may be visible. In severe cases and in secondary Raynaud's phenomenon, gangrene of the distal digits may occur, though it is uncommon.

Nailfold capillaroscopy is extremely helpful in diagnosing cases of secondary Raynaud's phenomenon.[10,11] It is normal in primary disease, whereas in scleroderma and dermatomyositis, enlarged capillary loops with areas of capillary dropouts are seen. In mixed connective tissue disease, bushy capillary formations are more commonly seen.

Clinical differentiation from a normal cold-induced acrocyanosis can be made easily in fair-skinned patients, since the typical color changes are absent. In dark-skinned patients, pointers away from a diagnosis of Raynaud's phenomenon are involvement of whole hands and feet and not just the digits, more common involvement of feet and equal sex distribution.

In all patients with Raynaud's phenomenon, an underlying cause should be looked for thoroughly (Box 4). History of trauma, smoking, drug exposure, and collagen vascular diseases should be carefully taken. All peripheral pulses should be palpated and blood pressure taken in all extremities. Blood investigations are guided by history and examination findings, but tests to rule out collagen vascular diseases and hypercoagulable states should be undertaken in most, if not all cases. Chest X-ray to rule out thoracic rib and clinical testing for thoracic outlet syndrome should also be done. Biochemistry and urinalysis should also be performed. A vascular surgery referral may be needed in many cases, especially if ulcers or gangrene is present. Only after a thorough workup, should a diagnosis of primary Raynaud's disease be made.

> **Box 4: Causes of Raynaud's phenomenon**
> - Vascular causes: Connective tissue diseases, obstructive arterial diseases
> - Trauma: Jackhammer operators, typists, and pianists
> - Drugs: Beta blockers, bleomycin, vinblastine, clonidine, bromocriptine, and ergot derivatives
> - Neurologic causes: Thoracic outlet syndrome, hemiplegia, multiple sclerosis, and reflex sympathetic dystrophy
> - Hematologic causes: Polycythemia, cryoglobulinemia/cryofibrinogenemia, and macroglobulins
> - Others: Intra-arterial injections, hypothyroidism, and vinyl chloride disease

Common sense precautions such as avoidance of cold exposure, wearing loose and warm clothing, cessation of smoking, and avoidance of trauma should be taken in all patients. The underlying disease should be effectively treated in secondary cases. Avoidance of precipitating drugs should be ensured.

Drug treatment is needed in all symptomatic patients and oral vasodilators are the cornerstone of therapy. All calcium channel blockers except verapamil are useful, with long-acting molecules/formulations being preferred. Prazosin is helpful in some cases and sublingual or topical nitrates may be helpful in combination with other drugs, as are drugs like pentoxifylline and antiplatelet agents. Angiotensin receptor antagonists (telmisartan, valsartan) and phosphodiesterase-5 inhibitors (e.g., sildenafil, tadalafil) have been reported to be helpful in treating recalcitrant cases. Parenteral prostacyclin is reported to be useful in averting impending gangrene.

Calcinosis Cutis

Calcinosis cutis (CC) term is used when there is deposition of calcium into the skin. It is classified into

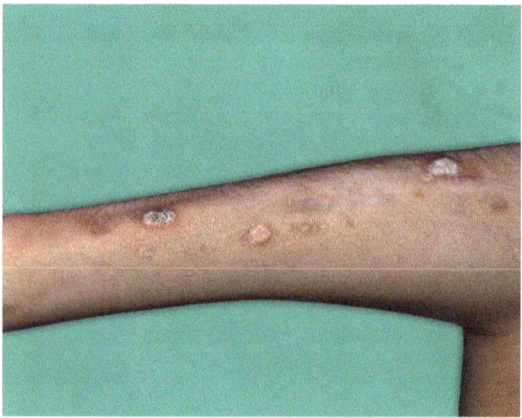

FIGURE 11: Whitish plaques of calcinosis cutis in a dermatomyositis patient.

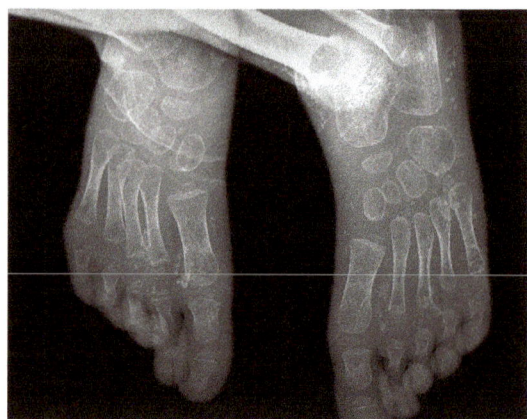

FIGURE 13: X-ray showing patchy cutaneous calcinosis over feet in juvenile DM patient.

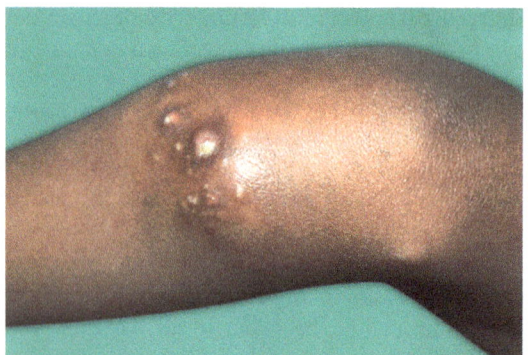

FIGURE 12: Calcinosis cutis in a systemic sclerosis patient.

four major types—(i) idiopathic, (ii) metastatic, (iii) dystrophic and (iv) iatrogenic. Calcinosis cutis seen in rheumatologic disorders falls into the dystrophic group primarily.[12,13] It is an important feature of dermatomyositis (Figs 11 and 12) and can also be seen in systemic sclerosis (SSc) and sometimes lupus panniculitis, lupus erythematosus, and mixed connective tissue disease.

Dystrophic CC occurs in tissues with altered architecture because of tissue damage. Calcinosis cutis is more common and has early onset in juvenile DM compared to adult DM patients. Affected areas are extremities as well as the trunk. Dystrophic CC in DM patients can be a localized cutaneous nodule, subcutaneous tumoral deposits or intramuscular, and fascial calcification. Also CC is more commonly a feature of limited cutaneous SSc, occurs after a protracted period of disease activity, involves extremities and trauma prone sites, and lesions are often small and involve localized areas of hand and feet (Fig. 13). Calcinosis cutis is uncommon in systemic lupus erythematosus (SLE) but can occur in lupus panniculitis. Complications associated with CC include ulceration, secondary infection, and restriction of joint mobility. Treatment of CC is difficult.

REFERENCES

1. Micheletti RG, Werth VP. Small vessel vasculitis of the skin. Rheum Dis Clin North Am. 2015;41:21-32.
2. Piette WW. The differential diagnosis of purpura from a morphologic perspective. Adv Dermatol. 1994;9:3-23.
3. Stevens GL, Adelman HM, Wallach PM. Palpable purpura: an algorithmic approach. Am Fam Physician. 1995;52:1355-62.
4. Goeser MR, Laniosz V, Wetter DA. A practical approach to the diagnosis, evaluation, and management of cutaneous small-vessel vasculitis. Am J Clin Dermatol. 2014;15:299-306.
5. Gupta R, Gautam RK, Bhardwaj M, Chauhan A. A clinical approach to diagnose patients with localized telangiectasia. Int J Dermatol. 2015;54:e294-301.
6. Gibbs MB, English JC 3rd, Zirwas MJ. Livedo reticularis: an update. J Am Acad Dermatol. 2005;52:1009-19.
7. Llamas-Velasco M, Alegría V, Santos-Briz Á, Cerroni L, Kutzner H, Requena L. Occlusive Nonvasculitic Vasculopathy: A Review. Am J Dermatopathol. 2016; [Epub ahead of print].
8. Hughes M, Herrick AL. Raynaud's phenomenon. Best Pract Res Clin Rheumatol. 2016;30:112-32.
9. Wigley FM, Flavahan NA. Raynaud's Phenomenon. N Engl J Med. 2016;375:556-65.
10. Cutolo M, Sulli A, Smith V. How to perform and interpret capillaroscopy. Best Pract Res Clin Rheumatol. 2013;27:237-48.
11. Fueyo-Casado A, Campos-Muñoz L, Pedraz-Muñoz J, Conde-Taboada A, López-Bran E. Nailfold dermoscopy as screening in suspected connective tissue diseases. Lupus. 2016;25:110-1.
12. Gutierrez A Jr, Wetter DA. Calcinosis cutis in autoimmune connective tissue diseases. Dermatol Ther. 2012;25:195-206.
13. Valenzuela A, Chung L. Calcinosis: pathophysiology and management. Curr Opin Rheumatol. 2015;27:542-8.

CHAPTER 3

Dermatopathology of Rheumatologic Diseases

Rajiv Joshi

INTRODUCTION

Several rheumatologic diseases present with skin manifestations which may be either the presenting features of the disease before other systemic manifestations are evident or may be used for diagnosis by a skin biopsy. Most rheumatologic diseases present with dermatological findings that may be either specific to the disease (specific skin lesions) or conditions that represent known clinicopathological entities like vasculitis, erythema nodosum, etc., which are considered as nonspecific skin lesions.

This chapter explores in brief, the dermatopathological findings of specific skin lesions in the commonly seen rheumatologic diseases.[1] For the sake of brevity, clinical findings are not elaborated here and the reader is referred to the chapters that deal with the individual diseases elsewhere in this book.

CUTANEOUS LUPUS ERYTHEMATOSUS

Skin lesions in lupus erythematosus (LE) may be broadly divided into those that are specific and diagnostic for the disease and nonspecific manifestations like vasculitis, vaso-occlusive conditions, Raynaud's phenomenon, and non-cicatricial hair loss which are distinct entities by themselves and are not specific for LE.

Lupus-specific skin lesions are broadly subdivided into acute, subacute, and chronic cutaneous lesions which often correlate well with the presence or absence of systemic activity of the disease. Acute malar (butterfly) rash is most common in patients with active systemic lupus while the subacute polycyclic-psoriasiform rash is common in patients with the subset of LE with positive anti-Ro/La antibodies. Likewise chronic cutaneous LE or discoid lesions (DLE) are usually not associated with systemic involvement or activity.

PATTERN OF INFLAMMATION

Histological evaluation of a skin biopsy starts with assessment of the pattern of inflammation which, in LE, is that of a lymphocytic inflammation with superficial and deep perivascular and periadnexal lymphocytic infiltrates which may vary in density from sparse to dense, at times even nodular. This lymphocytic infiltrate of skin is a common pattern for conditions other than LE which includes Jessner's lymphocytic infiltrate, polymorphous light eruption, lymphocytoma cutis, and lymphoma of the skin. Epidermal changes are useful in differentiating LE from the other conditions but in an expression of LE called tumid LE, no epidermal changes are seen and the condition then is diagnosed on the basis of finding of dermal mucin.

A lichenoid infiltrate of lymphocytes resembling lichen planus may be seen and differentiation from lichen planus can be made if there is basement membrane thickening or mucin in the reticular dermis or a deep perivascular and periadnexal infiltrate of lymphocytes.

Skin in Rheumatologic Diseases

Although LE in general is a lymphocytic inflammation of skin, early lesions like the malar rash of acute systemic lupus erythematos (SLE) often show presence of neutrophils scattered in the upper dermis or lined up just beneath the basal layer of the epidermis.[2] This may be accompanied by karyorrhexis of lymphocytes.

EPIDERMAL CHANGES IN LUPUS ERYTHEMATOSUS

The epidermis is usually flat or atrophic at least focally and shows vacuolar-interface changes with basal cell vacuolization and smudging of the dermoepidermal junction (Figs 1 and 2). Few colloid bodies are often seen at the dermoepidermal junction or in the upper papillary dermis. Longstanding lesions of DLE show at least focally a thickened basement membrane that appears as a broad homogenous pink band which stains bright red with periodic acid-Schiff (PAS) stain (Fig. 3). Basement membrane thickening is also seen to involve follicular infundibula and is highly specific for LE and dermatomyositis.

Uncommon findings include parakeratosis and numerous necrotic keratinocytes scattered throughout the spinous layers (Figs 4 and 5) and then the differential diagnoses (DDs) include erythema multiforme, pityriasis lichenoides, and varioliformis acuta and drug eruption. Confluent

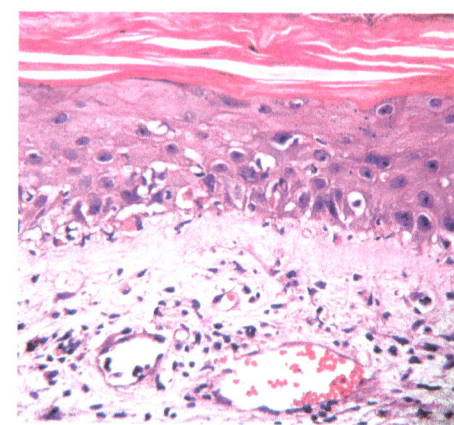

FIGURE 2: Subacute cutaneous lupus erythematosus, flat epidermis with basal cell vacuolization, several individually necrotic keratinocytes at the dermoepidermal junction, parakeratosis and dermal telangiectasia and lymphocytic infiltrate. H&E, 400x.

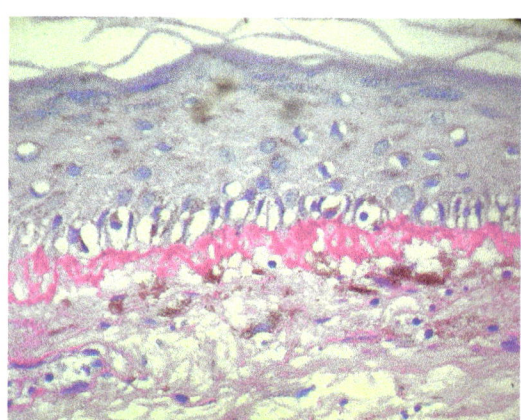

FIGURE 3: Lupus erythematosus, thickened basement membrane stained bright pink by PAS stain. periodic acid-Schiff 400x.

basal cell vacuolization with necrosis of epidermis may be seen in acute, rapidly spreading lesions of LE that resemble toxic epidermal necrolysis.

DERMAL CHANGES

Dermal mucin deposits, seen as bluish-gray stringy material between collagen of the upper and mid-reticular dermis, is a finding that has great diagnostic value in LE (Fig. 6). The amount of mucin may vary from sparse and barely recognizable to large pools that widely separate

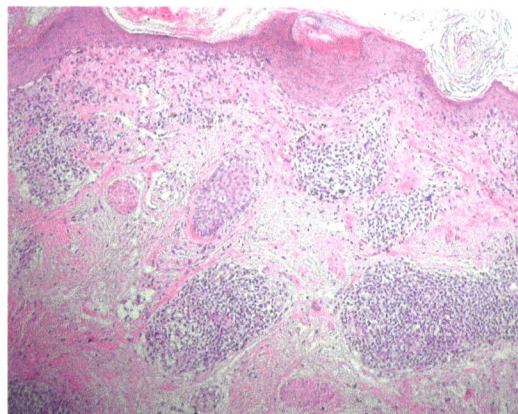

FIGURE 1: Lupus erythematosus showing flat epidermis with basal cell vacuolization and subepidermal clefts, a nodular perivascular and periadnexal lymphocytic infiltrate in the dermis. H&E, 100x.

Dermatopathology of Rheumatologic Diseases

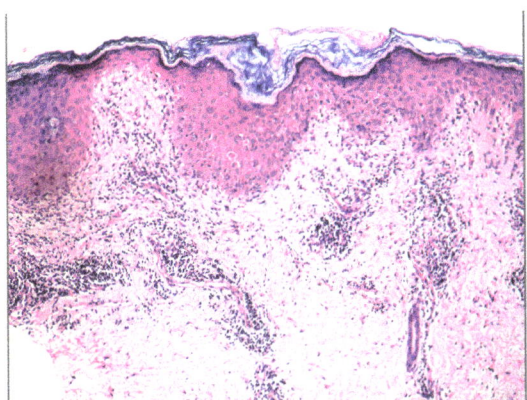

FIGURE 4: Lupus erythematosus, epidermal hyperplasia with many necrotic keratinocytes scattered in spinous zone with mild parakeratosis. Differential diagnoses includes drug reaction and erythema multiforme. H&E, 100x.

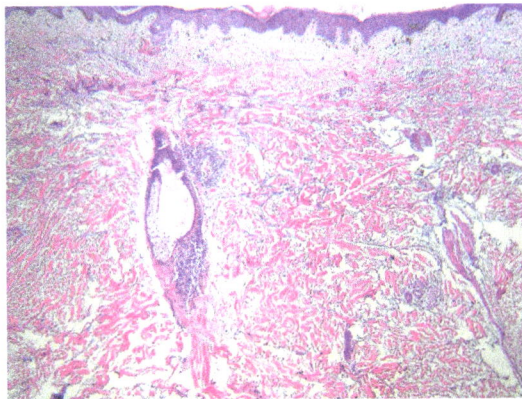

FIGURE 6: Lupus erythematosus, high power showing many scattered necrotic keratinocytes with interface changes and dermal lymphocytic infiltrate. H&E, 400x.

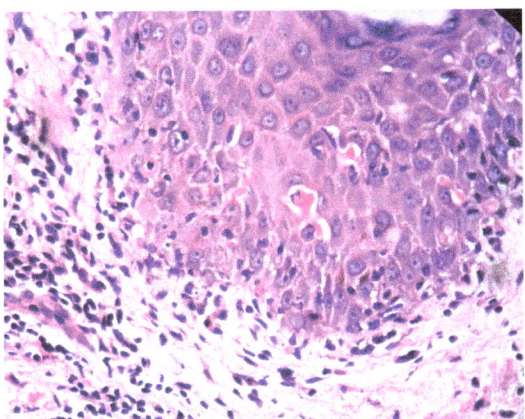

FIGURE 5: Lupus erythematosus, melanophages in the papillary dermis with abundant bluish-gray stringy mucin seen interstitially in the reticular dermis. H&E, 400x.

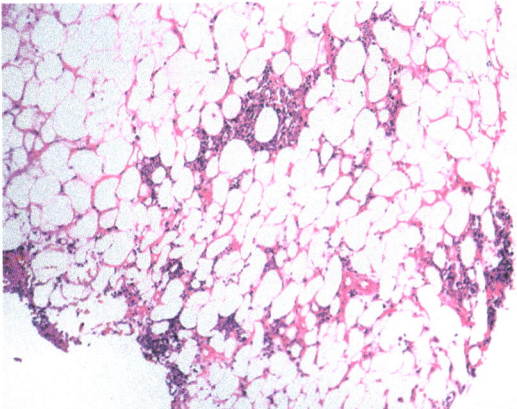

FIGURE 7: Lupus profundus, patchy lobular inflammation with mainly lymphocytes. H&E, 100x.

collagen bundles. Finding of dermal mucin in the absence of epidermal changes helps in the diagnosis of tumid LE and to differentiate it from the other lymphocytic infiltrates of the skin.

The papillary dermis is usually thickened and may be sclerotic and edematous and has a scattered lymphocytic infiltrate with melanophages. The infiltrate at times may be dense and lichenoid and resemble lichen planus. Longstanding lesions show a very sparse infiltrate but often have dilated telangiectases in the papillary dermis.

"Panniculitis (lupus profundus)" may be seen in LE and shows lobular lymphocytic panniculitis with diffuse lymphocytic infiltrates in the subcutaneous fat lobules (Figs 7 and 8).

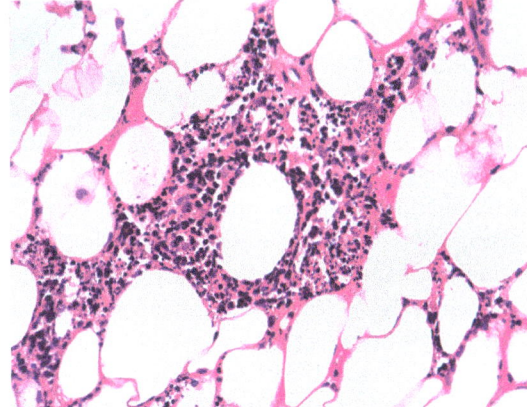

FIGURE 8: Lupus profundus, high magnification showing karyorrhexis of lymphocytes. H&E, 400x.

Lymphocytic nuclear dust is common and few plasma cells may be seen. Some cases show formation of lymphoid follicles and some may show areas of necrosis with histiocytes with engulfed nuclear debris (periempolesis) with marked nuclear atypia. Lymphomatoid lupus panniculitis has to be differentiated from the more serious subcutaneous panniculitis like T-cell lymphoma (SCPTCL). If there are accompanying epidermal and/or dermal changes of LE, diagnosis of lupus profundus is easily made.

Clinically, lupus profundus is seen mainly in women in their 3rd to 5th decades who present with deep-seated hard nodules on face, buttocks, arms and which may ulcerate leaving unsightly scars.

FOLLICULAR INVOLVEMENT IN LUPUS ERYTHEMATOSUS

Chronic LE lesions on the scalp result in scarring alopecia due to destruction of hair follicles. The follicular infundibula show interface changes with thinning of the follicular walls and keratin plugs. Long-standing lesions progress to complete destruction of the follicles and their replacement by vertically oriented fibrotic tracts that contain thick collagen and some lymphocytic infiltrate. Intact muscles of hair erection are often seen at the bases of these fibrotic tracts.

UNCOMMON CUTANEOUS PRESENTATIONS OF LUPUS ERYTHEMATOSUS

Bullous Lupus Erythematosus

Bullae in patients with SLE may present as blisters arising on a background of erythema resembling pemphigoid or small vesicles as seen in dermatitis herpetiformis (DH). Biopsy of a vesicle shows a subepidermal blister filled with numerous neutrophils or papillary neutrophilic microabscesses as seen in DH and the histological DDs include linear IgA disease and epidermolysis bullosa acquisita. Direct immunofluorescence (DIF) shows linear deposits of IgG and IgM at the dermoepidermal junction.

Lymphomatoid Lupus Erythematosus

Dense infiltrates of lymphoid cells with some atypia may be seen in cutaneous lesions of LE and may be mistaken for lymphoma.

Various histological patterns have been described under this entity:
- Folliculotropic lymphomatoid LE: It has dense perifollicular infiltrates of lymphocytes and clinically presents as follicular papules on face
- Lichenoid pattern with a dense band like infiltrate of lymphoid cells, with some epidermotropism and atypia of lymphocytes that may resemble cutaneous T-cell lymphoma
- Angioimmuno proliferative lesions
- Panniculitis with dense infiltrates of sometimes atypical lymphoid cells that resembles SCPTCL.

Drug-induced Lupus Erythematosus

Several classes of drugs are known to induce LE like eruption and the histology generally is the same as idiopathic LE with vacuolar-interface dermatitis and atrophy of the epidermis.[3] Many individually necrotic keratinocytes, parakeratosis, and dermal eosinophils are suggestive of a drug-induced eruption.

Chilblain Lupus Erythematosus

Patients with LE may present in cold and damp environments with painful violaceous and red nodules on the hands and feet. Histology may not show typical interface dermatitis of lupus but instead show marked subepidermal edema with a dense superficial and deep perivascular infiltrate of lymphocytes.

DERMATOMYOSITIS

Histopathologic changes in dermatomyositis are very similar to those seen in LE and biopsies taken from erythematous patches or plaques show pauci-cellular vacuolar-interface dermatitis with atrophy of the epidermis and numerous dilated thin-walled telangiectases in the papillary dermis (Figs 9 and 10). Like LE, dermatomyositis also has thickening of the basement membrane that may be demonstrated very elegantly by a PAS stain. Mucin deposits too are seen in dermatomyositis

Dermatopathology of Rheumatologic Diseases

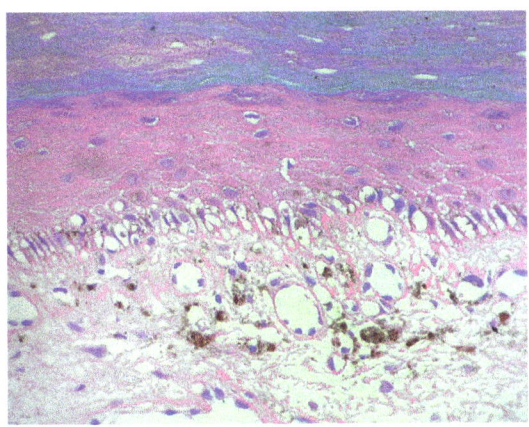

FIGURE 9: Dermatomyositis, basal cell vacuolization, dermal melanophages, telangiectases, note paucity of lymphocytes. H&E, 400x.

Gottron's papules which are erythematous papules that arise typically on the dorsae of knuckles of hands but also on bony prominences like elbows, show interface changes of basal cell vacuolization with hyperplasia of the epidermis. Late lesions may show flattening or even atrophy of the epidermis.

Mechanic's hands are distinctive skin changes seen in dermatomyositis which present with a cracked fissured appearance of skin, of the fingers, of the hands and may be mistaken for hand eczema. A biopsy from such lesions shows psoriasiform epidermal hyperplasia with scatter of several individually necrotic keratinocytes in the mid- and upper-spinous layers with some parakeratosis of the thick keratin layer. No basal cell vacuolization is seen (Figs 11 and 12).

Differentiation of dermatomyositis from cutaneous LE can be difficult on histology alone but pointers to the diagnosis of LE include a superficial and deep lymphocytic infiltrate that is fairly dense, mucin that is more abundant and a positive DIF test that shows a positive lupus band test with linear deposits of immunoglobulins, usually IgG and IgM at the dermoepidermal junction. Direct immunofluorescence is consistently negative in dermatomyositis.

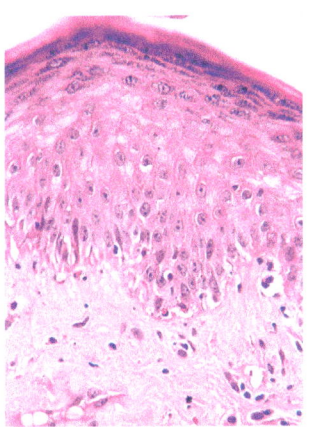

FIGURE 10: Dermatomyositis, subtle interface changes with individually necrotic keratinocytes and a thickened granular layer. Such changes are also seen in graft versus host disease. H&E, 400x.

but are very scant and may not be seen easily on hematoxylin (H) and eosin (E) stained sections. In general, the inflammatory infiltrate is very scant in lesion of dermatomyositis.

If the biopsy is from a clinically poikilodermatous lesion, the histologic findings reflect the changes of poikiloderma, namely, a lichenoid infiltrate of lymphocytes admixed with variable number of melanophages and dilated thin-walled telangiectases.

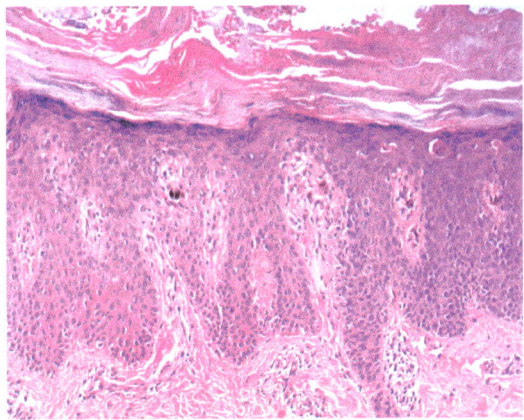

FIGURE 11: Mechanic's hands in dermatomyositis, psoriasiform hyperplasia with parakeratosis and scattered individually necrotic keratinocytes in the upper spinous zone. H&E, 100x.

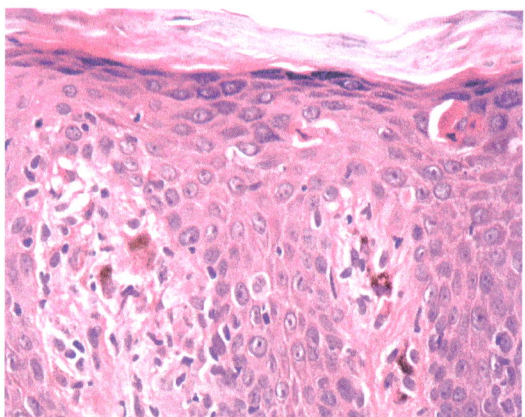

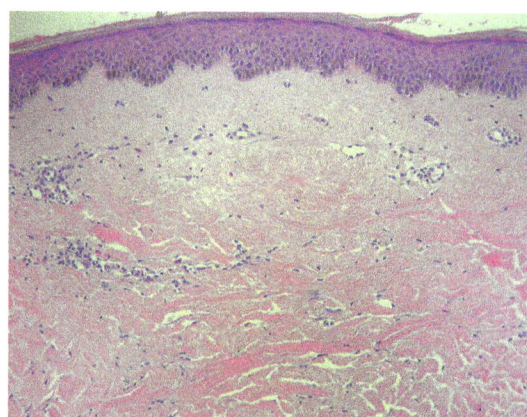

FIGURE 12: Mechanic's hands, high magnification showing scattered individually necrotic keratinocytes in upper spinous zone and papillary dermal melanophages. H&E, 400x.

FIGURE 14: Morphea, sclerotic hyalinized collagen with interstitial infiltrate of lymphocytes and few eosinophils. H&E, 100x.

SCLERODERMA

The histological findings of morphea (localized scleroderma) and systemic sclerosis (SSc) are similar but are best appreciated in morphea which is the prototype of sclerosing dermatitis. In SSc the early edematous phase has findings very similar to morphea, however, as the lesions age the findings become less specific and in late long-standing scleroderma may be totally nonspecific.

Morphea in all its clinical variants shows in early and active lesions a sparse mixed cell infiltrate of lymphocytes and plasma cells accompanied by few eosinophils (Figs 13 and 14).

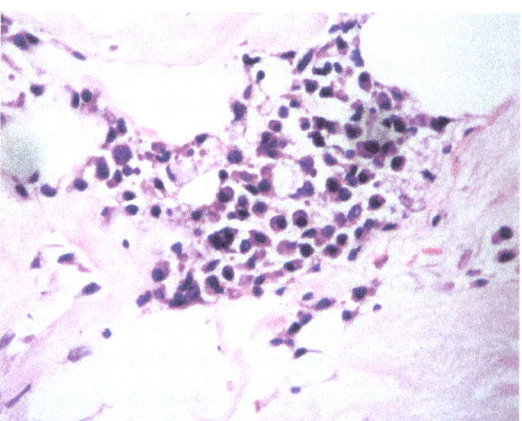

FIGURE 15: Morphea, plasma cell infiltrate with sclerotic collagen. H&E, 400x.

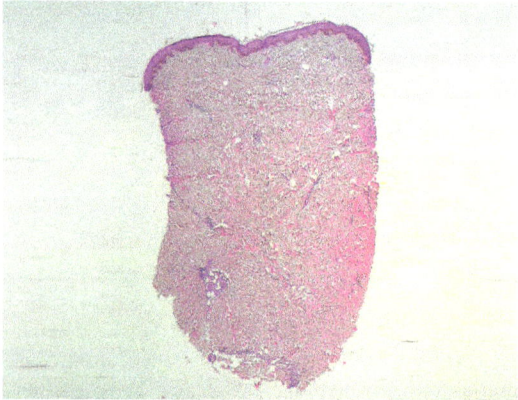

FIGURE 13: Morphea, square outline of biopsy due to thickened sclerotic collagen, prominent melanin in the basal layer of the epidermis and marked paucity of adnexal structures. H&E, 40x.

The infiltrate is in perivascular and interstitial locations and is more pronounced in the lower parts of the dermis and the dermal-subcutaneous junction. Perineural infiltrates of plasma cells are quite characteristic in morphea but are not seen in all cases (Fig. 15). In cases of deep morphea (morphea profunda), the infiltrate is also seen to involve the thickened fibrous septae of the subcutaneous fat tissue leading to a sclerotic septal panniculitis. As the lesions develop, the infiltrate can become denser and at times nodular collections of lymphocytes and plasma cells may be seen in the deep dermis at the dermal-subcutaneous junction.

Dermatopathology of Rheumatologic Diseases

Sclerosis of collagen is the histological characteristic of morphea and in well-developed lesions, gives the biopsy a square outline due to dense hyalinized collagen of the reticular dermis that does not show any spaces between the collagen bundles. In older lesions, the sclerosis predominates and the inflammatory infiltrate may be very sparse and is mostly interstitial in location. Occasionally, abundant mucin may be seen in interstitial location in the upper and mid-reticular dermis and may be mistaken for a lesion of cutaneous LE. The epidermis in most cases if flattened and shows prominent melanin in the basal layer which correlates clinically with the hyperpigmented appearance of most lesions of morphea.

Eosinophilic fasciitis (Schulman's syndrome) is considered by some to be part of the spectrum of morphea in which the inflammation is centered on the fascia and deep dermis and subcutis and is accompanied by innumerable eosinophils.

"Lichen sclerosus" is a sclerotic dermatitis that involves the papillary dermis and has a very characteristic appearance in its fully developed stage (Fig. 16). The epidermis is flattened and may show mild basal cell vacuolization with a thickened laminated orthokeratotic stratum corneum.

The papillary dermis is edematous and may have extravasated erythrocytes and a scattered lympho-plasmacytic infiltrate in early lesions but with time gets sclerotic with pale homogenous collagen which pushes the infiltrate to the base of the sclerotic papillary dermis where it is often arranged in an interstitial and focally lichenoid manner. The reticular dermis in lichen sclerosus in contrast to morphea is normal and may be thinner than the thickened and sclerotic papillary dermis.

Lichen sclerosus occurs typically on the genitalia both in males and females but also may occur in extragenital locations. The histology is similar in all sites. In males, in the condition known as BXO (balanitis xerotica obliterans) vesicles, often hemorrhagic, occur on the glans and prepuce which histologically show features typical of lichen sclerosis with subepidermal blisters.

Lichen sclerosus of the female genitalia can be extremely pruritic and not uncommonly changes of rubbing similar to lichen simplex chronicus are seen and include a hyperplastic epidermis with a thick granular layer and a compact horny layer in addition to the typical dermal changes of sclerosis and a variably dense lymphoplasmacytic infiltrate with focal interface changes. Squamous cell carcinoma is a complication of long-standing genital lichen sclerosus.

In SSc biopsy of the salt and pepper pigmentation shows subtle interface changes of basal cell vacuolization with few colloid bodies and scattered melanophages in the upper papillary dermis (Fig. 17).

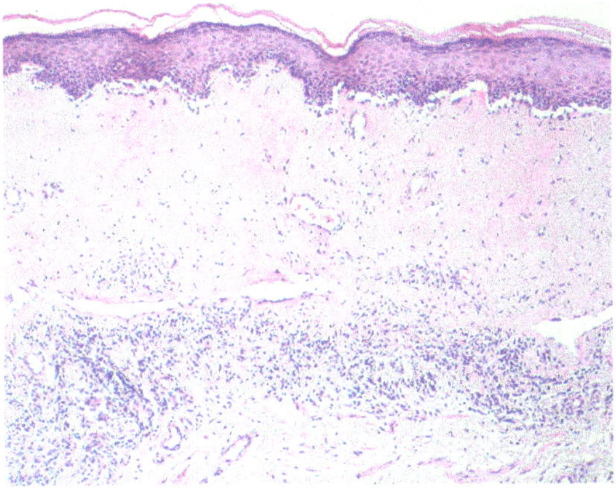

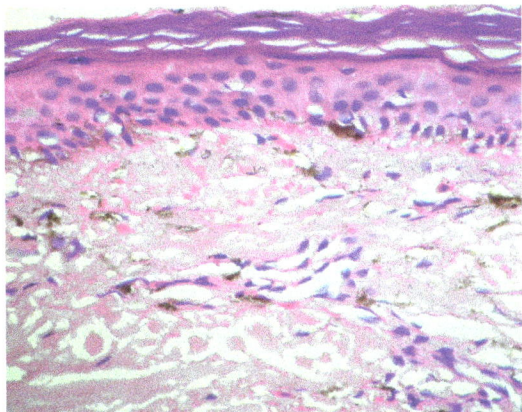

FIGURE 16: Lichen sclerosus, sclerotic collagen of upper dermis with telangiectases and a broad band like lymphocytic infiltrate at base of the sclerotic upper dermis. H&E, 100x.

FIGURE 17: Scleroderma, salt and pepper pigmentation, melanophages in papillary dermis with colloid bodies. H&E, 100x.

RHEUMATOID ARTHRITIS

Disease specific skin manifestations associated with rheumatoid arthritis include:
- Subcutaneous nodules:
  - Classical rheumatoid nodules (30% of patients)
  - Accelerated rheumatoid nodulosis
  - Rheumatoid nodulosis.

Rheumatoid nodules occur in both adult and juvenile rheumatoid arthritis and present as large, firm, asymptomatic, deep-seated masses over the elbow and other joints. Histologically, they present with large areas of necrobiosis with pink fibrin deposits surrounded by palisades of histiocytes and multinucleated giant cells. Traditionally three zones have been described: (i) Zone of central necrosis with fibrinoid changes, (ii) Surrounding cellular zone which has radially arranged histiocytes and giant cells, and (iii) Peripheral area consisting of thickened collagen that is concentrically arranged around the inner two zones. Long-standing lesions show mainly concentric scarring with disappearance of the central focus of necrosis and cellular infiltrates giving rise to a sclerotic nodule.

Rheumatoid necrobiotic-palisaded granulomas are usually much larger and located in the deep dermis or in the subcutis as compared to the smaller more superficial areas of necrobiosis seen in granuloma annulare. Also granuloma annulare shows bluish mucin in the center of the necrobiotic foci as compared to pink fibrin in rheumatoid nodules. The main differential diagnosis is subcutaneous granuloma annulare where it may be difficult to differentiate the two conditions on histologic findings alone.

Accelerated rheumatoid nodulosis occurs in patients with rheumatoid arthritis who have been on methotrexate and who while on therapy develop small subcutaneous nodules over fingers, elbows, and other bony prominences which disappear on stopping methotrexate. Histologically, they are similar to classical rheumatoid nodules.

Subcutaneous nodules are also common in rheumatic fever and they too clinically and histologically are similar to rheumatoid nodules.
- Rheumatoid vasculitis: Rheumatoid vasculitis involves both small- and medium-sized vessels and can affect several organs including the skin. Nailfold infarcts and leg ulcers are the usual clinical presentations. The pathology resembles that seen in polyarteritis nodosa with vessel wall damage by neutrophils and leukocytoclasia and fibrin deposits in vessel walls
- Neutrophilic dermatoses like Sweet's syndrome, pyoderma gangrenosum, rheumatoid neutrophilic dermatitis, and neutrophilic dermatosis of dorsum of hands may be seen in rheumatoid arthritis and histologically show features of a neutrophilic dermatosis with dense diffuse dermal infiltrates of neutrophils without vasculitis or abscess formation. Marked subepidermal edema may be seen in cases that resemble Sweet's syndrome
- Granulomatous dermatitides like interstitial granulomatous dermatitis and palisaded neutrophilic granulomatous dermatitis.[4]

Interstitial granulomatous dermatitis classically presents with indurated cord-like lesions on the trunk and axillae (rope sign) and histologically shows small foci of necrobiotic collagen with mild neutrophilic or eosinophilic debris and a sparse palisaded histiocytic infiltrate.

Palisaded neutrophilic granulomatous dermatitis on the other hand presents with crusted and umbilicated papules usually on elbows and are associated with rheumatoid arthritis and Churg-Strauss disease and histologically shows intense neutrophilic infiltrates with histiocytes scattered interstitially often with evidence of vasculitis.

There is an overlap between these entities and some authors believe that they represent either ends of a continuum of a single disease process. Another view is that these disorders represent a disease spectrum that manifests in the skin differently predicated on the balance between the humoral and cellular immune response. These interstitial granulomatous dermatitides have been associated not only with rheumatoid arthritis but with other autoimmune and lymphoproliferative diseases such as SLE, SSc, autoimmune hepatitis, hematologic malignancies and even drug reactions.

STILL'S DISEASE

Adult onset Still's disease (AOSD) is a symptom complex presenting with high fever, leukocytosis with neutrophilia, skin rash, and arthralgias. The typical skin rash of Still's disease is an evanescent faint Salmon-pink erythema commonly involving the extremities. Another skin manifestation associated with AOSD is a persistent rash of pruritic erythematous violaceous or brownish scaly or crusted papules on the trunk, neck, face and extensor aspects of extremities. The lesions may be arranged in bizarre linear patterns due to scratching by the patients. The persistent rash is described as persistent pruritic eruptions (PPEs) and various types of PPEs have been described in AOSD (lichenoid, urticarial, linear, dermographism like, dermatomyositis like, prurigo pigmentosa like and lichen amyloidosis like).[5]

HISTOPATHOLOGY

The evanescent pink rash shows a superficial perivascular infiltrate of lymphocytes and neutrophils.

The persistent lichenoid papules show epidermal hyperplasia with clusters of individually necrotic keratinocytes in the upper spinous as well as in the stratum corneum along with a superficial perivascular infiltrate of lymphocytes and scattered neutrophils. The combination of multiple necrotic keratinocytes in the upper epidermis and a dermal infiltrate of neutrophils is characteristic and differentiates this condition from other lichenoid and interface dermatitides.

SJÖGREN'S SYNDROME

The most common changes in Sjögren's syndrome are destruction of salivary and lachrymal glands which accounts for the xerostomia and dryness of conjunctiva.

A skin biopsy may help in the diagnosis and shows a mixed inflammatory cell infiltrate of lymphocytes with few or occasional plasma cells and histiocytes around salivary and sweat glands with mild necrosis of the glands.

REFERENCES

1. Ackerman AB, Chongchitnant N, Sanchez J, Guo Y, Benin B, Reichel M, et al. Histologic diagnosis of inflammatory skin diseases: An algorithmic method based on pattern analysis, 2nd ed. Philadelphia: Williams and Wilkins; 1997.
2. Crowson NA, Magro C. The cutaneous pathology of lupus erythematosus: A review. J Cut Pathol. 2001;28:1-23.
3. Joshi R. Interface dermatitis. Ind J Dermatol Venereo Leprol. 2013;79:349-59.
4. Chu P, Connolly MK, LeBoit PE. The histopathologic spectrum of palisaded neutrophilic and granulomatous dermatitis in patients with collagen vascular disease. Arch Dermatol. 1994;130:1278-83.
5. Lee JY, Hsu CK, Liu MF, Chao SC. Evanescent and persistent pruritic eruptions of adult-onset Still's disease: a clinical and pathologic study of 36 patients. Semin Arthritis Rheum. 2012;42:317-26.

CHAPTER 4

Immunodiagnostics in Rheumatologic Diseases

Sanat Phatak, Amita Aggarwal

INTRODUCTION

Laboratory tests play an important role in management of rheumatological diseases. They can be used to confirm or refute a diagnosis and in prediction of prognosis and response to treatment. However, as is true with laboratory tests in any other field of medicine, they must be used in the right clinical context. With unwarranted ordering, the same helpful tests can act as double-edged swords, adding confusion rather than clarity.

Immunodiagnostic tests used in rheumatologic illnesses include:
- Tests to measure inflammation
- Autoantibodies
- Miscellaneous tests: Complement levels, cryoglobulins.

MARKERS OF INFLAMMATION

Connective tissue disorders, especially in their active stages, are characterized by inflammation. The markers of inflammation include normochromic anemia, thrombocytosis, hyperferritinemia, and raised erythrocyte sedimentation rate (ESR) or C-reactive protein (CRP). In addition, the levels of albumin may be reduced. Among these ESR and CRP are used most often. The CRP rises quickly and comes down within a week after subsidence of inflammatory stimuli and its level can rise more than 100-fold, thus it is very sensitive to change with treatment. In contrast, ESR rises slowly and comes down over weeks. However, it is easy to do and cheap, thus can be used to monitor chronic inflammation.

AUTOANTIBODIES

Rheumatoid Factor

Rheumatoid factor (RF) is an autoantibody which recognizes Fc component of IgG. While in clinical practice IgM RF is measured, IgG and IgA RF isotypes are also present in patients with RA.

Measurement

Rheumatoid factor can be measured using latex agglutination and nephelometry. While the former is a simpler, less expensive method that can be carried out at the point of care, nephelometric analysis has the advantages of automation and quantification of the antibodies and has thus become standard of care. Rheumatoid factor should be expressed as international unit for ease of comparison across laboratories.

Clinical Utility

Classically, RF is used in the diagnosis of rheumatoid arthritis (RA). It is positive in 70–80% of patients with RA; however, it is not specific. Positive results for RF may be obtained in some healthy subjects as well as a host of other disorders (Table 1).[1]

When should RF be ordered? It should be ordered in a patient with polyarthritis or early arthritis where a diagnosis of RA is being

Immunodiagnostics in Rheumatologic Diseases

Table 1: Prevalence of rheumatoid factor	
Clinical disorder	RF positivity observed
Rheumatoid arthritis	70–80%
Sjögren's syndrome	40–60%
Systemic lupus erythematosus	20%
Mixed cryoglobulinemia	100%
Others: Autoimmune hepatitis Infections: Tuberculosis, infective endocarditis, viral hepatitis, bacterial infections Malignancy: Hematological and solid organ	15–20%
Healthy controls	5–10%

RF, rheumatoid factor.

considered. Presence of RF in such patients (inflammatory arthritis and palindromic rheumatism) increases the probability of progressing to overt rheumatoid arthritis and a need for early treatment. In a patient with RA, presence of RF suggests an aggressive disease with poor prognosis.[2] Rheumatoid factor is also useful in patients with suspected cryoglobulinemia or Sjögren syndrome.

Anticitrullinated Protein Antibodies

A relatively new test for rheumatoid arthritis, measures antibodies to citrullinated peptides and thus called "anticitrullinated peptide antibodies (ACPA)". It can be directed against multiple host antigens like filaggrin, vimentin, etc.

Measurement

It is measured by enzyme-linked immunosorbent assay (ELISA), thus it is easy to do. Second generation ELISA or anti-CCP2 (anti-cyclic citrullinated peptide) antibody test is the standard assay used in clinical practice.

Clinical Utility

Anticitrullinated peptide antibody has the advantage of being more specific (85–95%) for rheumatoid arthritis than RF, while maintaining a similar level of sensitivity. ACPA also predicts a more severe disease phenotype with increased risk of erosions, mortality and extra-articular features.[3] Current guidelines recommend testing for both antibodies in the diagnosis of RA as 5–10% of patients may have either RF or ACPA.

Antinuclear Antibodies

The term "antinuclear antibodies (ANA)" describe antibodies directed against different components of the cell nucleus. These include DNA and associated proteins like histones, RNA associated proteins, nucleolar proteins, centromere, etc.

Measurement

Indirect immunofluorescence (IIF) and ELISA are the most widely used methods. IIF is considered the gold standard and it shows the pattern of nuclear reactivity. Hep2 cells are the most commonly used substrate. These are cultured laryngeal squamous carcinoma cells, which have good sensitivity due to the larger size of their nuclei.[4] Newer Ro-transfected Hep2000 cells have the added advantage of detecting antibodies to Ro which can be missed sometime on Hep2 cells. The report should include the titer as well as the IIF patterns of ANA (Fig. 1) which can provide a clue to the nuclear antigen detected and thereby, the likely disease (Table 2).[5] IIF is inexpensive, sensitive and specific; however, it is time consuming and identification of the different patterns may be difficult for beginners.

In contrast ELISA is automated, quantifiable and easy to perform. ELISA has been shown to have acceptable sensitivity ranging between 70% and 100% when it was compared to IIF; the sensitivity drops at low titer positive ANAs. ELISA also has a high false positivity rate.[6]

Clinical Utility

Antinuclear antibodies should be ordered when clinical features suggest a diagnosis of connective tissue disorder such as SLE (malar rash, polyarthritis, serositis, nephritis, and cytopenias); systemic sclerosis (Raynaud's phenomenon, sclerodactyly, interstitial lung disease); Sjögren's syndrome (dryness of eyes and mouth, polyarthralgias, and renal tubular acidosis). It is also useful in diagnosing autoimmune hepatitis and predicting the risk of uveitis in juvenile idiopathic arthritis (JIA) and progression in isolated Raynaud's phenomenon.

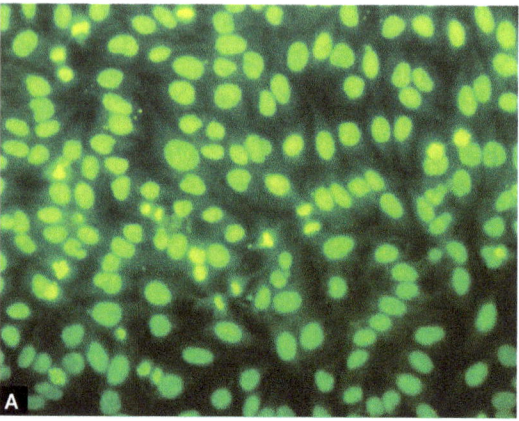
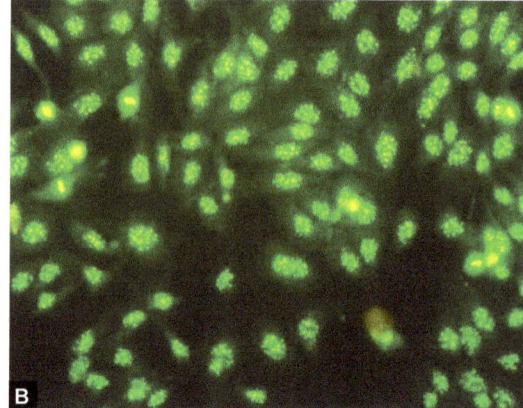

FIGURE 1: Antinuclear antibodies pattern on Hep2 cells. **A,** Homogeneous; **B,** Centromere.

Table 2: Antinuclear antibodies patterns and the probable antigenic targets		
ANA pattern	Antigens	Disease associated
Homogenous	Histone, dsDNA	SLE
Speckled	SSA, SSB, ribosomal P	SLE, Sjögrens
	Scl-70, RNP	Systemic sclerosis, MCTD
	Jo-1	Myositis
Centromere	CENP-A to E	Limited systemic sclerosis
Nucleolar	Pm/Scl, RNP	Systemic sclerosis, myositis

ANA, antinuclear antibodies; SLE, systemic lupus erythematosus; SSA, Sjögren's-syndrome-related antigen A; SSB, Sjögren's-syndrome-related antigen B; RNP, ribonucleoproteins; MCTD, mixed connective tissue disease; CENP, centromere proteins; dsDNA, double-stranded DNA.

Antinuclear antibodies are not recommended in the routine evaluation of joint pain, back pain or chronic fatigue. It should be remembered that elderly individuals and patients with infections, thyroiditis and other common diseases might have positive ANA with no clinical significance. Once positive, ANA need not be repeated periodically in patients with connective tissue disorders.

Antinuclear Antibodies Subspecificities

It is possible to characterize the actual nuclear antigens which are the target of antibodies.

- Anti double stranded DNA (dsDNA) antibodies: Antibodies directed against double-stranded DNA are specific for SLE (95%) and should be done in patients with suspected lupus where ANA is positive. ELISA is most commonly used as it is quantitative and cheap method. In contrast IIF using *Crithidia lucillae*, a hemoflagellate whose kinetoplast contains pure double-stranded DNA unadulterated by other nuclear antigens has a high specificity but is not quantitative.[7] The Farr assay is considered the most reliable method but it is cumbersome and carries the hazard of handling radioactivity[8]
- Antibodies to extractable nuclear antigens (ENA): Tissue extracts provided the actual nature of antigens present within the nucleus, Smith being the first to be identified. Now a large number of antigens have been identified, many of which have found their way into laboratory testing. Though not absolute, they display disease specificity and are therefore helpful in diagnosing the type of CTD (Table 3). In fact some diseases have come to be defined by their ENA specificities, the prototype being mixed connective tissue disease with antibodies to U1-RNP.

Antibodies to ENAs were originally described using gel precipitation assays.[9] ELISA and Western blotting have now replaced these older techniques. Popular assays utilize nitrocellulose paper with purified antigens blotted as dots (dot-blot assay) or as lines on a linear strip (line-blot assay). A blue-colored line produced by their binding to the specific antigen signifies the presence of autoantibodies in a test serum.[10] Usually, ENA is ordered in a patient with a positive ANA to characterize the type of CTD or in patients with Sjögren syndrome.

Table 3: Different extractable nuclear antigens specificities and disease association	
ENA	Disease association
Smith, ribosomal-P, nucleosome, histone	SLE
Ro/(SSA), La/(SSB)	SLE (subacute cutaneous lupus, neonatal lupus), Sjögren's syndrome
Scl-70, RNA polymerase III	Diffuse cutaneous systemic sclerosis
RNP	SSc, MCTD
CENP-A to E	Limited cutaneous SSc
Jo-1	Inflammatory myositis

ENA, extractable nuclear antigens; SLE, systemic lupus erythematosus; MCTD, mixed connective tissue disease; CENP, centromere proteinsSSc, systemic sclerosis; RNP, ribonucleoproteins.

Antineutrophil Cytoplasmic Antibodies

The ANCA are antibodies directed against primary granules of neutrophils, described in necrotizing vasculitides—now termed "ANCA associated vasculitis".

Measurement

Antineutrophil cytoplasmic antibodies can be detected using IIF and ELISA. IIF is performed on ethanol fixed neutrophils. Two separate patterns are discerned (Fig. 2): (1) cytoplasmic ANCA (c-ANCA) with fluorescence diffusely spread throughout the cytoplasm; (2) perinuclear ANCA (p-ANCA) shows fluorescence concentrated around the nucleus.[11] Though there are many antigenic targets serine protease proteinase-3 and myeloperoxidase are of clinical use, thus ELISA tests are available for them. IIF is more sensitive and is useful for screening, while ELISA is specific and is used for confirmation. It is recommended to do both IIF and ELISA to increase specificity.

Clinical Utility

The prevalence of ANCA in different disease varies from 30 to 80% (Table 4).[12]

Antineutrophil cytoplasmic antibodies should be ordered when features suggestive of necrotizing vasculitis are present such as pulmonary nodules, hemorrhage, pauci-immune glomerulonephritis, chronic otitis media, and chronic sinusitis, amongst others.[13] Indiscriminate use can lead to

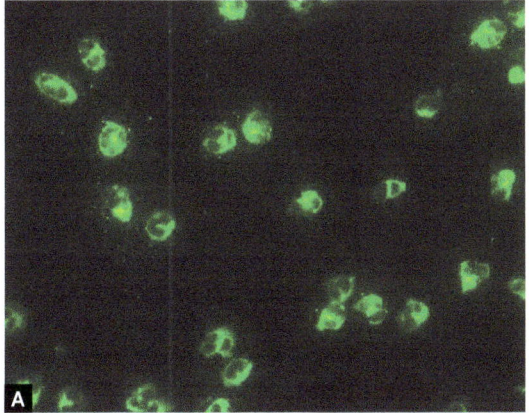
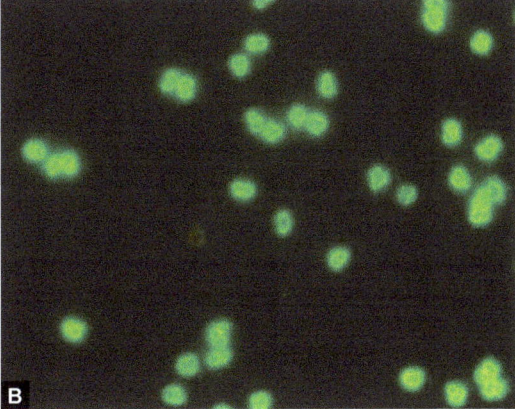

FIGURE 2: Antineutrophil cytoplasmic antibodies (ANCA) patterns on ethanol fixed human neutrophils. **A,** C-ANCA; **B,** P-ANCA.

Table 4: Prevalence of antineutrophil cytoplasmic antibodies in different diseases

Disease	Salient clinical features	IIF pattern	ELISA	Positivity (%)
Granulomatosis with polyangiitis, previously Wegener's granulomatosis	Upper respiratory involvement, pulmonary nodules, glomerulo-nephritis	c-ANCA	Proteinase-3 (PR-3)	60–80
Microscopic polyangiitis	Lower respiratory involvement (Alveolar hemorrhage), glomerulonephritis	p-ANCA	MPO	75
Eosinophilic granulomatosis with polyangiitis (EGPA, previously Churg-Strauss syndrome)	Reactive airways disease, peripheral eosinophilia, mononeuritis multiplex	p-ANCA	MPO	30–50

ANCA, antineutrophil cytoplasmic antibodies; IIF, indirect immunofluorescence; ELISA, enzyme-linked immunosorbent assay; MPO, myeloperoxidase.

high false positive rates, especially in IIF, due to antibodies to antigens other than MPO and PR3 like Ro, dsDNA, cathepsin, and lactoferrin. Common causes of ANCA positivity apart from AAV include other CTDs such as SLE, RA; infections such as tuberculosis, infective endocarditis and leprosy; inflammatory bowel disease; chronic liver disease-autoimmune hepatitis type 1; and malignancies like lymphoma. A positive ANCA report in these settings has no clinical utility.

MISCELLANEOUS TESTS

Complement Levels

Complement proteins are a highly conserved system of plasma and membrane proteins which play an important role in both innate and adaptive immunity. Its major role lies in effective clearance of immune complexes, opsonization of bacteria, and amplification of inflammatory response. Therefore, disorders characterized by immune complex deposition have reduced levels of complement due to a "mopping up" effect. A useful screening test for complement activation is the CH 50 (or total hemolytic complement assay) which demonstrates reduction in the level of any one of nine complement components. Antigenic assays for C3 and C4 are more commonly used and can be measured by nephelometry or turbidimetry.

Reduced complement levels are useful in SLE, cryoglobulinemia, and few forms of hypocomplementemic vasculitides such as urticarial vasculitis and rheumatoid vasculitis.[14] They are also useful in following up patients with lupus nephritis where low levels may signify flare, and Sjögren's syndrome where new onset fall in complement levels may be a harbinger for the development of lymphoma. Some patients may have inherited deficiencies of complement components and have an increased incidence of autoimmune diseases. The C3 and C4 are acute phase reactants and are raised in infections or inflammatory disorders, thus may be raised in patients with RA, etc.

Cryoglobulins

Cryoglobulins, as the name suggests, refers to proteins that precipitate at low temperature. They may be comprised of monoclonal immunoglobulins alone, or may be mixed with complement proteins. Three types of cryoglobulins have been described (Table 5).[15]

Cryoglobulinemias often present with palpable purpura, digital gangrene, arthritis, myalgias, and glomerulonephritis. Cryoglobulins are detected in sera, cooled to 4°C for 72 hours, and the precipitated proteins can then be quantified and characterized into subtypes.[16] Types II and III are called "mixed" cryoglobulinemia and testing will show presence of RF. Low levels of C4 with normal C3 are typical.

Table 5: Subtypes of cryoglobulins and their association

Type	Description	Disease associated	Symptomatology
Type I cryoglobulins	Monoclonal IgM or IgG	Monoclonal gammopathies—multiple myeloma, waldenstrom's macroglobulinemia, lymphomas, hepatitis C infection	Hyperviscosity and bland vessel thrombosis
Type II cryoglobulins	Monoclonal IgM with polyclonal IgG		Vasculitic manifestations (Immune complex deposition in blood vessels)
Type III cryoglobulins	Polyclonal IgG and polyclonal IgM	Infective, inflammatory disorders	

CONCLUSION

A large armamentarium of immunological tests is available to aid the physician in diagnosis and follow up of rheumatic diseases. Interpretation of these tests must be bolstered by appropriate clinical context. Inappropriate testing entails burden on laboratories, unnecessary referrals and further testing to confirm or refute diagnoses, thereby increasing healthcare costs.

REFERENCES

1. Nishimura K, Sugiyama D, Kogata Y, Tsuji G, Nakazawa T, Kawano S, et al. Meta-analysis: Diagnostic accuracy of anti-cyclic citrullinated peptide antibody and rheumatoid factor for rheumatoid arthritis. Ann Intern Med. 2007;146:797-808.
2. Guillemin F, Gerard N, van Leeuwen M, Smedstad LM, Kvien TK, van den Heuvel W, et al. Prognostic factors for joint destruction in rheumatoid arthritis: A prospective longitudinal study of 318 patients. J Rheumatol. 2003;30:2585-9.
3. Markatseli TE, Voulgari PV, Alamanos Y, Drosos AA, et al. Prognostic factors of radiological damage in rheumatoid arthritis: A 10-year retrospective study. J Rheumatol. 2011;38:44-52.
4. Cook L. New methods for detection of anti-nuclear antibodies. Clin Immunopathol. 1998;88:211-20.
5. Kumar Y, Bhatia A. Detection of antinuclear antibodies in SLE. Methods Mol Biol. 2014;1134:37-45.
6. Bizzaro N, Tozzoli R, Tonutti E, Piazza A, Manoni F, Ghirardello A, et al. Variability between methods to determine ANA, anti-dsDNA and anti-ENA auto-antibodies: a collaborative study with the biomedical industry. J Immunol Methods. 1998;219:99-107.
7. Slater NGP, Cameron JS, Lessof MH. The Crithidia luciliae kinetoplast immunofluorescence test in systemic lupus erythematosus. Clin Exp Immunol. 1976;25:480-6.
8. Farr RS. A quantitative immunochemical measure of the primary interaction between IxBSA and antibody. J Infect Dis. 1958;103:239-62.
9. Clark G, Reichlin M, Tomasi TB. Characterization of a soluble cytoplasmic antigen reactive with sera from patients with systemic lupus erythematosus. J Immunol. 1969;102:107-22.
10. Damoiseaux J, Boesten K, Giesen J, Austen J, Tervaert JWC, et al. Evaluation of a Novel Line-Blot Immunoassay for the Detection of Antibodies to Extractable Nuclear Antigens. Ann NYA Sci. 2006;1050:340-7.
11. Savige JA, Paspaliaris B, Silvestrini R, Davies D, et al. A review of immuno-fluorescent patterns associated with antineutrophil cytoplasmic antibodies (ANCA) and their differentiation from other antibodies. J Clin Pathol. 1998;51:568-75.
12. Millet A, Pederzoli-Ribeil M, Guillevin L, Witko-Sarsat V, Mouthon L, et al. Antineutrophil cytoplasmic antibody-associated vasculitides: Is it time to split up the group? Ann Rheum Dis. 2013;72:1273-9.
13. Savige J, Gillis D, Benson E, Davies D, Esnault V, Falk RJ, et al. International consensus statement on testing and reporting of antineutrophil cytoplasmic antibodies (ANCA). Am J Clin Pathol. 1999;111:507-13.
14. Gorevic PD. Rheumatoid factor, complement, and mixed cryoglobulinemia. Clin Dev Immunol. 2012;2012:439018.
15. Ramos-Casals M, Stone JH, Cid MC, Bosch X, et al. The cryoglobulinaemias. Lancet. 2012;379:348-60
16. Motyckova G, Murali M. Laboratory testing for cryoglobulins. Am J Hematol. 2011;86:500-2.

CHAPTER 5

Chronic Cutaneous and Subacute Cutaneous Lupus Erythematosus

Garima, Dipankar De, Sanjeev Handa

INTRODUCTION

Lupus erythematosus (LE) is the term designated to a spectrum of autoimmune diseases that are linked together by immunity against ribonucleoproteins and nucleosomes but having diverse clinical manifestations varying from mild isolated skin involvement in discoid LE (DLE) to life-threatening systemic involvement in systemic LE (SLE). Any subtype of cutaneous LE may be associated with SLE, which is a conglomeration of clinical manifestations, both cutaneous and systemic. Cutaneous lupus erythematosus (CLE) includes chronic cutaneous lupus erythematosus (CCLE), subacute cutaneous lupus erythematosus (SCLE), and acute CLE (ACLE). Though subtypes of CLE can be differentiated clinically, sometimes it may be difficult clinically and even histologically. This chapter will deal with the former two types only. A clear understanding of pattern of skin involvement can provide a clue to the risk of progression of disease and associated systemic involvement.

HISTORY

The term *lupus* (Latin for 'wolf') was first used during the Middle Ages to describe erosive skin lesions evocative of a wolf's bite. Due to early diagnosis and prompt treatment, these manifestations are unseen today and classic derivation of the term may be of importance of yesteryears. The first description of lupus erythematosus was given by Biett and the terminologies and descriptions have evolved over the years. The cutaneous manifestations of LE have been classified by Gilliam and Sontheimer[1] into those lesions that show characteristic histological changes of LE (LE specific skin disease) and those that are not distinct for LE and/or may be seen as a feature of another disease process (LE nonspecific skin disease). The detailed classification is beyond the scope of this chapter. Box 1 depicts the LE specific skin diseases.

Box 1: Classification of lupus erythematosus specific skin diseases[1]

A. Acute cutaneous lupus erythematosus (ACLE)
   - Localized ACLE
   - Generalized ACLE
B. Subacute cutaneous lupus erythematosus (SCLE)
   - Annular SCLE
   - Papulosquamous SCLE
C. Chronic cutaneous lupus erythematosus
   - Classical discoid lupus erythematosus (DLE)
   - Localized DLE
   - Generalized DLE
   - Hypertrophic cutaneous lupus erythematosus
   - Lupus profundus/lupuspanniculitis
   - Lupus erythematosus tumidus
   - Chilblain LE
   - Lichenoid DLE
   - Mucosal DLE
     ○ Oral
     ○ Conjuctival
   - Other uncommon variants

Chronic Cutaneous and Subacute Cutaneous Lupus Erythematosus

EPIDEMIOLOGY

Women are preferentially affected in CCLE in 2–3:1 ratio with the onset of disease typically occurring in second to fourth decade of life. Only 5% of patients present before 15 years of age or in the eighth decade of life. Discoid LE is slightly more common in African Americans than in whites or Asians.[2] Chronic cutaneous lupus erythematosus is present in 15–30% of SLE populations and approximately 5% of patients with isolated localized DLE subsequently develop SLE. Subacute cutaneous lupus erythematosus has been reported mostly in middle aged women aged 15–40 years and make up approximately 10–15% of the LE population.[2]

PATHOGENESIS

There are various studies demonstrating the combination of cellular and molecular events in pathogenesis of LE. However, a complete understanding of the diverse pathophysiological mechanisms of LE specific skin diseases does not exist as their pathogenesis is inextricably intertwined with SLE pathogenesis. Lupus erythematosus is a disorder in which the interplay between nonmodifiable factors (susceptibility genes, hormones, etc.) and modifiable factors (e.g., ultraviolet (UV) radiation, viruses, drugs etc.) leads to loss of self-tolerance and induction of autoimmunity. This is then succeeded by activation and expansion of the immune system resulting in tissue damage.

Nonmodifiable Factors

Genetic Factors

Cutaneous lupus erythematosus appears to follow a polygenic inheritance pattern. Recent genetic association studies have identified a number of genes that confer disease risk for CLE. Major genetic associations with DLE include the human leukocyte antigen (HLA)-A1, B8, DR3, B7, and DR2 haplotypes[3] and those with SCLE are HLA-A1, B8, DR3, DQ2, DRw52, and C4 null.[4] Additionally, SCLE is closely associated with the HLA haplotype DRB1*0301-B*086 which includes the 308A tumor necrosis factor-alpha (TNF-α) promoter polymorphism, which is associated with increased UV-induced TNF-α production in keratinocytes.[5] Many genetic regions outside the major histocompatibility complex region, for example genes encoding cytokines, their receptors, adhesion molecules, antioxidant enzymes, and apoptosis also increase the susceptibility to CLE[6-9] (Flowchart 1).

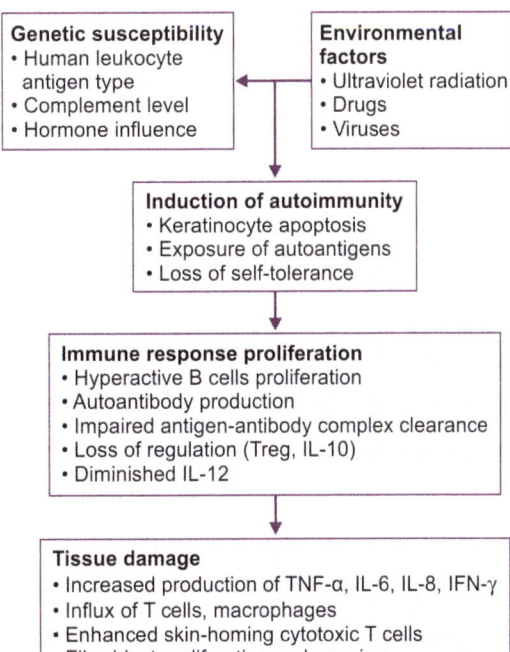

FLOWCHART 1: Steps in pathogenesis of discoid lupus erythematosus/subacute cutaneous lupus erythematosus.

Hormonal Factors

It has been observed that female predilection in CCLE is not as marked as in SLE. There is paucity of studies which explain slightly higher risk of SCLE in females. The potential causes of female predilection for SLE include the effects of estrogen and its hydroxylation, decreased androgen levels, hyperprolactinemia, and differences in gonadotropin-releasing hormone signaling.[10] In CLE, estrogen facilitates the interaction between keratinocytes expressing autoantigens and autoantibodies like anti-Ro and anti-La.[11] However, the pathogenesis and roles of hormones is not very clear in CCLE.

Infectious Agents

Infection by alpha-viruses, such as *Sindbis*, rubella and *Cytomegalovirus* has been associated with CLE. They act by inducing cell surface expression of Ro and related autoantigens in host cells which are undergoing virus-induced apoptosis.[12] However, no concrete evidence has been found in this regard.

Modifiable Factors

Ultraviolet Light

Genetic predisposition in itself is not sufficient to produce the disease. The induction of autoimmunity in such patients is often triggered by some inciting events, like UV light exposure, trauma, stress, drugs, infections, and other nonspecific factors. Deoxyribonucleic acid and protein mainly absorb ultraviolet B (UVB), which may explain why UVB might contribute more to the immunopathogenesis of inflammatory response. It has been hypothesized that UV-induced apoptosis, externalization of autoantigens, and activation of cytokine cascades play important roles. The UVB irradiation induces externalization of Ro autoantigen to the cell surface membrane of keratinocytes.[13] The Ro antigen is a nucleoprotein complex that has nuclear, cytoplasmic and plasma membrane localization at different stages in the cell cycle which is influenced by exposure of keratinocytes to UV radiation.[14] The externalization of autoantigens allows circulating autoantibodies to gain access to these autoantigens. Increased cytokine and chemokine release are often associated with UV irradiation of keratinocytes and other cells.[15] These cytokines and chemokines, such as IFN-γ, TNF-α, Interleukin-1 (IL-1), IL-10, and IL-17, may contribute to the initiation and amplification of the inflammatory process. The Ro52 antigen, which is upregulated in CLE lesions, is associated with enhanced keratinocyte apoptosis and impaired phagocytosis.[16] Also, defective Ro function drives autoimmune tissue inflammation via the IL-23/Th17 pathway which is a relatively recent finding.[17] Although anti-Ro and anti-La antibodies are closely associated with CLE, other autoantibodies may also be implicated in CLE. Anti-annexin 1 antibodies which is believed to interact with anti-La antibodies, to export La antigens to the surface of apoptotic cells have been observed in high percentage of patients with DLE.[18,19] Antibodies against complements like anti-C1q have been observed in CLE patients.[20] In addition to forming immune complexes, antibodies cause tissue damage by antibody-dependent cellular cytotoxicity.[21]

Drugs

Various drugs can induce CLE like lesions owing to their photosensitizing properties, which may then induce CLE lesions via isomorphic response in predisposed individuals. They also cause an increase in keratinocyte apoptosis, exposure of previously intracellular peptides on epidermal cell surfaces, and enhance proinflammatory cytokines such as TNF-α and IFN-γ. The existence of drug-induced DLE has often been questioned since the first reports of DLE-like lesions following treatment with fluorouracil, chemotherapeutic agents (tegafur, uracil-tegafur) and the TNF-α antagonists (infliximab and etanercept) appeared.[22] Drug-induced SCLE has been most commonly linked to antihypertensive drugs like hydrochlorothiazide, calcium channel blockers, beta blockers, and angiotensin converting enzyme inhibitors. Antifungals (terbinafine and griseofulvin) and chemotherapeutic drugs (docetaxel, paclitaxel, tamoxifen, and capecitabine) are the other two major groups of drugs associated with SCLE. Other drugs less commonly reported to precipitate SCLE include antihistamine (ranitidine, pheniramine, and cinnarizine), statins (simvastatin and pravastatin), proton pump inhibitors (lansoprazole), antiepileptics (carbamazepine and phenytoin), biologics (etanercept and efalizumab), immunomodulators (leflunomide, interferon α and β), nonsteroidal anti-inflammatory drugs (naproxen, piroxicam), and dermatological phototherapy.[23]

Immune Response

Chronic cutaneous lupus erythematosus is primarily a Th1 immune mediated immune disease. Scarring skin lesions of DLE are characterized by high numbers of skin-homing CD8+ cytotoxic lymphocytes associated with strong expression of the type I IFN-induced protein MxA. The role of Th17 cells in the pathogenesis of CLE has been increasingly recognized. The Th17 cells are regarded as major inducers of tissue inflammation and autoimmunity and they are able to exaggerate the response of Th1 and Th2 cells. In CLE patients, a skin specific defect in natural regulatory T cells (Tregs) with characteristic expression of CD4, CD25, and Foxp3 has been observed, unlike SLE where a generalized defect is seen.[24] The TNF-α is a major cytokine involved in the pathogenesis of SCLE. It serves as a growth factor for B cells and is involved in the production of antibodies. The IL-6, IL-10, IL-12, IL-17, and IL-18 have been implicated in the immunopathogenesis of CLE.[25]

Smoking

Associations between smoking and CLE are still under investigation. Previous studies have suggested that CCLE, particularly DLE and lupus erythematosus tumidus (LET), is more common in smokers.[26] Smoking induces dose-dependent cell death signaling, lower doses cause apoptosis whereas higher doses induce necrosis.[27]

CLINICAL FEATURES

CHRONIC CUTANEOUS LUPUS ERYTHEMATOSUS

It is important to distinguish among the subtypes of LE specific skin disease because the type of skin involvement in LE can predict presence of SLE or pattern of its activity. The designations acute, subacute, and chronic CLE are not related to duration of individual lesions but predict possibility of underlying SLE. For example, ACLE almost always occurs in the setting of SLE, whereas CCLE often occurs in the absence of SLE or in the presence of mild smoldering SLE. Subacute cutaneous lupus erythematosus occupies an intermediate position. It is not uncommon to see more than one subtype of LE specific skin disease in the same patient and occasionally it may be difficult to differentiate them clinically.

DISCOID LUPUS ERYTHEMATOSUS

Classical Discoid Lupus Erythematosus

It is the most common clinical variant of CCLE (Fig. 1) and involves the sun-exposed sites like face, V-region of the neck, and extensor surfaces of the arms, but it can also affect photoprotected sites like scalp (Fig. 2), retroauricular area (Fig. 3), trunk (Fig. 4), palmoplantar region (Fig. 5) or the inguinal folds. Early lesions are characterized by erythematous to violaceous papules and plaques with overlying adherent scale (Fig. 6). This scaling may extend into dilated hair follicles (follicular plugging) and on removal, keratotic spikes are seen on the undersurface of scale referred as the carpet tack sign. This sign is also seen in seborrheic dermatitis and pemphigus foliaceus but on removal of scale bleeding may be seen in DLE due to presence of adherent scale unlike the other two, where the scales are loose.[28] The lesions typically expand with erythema and hyperpigmentation at the periphery leaving hallmark atrophic central scarring, telangiectasia, and hypopigmentation (Fig. 7). A symmetric butterfly-shaped DLE plaque can be seen on the malar areas of the face

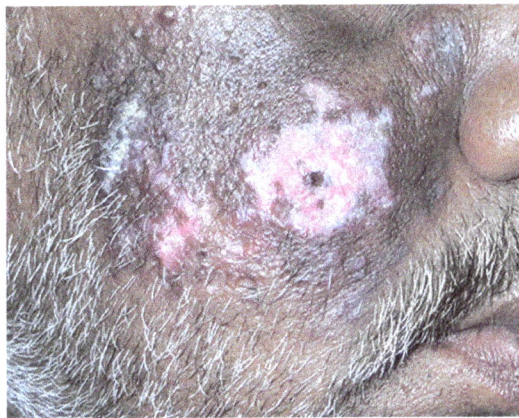

FIGURE 1: Discoid lupus erythematosus plaque over right cheek.

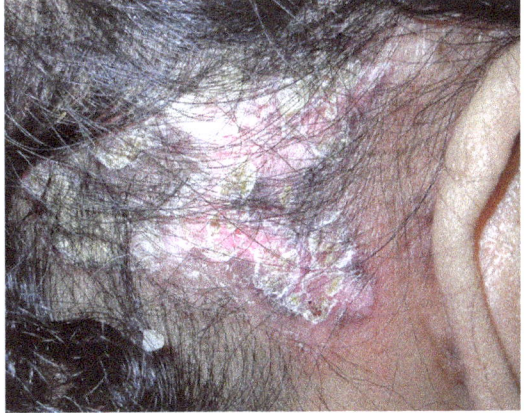

FIGURE 2: Discoid lupus erythematosus lesion over scalp showing scaling, central depigmentation, and peripheral hyperpigmentation, leading to scarring alopecia.

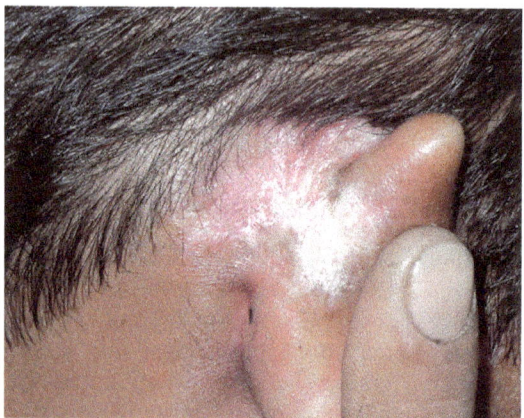

FIGURE 3: Psoriasiform discoid lupus erythematosus plaque over retroauricular area.

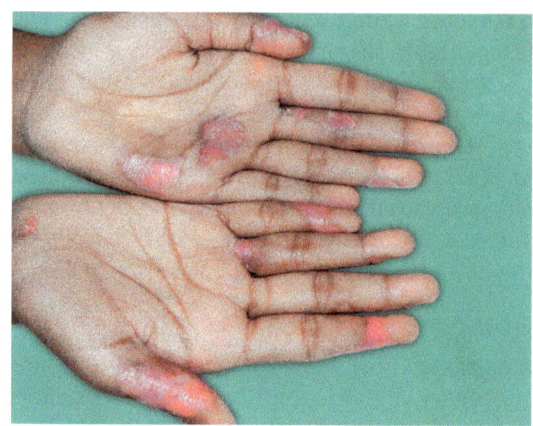

FIGURE 5: Discoid plaques over both palms.

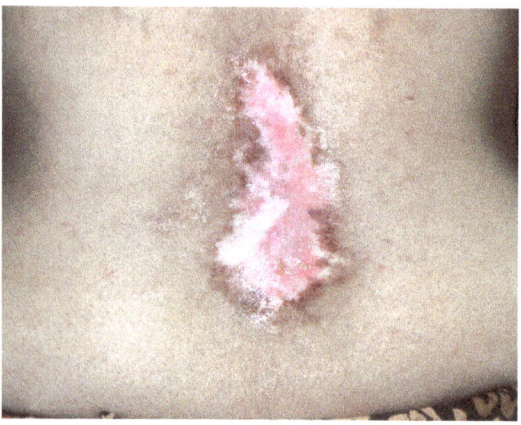

FIGURE 4: Chronic cutaneous lupus erythematosus plaque on lower back.

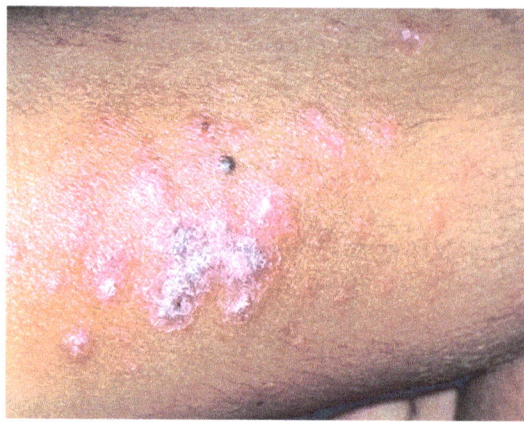

FIGURE 6: Early discoid lupus erythematosus lesion: well-defined erythematous to violaceous papules to plaques with adherent scaling and central atrophy. It is difficult to diagnose the lesion at this stage.

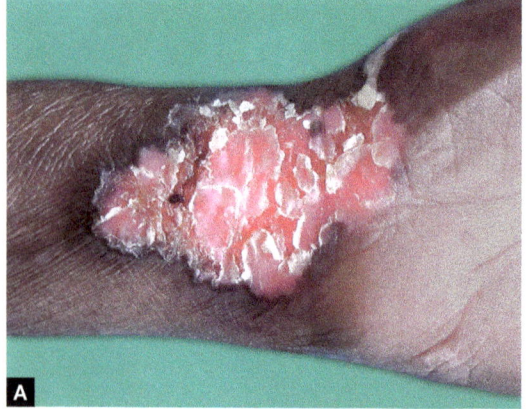

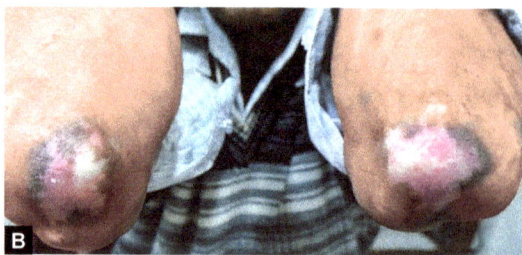

FIGURE 7: A, Hyperkeratotic discoid lupus erythematosus plaque over flexor aspect of wrist; **B,** Healed discoid lupus erythematosus lesions over both elbow with central eythema and hypopigmentation and peripheral hyperpigmentation (Koebner's phenomena).

and bridge of the nose sparing nasolabial folds (Fig. 8) similar to the lesions of ACLE. They can be differentiated by the presence of induration and adherent scaling in DLE. In Indians, DLE can also present as an isolated areas of macular hyperpigmentation (Fig. 9) or as small papular lesions with atrophic centre.[29]

Disseminated Discoid Lupus Erythematosus

It denotes widespread distribution on the trunk and limbs apart from face (Fig. 10) and is more common in women and smokers. It is often persistent, resistant to therapy and is associated with severe psychological upset. The distinction between localized and generalized DLE has prognostic implications, since the risk of developing SLE is only 5% in the former while it is 20% in the latter.[30] The appearance may sometimes be indistinguishable from the papulosquamous type of SCLE; however, presence of scarring suggests DLE.

Site Specific Lesion

Discoid lupus erythematosus lesions can appear in photo-protected areas like scalp (Fig. 11), ears

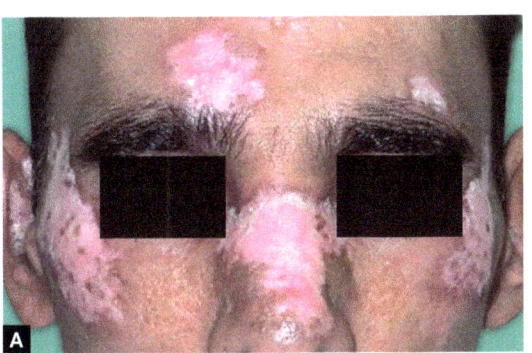
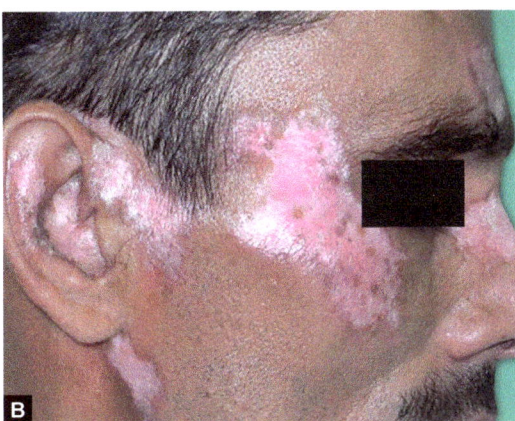

FIGURE 8: Discoid rash in butterfly distribution involving the bridge of nose and malar area.

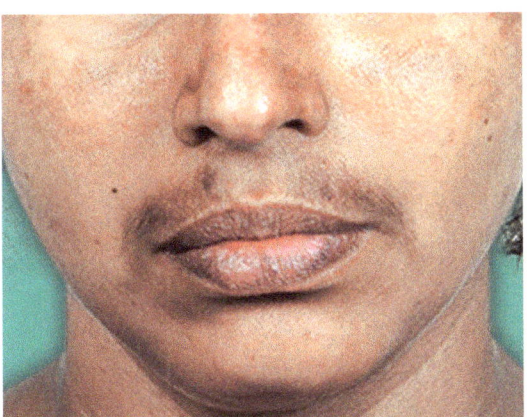
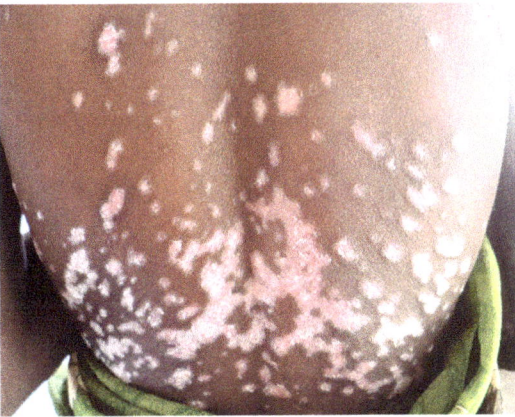

FIGURE 9: Discoid lupus erythematosus with only pigmentary abnormality; discoid lupus erythematosus lesions over left eyebrow and bilateral zygomatic area presenting with only hyperpigmentation and minimal follicular plugging in a few areas. Discoid lupus erythematosus lesions can also be appreciated over lower lip.

FIGURE 10: Disseminated discoid lupus erythematosus; erythematous to violaceous plaques present over the lower back.
Note: most lesions present in sari-exposed area over lower back unlike subacute cutaneous lupus erythematosus where upper back is more commonly involved.

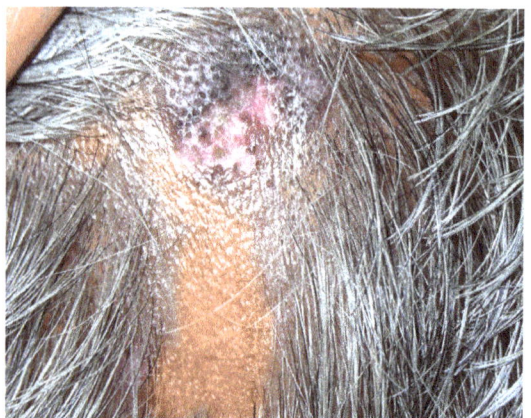

FIGURE 11: Classical discoid lupus erythematosus plaque over scalp showing dilated follicular ostia, prominent follicular plugging and cicatricial alopecia.

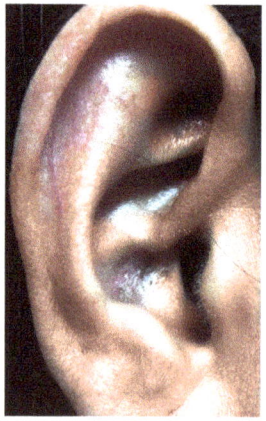

FIGURE 12: Shuster's sign: follicular plugging present in the concha of the right ear.

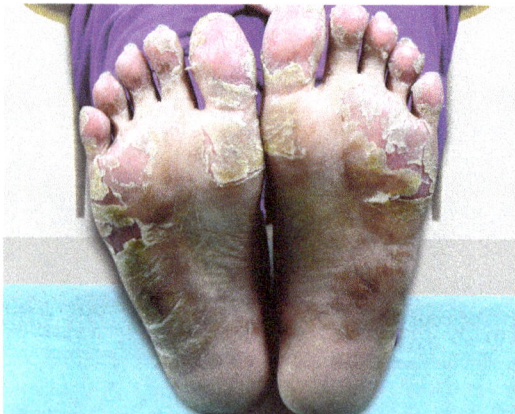

FIGURE 13: Discoid lupus erythematosus lesions over bilateral feet; scaly erythematous plaques with minimal atrophy present predominantly over forefoot and toes.

(Fig. 12), trunk, genitalia, palms, soles (Fig. 13). This suggests that the lesions can follow any form of trauma to the skin (Koebner's phenomenon) (Fig. 14).[31] In a series by Rowell and Goodfield,[32] they observed that DLE lesions were initiated by trauma in 11% of patients, sunburn in 5%, infection in 3%, and exposure to cold in 2%. Scalp is involved in approximately 60% patients of DLE and in approximately 10% of cases scalp is the only involved site (Fig. 15). It commonly presents as irreversible scarring alopecia[33] secondary to destruction of hair follicles, and rarely can be very extensive (Fig. 16).

Involvement of ears (Fig. 17) or tip of nose and scalp (Fig. 18) can lead to scarring and mutilations, with considerable disfigurement.

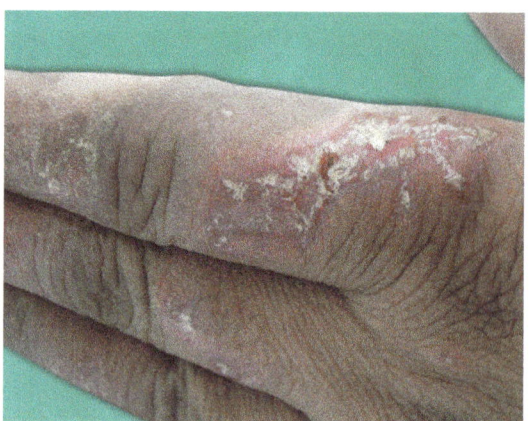

FIGURE 14: Linear discoid lupus erythematosus plaque appeared over the site of trauma from knife.

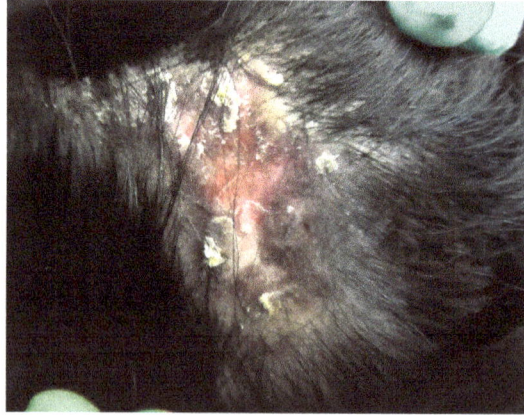

FIGURE 15: Scalp discoid lupus erythematosus; erythematous atrophic plaque with adherent scaling and both hypo and hyperpigmentation.

Chronic Cutaneous and Subacute Cutaneous Lupus Erythematosus

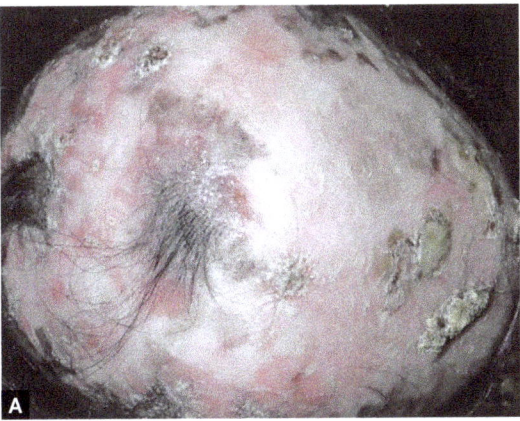
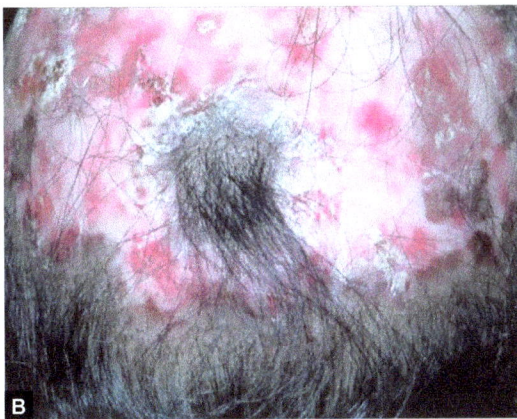

FIGURE 16: Extensive scalp discoid lupus erythematosus involving entire vertex and occipital area leading to extreme disfigurement.

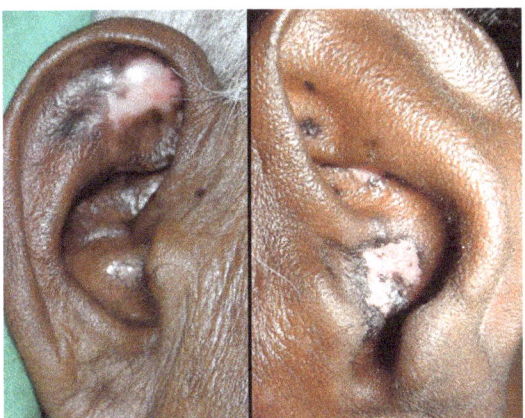

FIGURE 17: Classical discoid lupus erythematosus plaque involving the ear lobes.

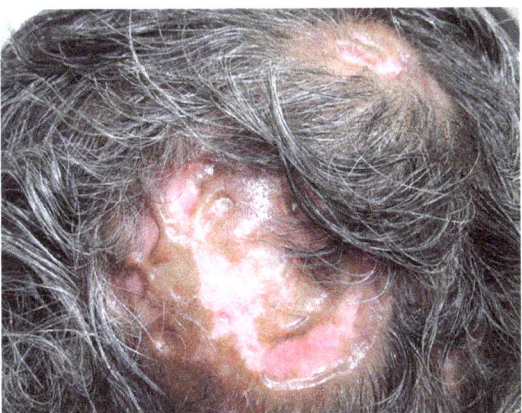

FIGURE 18: Scalp discoid lupus erythematosus healing with marked atrophy and scarring.

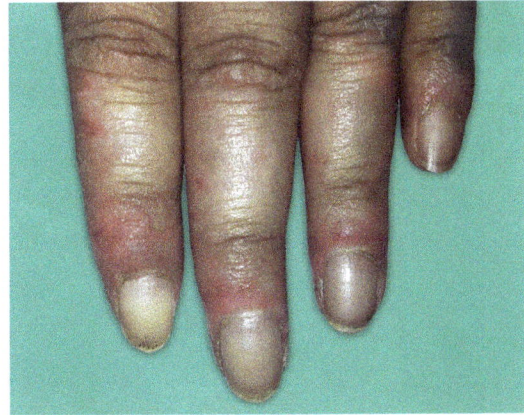

FIGURE 19: Erythematous painful plaques present over the tips of fingers.

Note: The nail fold capillary thrombosis, splinter hemorrhages in nail, and spindling of digits.

Fingers and toes may rarely show atrophic spindling with patchy erythema (Fig. 19), nail dystrophy, and terminal resorption on X-rays. Discoid LE of the palms (Fig. 20) and soles (Fig. 21) can present as classical discoid lesions or as painful to asymptomatic erythematous (Fig. 22) to violaceous plaques. Often, patient develop painful erosion and ulceration in violaceous plaques over extremities (Fig. 23) which may heal with contracture formation (Fig. 24). Nail involvement is uncommon and various nail changes reported in DLE include nail plate dystrophy with pitting, horizontal and longitudinal ridging, leukonychia striata,

Skin in Rheumatologic Disease

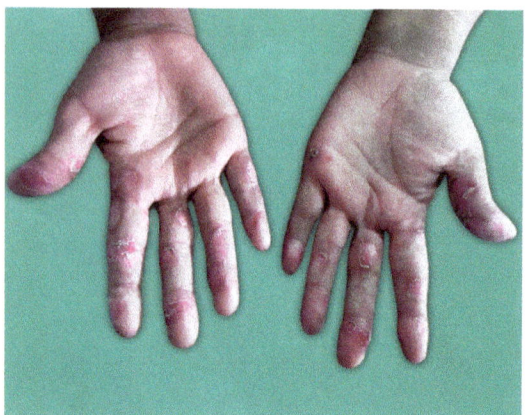

FIGURE 20: Discoid lupus erythematosus lesions over both palms.

onycholysis, clubbing, nail bed erythema, telangiectasias, and pterygium unguis. Periungual telangiectasias and erythema of the proximal nail fold are significant cutaneous findings that suggest progression to systemic disease in DLE patients.[34]

Rare Variants

Follicular DLE is characterized by follicular erythematous papules which is commonly located on the elbow region. Lupus erythematosus comedonicus simulates acneiform lesions and comedo-like structures on the seborrheic areas of the face (chin, nasolabial folds, ears, and scalp).[35] In LE vermiculatus (Fig. 25), tiny

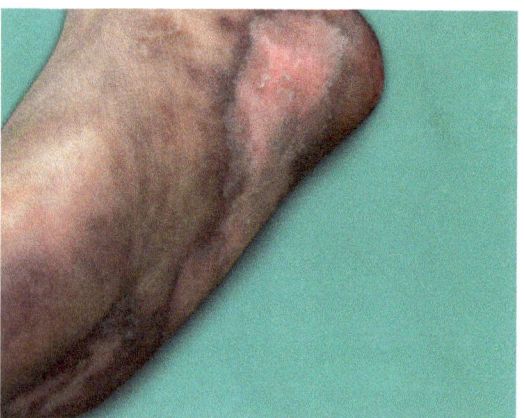

FIGURE 21: Discoid lupus erythematosus lesion over sole in a patient on treatment; scaling has reduced but the pigmentary changes and erythema is persisting.

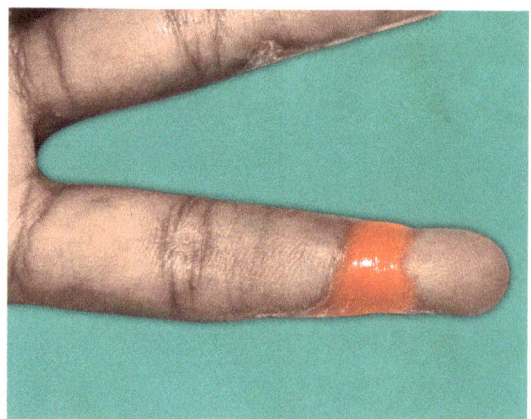

FIGURE 22: Erythematous chronic cutaneous lupus erythematosus plaque encircling the right index finger.

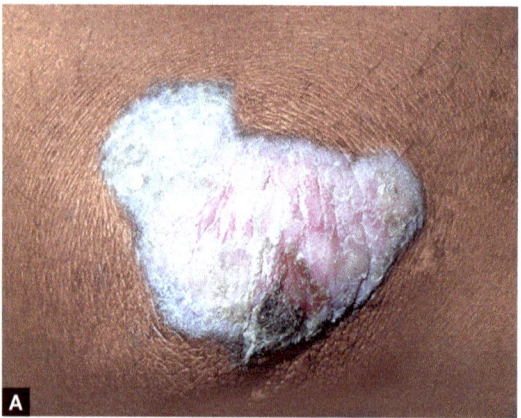

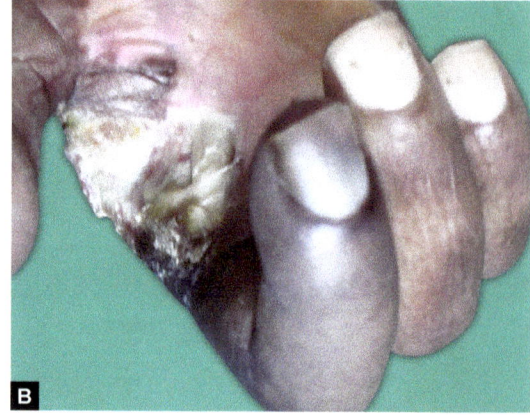

FIGURE 23: A, Erosion over the lichenoid hypertrophic plaque of discoid lupus erythematosus on right elbow; **B,** ulcerated and infected discoid lupus erythematosus plaque on right palm with gangrenous changes in right index finger.

Chronic Cutaneous and Subacute Cutaneous Lupus Erythematosus

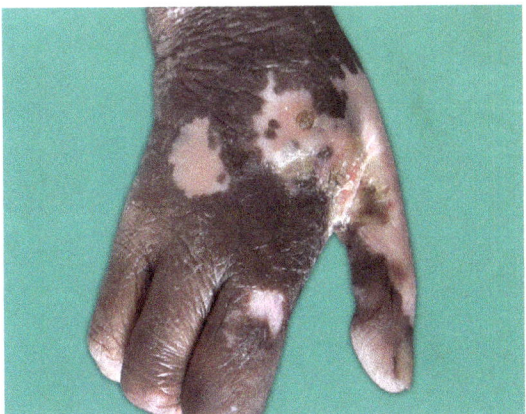

FIGURE 24: Contracture following healing of ulcerated discoid lupus erythematosus plaque in web space of right hand.

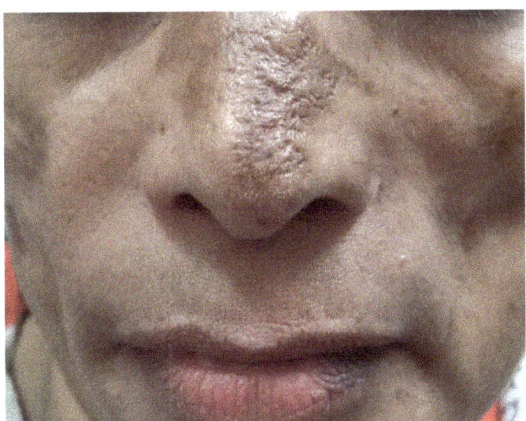

FIGURE 25: Lupus erythematosus vermiculatus with lupus erythematosus profundus; well-defined hyperpigmented plaque over the nose with multiple small pitted scars suggestive of lupus erythematosus vermiculatus. There is subcutaneous tissue atrophy with minimal hyperpigmentation present over both cheeks suggestive of a past lupus erythematosus profundus lesion. Discoid lupus erythematosus lesions also present over lower lip.

atrophic lesion without erythema or follicular plugging are present which resemble pitted scars or atrophoderma vermiculata. Lupus erythematosus linearis is LE lesions following the lines of Blaschko which may be present on trunk, arms, or legs.[36] Lupus erythematosus hemorrhagicus presents with purpura or petechial lesions. Telangiectatic variant presents with persistent, reticulate telangiectasia on the face, neck, ears, arms, legs, and dorsum of hands and feet. In addition, DLE mimicking tinea faciei or chronic cutaneous granulomatous disease has been reported.[37] Multiple cutaneous horns have also been reported as presenting feature of DLE.[38] Rarely DLE can present in unilateral distribution over face (Fig. 26) and can also appear over vitiligo patches (Fig. 27).

Mucous Membrane Discoid Lupus Erythematosus

Mucosal involvement can be observed in 25% of patients with CCLE.[39] Mucosal involvement do not reflect systemic manifestation or high disease activity. Lips (Fig. 28) and buccal mucosa (Fig. 29) are most commonly affected followed by palate, alveolar processes, and tongue. Rarely nasal, conjunctival, and anogenital mucosa are involved. Individual lesions begin as acutely painful, erythematous patches, which later form chronic plaque with a sharp margin and irregularly scalloped white border with radiating white striae (Fig. 30). The center of these plaques atrophies, ulcerates and heals with scarring. Discoid LE can present as diffuse cheilitis on the more sun-exposed lower lip causing pain and discomfort to the patient.[40] Nasal septum perforation due to generalized DLE has been observed. Lower eyelids particularly outer one-third involvement can be observed in the form of erythema, infiltration, and mild scaling (Fig. 31). Isolated lower lid involvement may simulate blepharitis and often delays diagnosis of DLE.[41] Discoid LE may also present with conjunctival scarring, loss of eyelashes, ectropion, symblepharon, superficial punctate keratopathy, and stromal keratitis.[42]

Systemic Involvement

Approximately, 5% of patients with localized DLE and 20% patients with generalized DLE subsequently develop SLE.[30] Risk factors suggesting increased risk of developing SLE in DLE patients are generalized lymphadenopathy, LE nonspecific skin lesions such as vasculitis (Fig. 32), diffuse nonscarring alopecia, periungual nail fold telangiectasia, Raynaud phenomenon and laboratory abnormalities like unexplained anemia, marked leukopenia, false-positive

Skin in Rheumatologic Disease

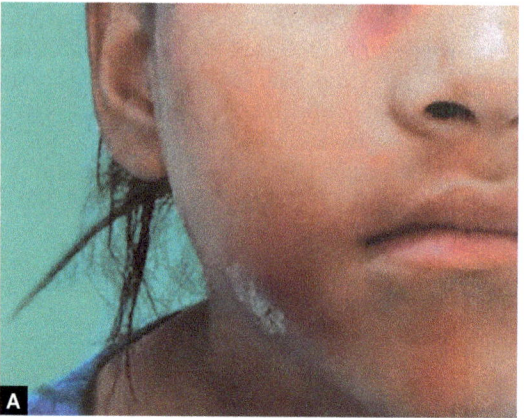
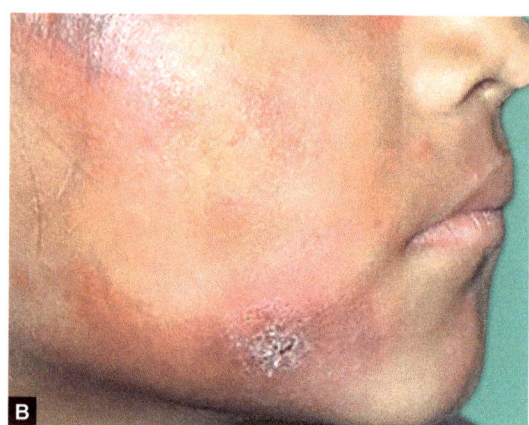
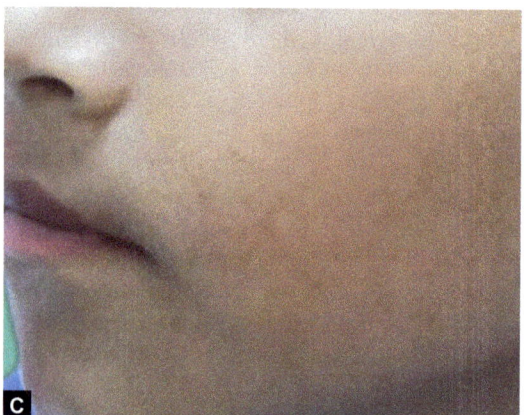

FIGURE 26: Unilateral discoid lupus erythematosus rash localized to right half of the face in a young female child; lesion are in the form of erythematous infiltrated plaques with follicular plugging, while the pigmentary changes are minimal in the form of central hyperpigmentation.

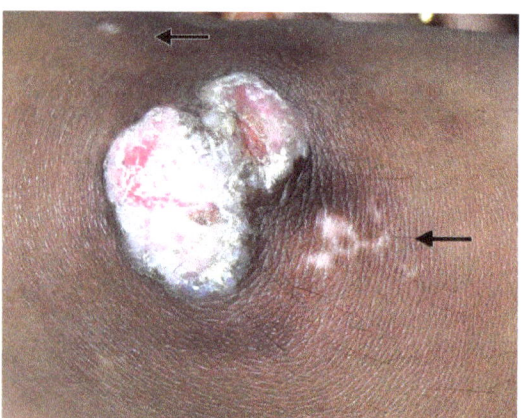

FIGURE 27: Hypertrophic discoid lupus erythematosus lesion appeared over a vitiligo patch on right elbow following treatment with topical PUVA sol. Small vitiligo patches (black arrow) visible in the vicinity of discoid lupus erythematosus plaque.

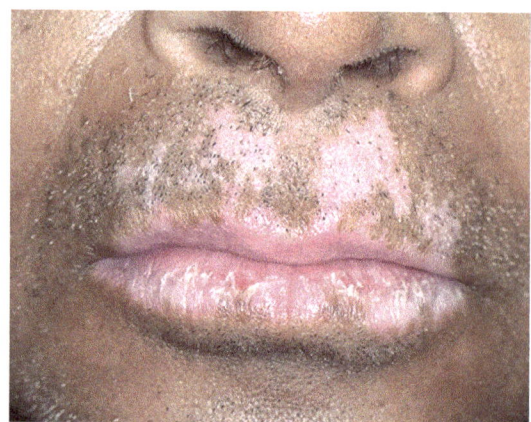

FIGURE 28: Lip discoid lupus erythematosus; erythematous to violaceous plaques present over both lips (lower > upper) with minimal superficial ulceration and atrophy in the central part of the lower lip.

Chronic Cutaneous and Subacute Cutaneous Lupus Erythematosus

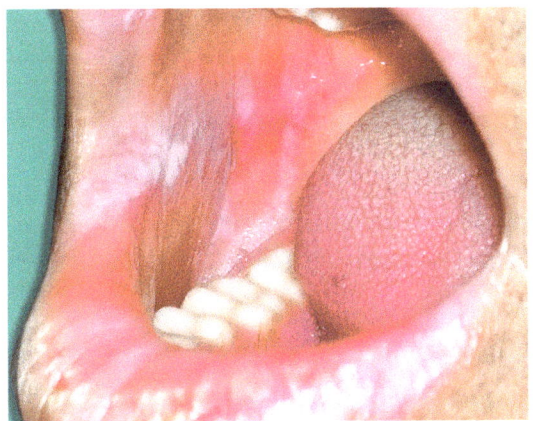

FIGURE 29: Mucosal discoid lupus erythematosus resembling oral Lichen planus; erythematous to violaceous plaque present over lower lip and buccal mucosa. Predominant involvement of lower lip, presence of adherent scaling and no wickham's striae can be helpful in differentiating the two.

tests for syphilis, persistently positive high antinuclear antibody (ANA) titer, anti-single stranded DNA antibody, hypergammaglobulinemia, elevated erythrocyte sedimentation rate (ESR) (>50 mm/hour), positive sun-protected nonlesional lupus band test, and elevated levels of soluble Interleukin-2 (IL-2) receptor.[43] Roughly 25% of patients with SLE develop DLE lesions sometime during the course of their disease and these patients often have less severe systemic involvement.[44]

Differential Diagnoses

Common differential diagnoses for DLE include chronic discoid dermatitis, psoriasis, hypertrophic lichen planus, lupus vulgaris, tinea incognito, Bowen's disease, (Fig. 33) and sarcoidosis, from which it can be differentiated

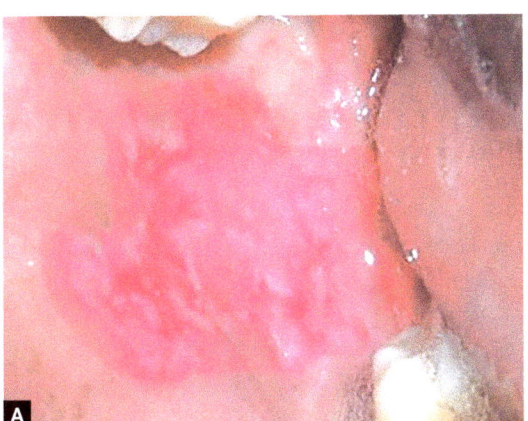
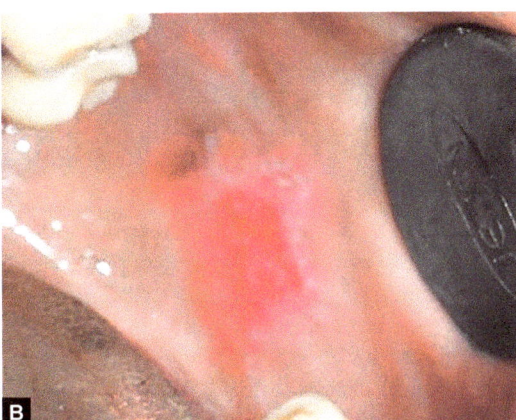

FIGURE 30: Classical mucosal discoid lupus erythematosus involving buccal mucosa in the form of erythematous ulcerated central plaques with irregularly scalloped white border with radiating white striae.

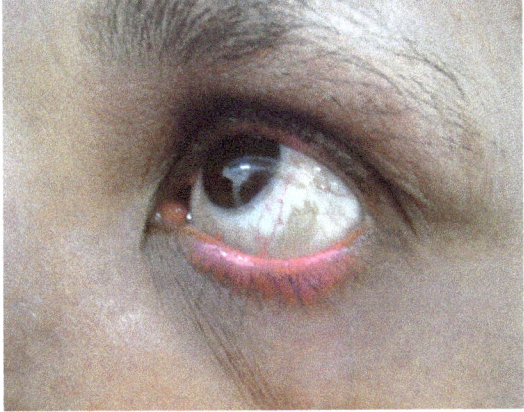

FIGURE 31: Discoid lupus erythematosus plaque involving the left lower eyelid.

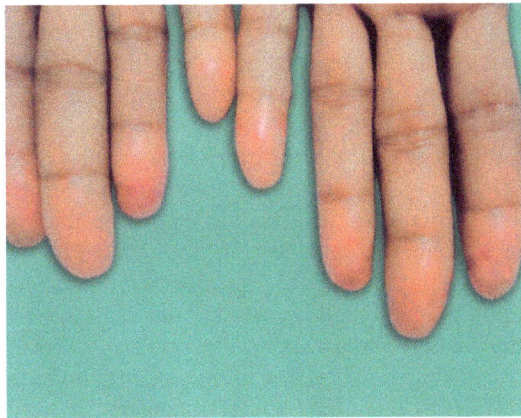

FIGURE 32: Vasculitic lesion over finger tips in a discoid lupus erythematosus patient.

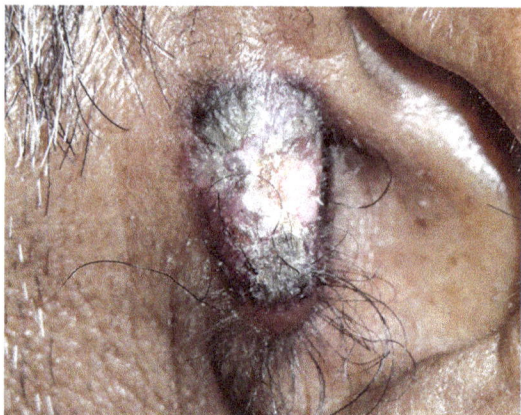

FIGURE 33: Bowen's plaque over left ear tragus resembling discoid lupus erythematosus.

clinically, by its characteristic clinical findings. Differential diagnoses of mouth ulcers include common conditions such as oral lichen planus, aphthous ulcer, herpetic and traumatic ulcer, autoimmune diseases like pemphigus, Behcet's disease, Wegener's granulomatosis, and squamous cell carcinoma.

Histopathology

Characteristic microscopic features of DLE are hyperkeratosis with follicular plugging, thinning, or flattening of the epidermis with interface dermatitis. In addition, there is basement membrane thickening and interstitial mucin deposition in dermis. Initially, there is only fine fibrillar reduplication of basal lamina visible only in special stains which progresses to form a broad eosinophilic homogenous band of basement membrane. Lesions of DLE are characterized by an interface dermatitis involving the follicles and epidermis accompanied by a moderate to heavy superficial and deep perivascular and periappendageal lymphocytic infiltrate. The infiltrate extends into the basal layer keratinocytes of adnexae and of the interfollicular epidermis. The dermal infiltrate is composed predominantly of lymphocytes with few macrophages. Plasma cells are prominent in oral lesions. Chronic lesions have gradual replacement of this infiltrate by dermal fibroplasia. In scalp, scarring alopecia may occur with reduction in sebaceous glands and the lymphocytic infiltrate which is maximal around the mid-follicle at the level of the sebaceous gland (also refer Chapter 3: Dermatopathology of Rheumatologic Diseases).

Immunofluorescence

Linear or granular deposits of several immunoglobulins (IgG, IgM, and IgA) and complement C3 are found along the dermoepidermal junction in 80–90% patients. This lesional lupus band is particularly prominent around the hair follicles and positivity is more in older lesions (>6 weeks).[45] It is more frequent on the face and in untreated lesions, but is rare on the trunk and non-sun-exposed sites.[46] Immunoreactants are also found in oral mucosa and the conjunctiva.[47] The C1q deposits are found in approximately 30% of patients with DLE and its presence indicates increased risk of developing SLE.[48] In addition, properdin deposition has been demonstrated at the dermal-epidermal junction in 70% of lesions indicating complement activation with C3, C4.[49] The presence of immune deposits around the hair follicle serves as an important clue to differentiate scarring alopecia caused by DLE from other causes.[50]

Dermoscopy

Very little work has been done in dermoscopy of DLE. Perifollicular whitish halo, follicular keratotic plugs, and telangiectasias are the most common dermoscopic findings in DLE.[51]

Other Investigations

Antinuclear antibodies are present in low titer in 30–40% of patients with DLE. The homogeneous type of ANA is more frequent than speckled type. Antinuclear antibody is more common in older patients, long standing lesions and extensive involvement.[52] Antibodies to single-stranded DNA occur in nearly 20% and indicate widespread and progressive disease.[53] Low titer anti-Ro and La antibodies may be seen in 10% of patients.[54] Other laboratory abnormalities seen in DLE are anemia, leukopenia or thrombocytopenia, raised ESR, raised serum globulin, positive Coombs test, positive cryoglobulins, positive cold agglutinins, false-positive syphilis serology, and positive anticardiolipin antibodies (mainly IgM).

OTHER CLINICAL VARIANT OF CHRONIC CUTANEOUS LUPUS ERYTHEMATOSUS

Hypertrophic/Verrucous Variant of Chronic Cutaneous Lupus Erythematosus

It is a rare variant of CCLE in which there is marked hyperkeratosis (Fig. 34). The most commonly affected sites are face (Fig. 35), extremities, and upper back. The entity lupus erythematosus hypertrophicus et profundus appears to represent a rare form of hypertrophic CCLE, affecting the face with the additional features of violaceous to erythematous, indurated, rolled borders, and striking central, crateriform atrophy. However, it doesn't have LE panniculitis on histopathology. Patients with hypertrophic CCLE probably do not have a greater risk for developing SLE than do patients with DLE lesions. Histopathology is also similar to DLE with more marked hyperkeratosis and epidermal hyperplasia resembling squamous cell carcinoma at times. The risk of malignant transformation (Fig. 36) in DLE lesion is 3.3%.[55] In DLE lesions, lack of protective melanin leads to more skin exposure to the UVB which inactivates the *p53* tumor suppressor gene.[56] In addition, immunosuppressive and cytotoxic therapy of DLE with agents such as azathioprine, cyclophosphamide, and cyclosporine can lead to malignancy. The long-term prognosis of

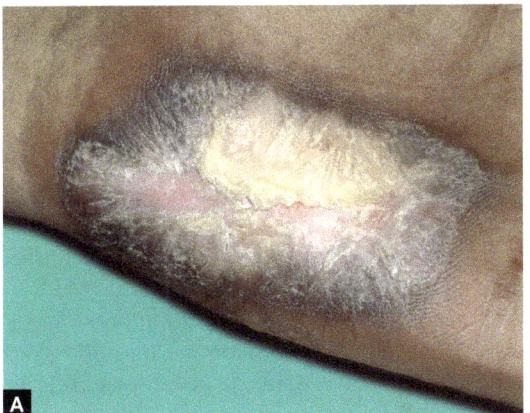
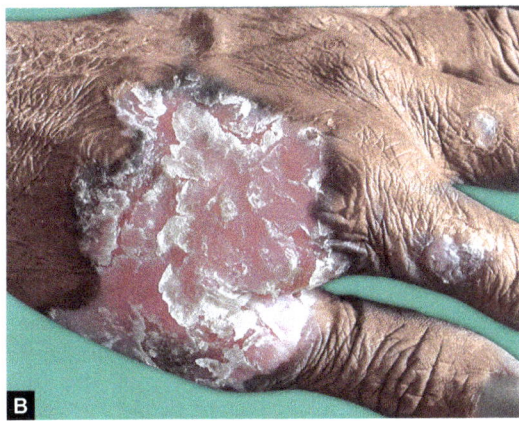

FIGURE 34: A, Verrucous chronic cutaneous lupus erythematosus over left hand; hyperkeratotic well-defined plaque present over left hand with hyperpigmentation and follicular plugging; **B,** Hyperkeratotic chronic cutaneous lupus erythematosus plaque over dorsum of left hand.

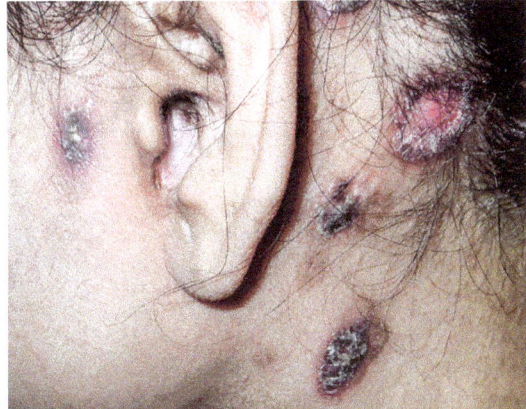
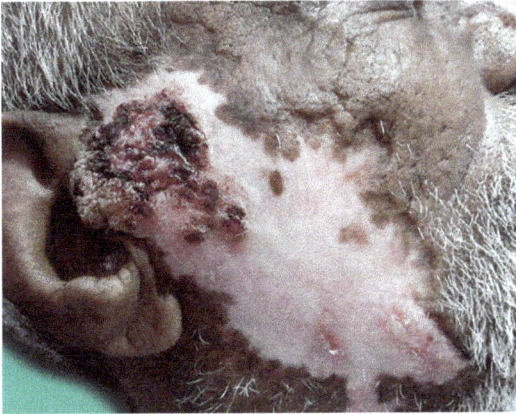

FIGURE 35: Hyperkeratotic chronic cutaneous lupus erythematosus plaque over neck and face.

FIGURE 36: Squamous cell carcinoma arising over the preauricular area in a discoid lupus erythematosus lesion.

such cases is varied. The risk of SCC is slightly higher in hypertrophic DLE than classic DLE owing to the chronicity of the disease. It is more difficult to diagnose squamous cell carcinoma in verrucous DLE due to marked epidermal hyperplasia. Squamous cell carcinoma arising in DLE is regarded as a locally aggressive but low-grade carcinoma. A single study reported local recurrences in about 20% and metastasis in 30% cases.[57]

Lichenoid Discoid Lupus Erythematosus/Lupus Planus

It denotes a morphological DLE variant resembling lichen planus. The existence of an overlap syndrome of lichen planus and DLE is questionable and many authors believe it is merely coexistence of two skin diseases.

Chilblain Lupus Erythematosus

This subtype of CCLE is more frequent in women. The lesions commonly involve dorsal and lateral parts of the hands (Fig. 37) and feet, ears, nose, elbows, knees, and calves. Lesions initially develop as violaceous to erythematous papules and plaques on the toes, fingers, or other sites, precipitated by cold, damp climates and are clinically and histologically similar to idiopathic chilblains (pernio). Gradually, the lesions develop into scarred atrophic plaques with associated telangiectasia. Patients with chilblain LE often have typical DLE lesions elsewhere on the body. The pathogenesis is not fully known but microvascular injury secondary to exposure to cold and possible hyperviscosity from immunologic abnormalities may play a role.[58] Another possibility is that chilblain LE begins as a classic acral cold induced chilblain with subsequent koebnerization of DLE lesions on them, thus explaining the spectrum of clinicohistologic findings. Ulceration and necrosis often occurs on the extremities (Fig. 38). A criterion has been proposed by Su et al. for diagnosis of chilblain LE lesion.[59] Major criteria include (i) cold-induced or cold-aggravated lesions in acral locations and (ii) evidence of LE on histopathology or direct immunofluorescence. Minor criteria include (i) the coexistence of SLE or other manifestations of CLE, (ii) positive response to LE therapy, and (iii) negative results of cryoglobulin and cold agglutinin studies. The diagnosis of chilblain LE may be affirmed if the patient fulfills both major criteria and at least one of the minor criteria. Histopathology and immunofluorescence are almost similar to that of DLE. Additionally, lymphocytic vasculitis and fibrin deposition in dermal blood vessel may be observed. The risk of developing SLE in chilblain LE is estimated to be approximately 20%. Persistence of lesions beyond the cold months, a positive ANA, or presence of one or the other American College of Rheumatology [ACR, formerly ARA (American Rheumatism

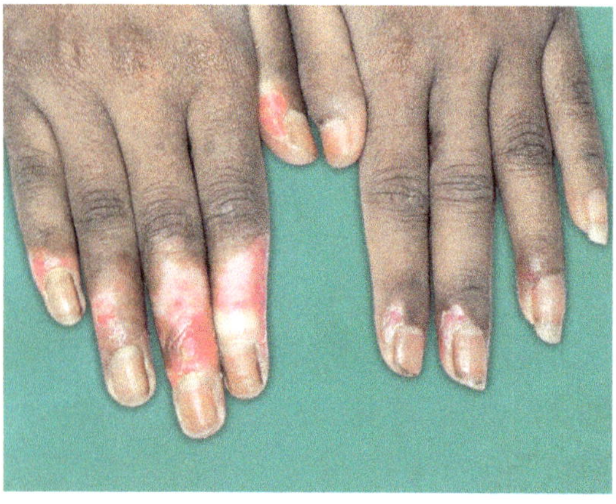

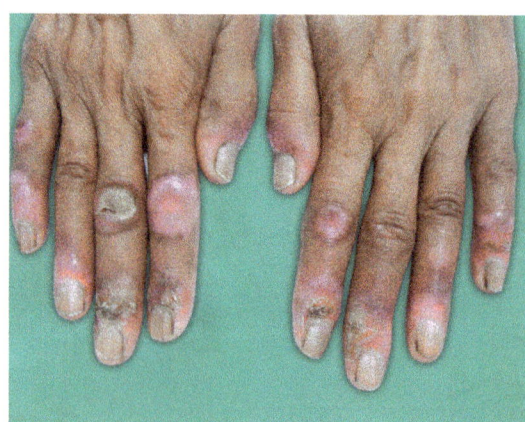

FIGURE 37: Chilblain lupus erythematosus lesions over the finger tips.

FIGURE 38: Chilblain lupus erythematosus lesion over fingers with ulcerations in lesion over nail folds; classical discoid lesion visible more proximally over the fingers.

Association)] criteria for SLE at the time of diagnosis of chilblain LE helps to distinguish chilblain LE from idiopathic chilblains (Fig. 39).[60] Some patients with chilblain LE present with a polyclonal hypergammaglobulinemia and a positive rheumatoid factor RF. In addition, anti-dsDNA or anti-Ro antibodies have often been detected in these patients. Differential diagnosis includes perniosis, cutaneous sarcoidosis, vasculitis, cryoglobulinemia, and cryofibrinogenemia.

Lupus Erythematosus Profundus/Kaposi-Irgang Disease/Lupus Panniculitis

It is a rare variant of CCLE in which pathologic changes occur primarily in the lower dermis and subcutaneous tissue. It is more common in middle-aged women and predominantly affects fat bearing areas like face (Fig. 40), shoulder, arm, trunk, back, buttocks, and thighs (Fig. 41).[61] Early lesions are characterized by single or multiple 1–3 cm sharply defined, persistent, and asymptomatic to painful subcutaneous plaques or nodules.[30] Gradually, overlying skin becomes attached to the subcutaneous nodule producing a deep depression. Overlying skin may be normal but majority (70%) of patients has atrophy, erythema, poikiloderma, or classic DLE lesion. Lupus erythematosus profundus (LEP) designates the set of patients who have both LE panniculitis with DLE lesions on the top of them, and LE panniculitis refers to those having only subcutaneous involvement.[62] The course is usually chronic and characterized by periods of remission and exacerbation. Dystrophic calcifications or ulcerations may occur within older lesions. Lupus erythematosus profundus of the breast may produce nodules that can mimic carcinoma, clinically, radiologically and often histopathologically and is referred to as lupus mastitis.[63] Lupus erythematosus tumidus can affect the periorbital tissues and cause severe localized edema and scarring.[64] Lesions on the face produce marked disfigurement due to lipoatrophy. Linear lupus panniculitis of the scalp presenting as alopecia along Blaschko's lines has been observed in few Asian population.[65]

Histology shows typically lobular panniculitis with lymphocytes, histiocytes, and plasma cells in deep dermis and subcutaneous tissue along with perivascular infiltrates of lymphocytes, vessel wall thickening, fibrinoid, degeneration of collagen, and mucin deposits in the lower dermis and zones of hyaline adipocyte necrosis which gradually become replaced by sclerotic tissue. Often lymphocytic vasculitis is also seen. Interface changes are absent. Immunofluorescence findings are similar to classic DLE except

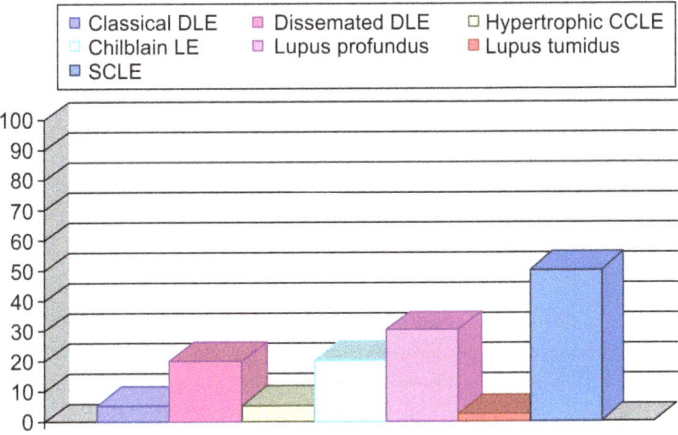

FIGURE 39: Prognosis of chronic cutaneous lupus erythematosus and subacute cutaneous lupus erythematosus. Percentage of patients developing systemic lupus erythematosus or fulfilling American Rheumatism Association (ARA) criterion of systemic lupus erythematosus among different types of chronic cutaneous lupus erythematosus and subacute cutaneous lupus erythematosus.

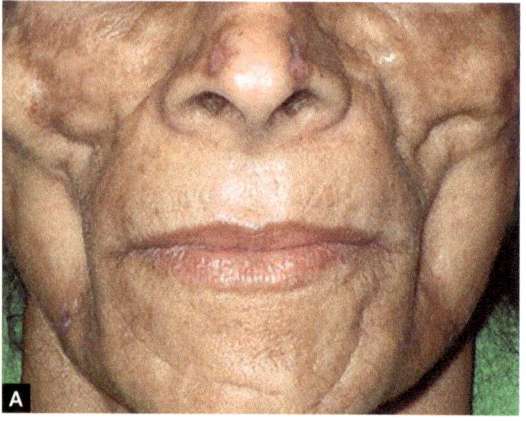
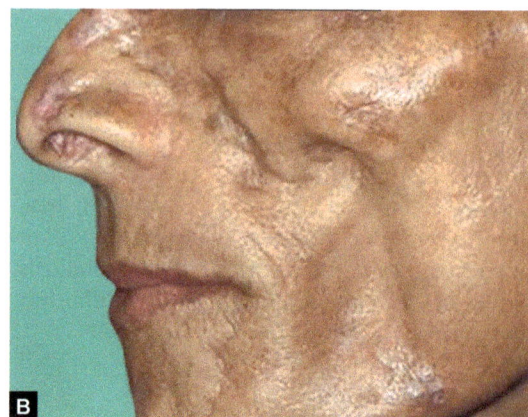
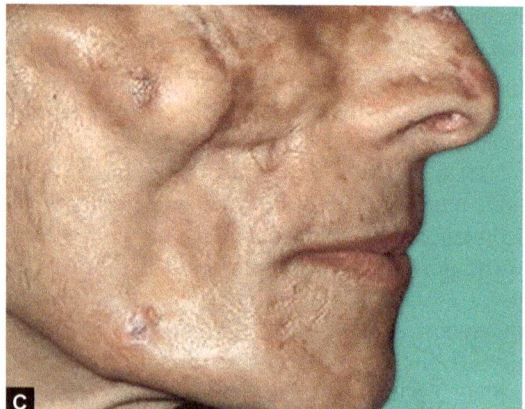

FIGURE 40: Lupus profundus and panniculitis of face resulting in marked atrophy and disfigurement; classical discoid lesion overlying the atrophic area can be seen on the nose and cheek.

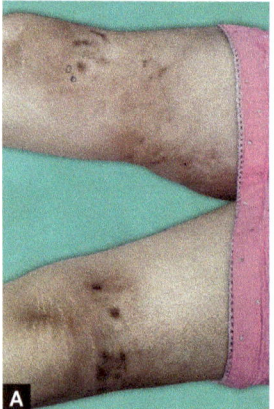
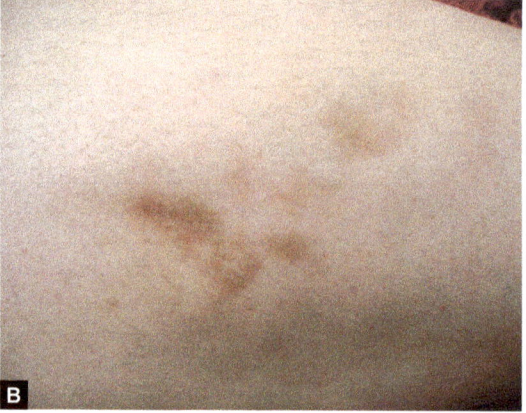

FIGURE 41: A, Lupus profundus. Large well defined painful indurated subcutaneous noduloplaque present over both thighs with overlying skin having hyperpigmentation, atrophy and follicular plugging in a few areas; **B,** Lupus profundus plaques over thigh and overlying skin showing mild erythema and brownish discoloration.

in LEP, immune complexes deposition can be demonstrated in deep dermal vessels.[66] Approximately 30% of patients of LEP meet 4 ACR criteria for a diagnosis of SLE, but systemic disease is rare in them.[67] Approximately 3% of patients with SLE suffer from LEP.[30] Differential diagnoses

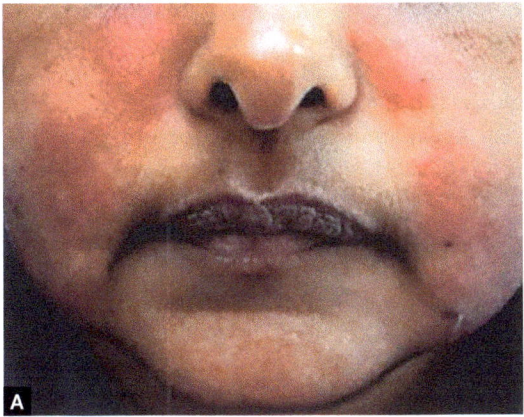
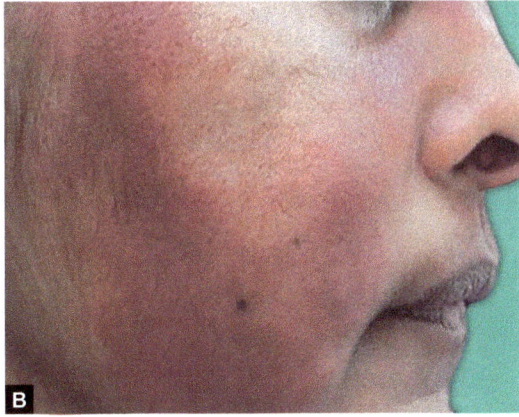

FIGURE 42: Lupus tumidus; erythematous painless succulent plaque over both cheeks in a female patient.

include glucocorticosteroid induced lipoatrophy, morphea profundus, subcutaneous panniculitis like T cell lymphoma, subcutaneous sarcoidosis, eosinophilic fasciitis, infective (deep fungal/mycobacterial) panniculitis, and traumatic panniculitis.

Lupus Erythematosus Tumidus

It is rare form of CCLE which presents with marked photosensitivity without much scarring. The succulent appearance of the lesions and the absence of clinically visible epidermal involvement (Fig. 42) are the most important clinical features of this subtype. Unlike other forms of CCLE, it is more common in middle aged males (Fig. 43) particularly smokers. Early lesions present as succulent, urticaria-like, single or multiple smooth surfaced plaques with a bright erythematous or violaceous hue.[58] Differential diagnosis includes polymorphous light eruption, Jessner's lymphocytic infiltration of the skin, urticaria, granuloma faciale, urticarial vasculitis, and pseudolymphoma. Histologically, it presents with patchy lymphocytic infiltrates in the dermis and increased mucin deposits between the collagen fibers. The epidermis and the subcutaneous tissue are usually not involved unlike other forms of CCLE. In long-lasting lesions, usually there is deposition of IgG and IgM along the basement membrane.[24] In a blinded comparison of histopathology of tumid lupus and Jessner's lymphocytic infiltrate, there

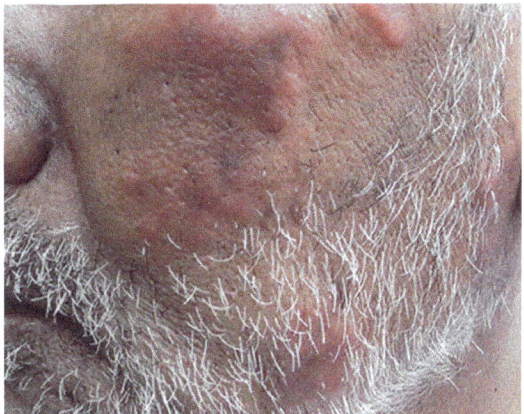

FIGURE 43: Lupus tumidus plaque over cheek in a male patient.

were only few differences between the two.[68] Mild epidermal atrophy and focal thickening of the dermoepidermal junction were more common in tumid lupus. Lymphocytic infiltrate was less dense in tumid lupus than in Jessner's lymphocytic infiltrate. Few authors believe that tumid lupus, Jessner's lymphocytic infiltrate, are both similar and represent dermal variants of LE specific skin disease.

SUBACUTE CUTANEOUS LUPUS ERYTHEMATOSUS

Subacute cutaneous lupus erythematosus is clinically characterized by recurrent, nonscarring skin lesions occurring in a symmetrical photodistributed pattern and comprises of approximately 10% of patients with LE.[69] Patients with SCLE are highly photosensitive and lesions usually occur above the waist and particularly around the V-area of the neck, upper chest and back, and shoulders as well as the extensor aspects of the arms and hands. Lesions begin as erythematous mildly scaly papules which rapidly coalesce to form plaques. They heal with postinflammatory dyspigmentation and telangiectasia. Patients have either nonscarring papulosquamous (two-thirds) (Fig. 44) or annular polycyclic (one-third) lesions (Fig. 45) and rarely, both simultaneously. The morphological variants of SCLE do not carry

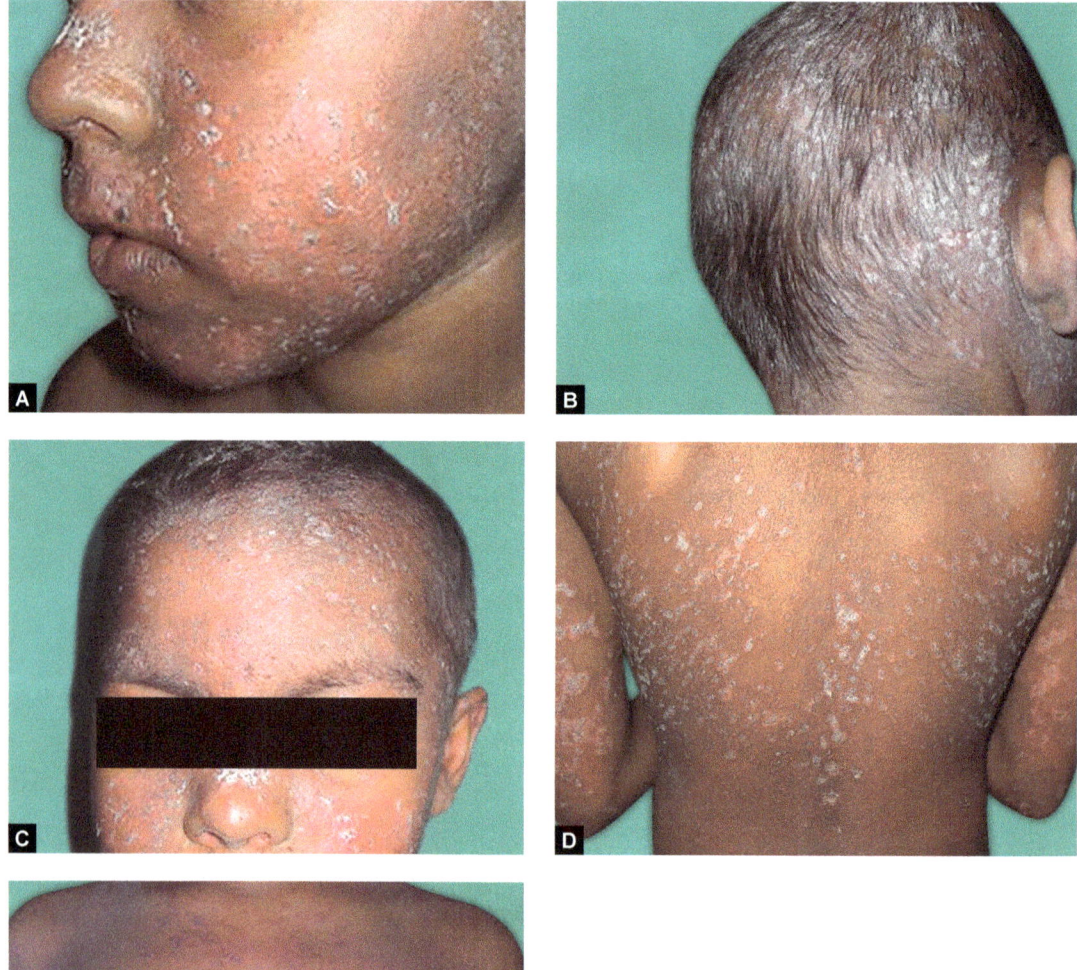

FIGURE 44: Psoriasiform subacute cutaneous lupus erythematosus rash in a male child affecting the scalp, face, and trunk. Violaceous hue, ill defined lesion, prominent involvement of upper trunk alone, and central hypopigmentation helps to differentiate from psoriasis.

Chronic Cutaneous and Subacute Cutaneous Lupus Erythematosus

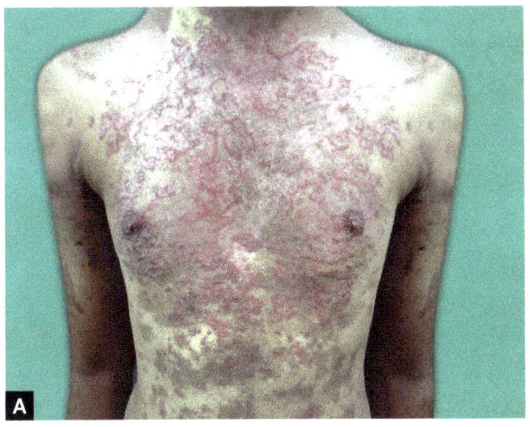
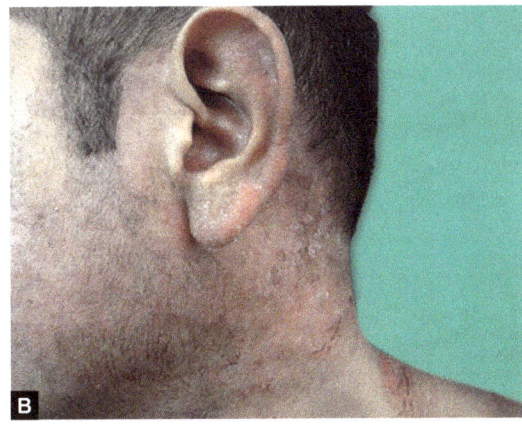

FIGURE 45: A, Subacute cutaneous lupus erythematosus: polycyclic erythematous plaques with minimal scaling and no atrophy present over the upper trunk healing with hyperpigmentation. Similar lesions present over both arms and face; **B,** Subacute cutaneous lupus erythematosus face: erythematous plaques with minimal scaling and mild atrophy present over right side of face, ear, and neck. Here lateral side of face is more involved than central face unlike systemic lupus erythematosus.

prognostic implications. Absence of induration and atrophic scarring helps to distinguish SCLE from DLE. The borders of plaques may rarely show vesiculation and crusting and occasionally bullae formation owing to intense injury to basal layers of epidermis. This presentation may mimic Stevens-Johnson syndrome or toxic epidermal necrolysis. Occasionally, SCLE lesions may present initially with an appearance of erythema multiforme, similar to Rowell syndrome (erythema multiforme-like lesions occurring in patients with SLE in the presence of La autoantibodies). Rarely, SCLE presents with acral, exfoliative, erythrodermic, pityriasiform, or exanthematous variants. Patients with SCLE may also develop localized facial lesions similar to acute LE.[70] However, acute LE skin lesions tend to be more transient, edematous, less scaly, and heal without any pigmentary changes. Acute LE lesions affect central area of face whereas SCLE lesions affect lateral part of face more commonly with sparing of central face and malar area. It may rarely present with papular mucinosis like lesions on these sites.

Systemic Involvement

About 50% of patients meet formal ACR criteria for SLE, but only 10-15% develops systemic symptoms, arthralgias being more frequent. Rarely mild renal or cerebral involvement is observed. This subgroup of patients is marked by the presence of papulosquamous SCLE, facial involvement, high-titer ANA, leukopenia, and/or antibodies to dsDNA.[71]

Differential Diagnoses

Differential diagnoses of annular SCLE include pityriasis rosea, tinea corporis, granuloma annulare, dry discoid eczema, erythema marginatum, erythema annulare centrifugum, and erythema gyratum. The papulosquamous variant of SCLE resembles psoriasis, lichen planus, pityriasis rosea, pityriasis rubra pilaris, mycosis fungoides, and polymorphous light eruption.

Histopathology

In SCLE, there is marked epidermal atrophy with interface dermatitis, dermal edema, and mucin deposition. Sparse perivascular and periadnexal mononuclear infiltrate is mainly localized to upper one-third of the dermis. Colloid bodies and epidermal necrosis are present in more than 50% of patients especially in those with Ro autoantibodies. Histopathologically, SCLE can be differentiated from DLE by the presence of more epidermal atrophy and less hyperkeratosis, basement-membrane thickening, follicular plugging, and dense inflammatory infiltration.[72] The histopathological differences between the two has been summarized in table 1.[73]

Skin in Rheumatologic Disease

Table 1: Histopathological differences between discoid lupus erythematosus and subacute cutaneous lupus erythematosus[73]

Histological features	Discoid lupus erythematosus	Subacute cutaneous lupus erythematosus
Hyperkeratosis	Marked	Minimal
Follicular plugging	Marked	Minimal
Vacuolar alteration in basal keratinocytes	Marked	Less marked
Basement membrane thickening	Marked	Less marked
Loss of appendages	Present	Less common
Superficial and deep perivascular infiltrate	Marked	Less marked
Mucin deposition in reticular dermis	Present	Present
Slender fibrocytes in upper dermis	Common	Minimal

Immunofluorescence

Dust-like particulate deposition of IgG and complements in and around basal epidermal keratinocytes is found in approximately 60% of patients. It is more frequent in papulosquamous (88%) than annular lesions (29%).[71] A granular fluorescence is seen in some patients with SCLE in the cytoplasm and nuclei of basal keratinocytes which is caused by binding of anti-Ro or La antibodies to their cytoplasmic or nuclear antigens, respectively. This feature is not seen in CCLE.[72]

Laboratory Abnormalities

Antinuclear antibodies are present in 60–80% of patients with SCLE, and rheumatoid factor is present in approximately one-third. The laboratory markers for SCLE are the presence of anti-Ro (70–90%) and, less commonly, anti-La (30–50%) autoantibodies. Other autoantibodies in patients with SCLE include false-positive serological tests for syphilis VDRL/RPR (7–33%), anticardiolipin (10–16%), antithyroid (18–44%), anti-Sm (10%), anti-dsDNA (10%), and anti-U1 ribonucleoprotein (10%).[72]

PREVENTION AND MANAGEMENT

While treating CLE, aim is to prevent the formation and progression of lesions and to improve the appearance of skin through a combination of patient education, topical and systemic therapies. Patients are advised to avoid excessive heat, sun exposure, and causative drugs. Overwork, mental stress, and fatigue are often factors involved in the deterioration of the disease, and patients with facial scarring often suffer severe psychological upset and depression. For this subset of patients, psychological support is very important and they should be counseled to avoid smoking. Strict adherence to sunscreens is a critical component of therapy, as both UVA and UVB irradiation (UVB > UVA) has been shown to induce CLE lesions.[74] Adequate amounts (2 mg/cm^2) of sunscreens with a high sun protection factor (SPF) 50+ should be applied 20–30 minutes prior to expect exposure should be reapplied every 2–3 hours. Almost all sunscreens provide protection against UVB with good SPF factor but very few provide protection against UVA also with PA++ or +++ rating. Physical sunscreens such as titanium dioxide or zinc oxide provide particularly a good broad-spectrum protection. Few patients experience photosensitivity behind glass windows like during driving, through which UVA rays are penetrable, and in these cases, UV-blocking films can be applied and sunscreens effective against UVA should be used.[55] Klein et al. analyzed the role of UV emitting indoor fluorescent light bulbs in exacerbation of photosensitive diseases and they concluded that the lowest UV irradiance should be used to minimize cumulative dose of UV radiations.[75] Some compact fluorescent bulbs emit more UVB than incandescent bulbs and LED lights and in CLE patients latter should be preferred.[76] In addition to sunscreen, importance of other physical protection measures like umbrella, hats, protective clothing, and behavioral modification to avoid sun-exposure between 10 am and 4 pm should be emphasized. A major concern in these patients is cosmetic, so camouflage creams and artificial hair prosthetics can be advised based on patient's concerns and disease status.

Topical Therapies

Topical therapy, including steroids and/or calcineurin inhibitors, is the mainstay of treatment in cutaneous lesions of LE.

Topical and Injectable Corticosteroids

They are the most frequently used medications in treatment of CLE lesions worldwide. While advising topical steroids to these patients, potency and vehicle are the two important considerations. Low-potency steroids, such as desonide 0.05% or clobetasone butyrate 0.05% can be used for thin-skin areas, including the face and groin. Mid-potency steroids, such as mometasone are appropriate for the trunk and extremities. For thick skin areas, including the scalp, palms, and soles, high-potency steroids, such as clobetasol propionate should be advised. Topical steroids are often prescribed as creams, as they are more tolerable but patients with severe disease may require ointments. Foams and lotions are appropriate for lesions on the scalp. Due to the various side effects of topical steroids which are similar to cutaneous sequelae of DLE, such as atrophy, telangiectasia, hypopigmentation etc., the lowest potency steroids should be used for the shortest duration possible. Intralesional injection of triamcinolone (5–10 mg/mL) is particularly useful to treat chronic lesions, hyperkeratotic lesions, and those that do not respond adequately to topical steroids. Lesions at particular sites, e.g., the scalp and the leg may benefit from intralesional steroids.

Calcineurin Inhibitors

Calcineurin inhibitors like tacrolimus and pimecrolimus have emerged as an alternative topical option for various CLE subtypes. Although slow acting, they are free of the inherent side effects of steroids like atrophy. In a double-blind, randomized-controlled trial, half the face of 20 DLE patients was treated with tacrolimus 0.1% ointment and the other half with clobetasol propionate 0.05% ointment. The two ointments showed equal efficacy, however, 61% of patients developed telangiectasias on the clobetasol treated side as early as week 3, indicating that tacrolimus may be a better option in cosmetically important areas.[77] Pimecrolimus has the same functional activity as tacrolimus, but is more lipophilic, has higher epidermal affinity, lower penetration into the skin, and lower resorption.[78]

Topical Retinoids

Retinoids like tazarotene and tretinoin have been used in treatment of hyperkeratotic DLE lesions and have been found to be beneficial. However, there are not many studies to validate this.[79]

Other Topical Drugs

Imiquimod is an immunomodulator drug which has been tried in recalcitrant lesion of DLE. Gul et al. successfully treated generalized DLE with 5% imiquimod cream applied to lesions once a day three times a week. After 20 applications all of the lesions regressed significantly.[80] Another topical agent used is R-salbutamol. It is a β2-adrenergic receptor agonist used in treatment of asthma. A multicenter randomized-controlled trial investigated the use of R-salbutamol in the treatment of DLE and found statistically significant improvements in pain, itch, scaling, ulceration, and global assessment as compared to placebo. There was however no significant change in the cutaneous disease severity.[81]

Systemic Therapies

Systemic therapies are indicated in patients with extensive involvement or in cases refractory to topical treatment. Extracutaneous manifestations, such as arthritis, also require the use of systemic therapy. When systemic treatments are prescribed, topical agents are often continued as adjunctive therapy. Presently, there are no medications specifically approved for the treatment of CLE. The drugs used for the treatment of the various subtypes of CLE are generally also used for the treatment of SLE, with the exception of thalidomide.

Antimalarials

Oral antimalarials are considered first-line systemic therapy for all CLE subtypes. Hydroxychloroquine, chloroquine, and quinacrine are currently used antimalarials in CLE. Antimalarials can take upon 2–3 months for maximum efficacy, and therefore patients are often bridged with topicals and intralesional injections. The exact mechanism of action of antimalarials is still not completely understood. It consists of a number of interrelated anti-inflammatory and immunomodulatory effects that include photoprotection, lysosomal stabilization, suppression of antigen presentation, inhibition of prostaglandin, cytokine synthesis, and endosomal toll-like receptor signaling, limiting B cell and dendritic cell activation. Patients who smoke often have severe CLE and are more refractory to treatment with antimalarials. Hence, all patients should therefore be counseled for smoking cessation.[82] Major side effects of antimalarials include ocular toxicity, xerosis, exanthematous or lichenoid drug eruptions, urticaria, blue-gray skin hyperpigmentation, gastrointestinal upset, myopathy, cardiomyopathy, and rare central nervous system side effects (dizziness, headache, insomnia, psychosis, seizures). Quinacrine can cause yellow discoloration of skin, sclera, and bodily fluids and aplastic anemia. Regular retinopathy screening for patients on antimalarials is ideal to prevent its toxicity.[83]

Systemic Corticosteroids

Long-term therapy with systemic corticosteroids is avoided in CLE patients due to the well-known risks of developing diabetes, osteoporosis, Cushing's syndrome etc. Avascular necrosis of femoral head has been reported in patients treated with systemic corticosteroids. Patients who fail antimalarial combinations are often also refractory to other systemic treatments. In such treatment unresponsive patients with severe disease, short duration treatment with prednisone at 0.5–1.0 mg/kg/day may be used which can be tapered over 2–4 weeks.[84]

Immunosuppressants

They are mostly used in patients nonresponsive to antimalarials.[85] Methotrexate is recommended in a dose of 7.5–25 mg once a week.[86] A retrospective analysis of 43 treatment-refractory CLE patients treated with oral or subcutaneous methotrexate observed improvement in 98% of cases.[87] Azathioprine is the prodrug of 6-mercaptopurine, a purine antimetabolite with cytotoxic and immunosuppressive activity attributed to the disruption of nucleic acids in the S-phase of the cell cycle. Therapeutic doses range between 1–2.5 mg/kg body weight/day.[88] Mycophenolate mofetil (MMF) is a specific, noncompetitive, reversible inhibitor of inosine monophosphate dehydrogenase. Decreased activity of this enzyme affects proliferation of B and T lymphocytes and directly induces apoptosis of activated T lymphocytes. It has been found to be effective in treating all CLE subtypes.[89] Mycophenolate mofetil is well tolerated and clinical results are achieved in 1–2 months with doses from 1–3 g/day. Other immunosuppressive drugs that have been used in CLE are cytarabine, cyclophosphamide, and cyclosporine.[90]

Other Immunomodulators

Dapsone is a sulfone that inhibits dihydrofolic acid synthesis and exhibits both antibiotic and anti-inflammatory properties. Dapsone (25–150 mg/day) is effective in treatment of bullous LE, lupus panniculitis, SCLE, and DLE. The combined results of three case series of 55 CLE patients treated with dapsone demonstrated a 55% improvement rate.[91] Thalidomide acts by inhibiting the synthesis of TNF-α and UVB-induced keratinocyte apoptosis. Its therapeutic doses range from 50–100 mg/day. Multiple case series support the use of thalidomide in CCLE and SCLE (Flowchart 2)[92] Lenalidomide is a structural analog of thalidomide with more potent immunomodulatory effects and lower risk of polyneuropathy. Side effects are similar to those of thalidomide, but generally milder. It has been found to be beneficial in patients of CLE.[93] Clofazimine is an antibiotic with anti-inflammatory and immunosuppressive activity traditionally used in the treatment of leprosy. A randomized, double-blind, controlled trial

Chronic Cutaneous and Subacute Cutaneous Lupus Erythematosus

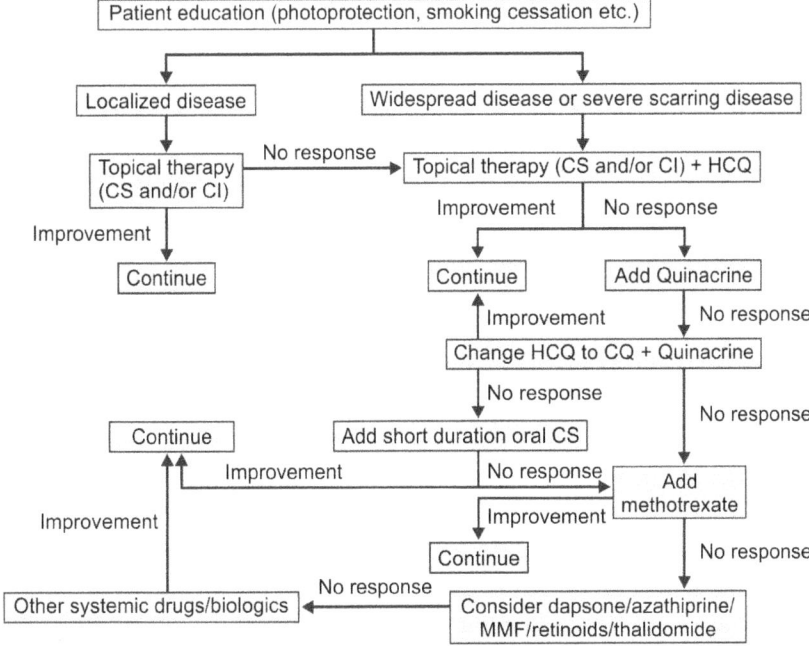

CS, corticosteroids; CI, calcineurin inhibitors; HCQ, hydroxychloroquine; CQ, chloroquine; MMF, mycophenolate mofetil.

FLOWCHART 2: Treatment algorithm of chronic cutaneous lupus erythematosus and subacute cutaneous lupus erythematosus.[92]

compared clofazimine (100 mg/day) with chloroquine (250 mg/day) in 33 patients with SLE with active skin lesions (ACLE, SCLE, localized and disseminated DLE). It was observed that complete response was seen in 18.8% of patients treated with clofazimine as compared with 41.2% of patients treated with chloroquine, but the difference was not significant.[94] These findings suggest that clofazimine may be equally effective as chloroquine in controlling cutaneous lesions in patients with SLE. Auranofin has been used in treatment of cutaneous LE.[95] Danazol is a testosterone derivative used to treat endometriosis, fibrocystic breast disease, and hereditary angioneurotic edema. It suppresses the pituitary-ovarian axis and may decrease immunoglobulin levels. Oral danazol has been used effectively to treat patients with DLE associated with premenstrual exacerbations.[96] Cefuroxime axetil resulted in the clearing of skin lesions in three patients with SCLE at a dose of 500 mg daily.[97]

Oral Retinoids

Oral retinoids can be used as second-line therapy in LE. Acitretin has been shown to be effective in half of CLE patients in a randomized-controlled trial,[98] while isotretinoin's efficacy has been seen in multiple case reports.[99] Kuhn et al. recently reported successful off-label treatment of various CLE subtypes with alitretinoin.[100]

Biologics

Rituximab is a chimeric monoclonal antibody against CD20 and induces depletion of B cells through both antibody dependent and independent pathways. It has shown efficacy in few cases with refractory SCLE.[86] Usmani and Goodfield[101] reported good to excellent response in 12 out of 13 patients with DLE who were treated with efalizumab, a monoclonal antibody directed against CD11a. Treatment with intravenous immunoglobulin (IVIG) has been reported to show beneficial effects in a 2-day course (1 g/kg/day) every 4 weeks in 5 patients with refractory extensive long-lasting DLE with facial lesions.[102] High-dose IVIG at 1 gm/kg/day for 2 consecutive days monthly has been used by Goodfield et al.[103] in 12 patients, who had failed multiple previous therapies. In few case reports there was no response to IVIG.[104] As a corollary of efficacy of thalidomide by its anti-TNF-α effects, it can be presumed that infliximab, adalimumab, or etanercept might also prove to be of benefit to patients with cutaneous LE. However, these agents have been associated with the development of drug-induced SLE and SCLE. Prinz and colleagues have used chimeric CD4 monoclonal antibody infusions in five patients with severe, refractory cutaneous LE.[105]

Physical Treatments

Various physical modalities used for CLE include laser therapy, cryotherapy, and dermabrasion. Cryotherapy can be used as a treatment option for DLE lesions that are resistant to local or systemic therapy.[106] The efficacy of pulsed-dye and argon laser has been shown in several case reports and series. An open prospective study of 12 DLE patients treated with pulsed-dye laser demonstrated efficacy after 6 weeks of treatment.[107] Purpura, pain, and postinflammatory pigmentary changes are reported side effects of treatment. UV radiation is a well-known trigger factor of CLE and may even lead to exacerbation of systemic symptoms. Interestingly, it has been observed by some groups that low-dose UVA1 can be used to treat skin lesions in CLE as it causes UV-hardening of skin, particularly in photosensitive CLE subset. In a retrospective study of home-based UVB hardening therapy, patients were able to gradually increase their monthly UVB dose and maintained their increased UVB tolerance over a longer period of time. A majority also reported an improved tolerance for environmental UV radiation, indicating its potential use in CLE.[108,109]

Since postinflammatory depigmentation is a significant concern in those with darker skin type, non-cultured epidermal cell suspension procedure (Fig. 46) can be performed once the disease is not active.

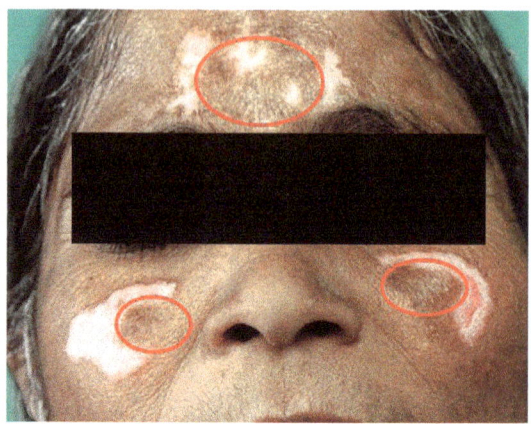

FIGURE 46: Significant postinflammatory depigmentation over the cheeks and chin in a 55-year lady, partially improved with non-cultured epidermal cell suspension technique.

OUTCOME MEASURES

Cutaneous Lupus Erythematosus Area and Severity Index (CLASI) were developed in 2005 as a means of assessing cutaneous activity and tissue damage in patients with CLE.[92] The CLASI provides a quantitative measure of the skin-specific burden of disease. The CLASI is a simple, single-page tool wherein each part of the body, from the scalp to the feet, is listed separately. It also has sections focusing on mucous membrane involvement and alopecia. For the activity score, points are given for the presence of erythema, scale, mucous membrane lesions, recent hair loss, and inflammatory alopecia. For the damage score, points are given for the presence of dyspigmentation, scarring, and scarring alopecia. For both activity and damage, higher scores are awarded for more severe manifestations. In 2010, the CLASI was revised, known as RCLASI by increasing the accuracy of existing parameters, such as scaling or hypertrophy and dyspigmentation, and by adding several new adjusted parameters, such as edema or infiltration and subcutaneous nodule or plaque.[110]

CONCLUSION

Chronic cutaneous lupus erythematosus is a chronic scarring and potentially disfiguring disease seen in all parts of the world with high morbidity. Hence, early diagnosis and appropriate treatment are important. Correct identification and diagnosis of subtypes of CCLE helps in determination of prognosis of disease and also in predicting systemic involvement. There are several forms of treatment that are effective but there are too few properly conducted randomized trials. Clinicians at present can chose different treatment modalities based on their own experience and judgment. There is a need for further large randomized-controlled trial to assess the effectiveness and safety of one form of treatment compared with another. Since CCLE and SCLE patients have a definite but variable risk of developing SLE, a regular follow up and risk assessment form an integral part of therapy in these patients.

REFERENCES

1. Gilliam JN, Sontheimer RD. Distinctive cutaneous subsets in the spectrum of lupus erythematosus. J Am Acad Dermatol. 1981;4:471-5.
2. Damm J, Sonnischen N. Clinical examinations of chronic discoid lupus erythematosus. Dermatol Wochenschr. 1964;150:268.
3. Millard TP, McGregor JM. Molecular genetics of cutaneous lupusverythematosus. Clin Exp Dermatol 2001;26:184-91.
4. Fischer GF, Pickl WF, Fae I, et al. Association between chronic cutaneous lupus erythematosus and HLA class II alleles. Hum Immunol 1994;41:280-4.
5. Werth VP, Zhang W, Dortzbach K, et al. Association of a promoter polymorphism of tumor necrosis factor-alpha with subacute cutaneous lupus erythematosus and distinct photoregulation of transcription. J Invest Dermatol. 2000;115:726-30.
6. Osmola A, Namysl J, Jagodzinski PP, et al. Genetic background of cutaneous forms of lupus erythematosus: update on current evidence. J Appl Genet. 2004;45:77-86.
7. Pickering MC, Fischer S, Lewis MR, et al. Ultraviolet-radiation-induced keratinocyte apoptosis in C1q-deficient mice. J Invest Dermatol 2001;117:52–8.
8. Werth VP. Cutaneous lupus: insights into pathogenesis and disease classification. Bull NYU Hosp Jt Dis 2007;65:200-4.
9. Lee-Kirsch MA, Gong M, Schulz H, et al. Familial chilblain lupus, a monogenic form of cutaneous lupus erythematosus, maps to chromosome 3p. Am J Hum Genet 2006;79:731-7.
10. Sakabe K, Yoshida T, Furuya H, et al. Estrogenic xenobiotics increase expression of SS-A/Ro autoantigens in cultured human epidermal cells. Acta Derm Venereol 1998;78:420-3.
11. Cutolo M, Sulli A, Capellino S, et al. Sex hormones influence on the immune system: basic and clinical aspects in autoimmunity. Lupus 2004;13:635-8.
12. Zhu J. Cytomegalovirus infection induces expression of 60 KD/Ro antigen on human keratinocytes. Lupus. 1995;4:396-406.
13. Furukawa F, Kashihara-Sawami M, Lyons MB, et al. Binding of autoantibodies to the extractable nuclear antigens SS-A/Ro and SS-B/La is induced on the surface of human keratinocytes by ultraviolet light (UVL): implications for the pathogenesis of photosensitive cutaneous lupus. J Invest Dermatol 1990;94:77-85.
14. Norris DA. Pathomechanisms of photosensitive lupus erythematosus. J Invest Dermatol. 1993;100:58S-68S.
15. Caricchio R, McPhie L, Cohen PL. Ultraviolet B radiation-induced cell death: critical role of ultraviolet dose in inflammation and lupus autoantigen redistribution. J Immunol. 2003;171:5778-86.
16. Oke V, Wahren-Herlenius M. The immunobiology of Ro52 (TRIM21) in autoimmunity: a critical review. J Autoimmun 2012;39:77-82.
17. Espinosa A, Dardalhon V, Brauner S, et al. Loss of the lupus autoantigen Ro52/Trim21 induces tissue inflammation and systemic autoimmunity by disregulating the IL-23-Th17 pathway. J Exp Med. 2009;206:1661-71.
18. Kretz CC, Norpo M, Abeler-Dorner L, et al. Anti-annexin 1 antibodies: a new diagnostic marker in the serum of patients with discoid lupus erythematosus. Exp Dermatol 2010;19:919-21.
19. Neufing PJ, Clancy RM, Jackson MW, et al. Exposure and binding of selected immunodominant La/SSB epitopes on human apoptotic cells. Arthritis Rheum. 2005;52:3934-42.
20. Hegazy A, Barakat AF, Gayyar MA, et al. Prevalence and clinical significance of anti-C1q antibodies in cutaneous and systemic lupus erythematosus. Egypt J Med Hum Genet. 2012;13:167-71.
21. Yoshimasu T, Hiroi A, Ohtani T, et al. Comparison of anti 60 and 52 kDa SS-A/Ro antibodies in the pathogenesis of cutaneous lupus erythematosus. J Dermatol Sci. 2002;29:35-41.
22. Marzano AV, Vezzoli P, Crosti C. Drug-induced lupus: an update on its dermatologic aspects. Lupus. 2009;18:935-40.
23. Lowe GC, Henderson CL, Grau RH, et al. A systematic review of drug-induced subacute cutaneous lupus erythematosus. Br J Dermatol. 2011;164:465-72.
24. Kind P, Lehmann P, Plewig G. Phototesting in lupus erythematosus. J Invest Dermatol 1993;100:53S-57S.
25. Franz B, Fritzsching B, Riehl A, et al. Low number of regulatory T cells in skin lesions of patients with cutaneous lupus erythematosus. Arthritis Rheum. 2007;56:1910-20.
26. Postal M, Appenzeller S. The role of Tumor Necrosis Factor-alpha (TNF-α) in the pathogenesis of systemic lupus erythematosus. Cytokine. 2011;56:537-43.
27. Miot HA, Bartoli Miot LD, Haddad GR. Association between discoid lupus erythematosus and cigarette smoking. Dermatology 2005;211:118–22.
28. Böckle BC, Sepp NT. Smoking is highly associated with discoid lupus erythematosus and lupus erythematosus tumidus: analysis of 405 patients. Lupus. 2015;24:669-74.

29. Kangle S, Amladi S, Sawant S. Scaly signs in dermatology. Indian J Dermatol Venereol Leprol 2006;72:161-4.
30. Costner MI, Provost TT. Lupus Erythematosus. Cutaneous Manifestations of Rheumatic Diseases. In: Sontheimer RD, Provost TT (Eds). Lippincott Williams and Wilkins; 2003. pp. 15-64.
31. Ueki H. Köbner phenomenon in lupus erythematosus. Hautarzt 1994;45:154-16.
32. Rowell NR, Goodfield MJD. The connective tissue diseases. Textbook of Dermatology, 5th edition. In: Champion RH, Burton JL, Ebling FJG (Eds) Blackwell Scientific Publication Oxford; 1992. pp. 2163-2225.
33. Sontheimer RD. The lexicon of cutaneous lupus erythematosus—a review and personal perspective on the nomenclature and classification of the cutaneous manifestations of lupus erythematosus. Lupus. 1997;6:84-95.
34. Rothfield N, Sontheimer R, Bernstein M. Lupus erythematosus: systemic and cutaneous manifestations. Clin Dermatol. 2006;24:348-62.
35. Farias DF, Gondim RM, Redighieri IP, et al. Comedonic lupus: a rare presentation of discoid lupus erythematosus. An Bras Dermatol. 2011;86:S89-91.
36. Verma SB, Wollina U. Chronic disseminated discoid lupus erythematosus with linear lesions following Blaschko's lines on forearm and hand. J Dtsch Dermatol Ges. 2012;10:129-30.
37. Nakamura S, Yamada T, Umemoto N, et al. Cheek and periorbital peculiar discoid lupus erythematosus: rare clinical presentation mimicking tinea faciei, cutaneous granulomatous disease or blepharitis. Case Rep Dermatol. 2015;7:56-60.
38. Chowdhury J, Kumar P, Gharami RC. Multiple cutaneous horns due to discoid lupus erythematosus. Indian J Dermatol Venereol Leprol. 2014;80:461-2.
39. Botella R, Alfonso R, Silvestre JF, et al. Discoid lupus erythematosus-like lesions and stomatitis. Arch Dermatol 1999;135:847-850.
40. Ranginwala AM, Chalishazar MM, Panja P, et al. Oral discoid lupus erythematosus: A study of twenty-one cases. J Oral Maxillofac Pathol. 2012;16:368-73.
41. Zheleva D, Darlenski R, Obreshkova E, et al. Unilateral eyelid involvement as single presentation of discoid lupus erythematosus: a clinical conundrum. Acta Dermatovenerol Croat. 2015;23:48-51.
42. Afshari NA, Afshari MA, Foster CS. Inflammatory conditions of the eye associated with rheumatic diseases. Curr Rheumatol Rep 2001;3:453-8.
43. Chong BF, Song J, Olsen NJ. Determining risk factors for developing systemic lupus erythematosus in patients with discoid lupus erythematosus. Br J Dermatol. 2012; 166:29-35.
44. Tebbe B. Clinical course and prognosis of cutaneous lupus erythematosus. Clin Dermatol. 2004;22:121-4.
45. Prystowsky SD, Gilliam JN. Discoid lupus erythematosus as part of a larger disease spectrum. Correlation of clinical features with laboratory findings in lupus erythematosus. Arch Dermatol 1975;111:1448-52.
46. Weigand DA. Lupus band test: anatomic regional variations in discoid lupus erythematosus. J Am Acad Dermatol 1986;14:426-8.
47. Burge SM, Frith PA, Millard PR, et al. The lupus band test in oral mucosa, conjunctiva and skin. Br J Dermatol 1989;121:743-52.
48. Leibowitch M, Droz D, Noel LH, et al. C1q deposits at the dermoepidermal junction: a marker discriminating for discoid and systemic lupus erythematosus. J Clin Immunol 1981;2:119-24.
49. Schrager MA, Rothfield NF. Pathways of complement activation in chronic discoid lupus. Arthritis Rheum 1977;20:637-45.
50. Amato L, Mei S, Massi D, et al. Cicatricial alopecia; a dermatopathologic and immunopathologic study of 33 patients (pseudopelade of Brocq is not a specific clinicopathologic entity). Int J Dermatol 2002;41:8-15.
51. Lallas A, Apalla Z, Lefaki I, et al. Dermoscopy of discoid lupus erythematosus. Br J Dermatol. 2013;168:284-8.
52. Beck JS, Rowell NR. Discoid lupus erythematosus. Q J Med. 1966;35:119-36.
53. Callen JP, Fowler JF, Kulick KB. Serologic and clinical features of patients with discoid lupus erythematosus: relationship of antibodies to single-stranded deoxyribonucleic acid and of other anti-nuclear antibody subsets to clinical manifestations. J Am Acad Dermatol 1985;13:748–55.
54. Lee LA, Roberts CM, Frank MB, et al. The antibody response to Ro/SSA in cutaneous lupus erythematosus. Arch Dermatol. 1994;130:1262-8.
55. Millard LG, Barker DJ. Development of squamous cell carcinoma in chronic discoid lupus erythematosus. Clin Exp Dermatol. 1978;3:161-6.
56. Gervin CM, McCulla A, Williams M, et al. Dysfunction of p53 in photocarcinogenesis. Front Biosci 2003;8:S715-7.
57. Sulica VI, Kao GF. Squamous-cell carcinoma of the scalp arising in lesions of discoid lupus erythematosus. Am J Dermatopathol 1988;10:137-41.
58. Mascaro JM, Herrero C, Hausmann G. Uncommon cutaneous manifestations of lupus erythematosus. Lupus. 1997;6:122-31.
59. Su WP, Perniciaro C, Rogers RS, et al. Chilblain lupus erythematosus (lupus pernio): clinical review of the Mayo Clinic experience and proposal of diagnostic criteria. Cutis. 1994;54:395-9.
60. Viguier M, Pinquier L, Cavelier-Balloy B, et al. Clinical and histopathologic features and immunologic variables in patients with severe chilblains. A study of the relationship to lupus erythematosus. Medicine (Baltimore) 2001;80:180-8.
61. Martens PB, Moder KG, Ahmed I. Lupus panniculitis: clinical perspectives from a case series. J Rheumatol. 1999; 26:68-72.
62. Balabanova MB, Mateev GS, Obreshkova EW, et al. Lupus erythematodes hypertrophicus et profundus. Z Hautkr 1992; 67:812-15.
63. Kinonen C, Gattuso P, Reddy VB. Lupus mastitis: an uncommon complication of systemic or discoid lupus. Am J Surg Pathol. 2010;34:901-6.

64. Sheehan-Dare RA, Cunliffe WJ. Severe periorbital oedema in association with lupus erythematosus profundus. Clin Exp Dermatol 1988;13:406-7.
65. Chen YA, Hsu CK, Lee JY, et al. Linear lupus panniculitis of the scalp presenting as alopecia along Blaschko's lines: a distinct variant of lupus panniculitis in East Asians? J Dermatol 2012;39:385-8.
66. Dammert K. Lupus erythematosus hypertrophicus et profundus. Acta Derm Venereol. 1971;51:315-6.
67. Kuhn A, Sticherling M, Bonsmann G. Clinical manifestations of cutaneous lupus erythematosus. J Dtsch Dermatol Ges. 2007;5:1124-37.
68. Lipsker D, Mitschler A, Grosshans E, et al. Could Jessner's lymphocytic infiltrate of the skin be a dermal variant of lupus erythematosus? An analysis of 210 cases. Dermatology. 2006;213:15-22.
69. Sontheimer RD, Thomas JR, Gilliam JN. Subacute cutaneous lupus erythematosus: a cutaneous marker for a distinct lupus erythematosus subset. Arch Dermatol 1979;115:1409-15.
70. Fabbri P, Bernacchi E, Neri R. [Subacute cutaneous lupus erythematosus. Review of the literature and immunological studies of 11 patients. G Ital Dermatol Venereol. 1990;125:329-36.
71. Sontheimer RD, Maddison PJ, Reichlin M, et al. Serologic and HLA associations in subacute cutaneous lupus erythematosus, a clinical subset of lupus erythematosus. Ann Intern Med. 1982;97:664-71.
72. David-Bajar KM, Bennion SD, DeSpain JD, et al. Clinical, histological, and immunofluorescent distinctions between subacute cutaneous lupus erythematosus and discoid lupus erythematosus. J Invest Dermatol. 1992;99:251-7.
73. David-Bajar KM, Davis BM. Pathology, immunopathology and immunohistochemistry in cutaneous lupus erythematosus. Lupus 1997;6:145-57.
74. Kuhn A, Sonntag M, Richter-Hintz D, et al. Phototesting in lupus erythematosus: a 15-year experience. J Am Acad Dermatol. 2001;45:86-95.
75. Klein RS, Werth VP, Dowdy JC, et al. Analysis of compact fluorescent lights for use by patients with photosensitive conditions. Photochem Photobiol. 2009;85:1004-10.
76. Sayre RM, Dowdy JC, Poh-Fitzpatrick M. Dermatological risk of indoor Ultraviolet exposure from compact fluorescent light or use by patients with photosensitive conditions. Photochem Photobiol. 2009;85:1004-10.
77. Tzung TY, Liu YS, Chang HW. Tacrolimus vs. clobetasol propionate in the treatment of facial cutaneous lupus erythematosus: a randomized, double-blind, bilateral comparison study. Br J Dermatol 2007;156:191-2.
78. Kreuter A, Gambichler T, Breuckmann F, et al. Pimecrolimus 1% cream for cutaneous lupus erythematosus. J Am Acad Dermatol 2004;51:407-10.
79. Edwards KR, Burke WA. Treatment of localized discoid lupus erythematosus with tazarotene. J Am Acad Dermatol 1999;41:1049-50.
80. Gul U, Gonul M, Cakmak SK, et al. A case of generalized discoid lupus erythematosus: successful treatment with imiquimod cream 5%. Adv Ther. 2006;23:787-92.
81. Jemec GB, Ullman S, Goodfield M, et al. A randomized controlled trial of R-salbutamol for topical treatment of discoid lupus erythematosus. Br J Dermatol. 2009;161: 1365-70.
82. Ezra N, Jorizzo J. Hydroxychloroquine and smoking in patients with cutaneous lupus erythematosus. Clin Exp Dermatol 2012;37:327-34.
83. Marmor MF, Carr RE, Easterbrook M, et al. Recommendations on screening for chloroquine and hydroxychloroquine retinopathy: a report by the American Academy of Ophthalmology. Ophthalmology. 2002;109:1377-82.
84. Kuhn A, Ruland V, Bonsmann G. Cutaneous lupus erythematosus: update of therapeutic options part 1. J Am Acad Dermatol 2011;65:e179-93.
85. Wenzel J, Brahler S, Bauer R, et al. Efficacy and safety of methotrexate in recalcitrant cutaneous lupus erythematosus: results of a retrospective study in 43 patients. Br J Dermatol. 2005;153:157-62.
86. Kuhn A, Ruland V, Bonsmann G. Cutaneous lupus erythematosus: update of therapeutic options part 2. J Am Acad Dermatol. 2011;65:e195-213.
87. Kreuter A, Tomi NS, Weiner SM, et al. Mycophenolate sodium for subacute cutaneous lupus erythematosus resistant to standard therapy. Br J Dermatol 2007;156:1321–7.
88. Tsokos GC, Caughman SW, Klippel JH. Successful treatment of generalized discoid skin lesions with azathioprine. Its use in a patient with systemic lupus erythematosus. Arch Dermatol 1986;121:1323-5.
89. Ashinoff R, Werth VP, Franks AG Jr. Resistant discoid lupus erythematosus of palms and soles: successful treatment with azathioprine. J Am Acad Dermatol 1988;19:961-5.
90. Yell JA. Burge SM. Cyclosporin and discoid lupus erythematosus. Br J Dermatol 1994;131:132-3.
91. Chang AY, Werth VP. Treatment of cutaneous lupus. Curr Rheumatol Rep 2011;13:300-7.
92. Albrecht J, Taylor L, Berlin JA, et al. The CLASI (Cutaneous Lupus Erythematosus Disease Area and Severity Index): an outcome instrument for cutaneous lupus erythematosus. J Invest Dermatol. 2005;125:889-94.
93. Braunstein I, Goodman NG, Rosenbach M, et al. Lenalidomide therapy in treatment-refractory cutaneous lupus erythematosus: histologic and circulating leukocyte profile and potential risk of a systemic lupus flare. J Am Acad Dermatol. 2012;66:571-82.
94. Bezerra EL, Vilar MJ, da Trindade Neto PB, et al. Doubleblind, randomized, controlled clinical trial of clofazimine compared with chloroquine in patients with systemic lupus erythematosus. Arthritis Rheum 2005;52:3073-8.
95. Stenjker B. Auranofin in the treatment of discoid lupus erythematosus. J Dermatol Treat 1991;2:27-9.
96. Torrelo A, Espana A, Medina S, et al. Danazol and discoid lupus erythematosus. Dermatologica. 1990;181:239

97. Rudnicka L, Szymanska E, Walecka I, et al. Long-term cefuroxime axetil in subacute cutaneous lupus erythematosus. A report of three cases. Dermatology. 2000;200:129-31.
98. Jessop S, Whitelaw DA, Delamere FM. Drugs for discoid lupus erythematosus. Cochrane Database Syst Rev. 2009 Oct 7;(4):CD002954.
99. Chang AY, Piette EW, Foering KP, et al. Response to antimalarial agents in cutaneous lupus erythematosus: a prospective analysis. Arch Dermatol. 2011;147:1261-7.
100. Kuhn A, Patsinakidis N, Luger T. Alitretinoin for cutaneous lupus erythematosus. J Am Acad Dermatol. 2012;67:e123-6.
101. Usmani N, Goodfield M. Efalizumab in the treatment of discoid lupus erythematosus. Arch Dermatol. 2007;143:873-7.
102. Piette JC, Frances C, Roy S, et al. High-dose immunoglobulins in the treatment of refractory cutaneous lupus erythematosus. Open trial in 5 cases. Arthritis Rheum. 1995;38:304.
103. Goodfield M, Davison K, Bowden K. Intravenous immunoglobulin (IVIg) for therapy-resistant cutaneous lupus erythematosus (LE). J Dermatolog Treat. 2004;15:46-50.
104. De Pita O, Bellucci AM, Ruffelli M, et al. Intravenous immunoglobulin therapy is not able to efficiently control cutaneous manifestations in patients with lupus erythematosus. Lupus 1997;6:415-7.
105. Prinz JC, Meurer M, Reiter C, et al. Treatment of severe cutaneous lupus erythematosus with a chimeric CD4 monoclonal antibody, cM-T412. J Am Acad Dermatol 1996;34:244-52.
106. Koch M, Horwath-Winter J, Aberer E, et al. [Cryotherapy in discoid lupus erythematosus (DLE)]. Ophthalmologe 2008;105:381-3.
107. Erceg A, Bovenschen HJ, van de Kerkhof PC, et al. Efficacy and safety of pulsed dye laser treatment for cutaneous discoid lupus erythematosus. J Am Acad Dermatol 2009;60:626-32.
108. Sanders CJ, Lam HY, Bruijnzeel-Koomen CA, et al. UV hardening therapy: a novel intervention in patients with photosensitive cutaneous lupus erythematosus. J Am Acad Dermatol 2006;54:479-86.
109. Okon LG, Werth VP. Cutaneous lupus erythematosus: diagnosis and treatment. Best Pract Res Clin Rheumatol. 2013;27:391-404.
110. Kuhn A, Meuth AM, Bein D, et al. Revised Cutaneous Lupus Erythematosus Disease Area and Severity Index (RCLASI): a modified outcome instrument for cutaneous lupus erythematosus. Br J Dermatol. 2010;163:83-92.

CHAPTER 6

Systemic Lupus Erythematosus

Ranjan Gupta, Amita Aggarwal

INTRODUCTION

Systemic lupus erythematosus (SLE) is an autoimmune disorder that can affect multiple organ systems. For the same reason, it is a challenging disease to diagnose and treat. The advances in treatment have significantly improved the outcome of patients with SLE. Skin being the largest organ of the body gets affected in almost 80–90% of patients with SLE and thus can serve as a clue to diagnose SLE.[1] Presence of systemic features and other organ affection along with laboratory abnormalities help in making a diagnosis of SLE.

EPIDEMIOLOGY

Systemic lupus erythematosus predominantly affects the females of child bearing age group with the female:male ratio of 9:1. However, female preponderance is less striking in young and elderly patients. This has been linked to influence of female sex hormones on the immune system or presence of extra X chromosome in females.[2] The prevalence of SLE seems to be increasing due to early diagnosis of milder cases and improved survival of patients. A recent population based study in the United States showed that age adjusted incidence and prevalence of SLE per 100,000 population were 5.5 and 72.8, respectively.[3] Persons of Asian and African-American descent have even higher incidence and prevalence of SLE. Children have higher risk of developing lupus nephritis and higher mortality compared to adult patients.

ETIOLOGY AND PATHOGENESIS

In SLE, multiple environmental factors (hormonal influences, ultraviolet light and retroviral infections) in a genetically susceptible host lead to disturbances of innate and adaptive immune system.[4] Defects in generation of apoptotic material and its clearance are important in generation of self-antigens like deoxyribonucleic acid (DNA) and nuclear antigens. Nuclear fragments are taken up by the antigen presenting cells and presented to the cells of adaptive immune system, i.e., T and B cells. The interaction between the two ultimately leads to production of antinuclear antibodies. These cells secrete a variety of cytokines leading to inflammation and tissue injury.

Further autoantibodies interact with self-antigens to form immune complexes (ICs). The clearance of ICs is impaired in SLE thus circulating ICs get trapped in small vessels and the capillaries. These ICs in turn activate complement cascade and enhances the inflammation at local site leading to various manifestations of the disease like skin rash, lupus nephritis, arthritis, and hemolytic anemia.

SYSTEMIC LUPUS ERYTHEMATOSUS CLASSIFICATION CRITERIA

As our knowledge about the disease presentation has expanded over years, the classification criteria for SLE have also evolved. The initial classification criteria proposed in 1982 had more weightage for clinical symptoms compared to laboratory features.[5] The latest 2010 SLICC criteria have not only expanded the laboratory features but have also made the section of clinical symptoms more comprehensive.[6] This shows that SLE is a disease with highly varied presentation and affects different organs in various combinations in different patients.

The 1982 American College of Rheumatology (ACR) classification criteria requires 4 out of 11 criteria to be met for classifying the patient as SLE. The ACR criteria includes four mucocutaneous manifestations, namely, photosensitivity, discoid lesions, oral ulcers, and malar rash. Thus a patient with only mucocutaneous manifestations may be misclassified as having SLE if they have all four manifestations.[7] However, less than one fifth of patients with cutaneous lupus erythematosus develop SLE within 3 years.[8] This suggests that a large proportion of patients may have only skin involvement as their clinical features which may not progress to become multi-organ systemic disease.

Clinical Features

Systemic lupus erythematosus has protean clinical manifestations, thus it is not possible to include every feature of lupus in this chapter. Chronic cutaneous and subcutaneous lupus erythematosus disease has been covered in another chapter and here an overview of the major manifestations of different organ system and rashes associated with systemic disease are being discussed in this chapter.

Presentation and course of the disease is variable in all the patients. In some cases, constitutional symptoms including fever, weight loss, anorexia, and malaise are more marked and skin involvement is milder. While in other cases skin involvement may be more prominent and extensive, but fatigue is a very common complaint by all the patients.

Renal Disease

Lupus nephritis (LN) affects almost 60–70% patients with SLE during lifetime and is present in almost 50% patients at first presentation itself.[9] The clinical manifestation can vary from asymptomatic proteinuria to rapidly progressive renal failure and includes hypertension, nephrotic syndrome, azotemia, and chronic renal failure. Urinary abnormalities (proteinuria and active sediment) define presence of renal involvement but the gold standard for diagnosis and treatment decisions is renal biopsy. Renal involvement has been classified into 6 classes on the basis of light microscopy and immunofluorescence findings.[10] If untreated, LN can lead to end-stage renal disease (ESRD), thus has important bearings on treatment decisions in SLE.[11] Lupus nephritis requires treatment with potent immunosuppressive drugs along with corticosteroids. In spite of best efforts, almost 5–10% patients with LN still develop ESRD after 10 years. Thus all patients with SLE need periodic urine examination and blood pressure measurements.

Nervous System

Neuropsychiatric systemic lupus erythematosus (NPSLE) consists of 19 distinct syndromes (12 central nervous system and 7 peripheral nervous system) as defined by ACR.[12] These can range from focal deficits like myelopathy and chorea to diffuse involvement in psychosis and acute confusional state. It is important to know that secondary causes like infections, metabolic abnormalities, and drug toxicity are more common than NPSLE and should always be excluded before making the diagnosis of NPSLE. There is no specific laboratory or imaging tests specific for diagnosis and the diagnosis is based upon thorough clinical evaluation with corroborating findings from serologic testing, cerebrospinal fluid (CSF) examination to exclude infection and neuroimaging using magnetic resonance imaging (MRI).[13]

Hematology

Systemic lupus erythematosus can affect all the three hematopoietic lineages. A large proportion of patients have anemia, lymphopenia, leucopenia, and mild thrombocytopenia. Before attributing cytopenias to disease activity, myelosuppressive effect of cytotoxic drugs and infections should always be excluded.

The most common cause of anemia in SLE is anemia of chronic disease. Other important cause of anemia in SLE is autoimmune hemolytic anemia (AIHA) which can predate the diagnosis of SLE by many years. Thrombotic microangiopathy in SLE can also present with intravascular hemolysis and should be thought of when patients have hemolytic anemia, thrombocytopenia, fever, renal, and/or neurologic involvement.

Leukopenia and lymphopenia occurs in almost 50% and 90% of SLE patients, respectively, over lifetime. Mild thrombocytopenia occurs in almost 50% SLE patients and like AIHA can predate the diagnosis of SLE by several years. Low level thrombocytopenia in SLE can also be due to antiphospholipid antibody (APLA) syndrome.[14]

Pulmonary

Pleuritis is the most common manifestation and occurs in nearly half the patients and it has good association with active disease in other organs as well. Diffuse alveolar hemorrhage is a rare life-threatening condition characterized by acute onset dyspnea, new radiographic chest infiltrates, cough with/without hemoptysis, and fall in hemoglobin. Another rare but potentially fatal manifestation is acute lupus pneumonitis characterized by fever, cough, hypoxemia, and chest infiltrates on radiograph. Other pulmonary manifestations include chronic interstitial lung disease, pulmonary arterial hypertension, and shrinking lung syndrome.[15]

Gastrointestinal

Abdominal pain is seen in almost half of lupus patients and can have varied etiology like SLE related causes, SLE nonrelated causes, infections, and drug toxicity. Systemic lupus erythematosus related causes include sterile peritonitis, mesenteric vasculitis, pancreatitis and intestinal pseudo-obstruction. Most of these manifestations occur during active phase of lupus. Chronic inflammation of liver can present as lupus hepatitis. Hepatic vascular disorders like Budd-Chiari syndrome and hepatic infarction have been reported in patients with coexistent antiphospholipid syndrome (APS).[16]

Cardiovascular

Pericarditis is the most frequent manifestation and affects almost 50% patients at some point during the disease course. Most of the pericardial effusions are small and asymptomatic. Rarely patients may present with cardiac tamponade. Myocarditis should be suspected in a patient having unexplained tachycardia, heart failure, and cardiomegaly. Asymptomatic valvular abnormalities may be seen in almost two-third of SLE patients and include Libman-Sacks endocarditis, valvular regurgitation, and stenosis. Mitral and aortic valve thickening is the most common valvular abnormality reported. The risk of myocardial infarction is 50-fold higher in lupus patients. Apart from the traditional risk factors like hypertension, diabetes, and exposure to steroids, SLE is an independent risk factor for atherosclerosis and coronary artery disease.[17]

Musculoskeletal

Arthritis occurs in almost 90% SLE patients during the course of disease. Classically, the arthritis is nonerosive and nondeforming but reducible deformities may occur in Jaccoud's arthropathy and 10% may have erosive disease.[18] Inflammatory myositis is seen in 5-8% patients. Steroids and statins may also cause myopathy in SLE. Systemic lupus erythematosus itself increases risk of avascular necrosis of bones and the incidence increases further in patients who use high dose glucocorticoids.

Mucocutaneous

Mucocutaneous involvement is seen in 80-90% of SLE patients. Gilliam et al. classified these lesions into lupus specific and lupus nonspecific based on histopathologic finding of interface dermatitis.[19] Lupus specific lesions have been subclassified into acute lupus erythematosus (ACLE), subacute lupus erythematosus (SCLE), and chronic cutaneous lupus erythematosus (CCLE). As SCLE and CCLE have already been discussed in the previous chapter, only ACLE is discussed here.

Acute lupus erythematosus can be either localized or generalized. Localized ACLE is popularly known as malar rash and refers to

Skin in Rheumatologic Diseases

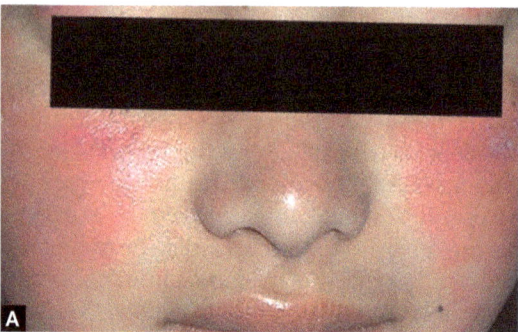 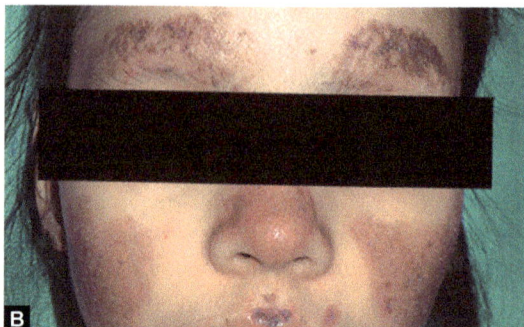

FIGURE 1: A, Malar rash on face; **B,** Discoid rash in butterfly distribution in a SLE patient.

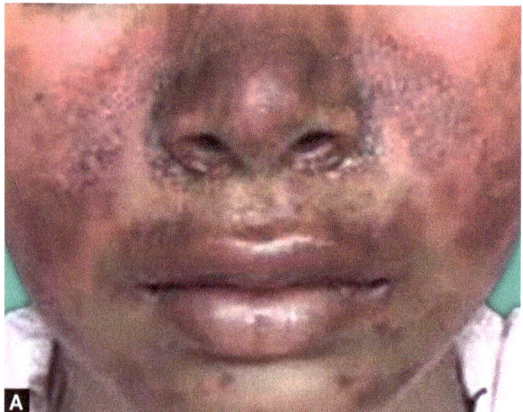 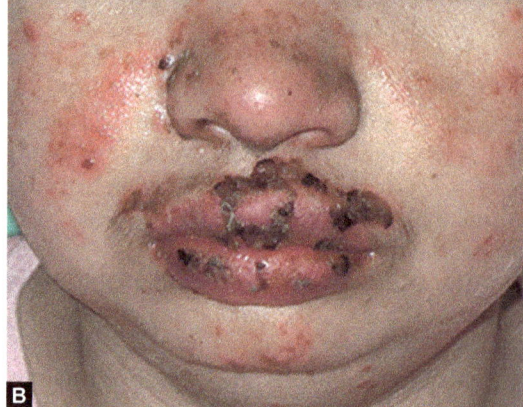

FIGURE 2: Severe malar rash on both cheek with erosions and crusting in two young female patients.

photosensitive erythematosus rash over both cheeks including the nasal bridge and sparing the nasolabial folds (Fig. 1). In addition, presence and severity of malar rash correlates with systemic disease activity. Severity of the rash can vary from mild erythema, scaling, and edema to more intense erythema, edema, erosions, and crusting (Fig. 2). Malar rash can be present in half of the patients at the time of diagnosis. Patients initially mistake it for sunburn.

Generalized ACLE is rarer and is also known as photosensitive lupus dermatitis (Fig. 3). It is characterized by more widespread symmetric eruption of maculopapular lesions involving face (Fig. 4), trunk (Fig. 5) and extensors of the limbs. The rash may be pruritic and photosensitive. In more severe forms of ACLE where cutaneous necrosis is severe, patient can develop toxic epidermal necrolysis, and erythema multiforme like lesions (Fig. 6).[20] The differential diagnosis of

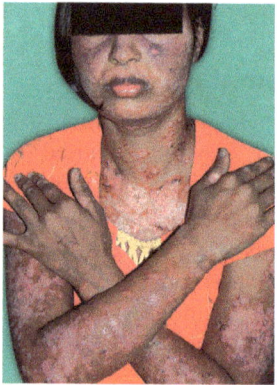

FIGURE 3: Generalized acute lupus erythematosus rash.

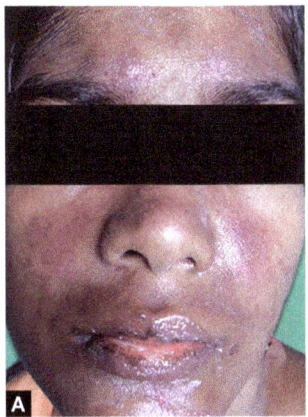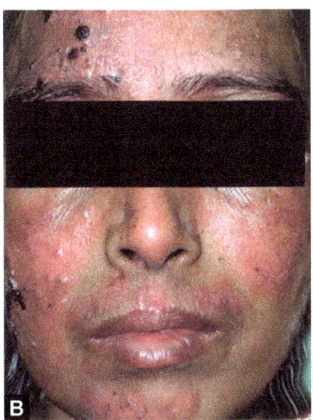

FIGURE 4: A, Generalized acute lupus erythematosus rash with diffuse facial involvement; **B,** Systemic lupus erythematosus patient with diffuse facial rash and herpes zoster over right half of face.

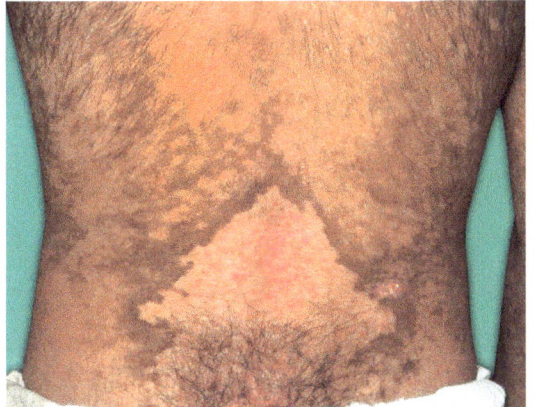

FIGURE 5: Maculopapular acute lupus erythematosus rash over trunk.

ACLE include photosensitive dermatitis, atopic dermatitis with photoaggravation, pemphigus erythematosus, and contact dermatitis.

Acute lupus erythematosus rash is often mistaken for a drug rash as palms and soles are also frequently involved (Fig. 7). On dorsum of hands, ACLE resembles the Gottron's rash of dermatomyositis but unlike dermatomyositis, the areas over the joints are spared (Fig. 8). Rarely Koebner phenomenon can be appreciated in ACLE rash (Fig. 9).

Other associated features are mucosal ulceration and hair loss.[1] Among all the mucosae, oral ulcers are the most common and can have gradual to more acute onset. They can occur anywhere on

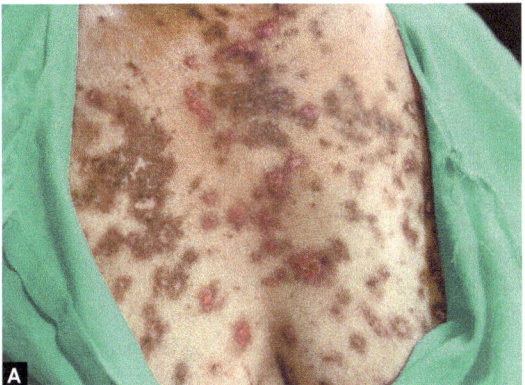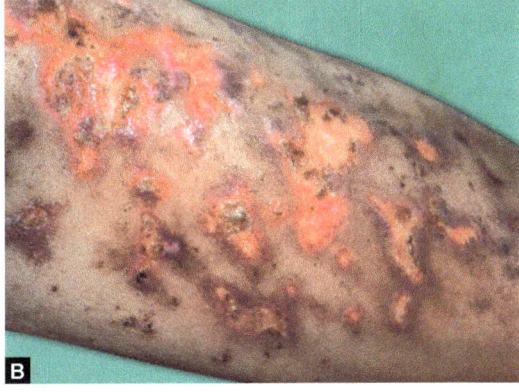

FIGURE 6: Crusted erosions and ulcers over chest and upper limb in a patient with toxic epidermal necrolysis-like systemic lupus erythematosus.

Skin in Rheumatologic Diseases

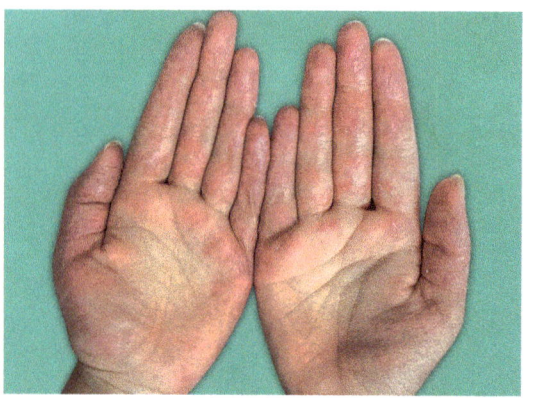

FIGURE 7: Acute lupus erythematosus rash over palms.

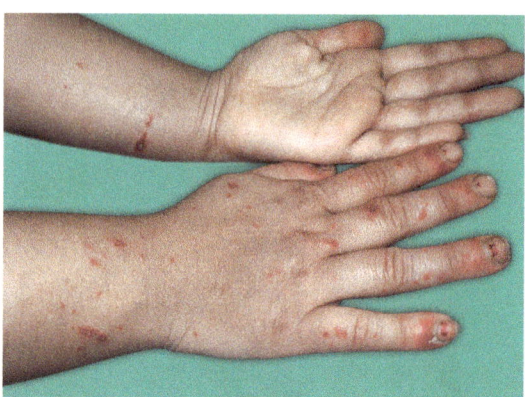

FIGURE 9: Acute lupus erythematosus lesions over acral areas and over sites of trauma (Koebner phenomenon).

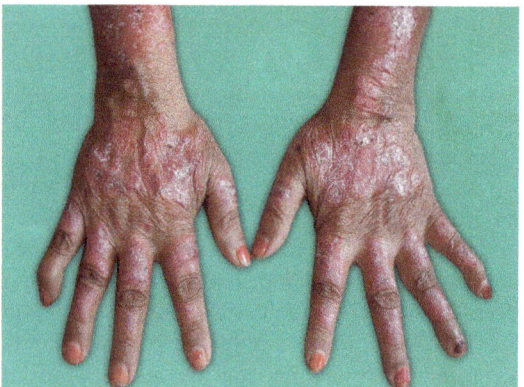

FIGURE 8: Acute lupus erythematosus rash on dorsum of hand sparing the skin over the joints.

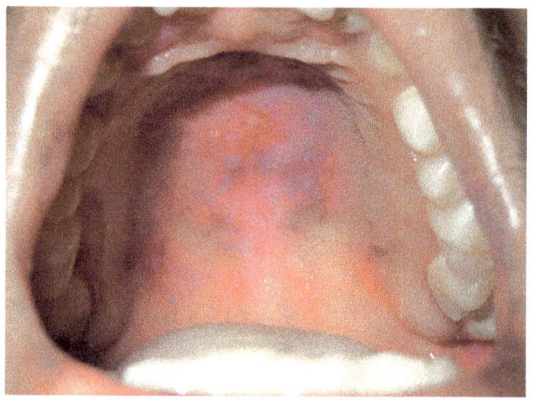

FIGURE 10: Palatal ulceration in a systemic lupus erythematosus patient.

the oral mucosa but commonly occur on the hard palate, vermilion border, and buccal mucosa. Acute oral lupus lesions commonly present as palatal red macules, ulcers, erosions, erythema, or petechiae (Fig. 10). They are usually painless and superficial.[21]

Hair loss in SLE patient can be due to lupus hair (Fig. 11), chronic telogen effluvium, effect of drugs, associated alopecia areata, or due to discoid lupus erythematosus (DLE) lesions over scalp (Fig. 12) leading to cicatricial alopecia. Lupus hair is coarse, dry, fragile, thin, short, and irregular in length.

Nails are involved in one-fourth of the patients but the changes are not specific. Commonly observed findings are nail fold capillary telangiectasia, nail plate pitting, ridging, onycholysis, and splinter hemorrhages.

Almost 36% SLE patients can have vasculitis which most commonly affects the small vessels but may also involve medium size vessels. Manifestations include punctate vasculitic lesions over extremities (Fig. 13), palpable purpurae (Fig. 14), livedo reticularis, urticarial vasculitis, and gangrene (Fig. 15). Less than 10% patients develop visceral vasculitis which may be organ or life-threatening.[22]

Rowell syndrome was originally described with DLE but now any lupus patient who develops erythema multiforme lesions (Fig. 16) in addition to specific lupus erythematosus lesions in an appropriate serological setting is labeled to be having Rowell syndrome. These patients test positive for rheumatoid factor, have speckled pattern antinuclear antibody (ANA), and anti-La/anti-Ro autoantibody.

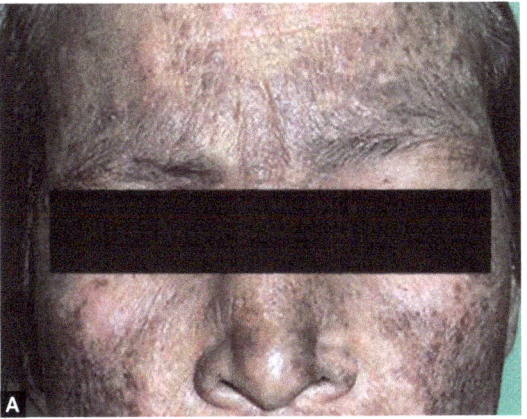 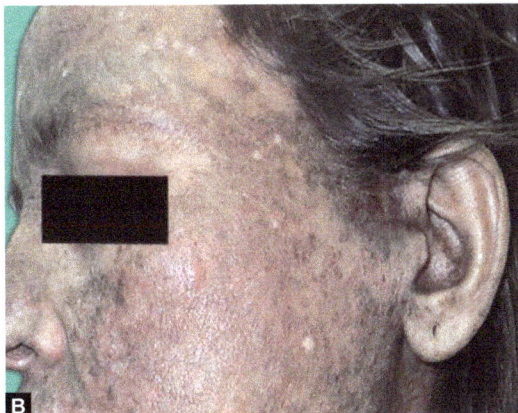

FIGURE 11: Lupus hair.

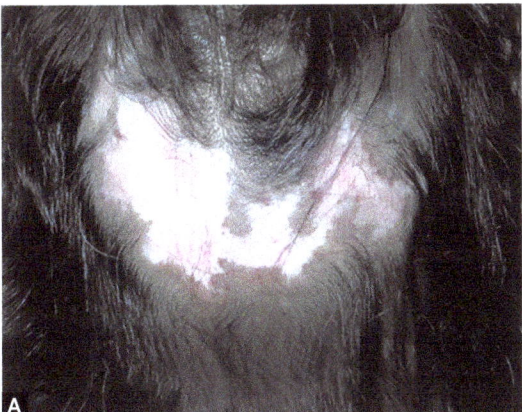 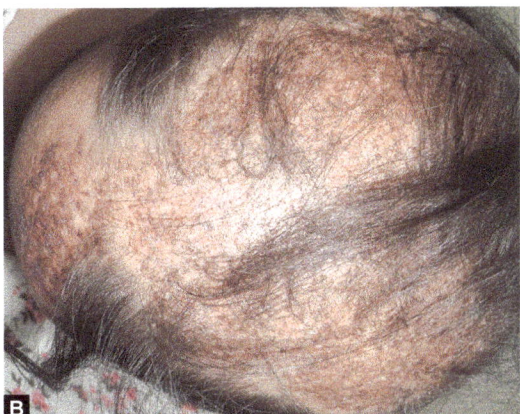

FIGURE 12: A, Discoid plaque over scalp leading to cicatricial alopecia and depigmentation in a systemic lupus erythematosus patient; **B,** Extensive DLE lesion over the scalp in a SLE patient leading to cicatricial alopecia.

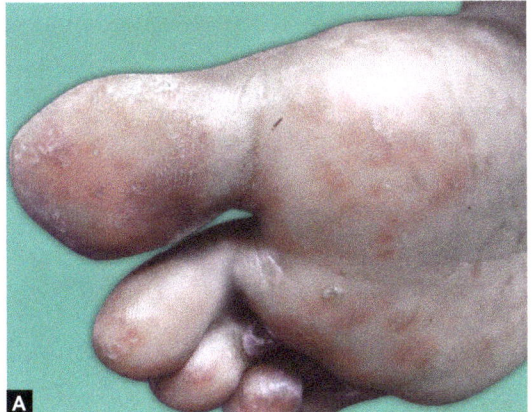 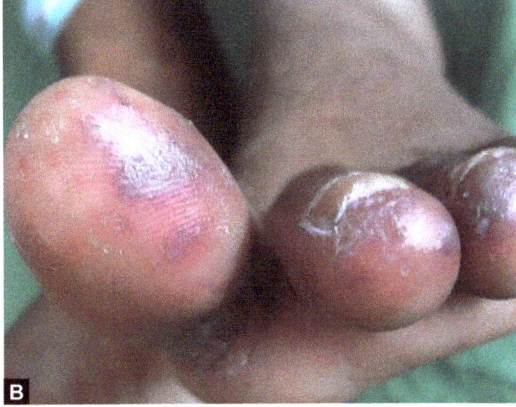

FIGURE 13: Chilblain lupus erythematosus and vasculitic lesion over extremities in a systemic lupus erythematosus patient.

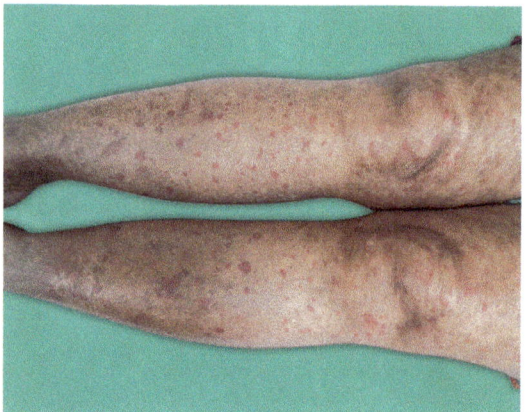

FIGURE 14: Leukocytoclastic vasculitis associated with systemic lupus erythematosus.

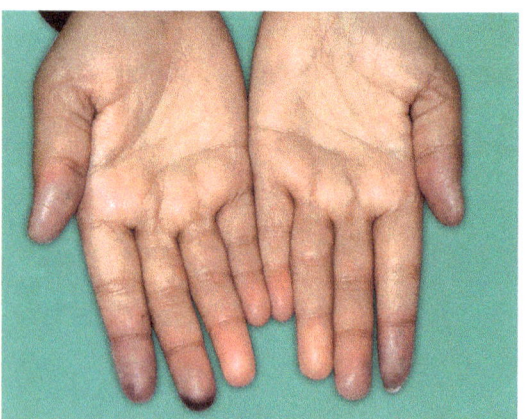

FIGURE 15: Finger tip gangrene in right middle finger along with pregangrenous changes in the tips of other fingers in a patient with vasculitis associated with systemic lupus erythematosus.

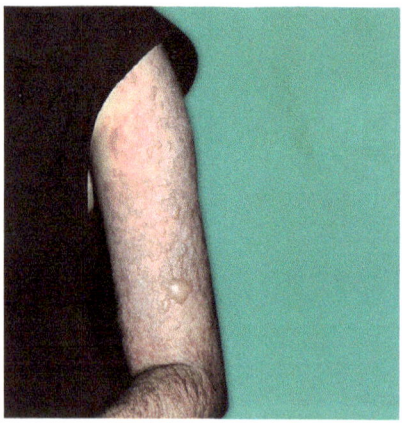

FIGURE 16: Bullous systemic lupus erythematosus.

Bullous lesions can occur in a SLE patient as a result of severe liquefaction degeneration of basal layer resulting in detachment of epidermis from dermis (Fig. 17). While some SLE patients go on to develop other immunobullous disorders including bullous pemphigoid, dermatitis herpetiformis, and epidermolysis bullosa acquisita.

Systemic lupus erythematosus patients can have CCLE lesions in almost one-third of the cases, more so in males and suggest a better prognosis (Figs 18 and 19). Acute lupus erythematosus lesions improve with treatment but often leave behind pigmentary changes. Postinflammatory hypopigmentation (Fig. 20) is more common, but those with darker skin color tend

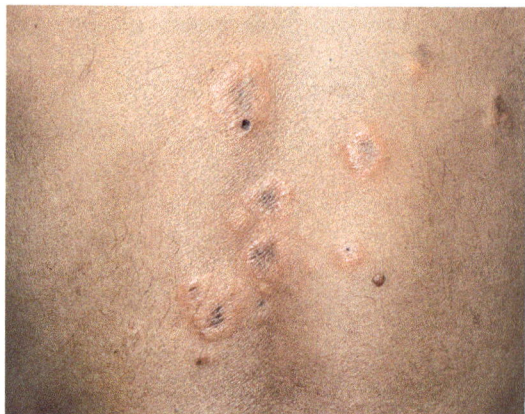

FIGURE 17: Rowell syndrome—edematous annular lesions with dusky center present over back in systemic lupus erythematosus patient.

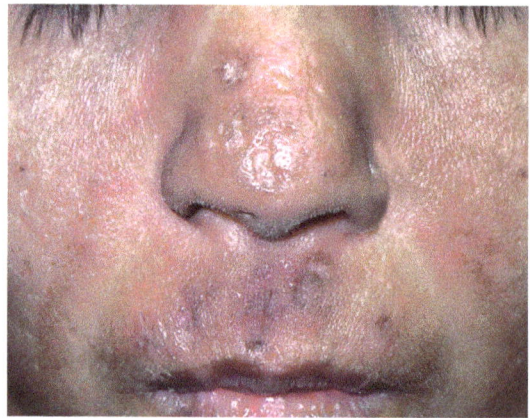

FIGURE 18: Discoid chronic cutaneous lupus erythematosus lesion over nose in a systemic lupus erythematosus patient.

Systemic Lupus Erythematosus

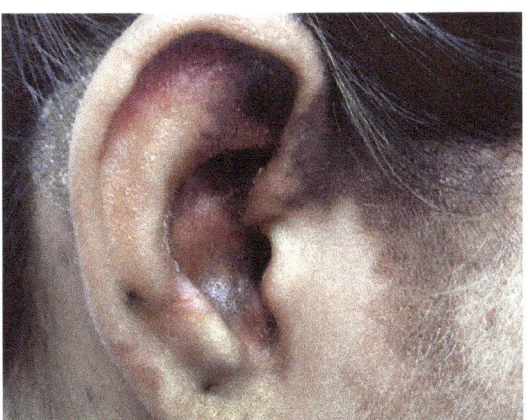

FIGURE 19: Pigmented erythematous macular discoid rash over pinna and pre and postauricular area.

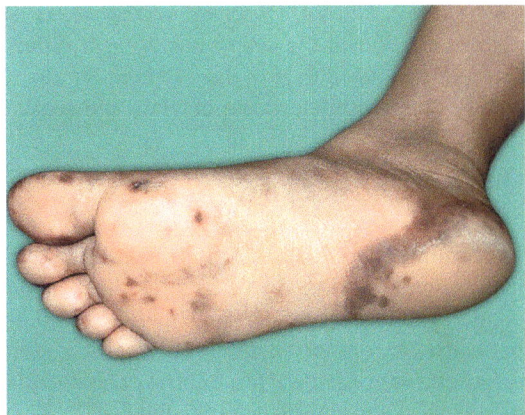

FIGURE 22: Systemic lupus erythematosus lesion over soles leaving behind postinflammatory hyperpigmentation.

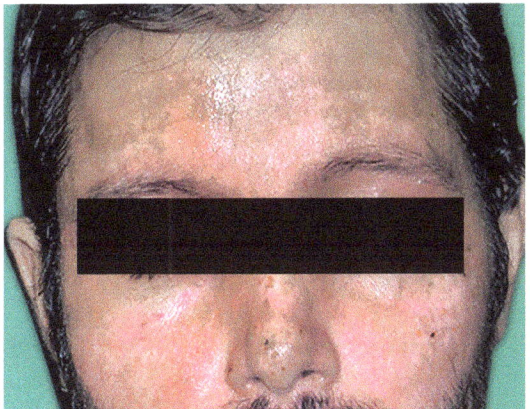

FIGURE 20: Systemic lupus erythematosus rash leaving postinflammatory hypopigmentation following treatment.

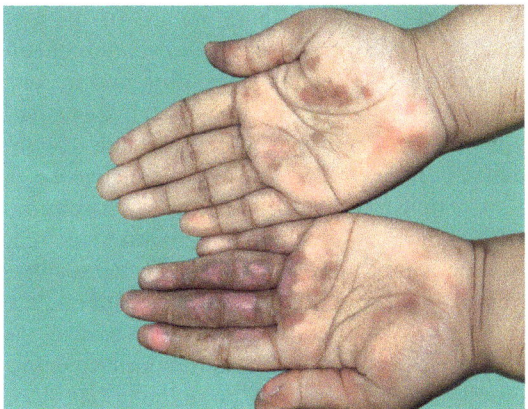

FIGURE 21: Systemic lupus erythematosus lesion over palms leaving behind postinflammatory hyperpigmentation.

to have postinflammatory hyperpigmentation (Figs 21 and 22).

Histological hallmark of lupus specific skin and mucosal lesions is interface dermatitis characterized by mononuclear cell infiltrate at the dermo-epidermal junction (Refer to chapter 3). Other features are liquefactive degeneration of basal layer, hyperkeratosis, perivascular, and periadnexal infiltrates.[23]

DRUG INDUCED LUPUS ERYTHEMATOSUS

Drug-induced lupus erythematosus occurs in older age group after taking the culprit drug for months to years. It is characterized by the presence of antihistone antibodies and absence of anti-DNA antibodies, renal and central nervous system involvement is uncommon, cutaneous involvement is in the form of bullous lesions or erythema multiforme, or vasculitis. All the patients developing drug-induced immunological abnormalities do not go down to full blown lupus syndromes, therefore, no need to discontinue drug in case of absence of signs and symptoms. Drugs commonly implicated are hydralazine, procainamide, isoniazid, diltiazem, and minocycline. Histopathological examination and direct immunofluorescence findings are similar to SLE, therefore, diagnoses is made based on temporal history of drug intake, serological test (antihistone antibody positivity, normal

C3/C4 level), and improvement within weeks of discontinuation of the suspected drug. It differs from drug induced flare of disease in SLE patient which occurs within few days of taking the drug.

DIAGNOSIS

The diagnosis of SLE is suspected based on history and examination in the setting of multisystem involvement. Simple investigations like blood counts can reveal anemia, leucopenia, lymphopenia, or thrombocytopenia. A raised serum creatinine or presence of proteinuria or hematuria may suggest asymptomatic renal disease.

Among the autoantibodies, antinuclear antibody is the screening test. It has 95–98% sensitivity, thus a negative test virtually excludes a diagnosis of SLE. However, ANA can be present in other connective tissue diseases as well. Once ANA is positive, antibodies to extractable nuclear antigen may further help in diagnosis. Anti-Sm antibodies if positive have very high specificity (95%) for SLE. In addition, antibodies to SS-A, SSB, and nRNP can be seen in 30–50% of patients with SLE. Anti-Ro/SS-A antibodies are seen in almost one-third of SLE patients and are associated with photosensitivity and subacute cutaneous lupus.

Anti-double stranded DNA (dsDNA) antibody is present in about 50–60% of patients and correlates with nephritis. Complement C3 and C4 levels are usually decreased in patients with SLE. Both anti-dsDNA and C3 and C4 levels are helpful in follow up of patients with SLE as they have moderate correlation with activity of disease.[24]

Anticardiolipin antibodies and lupus anticoagulant assay helps in looking for antiphospholipid antibodies, which correlate with livedo reticularis, digital gangrene, recurrent fetal loss, and arterial and venous thrombosis.

If renal disease is evident then kidney biopsy helps in knowing the degree of involvement and presence of chronicity if any. Active proliferative nephritis (Fig. 23) needs more aggressive therapy. Similarly, if neurological disease is present appropriate tests like nerve conduction, nerve biopsy, CSF examination, and MRI/computed tomography imaging of the relevant areas may be needed to know the type and extent of pathology (Box 1).

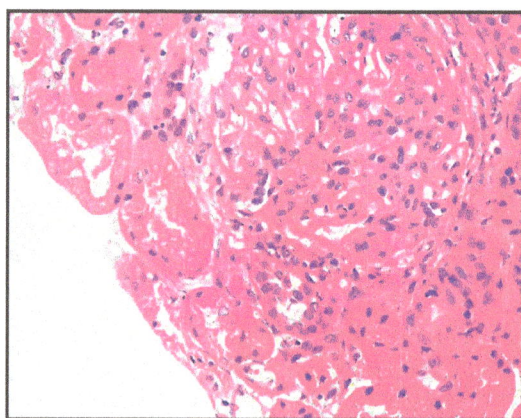

FIGURE 23: Class IV nephritis on kidney biopsy.

> **Box 1: Investigations in a systemic lupus erythematosus patient**
>
> - Complete hemogram including peripheral smear and erythrocyte sedimentation rate
> - Liver function tests, kidney function tests, serum electrolytes, urea
> - Antinuclear antibody, anti-double stranded deoxyribonucleic acid, C3, C4
> - Anticardiolipin antibodies and lupus anticoagulant
> - Direct coombs test
> - Renal biopsy in case of suspicion of involvement

TREATMENT

The management of a patient with SLE involves patient education, drugs, prevention of complications, etc. The first and foremost is patient education about nature of disease, need for regular drug therapy, prevention of sun exposure, stress, family issues, drug toxicity, etc. A physician needs to emphasize that if the patient and physician work together the outcome is bright and patient can lead a good and productive life.

Corticosteroids and hydroxychloroquine (HCQS) are the cornerstone therapy of SLE. Immunosuppressive drugs like cyclophosphamide (CYC), azathioprine, and mycophenolate (MMF) are indicated for severe disease or as steroid sparing agents. In addition, intravenous immunoglobulin, anti-CD20 antibody (RTX), or anti-B lymphocyte stimulator (belimumab) is used in special situations.

For minor organ disease like skin, joints, systemic features, mild cytopenias, or serositis, nonsteroidal anti-inflammatory drugs and HCQS is prescribed. If the response is inadequate, low dose prednisolone (0.25–0.5 mg/kg) may be added. For arthritis, weekly low dose methotrexate is a good choice.

Acute cutaneous lupus erythematosus usually resolves with the treatment for systemic manifestations and no specific therapy is required. Topical steroids and calcineurin inhibitors are useful in persistent or localized lesions. Local steroids with the mid potency are required for healing of skin lesions and should be used for the shortest duration possible. Calcineurin inhibitors have same efficacy without the adverse effects associated with steroids.[25] In widespread lesions, antimalarials (HCQS, chloroquine, and quinacrine) are the mainstay of therapy. Hydroxychloroquine has a more favorable profile compared to chloroquine in terms of retinopathy.[1] Since antimalarials take 2–3 months for their effects to come, oral steroids can be given during this time to bridge the gap. Other immunosuppressive drugs are reserved for resistant ACLE.

In patients with major organ diseases like nephritis, lung disease, or severe cytopenias, high dose prednisolone (1 mg/kg/day) along with immunosuppressive drugs is used to have effective control of inflammation and prevent irreversible damage. In organ or life-threatening diseases, intravenous methylprednisolone in a dose of 500–1,000 mg/day may be used for 1–3 days.

Treatment for nephritis (Flowchart 1) depends on the class of nephritis with class I and class II disease not requiring any special treatment except treatment for extra-renal disease. Class III and IV nephritis is treated with corticosteroids along with either CYC or MMF. Low dose CYC as 500 mg every 15 days for 6 doses is the preferred dose of CYC as it has less toxicity with equal efficacy[26] (Fig. 5). All patients need long-term maintenance therapy for 3–5 years. For membranous nephropathy, a 6-month course of corticosteroids along with MMF or CYC is given along with angiotensin receptor blockers to reduce proteinuria. A meticulous control of hypertension helps in preservation of renal function.[11]

In neurological disease, it is important to distinguish focal disease due to thrombosis related to APS and global disease related to antibodies. For focal disease related to APS, anticoagulants and antiplatelet agents are prescribed whereas for global dysfunction high-dose corticosteroids is used (Flowchart 2). Along with these, patients need symptomatic treatment for depression, seizures, psychosis, etc.[27]

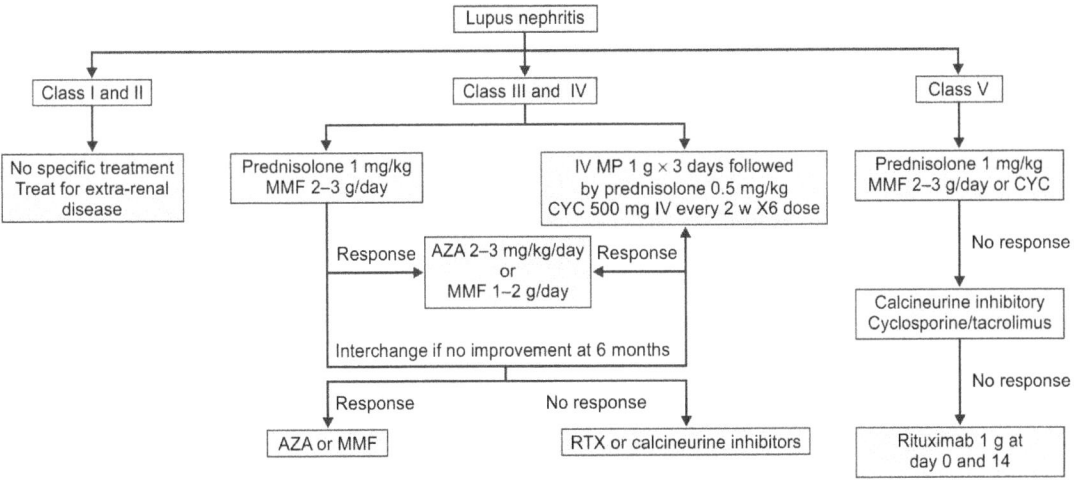

MMF, mycophenolate; IV, intravenous; MP, methylprednsiolone; CYC, cyclophosphamide; AZA, azathioprine; RTX, anti-CD20 antibody.

FLOWCHART 1: Algorithm showing management of lupus nephritis.

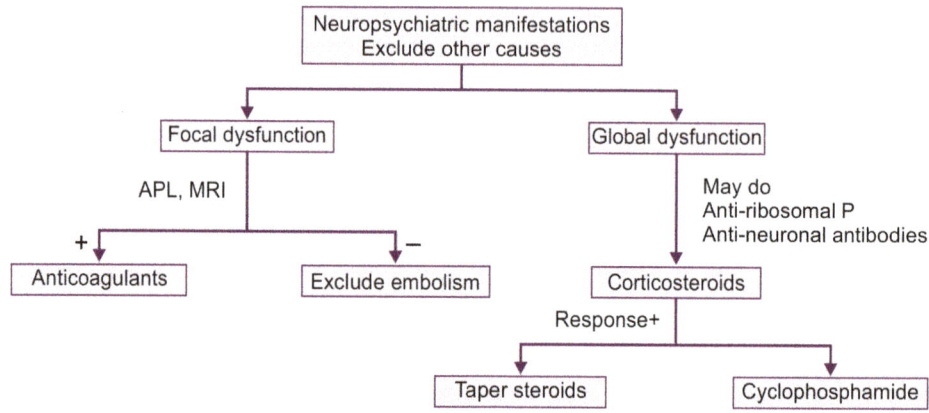

APL, antiphospholipid; MRI, magnetic resonance imaging.

FLOWCHART 2: Algorithm showing approach and management of central nervous system lupus.

Prevention of drug toxicity is an important issue as patients with SLE need long-term drugs. Corticosteroids should be prescribed in minimal possible dose for the shortest period of time depending on the clinical situation. Corticosteroids-sparing agents should be started early. Regular physical activity, and adequate calcium and vitamin D intake help reduce cardiovascular effects and osteoporosis. Patients on long-term steroids should have bone density measurement at periodic interval of 2-3 years.

Comorbidities like obesity, hypertension, and diabetes need adequate treatment to reduce risk of cardiovascular morbidity. As SLE affect women of child bearing age group, advice on family planning, pregnancy, delivery, etc. need to be discussed in detail with the patient. During pregnancy, combined care by a rheumatologist and obstetrician helps in improving outcome of pregnancy.

Disease activity measurement tools (e.g., Systemic Lupus Erythematosus Disease Activity Index or British Isles Lupus Assessment Group) are useful in follow up of patients with systemic disease. They are a composite scores of clinical and laboratory parameters. Same scale should be used at each visit. At every follow up visit simple tests like blood counts, serum creatinine, and urine analysis which are useful in assessing subclinical disease activity should be done.[28,29]

OUTCOME

Over the past two decades, mortality rates in lupus have decreased significantly with 10-15 years survival exceeding 85%. However, this has meant that patients have significant morbidity related to long-term corticosteroid and other drug use for infections, diabetes, and hypertension. In addition, damage due to diseases like avascular necrosis of hip, renal failure, cognitive decline, and arterial thrombosis also contributes to morbidity. Thus, to conclude, SLE is a treatable disease with good long-term outcome. Early diagnosis and meticulous follow up can further improve outcome.

REFERENCES

1. Patel P, Werth V. Cutaneous lupus erythematosus: a review. Dermatol Clin. 2002;20:373-85.
2. Lisnevskaia L, Murphy G, Isenberg D. Systemic lupus erythematosus. Lancet. 2014;384:1878-88.
3. Somers EC, Marder W, Cagnoli P, et al. Population-based incidence and prevalence of systemic lupus erythematosus: the Michigan Lupus Epidemiology and Surveillance program. Arthritis Rheumatol. 2014;66:369-78.
4. Wahren-Herlenius M, Dorner T. Immunopathogenic mechanisms of systemic autoimmune disease. Lancet. 2013;382: 819-31.
5. Tan EM, Cohen AS, Fries JF, et al. The 1982 revised criteria for the classification of systemic lupus erythematosus. Arthritis Rheum. 1982;25:1271-7.

6. Petri M, Orbai AM, Alarcón GS, et al. Derivation and validation of the Systemic Lupus International Collaborating Clinics classification criteria for systemic lupus erythematosus. Arthritis Rheum. 2012;64:2677-86.
7. Biazar C, Sigges J, Patsinakidis N, et al. Cutaneous lupus erythematosus: first multicenter database analysis of 1002 patients from the European Society of Cutaneous Lupus Erythematosus (EUSCLE). Autoimmun Rev. 2013;12:444-54.
8. Gronhagen CM, Fored CM, Granath F, et al. Cutaneous lupus erythematosus and the association with systemic lupus erythematosus: a population-based cohort of 1088 patients in Sweden. Br J Dermatol. 2011;164:1335-41.
9. Cameron JS. Lupus nephritis. J Am Soc Nephrol. 1999;10:413-24.
10. Weening JJ, D'Agati VD, Schwartz MM, et al. The classification of glomerulonephritis in systemic lupus erythematosus revisited. J Am Soc Nephrol. 2004;15:241-50.
11. Hahn BH, McMahon MA, Wilkinson A, et al. American College of Rheumatology guidelines for screening, treatment, and management of lupus nephritis. Arthritis Care Res (Hoboken). 2012;64:797-808.
12. The American College of Rheumatology nomenclature and case definitions for neuropsychiatric lupus syndromes. Arthritis Rheum. 1999;42:599-608.
13. Fanouriakis A, Boumpas DT, Bertsias GK. Pathogenesis and treatment of CNS lupus. Curr Opin Rheumatol. 2013;25:577-83
14. Fayyaz A, Igoe A, Kurien BT, et al. Haematological manifestations of lupus. Lupus Sci Med. 2015;3:e000078.
15. Kamen DL, Strange C. Pulmonary manifestations of systemic lupus erythematosus. Clin Chest Med. 2010;31:479-88.
16. Ebert EC, Hagspiel KD. Gastrointestinal and hepatic manifestations of systemic lupus erythematosus. J Clin Gastroenterol. 2011;45:436-41.
17. Miner JJ, Kim AH. Cardiac manifestations of systemic lupus erythematosus. Rheum Dis Clin North Am. 2014;40:51-60.
18. Ball EM, Bell AL. Lupus arthritis--do we have a clinically useful classification? Rheumatology (Oxford). 2012;51:771-9.
19. Gilliam JN, Sontheimer RD. Distinctive cutaneous subsets in the spectrum of lupus erythematosus. J Am Acad Dermatol. 1981;4:471-5.
20. Horne NS, Narayan AR, Young RM, et al. Toxic epidermal necrolysis in systemic lupus erythematosus. Autoimmun Rev 2006;5:160-4.
21. Jonsson R, Heyden G, Westberg NG, et al. Oral mucosal lesions in systemic lupus erythematosus--a clinical, histo-pathological and immunopathological study. J Rheumatol. 1984;11:38-42.
22. Barile-Fabris L, Hernández-Cabrera MF, Barragan-Garfias JA. Vasculitis in systemic lupus erythematosus. Curr Rheumatol Rep. 2014;16:440-447.
23. Kuhn A, Sonntag M, Ruzicka T, et al. Histopathologic findings in lupus erythematosus tumidus: review of 80 patients. J Am Acad Dermatol. 2003;48:901-8.
24. Kurien BT, Scofield RH. Autoantibody determination in the diagnosis of systemic lupus erythematosus. Scand J Immunol. 2006;64:227-35.
25. Okon LG, Werth VP. Cutaneous lupus erythematosus: diagnosis and treatment. Best Pract Res Clin Rheumatol. 2013;27:391-404.
26. Houssiau FA, Vasconcelos C, D'Cruz D, et al. Immuno-suppressive therapy in lupus nephritis: the Euro-Lupus Nephritis Trial, a randomized trial of low-dose versus high-dose intravenous cyclophosphamide. Arthritis Rheum. 2002;46:2121-31.
27. Bertsias GK, Ioannidis JP, Aringer M, et al. EULAR recommendations for the management of systemic lupus erythematosus with neuropsychiatric manifestations: report of a task force of the EULAR standing committee for clinical affairs. Ann Rheum Dis. 2010;69:2074-82.
28. Bombardier C, Gladman DD, Urowitz MB, et al. Derivation of the SLEDAI. A disease activity index for lupus patients. The Committee on Prognosis Studies in SLE. Arthritis Rheum. 1992;35:630-40.
29. Isenberg DA, Rahman A, Allen E, et al. BILAG 2004. Development and initial validation of an updated version of the British Isles Lupus Assessment Group's disease activity index for patients with systemic lupus erythematosus. Rheumatology (Oxford). 2005;44:902-6.

7 CHAPTER

Dermatomyositis

Aparna Palit

INTRODUCTION

Dermatomyositis (DM) is a multisystem collagen vascular disorder of multifactorial etiopathogenesis affecting any age group, the main plunge being upon the skin and muscles, and the prognosis is variable.

Dermatomyositis is relatively rare compared to other collagen vascular disorders. The first report of the disorder in English literature was early in 1863, reported by Wagner.[1] A probable pictorial depiction of the disease was available in French, artist Amedeo Modigliani's portrayal of a girl *fillette en bleu* (little girl in blue).[2] Nowadays, the understanding of the disease has achieved new dimensions clinically, pathogenetically, and management-wise.

CLASSIFICATION

Polymyositis and dermatomyositis (PM-DM) were considered a spectrum of disease included under the broad group of disorders idiopathic inflammatory myopathies (IIM). The original classification system for PM-DM group of disorders was proposed by Bohan and Peter in 1975.[3] With the recognition of a skin-limited variant, the "amyopathic dermatomyositis," a revised classification system has been proposed.[4,5,6] Both the classification systems have been presented in table 1.

Table 1: Classification of polymyositis and dermatomyositis[1,4-6]		
Classification for polymyositis and dermatomyositis (Bohan and Peter, 1975)	Revised classification system (Sontheimer, 1999)	
	Adult onset	Juvenile onset

• Group I: Polymyositis
• Group II: Dermatomyositis
• Group III: Malignancy associated polymyositis-dermatomyositis
• Group IV: Childhood onset polymyositis-dermatomyositis
• Group V: Collagen vascular disorder associated polymyositis-dermatomyositis
	• Classic polymyositis and dermatomyositis
	• Classic dermatomyositis with malignancy
	• Classic dermatomyositis with other connective tissue disorder overlap
	• Clinically amyopathic dermatomyositis (provisional/confirmed)*
	  ○ Amyopathic
	  ○ Hypomyopathic
		• Classic dermatomyositis
		• Clinically amyopathic dermatomyositis (provisional/confirmed)*
		  ○ Amyopathic dermatomyositis
		  ○ Hypomyopathic dermatomyositis

*Provisional: Biopsy-confirmed hallmark cutaneous features of dermatomyositis, without muscle weakness and with normal muscle enzymes for greater than or equal to 6 months. Confirmed: Same as provisional for ≥24 months.

ETIOLOGY AND PATHOGENESIS

There is an autoimmune response in genetically susceptible individuals to environmental insult. Microchimerism may be a possible etiological factor in the pathogenesis of juvenile dermatomyositis (JDM). The disease evolution is presumably through four phases:[5]

The Susceptibility Phase

Some individuals are genetically predisposed to develop DM. Identical twins may suffer from DM. Various human leukocyte antigen (HLA) associations have been recognized; the prominent ones being *HLA-A1, -C7, -B8, -C4AQ0, -C4B1, -DR3,* and *DQ2.* The *HLA-DR3* and *HLA-DRw52* positive individuals are prone to develop antisynthetase antibodies. Another factor depicting individual susceptibility is tumor necrosis factor-α (TNF-α)-308A promoter gene (TNF-α-308A) polymorphism, which determines disease chronicity, calcinosis, and high level of TNF in patients with JDM. Gene polymorphisms associated with low production of mannose-binding protein and genetic deficiency of complements 2 and 5 have also been reported in patients with DM.

The Induction Phase

In genetically susceptible individuals, there are various exogenous trigger-factors to precipitate the evolution of clinical features (Table 2). Single or multiple inciting factors may be operative in a given case.

The Expansion Phase

There is loss of normal immune regulation and expansion of autoreactive T cell lineage, as evidenced by diffuse T lymphocyte infiltrate in muscles and high level of soluble CD30. Various autoantibodies are produced at this phase (Table 3). In malignancy-associated DM, there may be detection of complement-fixing autoantibodies against the tumor cells. Myositis-related antigen expression in tumor cells may incite autoantibody formation against muscles.

Table 2: Trigger factors for dermatomyositis[5,7]

Environmental	Ultraviolet light (natural and artificial)
Infections	Coxsackie B virus, Echovirus, parvovirus B19, Epstein-Barr virus, human T cell leukemia virus-1, human immunodeficiency virus, *Toxoplasma gondii, Staphylococcus, Streptococcus*
Drugs causing myopathy	Corticosteroids, D-penicillamine, hydroxyurea, nonsteroidal anti-inflammatory drugs, quinidine, oral progesterone, tumor necrosis factor antagonists, zidovudine, lipid lowering drugs, retinoids, tamoxifen(?), alcohol
Primary malignancy (15–34%)	Lungs, breast, female genital tract, kidney, testis, rectum, nasopharyngeal carcinoma
Stress	Heavy muscular exercise

The Injury Phase

The autoantibodies against muscle antigens cause immune attack on the microvasculature of muscle; there is immune complex deposition, probably mediated by C5-C9 membrane attack complex. This results in ischemia and consequently muscle injury. The mechanism of cutaneous injury is less well-defined, but similar involvement of dermal microvasculature is the possible mechanism.

EPIDEMIOLOGY

Dermatomyositis is a ubiquitous disease affecting people of any race and color. It can occur at any age starting in infancy as well as in the elderly. Females suffer twice as commonly as males.[7] Adult DM starts 40 years onwards, with females presenting at an earlier age than males.[7]

CLINICAL FEATURES

Cutaneous lesions and muscle involvement may present simultaneously (60%) or one may precede the other.[5,7] Only cutaneous features are the presenting symptoms in 30% cases,

Skin in Rheumatologic Disease

Table 3: Various autoantibodies found in dermatomyositis[1,5,7,8]	
Myositis-specific autoantibodies	
Anti-tRNA synthetase enzymes	Jo-1 (20%), PL-7 (3%), PL-12 (3%), OJ, EJ
Anti-signal recognition particle (SRP) protein	SRP (5%)
Anti-helicase nuclear protein (Mi-2)	Mi-2 (15%)
Anti-p155/140 transcriptional protein (anti-TIF1γ)	20–80%
Anti-melanoma differentiation-associated gene 5 (MDA5)	–
Anti-nuclear matrix protein (NXP-2)	Anti-MJ (27%)
Other rare autoantibodies	Anti-FER, anti-KJ, anti-MAS
Myositis-associated autoantibodies	
• Antinuclear antibody (40%)	
• Anti-ssDNA (40%)	
• Anti-PM/Scl (PM-1) (40%)	
• Anti-U1-RNP (10%) and U2-RNP (1%)	
• Anti-Ro (15%)	
• Anti-Ku (3%)	
In juvenile dermatomyositis	
• Anti-synthetase antibodies (5–10%)	
• Anti-SRP (<5%)	
• Anti-Mi-2 (5%)	
• Anti-p155 (30%)	

Note: (%) indicates frequency of these autoantibodies in patients with dermatomyositis.

whereas the rest 10% present with muscle pain and weakness.[7] Amyopathic or hypomyopathic DM is a subset of the disease where muscle involvement is absent or minimal. Onset of the disease is usually insidious but though rarely, acute-onset, fulminant disease may occur.

Cutaneous Involvement

The cutaneous features of DM usually run a waxing and waning course, irrespective of the severity of the muscle disease. The initial nonspecific symptoms are usually photosensitivity, burning sensation and generalized pruritus.[5,6] More definite skin lesions appear gradually. The telltale colors of skin lesions of DM are reddish and violaceous in fair-skinned individuals (Fig. 1), while more purple (Fig. 2) in darker-skinned individuals.[9] The main skin lesions of DM have been categorized according to their diagnostic importance (Table 4). The characteristic description of each of these lesions follows.[5-7,10]

Gottron Papules

These are located symmetrically over the knuckles, dorsal aspects of finger-joints (Fig. 3), occasionally at the sides of fingers (Fig. 4) and around nailfolds. Toes, knees, and points of the elbows may be involved. Morphologically, these are violaceous, round, flat-topped papules with slight central depression (Fig. 5). Variable amount of scale may

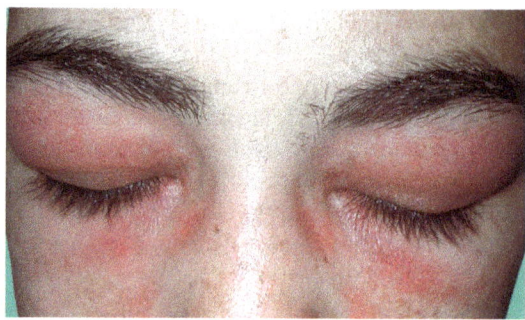

FIGURE 1: Heliotrope rash in a fair-skinned woman.
Courtesy: Department of Dermatology, Post-Graduate Institute of Medical Education and Research, Dr Ram Manohar Lohia Hospital, New Delhi.

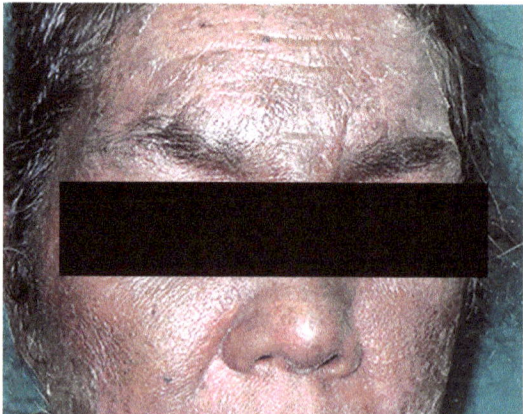

FIGURE 2: Dark purplish hue and background erythema of dermatomyositis rash involving whole face in a female with carcinoma ovary.

Table 4: Skin lesions of dermatomyositis, categorized according to diagnostic importance[5]	
Pathognomonic skin lesions	• Gottron papule • Gottron sign
Characteristic skin lesions	• Heliotrope rash • Periungual telangiectasias • Symmetric, macular erythema of dorsa of hands • Mechanics' hands
Skin lesions compatible with the diagnosis of dermatomyositis	• Poikiloderma atrophicans vasculare • Calcinosis cutis

be present over the lesions and telangiectasias may be appreciable. The lesions of some duration may appear shiny and atrophic (Fig. 6). In dark skin individuals these may resemble prurigo like lesions (Fig. 7). In some individuals these are present over the palmer aspect of the fingers and are called inverse Gottron papules (Fig. 8).

Gottron Sign

Symmetric, violaceous or erythematous plaques or atrophic macules over the bony prominences, like knuckles (Fig. 6), elbows (Fig. 9), knees (Fig. 10) and the malleoli.

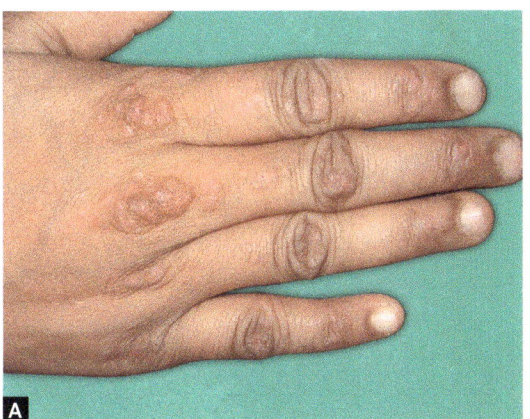
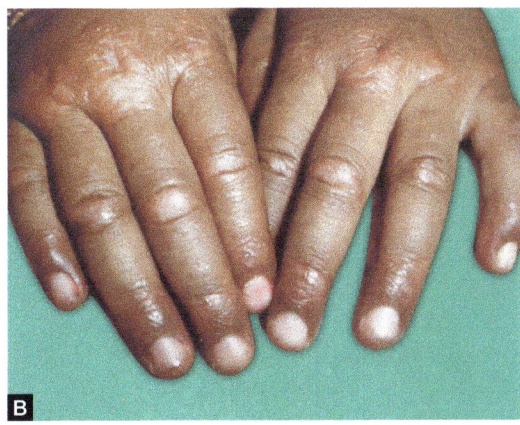

FIGURE 3: **A,** Gottron papules; **B,** Gottron's papules in a child with juvenile dermatomyositis.
Courtesy (Figure 3A): Dr BS Ankad, SN Medical College, Bagalkot, Karnataka.

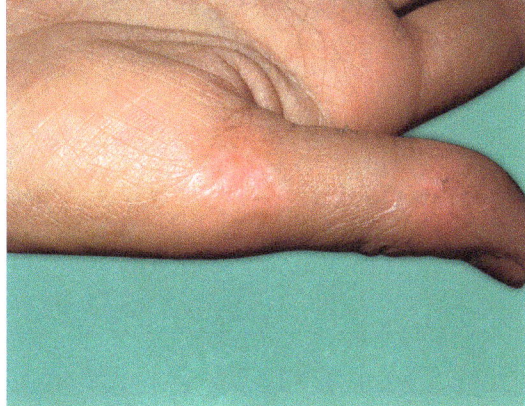
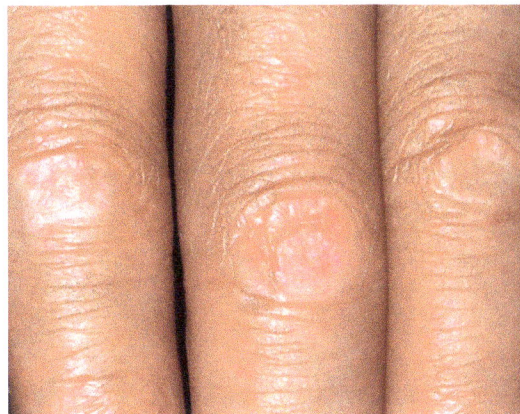

FIGURE 4: Gottron papules on side of the thumb.

FIGURE 5: Slight central depression at the center of Gottron papules.

Skin in Rheumatologic Disease

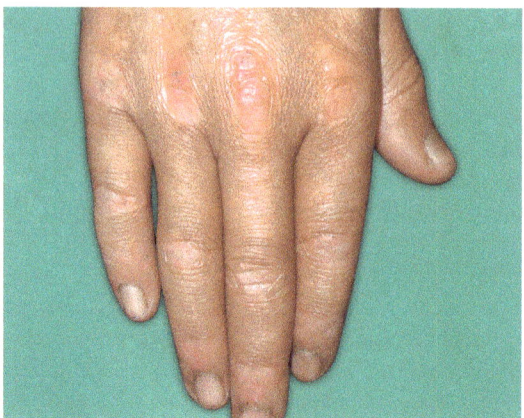

FIGURE 6: Shiny atrophic Gottron papules during healing phase.

Heliotrope Rash

It presents as symmetrical violaceous hue of the eyelids and periorbital region (30–60%)[7] with associated edema, better appreciable in fair-skinned individuals (Fig. 1). Sometimes the upper eyelid is selectively involved. It may spread diffusely to adjacent areas like forehead, temples, lateral root of the nose adjacent to the medial canthus of eyes (Fig. 11), and the cheeks.[6] Sometimes the color may be intense with a dusky appearance. In darker individuals, the color change may not be marked and only edema is representative of the lesion (Fig. 12). Periorbital edema may be an early finding and occasionally

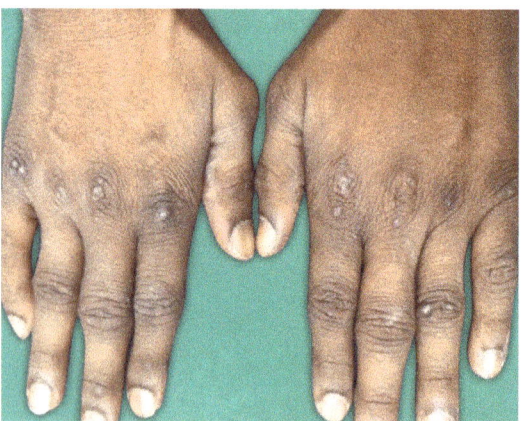

FIGURE 7: Prurigo-like Gottron papules.

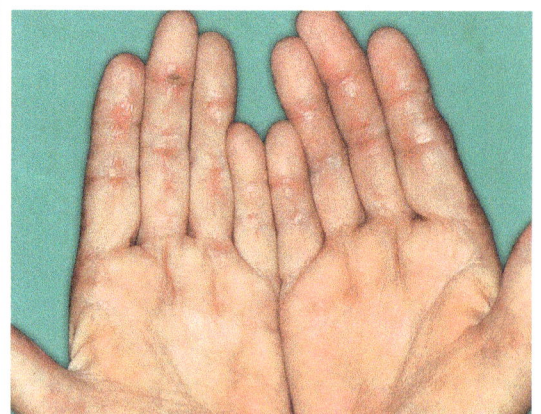

FIGURE 8: Inverse Gottron papules.

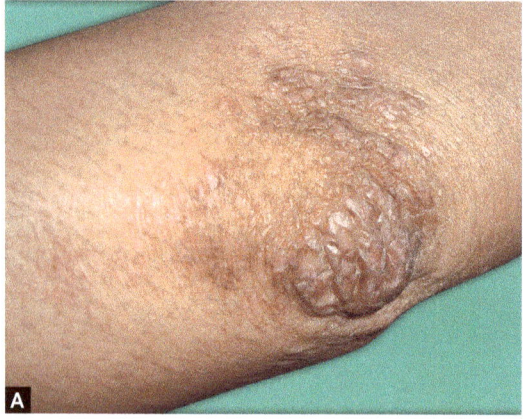

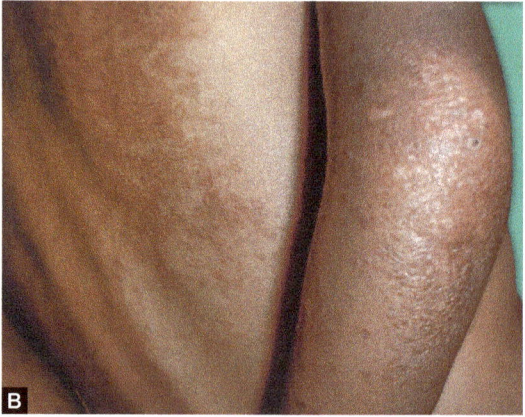

FIGURE 9: Gottron sign over elbow.

Courtesy (Figure 9A): Dr BS Ankad, SN Medical College, Bagalkot, Karnataka.

Dermatomyositis

long-lasting. While on therapy, the color fades away and the edema subsides, sometimes with residual pigmentation (Fig. 13).

Periungual Telangiectasia

Nail folds are erythematous and shiny, with easily visible capillaries on proximal nail folds. These are irregular, dilated, tortuous, and better appreciated with a lens or dermoscope (Fig. 14), but sometimes even seen through naked eyes (Fig. 15).[7] In absence of dermoscope at bedside, an ophthalmoscope or otoscope is helpful. The vascular patterns include capillary dilatations, loops, dropouts, and these are not specific as similar changes are observed in other collagen vascular disorders.[6] However, demonstration of periungual telangiectasias is of diagnostic importance in patients with DM when the initial presentation is only muscle weakness, to differentiate it from other idiopathic inflammatory myopathies (IIMs).[6] Periungual telangiectasias are more common in patients with pulmonary involvement, Raynaud's phenomenon and arthritis and hence, of prognostic value.[5,7]

The cuticles are thick, rough, ragged (moth-eaten appearance) (Figs 15 and 16), and often dystrophic with microvascular hemorrhage.[7]

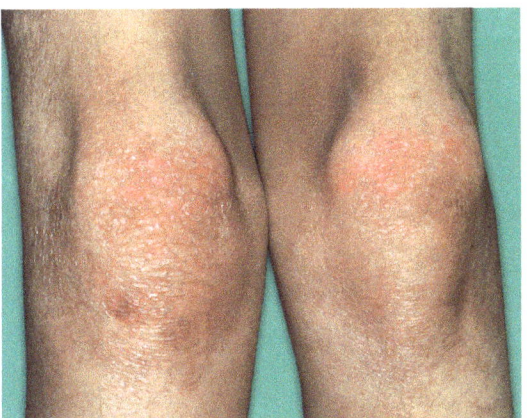

FIGURE 10: Gottron sign over knees.

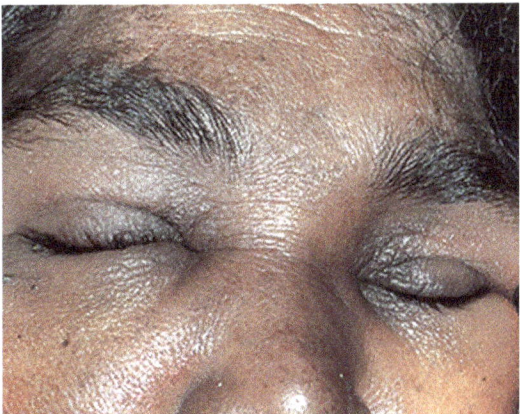

FIGURE 12: Heliotrope rash with prominent periorbital edema and mild erythema.

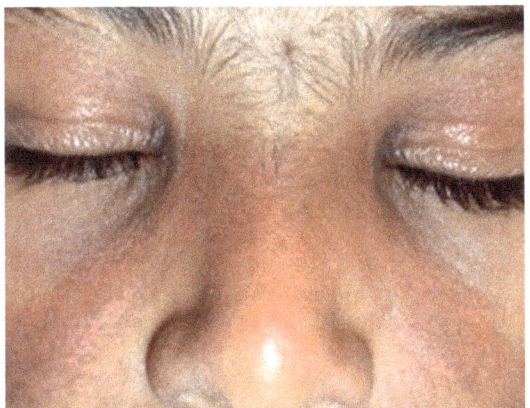

FIGURE 11: Edema of heliotrope rash and violaceous hue involving the medial canthus of eyes, lateral sides of root of nose and spreading to cheeks.

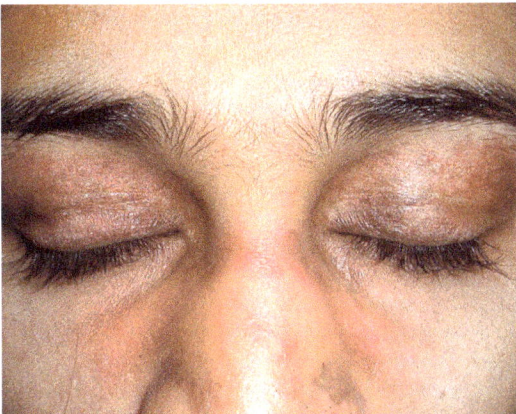

FIGURE 13: Subsiding heliotrope rash in a patient with dermatomyositis in remission.
Courtesy: Dr BS Ankad, SN Medical College, Bagalkot, Karnataka

Symmetric, Macular Erythema of Dorsa of Hands

There may be diffuse erythema of the bilateral dorsa of the hands. It may be linear or streaky distributed along the dorsa of fingers and extensor tendons on the back of hands.[5,7] In darker races, there may be linear hyperpigmentation representing this feature.[10]

Mechanics' Hands

There is hyperkeratotic, hyperpigmented fissuring on the palmar surface of the ulnar side of thumb and radial sides of index and middle fingers (Fig. 17).[5] The lesions are bilaterally symmetrical, nonpruritic and may simulate the dirty hands of laborers. Index finger is most commonly involved.[5] This feature may be an indicator of the presence of antisynthetase antibodies in the affected patient.[5,7]

Poikiloderma Atrophicans Vasculare

There are stages of evolution; the initial confluent macular violaceous erythema (CMVE) is often pruritic and distribution-wise designated as follows:
- Shawl sign: Confluent macular violaceous erythema distributed over upper back, neck, deltoid region, extensor aspects of arms and forearms, extending up to dorsa of hands and fingers simulating a shawl draped over body (Figs 18 and 19)

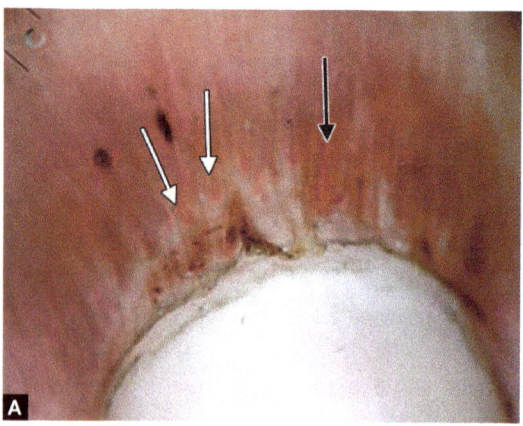
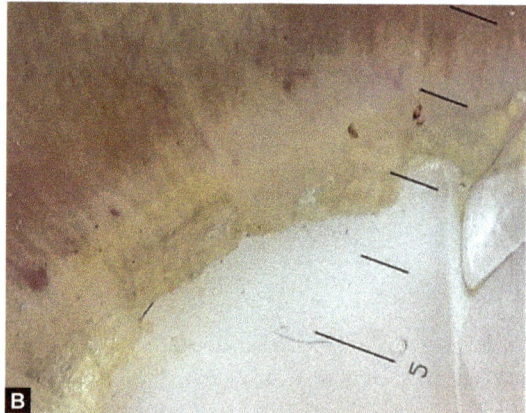

FIGURE 14: A, Dermoscopic findings of nail-fold erythema, telangiectasias, capillary loops (white arrow) and hemorrhage (black arrow); **B,** Dermoscopic finding of ragged cuticle (moth-eaten appearance) and periungual capillary dropout.
Courtesy: Dr BS Ankad, SN Medical College, Bagalkot, Karnataka.

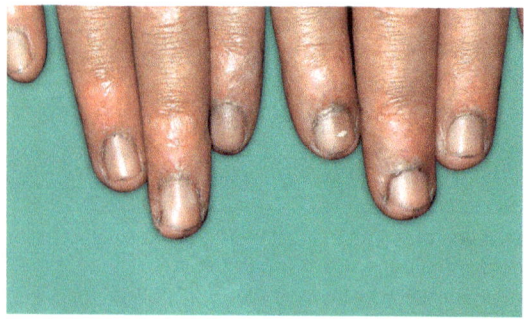

FIGURE 15: Periungual telangiectasia visible with naked eyes.

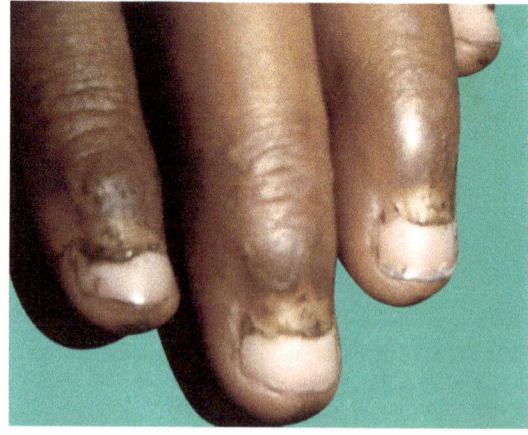

FIGURE 16: Thick, ragged cuticles in juvenile dermatomyositis.

- V sign: Confluent macular violaceous erythema distributed over front of the neck (Fig. 20)
- Holster sign: Confluent macular violaceous erythema distributed over the lateral aspect of buttocks and upper, outer thighs (Fig. 21).

With disease progression, the erythema is replaced by poikiloderma involving large body areas over neck, upper trunk, and proximal extremities symmetrically (Fig. 22). The poikilodermatous areas are indurated due to mucinous infiltration in the dermis. Diffuse scaling of these areas may follow, resulting in erythroderma and the ultimate healing is with patchy pigmentary changes (Fig. 23). Some patients may develop deep, irregular, retiform ulcers over the

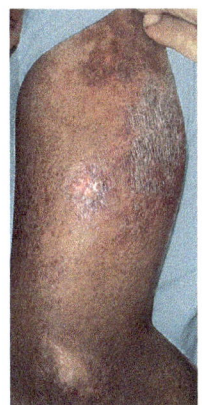

FIGURE 19: Shawl sign—confluent macular violaceous erythema over extensor of arm.

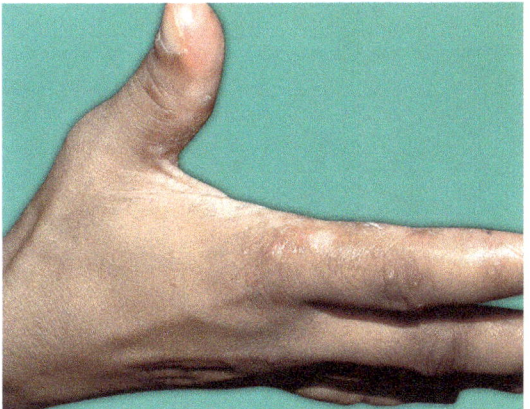

FIGURE 17: Mechanics hand.
Courtesy: Dr Neena Khanna, Professor, Department of Dermatology, All India Institute of Medical Sciences, New Delhi

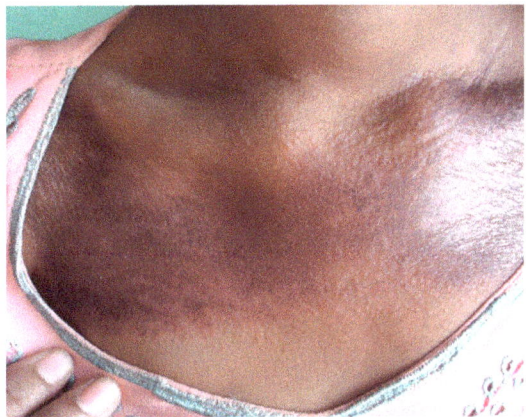

FIGURE 20: "V" sign in a case of dermatomyositis.

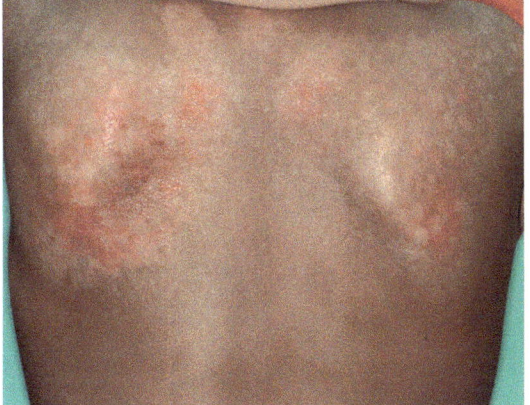

FIGURE 18: Shawl sign—confluent macular violaceous erythema over back.

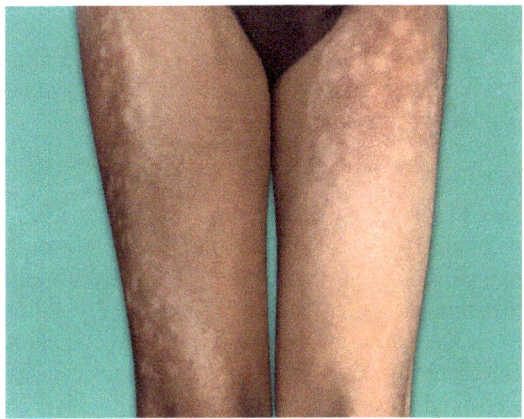

FIGURE 21: Holster sign.

Skin in Rheumatologic Disease

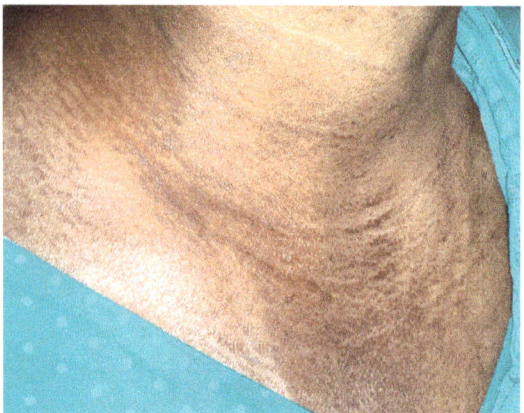

FIGURE 22: Poikiloderma over neck and trunk.
Courtesy: Professor Rama Murthy, Katuri Medical College, Andhra Pradesh.

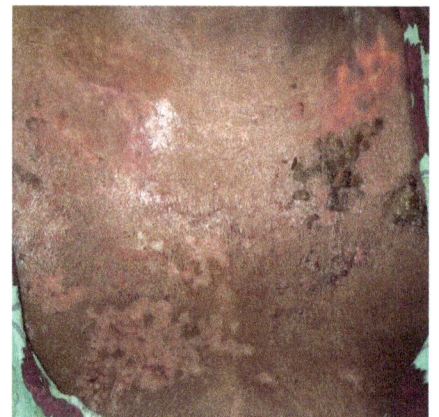

FIGURE 24: Retiform ulcers over poikilodermatous areas seen in severe dermatomyositis.

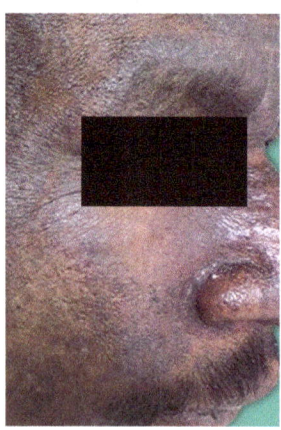

FIGURE 23: Patchy pigmentary changes of healed confluent macular violaceous erythema.

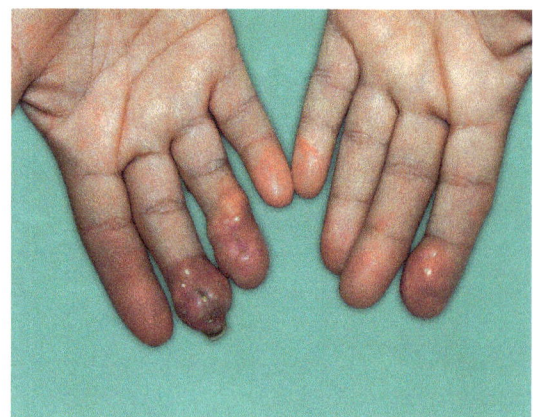

FIGURE 25: Severe periungual calcinosis cutis around finger joints.

poikilodermatous areas related to underlying vasculopathy (Fig. 24). These ulcers are indicative of poor prognosis.

Calcinosis Cutis

This is a common finding in JDM (30–70%), as compared to adults (10%).[7,8] Pressure points like elbows, knees, and buttocks are commonly involved as well as traumatized areas (Figs 25 to 27). Most common time of onset of calcinosis is 1–3 years, but may be seen at the disease-onset as well as after a span of 20 years.

The other common and uncommon cutaneous features of DM are presented in table 5.

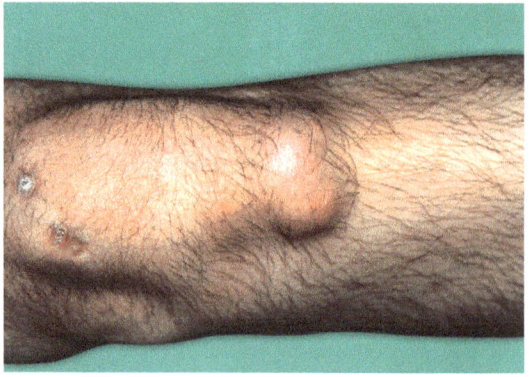

FIGURE 26: Severe cutaneous calcinosis around knee joint in an adult patient with dermatomyositis.

Dermatomyositis

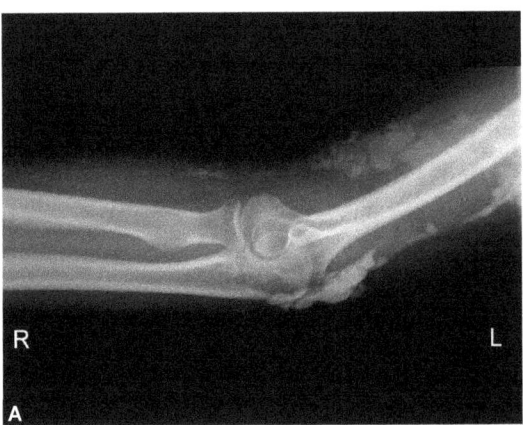
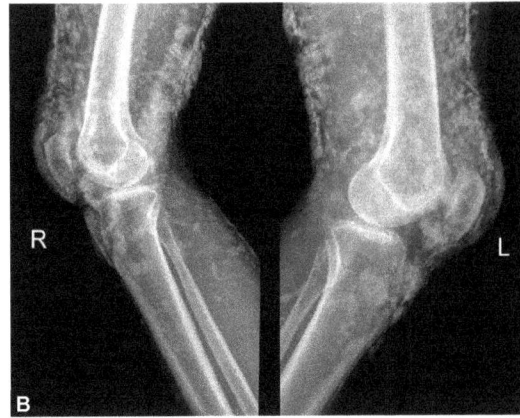

FIGURE 27: X-ray showing calcinosis around elbow and knee joints.

Table 5: Other cutaneous features of dermatomyositis[5-7,10]	
Cutaneous feature	**Comment**
Photosensitivity	Found in one-third patients
Malignant erythema/ malignancy suffusion	Diffuse, deep-red erythema appearing over preexisting cutaneous eruption, in malignancy-associated dermatomyositis (Fig. 2)
Ulcer	Usually vasculitic, but may be multifactorial. Underlying panniculitis may result in ulcer. Deep penetrating cutaneous ulcers may be indicative of pulmonary involvement
Tender nodules	Present over buttocks and adjacent thighs, indicative of panniculitis. These ulcerate easily and calcinosis may be a sequelae
Livedo reticularis	May be associated with ulceration
Flagellate erythema	Streaky, violaceous, edematous, pruritic lesions on trunk
Tense vesiculobullous lesions	Occurs particularly at the sites of intense cutaneous inflammation. May be seen in malignancy associated dermatomyositis
Raynaud's phenomenon	10% of adult patients, very rare in juvenile dermatomyositis
Scalp involvement (red, scaly scalp)	A common feature; erythema, atrophy and diffuse nonscarring alopecia may occur. Highly pruritic/burning sensation. Easily misdiagnosed as scalp psoriasis/ seborrhoeic dermatitis/lupus erythematosus
Follicular hyperkeratosis	–
Gingival telangiectasia	–
Acquired ichthyosis, edema of hands and forearms	–
Nasal septal perforation	–

Muscle Involvement

The extent of muscle involvement is unrelated to that of skin involvement and vice versa. The initial presentations are fatigue, weakness, and muscle ache. Gradually, symmetrical proximal limb muscle (triceps and quadriceps) weakness appear, as evident by difficulties in performing daily activities (Table 6). The involved muscles are tender in the active stage and later wasting and contracture is evident, especially in children.

Muscle involvement may be rapidly progressive resulting in severe weakness in few weeks. Calcification of the shoulder and hip-girdle muscles may occur and is more common in children (50%) as compared to adults (15%).[11] Calcified muscles show severe functional impairment in due course.

Functional assessment of involved proximal group of muscles can be undertaken by manual muscle testing (MMT) using 5-point scale (Medical Research Council).[11] However, other scoring systems are currently available (10-point scale) which in addition help to assess the ability to perform tasks.[11]

Systemic Involvement[5,7]

Some patients with DM may develop other systemic involvement. Pulmonary and joint involvements are the most common.

Constitutional Symptoms

Fever and malaise accompany muscle pain and occur early during illness.

Pulmonary

The predominant pulmonary involvement is interstitial pneumonitis (5-40%),[7] manifested by nonproductive cough, exertional dyspnea, and bibasilar crepitations. The presentation may be acute or insidious. There are other causes of pneumonia in these patients, like opportunistic infection, drug-induced (treatment with methotrexate), and aspiration due to reflux.

Gastrointestinal

Esophageal (50%) and intestinal diverticulosis may result due to weakness of the smooth muscles of the wall. Widespread vasculopathy in JDM may give rise to infarction and perforation of colonic wall.

Cardiovascular

Myocardial involvement occurs in one-third of the patients; myocarditis, followed by fibrosis and conduction defect is the sequelae. Pericarditis and effusion may occur.

Ocular

Retinitis may occur rarely as evident by ophthalmoscopic finding of fluffy exudates around the papillae and along the course of the veins.[7]

Renal

Renal involvement is very rare unlike systemic lupus erythematosus and scleroderma, but may occur due to acute, massive muscle injury resulting in myoglobinuria.[7]

Skeletal

Mild nonerosive symmetric arthritis may accompany the muscle disease and it is more common in JDM (20-65%). Knees, elbows, wrists, and fingers are commonly involved and patients may experience morning stiffness, simulating rheumatoid arthritis. Patients presenting with arthritis usually have pulmonary involvement. Joint effusions and recurrent bursitis around large joints (shoulder and hip) may occur.[7]

Table 6: Various functional impairments in patients with dematomyositis and the muscles involved[5-7]

Functional impairment	Group of muscles involved
Difficulty in climbing stairs. Inability to rise to feet from sitting/squatting position	Hip-girdle muscles
Difficulty in combing hair. Inability to bring down objects kept in a high rack	Shoulder-girdle muscles
Drooping of neck	Extensors of neck
Dysphagia	Pharyngeal and esophageal (upper one-third) muscles
Reflux	Upper and mid-esophageal muscles
Difficulty in speech	Muscles of tongue
Hoarseness of voice	Laryngopharyngeal muscles
Difficulty in respiration	Intercostal and diaphragmatic muscles

Dermatomyositis

SPECIFIC SUBCATEGORIES OF DERMATOMYOSITIS

Juvenile Dermatomyositis

Juvenile dermatomyositis is a special category, pathologically characterized by intense vasculopathy of skin, muscle, and various other organs. Patients up to 18 years of age are designated as JDM (Fig. 28). These patients exhibit a double-peak in disease occurrence; in children below 4 years (25%) and again at 7 years onwards. However, the more common age of onset is between 7–8 years. The girl to boy ratio in JDM varies from 2–5:1 in various Western countries.

Specific HLA associations like *-B8* (white races), *-DRB1*0301, DQA1*0501,* and *DQA1*0301* are more common in JDM.[11] A rapidly progressive disease course has been encountered in 50% cases. Except a few, skin lesions are mostly similar to adult-onset DM (Figs 29 and 30), but systemic involvement is more frequent. Overall, the disease severity appears to be higher in JDM compared to adult disease because of the vasculopathic organ damage and higher occurrence of calcinosis (Fig. 31). Clinical features commoner in JDM as compared to adult-onset DM have been presented in table 7.

One quarter of JDM may progress to overlap syndromes. An overlap of JDM and scleroderma has been designated as *sclerodermatomyositis*. This condition is characterized by cutaneous features of both the conditions (Fig. 32) along

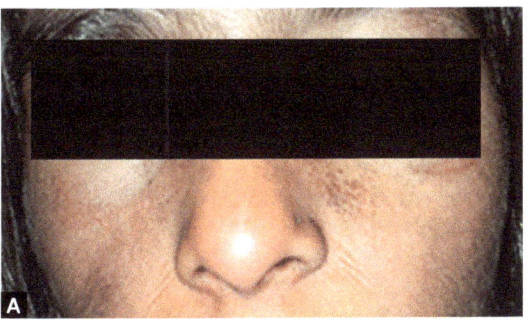
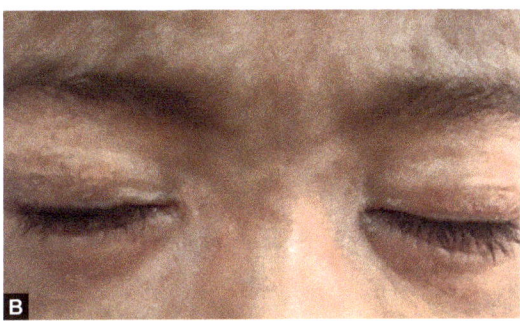

FIGURE 28: Juvenile dermatomyositis.

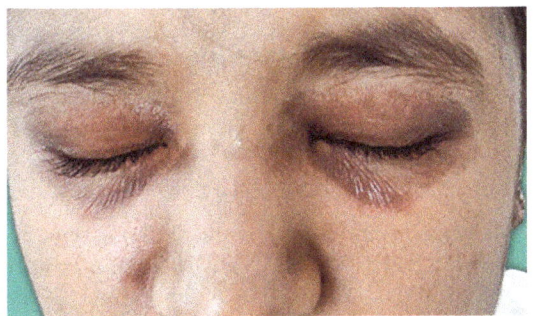

FIGURE 29: Heliotrope rash in a case of juvenile dermatomyositis.
Courtesy: Dr BS Ankad, SN Medical College, Bagalkot, Karnataka.

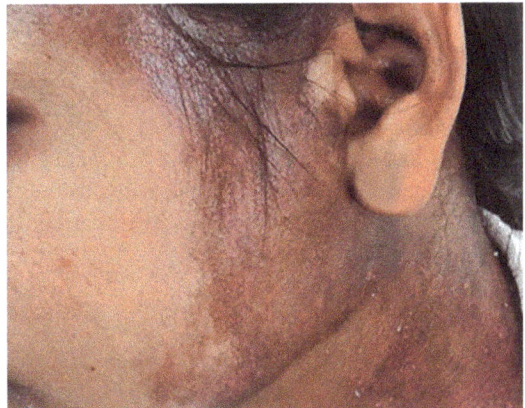

FIGURE 30: Confluent macular violaceous erythema in a case of juvenile dermatomyositis.
Courtesy: Dr BS Ankad, SN Medical College, Bagalkot, Karnataka.

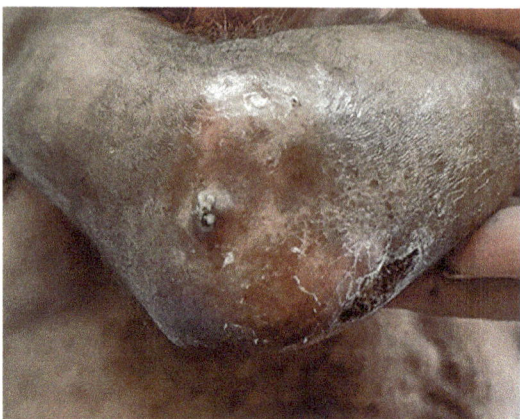

FIGURE 31: Calcinosis cutis and ulceration over elbow in juvenile dermatomyositis patient.

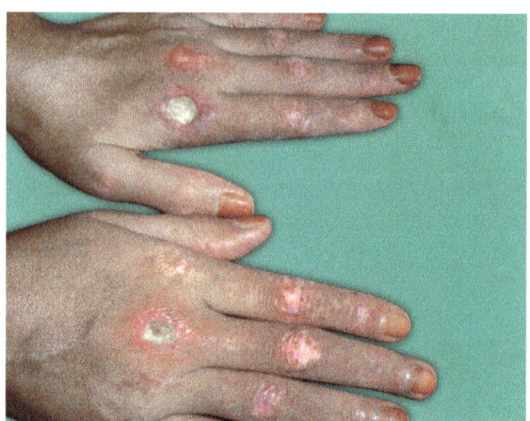

FIGURE 32: Gottron sign and vasculopathic skin ulcer over the knuckles in a case of sclerodermatomyositis.

Table 7: Clinical features commoner in juvenile dermatomyositis[11-13]

Organ involved	Clinical features more common in juvenile dermatomyositis
Skin	• Calcinosis cutis (two-third cases) • Hypertrichosis • Partial lipoatrophy • Cutaneous small vessel vasculitis • Ulcers (vasculitic)
Constitutional	• Low-grade fever is common
Joint	• Symmetric arthritis with joint contracture (<5% cases)
Gastrointestinal	• Acute abdomen due to bowel infarction and perforation
Others	• Calcification of muscles and areas of panniculitis

with myositis. The clinical features of DM are transient and there is gradual predominance of features of scleroderma. Systemic involvement is less frequent and the patients are treatment-responsive with a better prognosis.

Clinically Amyopathic Dermatomyositis

Cutaneous manifestations of DM often precede the myositis which may develop 3-6 months later. A subset of patients with DM may never develop muscle disease or it is minor or transient. This subset, also known as dermatomyositis siné myositis has been recognized as the entity, clinically amyopathic DM (Pearson, 1979). From different series of such patients, three variants can be distinguished (Sontheimer, 1991) as follows:[14]

1. Type 1: Only cutaneous features for 24 months or more
2. Type 2: Cutaneous features + subjective muscle pain and weakness, but absent laboratory evidence of muscle disease
3. Type 3: Cutaneous features + abnormal laboratory tests, but no muscle involvement demonstrable clinically.

Type 2 and 3 are categorized as hypomyopathic DM in recent time.

The occurrence is relatively higher among Asian population as compared to Europe and America.[5] Cutaneous manifestations are similar to the classic disease. Other systemic involvement may occur. Interstitial lung disease has been recorded in 13% of these patients, especially among Japanese population.[5] However, these patients are usually antisynthetase antibody negative and prone for high mortality.[5]

Malignancy-associated Dermatomyositis

This is encountered in people above 45 years of age, more so in the elderly, and such associations vary from less than 10% to more than 50%.[7] Ovarian carcinoma in females and gastric carcinoma and lymphoma in males are the most common underlying malignancies.[7] The cutaneous features are same as that of adult DM and the amyopathic variant may also have such association. The survival rate of malignancy-associated DM is lower than the other variants, probably related to the underlying tumor.

COMPLICATIONS

Complications are not very common in patients with DM, but relatively more common in JDM.

Various probable complications of DM have been listed in table 8.

DIAGNOSIS

Diagnostic criteria for DM, as proposed by Bohan and Peter (1976), are widely used (Box 1), though it is older considering the availability of magnetic resonance imaging of muscles and HLA assays at present. Both sensitivity and specificity of this criteria is approximately 90%.[6]

The pitfall of these criteria is that, diagnosis of amyopathic dermatomyositis is at a stake when this is used.[14] For these patients cutaneous features are given diagnostic importance; presence of 1–2 pathognomonic signs, with one or more characteristic sign and a suggestive skin histopathology (hematoxylin-eosin stained) are helpful in diagnosis of amyopathic dermatomyositis.[14] For JDM, the criteria remain same.

Various investigations are in use to evaluate a case of DM. These include laboratory tests like muscle enzymes, detection of autoantibodies, histopathology of skin and muscles, electromyography, and imaging of muscles.

Muscle Enzymes

Elevated level of creatine phosphokinase (CPK), the MM (muscle) isoenzyme, is the most important test for assessing extent of muscle involvement.[7] This may be high even prior to the development of muscle weakness. Serum aldolase (subtype A) is less sensitive and specific indicator of muscle damage as compared to CPK. Other muscle-related enzymes are glutamic oxaloacetic transaminase (GOT) and lactate dehydrogenase (LDH, isoenzymes 4 and 5), but specificity of these enzymes is further low. However, estimation of these enzymes should be considered to evaluate and follow up the patients with JDM, where a high CPK level is found in only two-third of the patients.[12]

In patients with features of active muscle disease but normal level of these enzymes, serial 24-hour urinary creatine excretion should be assessed to detect muscle damage.[7]

There may be spurious rise of muscle enzymes following strenuous exercise, intramuscular injection, insertion of electromyographic needle, or muscle biopsy.[7] Certain drugs and associated hypothyroidism may give rise to high CPK level.[5] Extra caution should be undertaken to rule out such factors before advising estimation of muscle enzymes.

Autoantibodies

The list of autoantibodies found in patients with DM and their frequency of occurrence has already

Table 8: Complications of dermatomyositis[5, 7]	
Respiratory	• Pulmonary hypertension and cor pulmonale from restrictive or interstitial lung disease • Respiratory failure resulting from muscle weakness • Aspiration pneumonia due to gastroesophageal reflux
Gastrointestinal	• Diverticular perforation, pneumatosis intestinalis and pneumoperitoneum • Colonic perforation in juvenile dermatomyositis
Cardiovascular	• Heart failure
Esophageal (dysphagia)	• Malnourishment in long-term and neglected cases
Ocular	• Visual loss (rare)
Infections	• Opportunistic pulmonary infection

Box 1: Bohan and Peter (1975) criteria for diagnosis of dermatomyositis

- Progressive symmetrical proximal muscle weakness
- Features of inflammatory myopathy in muscle biopsy
- Raised serum muscle enzymes
- Myopathic pattern in electromyography
- Typical cutaneous lesions of dermatomyositis

Note: Presence of criteria 5 is essential for diagnosis of dermatomyositis
   Definite diagnosis: Presence of 4 criteria
   Probable diagnosis: Presence of 3 criteria

been presented in Table 3. The specificity of these autoantibodies in diagnosing DM is variable. Presence of some of these autoantibodies is indicator of specific clinical features in patients with DM and is of prognostic value (Table 9).

Table 9: Clinical and prognostic significance of various autoantibodies in dermatomyositis[1,5,7,13]	
Autoantibodies	Clinical significance
Jo-1	• Antisynthetase syndrome* • Mechanics' hands • Carpal tunnel syndrome • Polymyositis
PL-7, PL-12, OJ, EJ	• Antisynthetase syndrome*
Signal recognition particle (SRP)	• Acute onset and fulminant course • Cardiac involvement • Very severe polymyositis • High creatine phosphokinase level
Mi-2	• Shawl sign and "V" sign • Nail-fold cuticular overgrowth • Carpal tunnel syndrome • Usually treatment-responsive
ANA	• Positivity in 80% cases of amyopathic dermatomyositis
Anti-p155	• "V" sign in adult-onset dermatomyositis • Nail-fold cuticular overgrowth • Adults, may be underlying carcinoma
Anti-U2 RNP	• Overlap with scleroderma
Anti-Ro, Anti-U1RNP	• Overlap syndromes
Anti-Ku	• Overlap with scleroderma • Raynaud's disease frequent • Arthralgia • Esophageal reflux
PM-Scl	• Overlap with scleroderma • Interstitial lung disease; may appear before detection of lung disease; prognostic importance • Arthritis in many cases • Raynaud's phenomenon • Calcinosis

*Antisynthetase syndrome: Combination of fever, interstitial pneumonia, polyarthritis and Raynaud's phenomenon. It is only partially responsive to treatment.

Usually a patient with DM expresses only one type of myositis-specific autoantibodies (MSA). Prevalence of these autoantibodies is also highly variable and hence, routine estimation of these during workup of a patient is of less diagnostic importance. This is more so for JDM, as very few children show presence of MSA or myositis-associated autoantibodies (MAA).[12] Recently, anti-p155 has been found to occur in approximately 30% cases of JDM, but the significance of its routine assessment is unclear. Usually appearance of MSA precedes the onset of myositis.

Histopathology

The histopathological features of both skin and muscle may be subtle and inconclusive (for detail, refer to Chapter 3).

Skin Biopsy

A classic skin lesion of DM may be biopsied and sent for histopathological examination and direct immunofluorescence study. The prominent histopathological features in acute stage are diffuse dermal edema and perivascular mixed-cellular infiltrate.[7] In Gottron's papules or other scaly lesions, epidermal changes like hyperkeratosis, acanthosis, and papillomatosis are observed. In skin lesions of some duration, thickening, homogenization, and sclerosis of dermal collagen and dermal mucin deposition are present. Dermal mucin deposition in the background of suggestive clinical features is indicative of DM, and this finding helps in differentiation from lesions of LE.[7] Direct immunofluorescence study reveals deposition of immunoglobulin G, immunoglobulin M, and C3 in half of the cases.[7]

Muscle Biopsy

Biopsy should be undertaken from a clinically weak and/or tender muscle. In absence of such features, ideally magnetic resonance imaging (MRI)-guided muscle biopsy should be undertaken as the involvement is highly focal. The usual histopathological features (Fig. 33) in affected muscles are as follows:[7]
• Degeneration and regeneration of muscle fibers; loss of transverse striations and hyalinization in early stage. In later stage, fragmentation and granular or vacuolar degeneration

Dermatomyositis

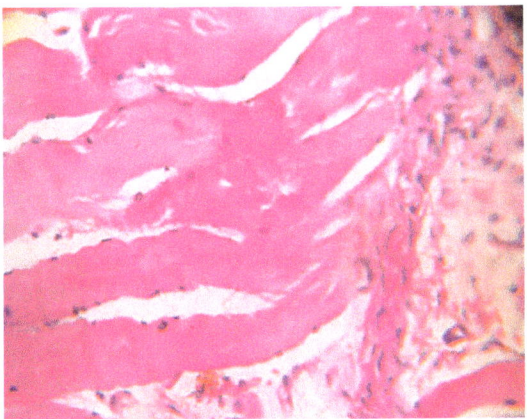

FIGURE 33: Histopathology of muscle (H&E stain, 40x) showing degeneration of muscle fibers with interstitial edema and inflammatory cells.

of the muscle fibers with basophilic staining is seen
- Perifascicular atrophy
- Perivascular lymphohistiocytic infiltrate
- Capillary injury; intense vasculopathy, as evidenced by eosinophilic intimal hyperplasia, fibrinous occlusion of vascular lumen and infarction may be seen in JDM
- Calcification of necrosed muscle may be observed.

Electromyography

The electromyography (EMG) findings from myopathic muscle fibers are as follows:[7]
- Increased insertional activity
- Increased spontaneous activity
- Myopathic pattern of motor-unit action potential
- Myopathic recruitment pattern.

In spite of utmost care taken to hit the affected muscle by biopsy or EMG, the clinician should be prepared to receive a normal report of muscle biopsy and/or normal EMG reading, as muscle involvement is extremely patchy.

Muscle Imaging

At present, MRI scan is the ultimate way to detect evidence of muscle inflammation. The advantages of this technique are:
- It is noninvasive
- Can be used for children
- Helps to perform muscle biopsy and EMG
- Usually considered as highly sensitive to detect muscle involvement.

Patchy areas of muscle inflammation can be detected with MRI easily.

Other imaging modalities to detect myopathy are power Doppler, gray-scale ultrasonography, and phosphorus-31-spectroscopy, but these are not as useful as MRI.[5,7]

Esophageal Screening

Video-fluoroscopic swallowing study helps to assess esophageal involvement and is of particular importance in JDM, as small children may not be able to express the swallowing difficulty.[13]

Other Investigations

All elderly patients presented with DM must be screened thoroughly for underlying malignancy both clinically and radiologically. In women, cervical pap smear should be undertaken.

PROGNOSIS, COURSE, AND SEQUELAE

Various prognostic factors in DM have been listed in table 10.

Table 10: Prognostic factors in dermatomyositis[5,7]

Poor prognostic factors	Good prognostic factor
- Underlying malignancy - Old age - Progressive muscle disease - Widespread cutaneous involvement of trunk - Deep, necrotic skin ulcers - Acute-onset interstitial lung disease - Dysphagia - Delay in initial diagnosis - Delay in starting therapy (>24 months) - Normal creatine phosphokinase level (pulmonary involvement/ underlying malignancy)	Presence of calcinosis

Course of DM is variable but prognosis is better as compared to other IIMs. Four distinct disease courses for DM have been recognized (Table 11). Equal proportions of patients are responsive and resistant to therapy and mortality is expected in 25% of the patients. Pulmonary infection, heart failure, metastatic underlying malignancy, and side effects of therapy are the common causes of death in patients with DM. In fulminant cases, death may occur by first year, but in others the disease activity settles down (burnt-out) over many years.

Episodes of recurrence may occur. In pregnant women, disease exacerbation is more common (50%) than remission (20%). In malignancy-associated cases, DM may resolve with effective treatment of the underlying tumor. Juvenile dermatomyositis has a better outcome in terms of disease remission and many patients may achieve it spontaneously.

Pigmentary changes and mild muscle weakness are the usual sequelae. Premature delivery and fetal loss (50%) are the consequences during pregnancy. Patients with JDM are left with crippling joint contracture and calcinosis.

DIFFERENTIAL DIAGNOSIS

As there is a variety of signs and symptoms in patients with DM, these can be mistaken with various other conditions at the initial period of illness. Clinical feature-wise differential diagnosis of DM has been presented in table 12.

Table 11: Disease course in dermatomyositis[11]	
Fulminant disease	Life-threatening events resulting in death
Monophasic	Single episode of the disease; patient is in clinical remission thereafter and achieve normalcy of laboratory parameters
Polycyclic (relapse–remission)	More than one episodes and patient is in remission in between episodes
Chronic (progressive)	The disease is only partially responsive to therapy progressive and failure to achieve remission after 24 months of diagnosis.

Note:
Remission: Stable improvement/normalization of muscle strength, normal creatine phosphokinase and/or lactate dehydrogenase level and disappearance of skin lesions.
Relapse: Reappearance of signs and symptoms of dermatomyositis after a remission of 6 months or more.

Table 12: Differential diagnosis of dermatomyositis[5-7,10]	
Clinical feature	**Differential diagnosis**
Photosensitivity and heliotrope rash	Systemic lupus erythematosus
	The rash is erythematous rather than violaceous, and in malar distribution unlike the periorbital location in dermatomyositis. Lesions are nonpruritic. The periorbital edema of heliotrope rash may simulate angioedema
Gottron's papules	Systemic lupus erythematosus
	The lesions of systemic lupus erythematosus usually spare the dorsal aspects of metacarpophalangeal and interphalangeal joints, where the Gottron's papules of dermatomyositis are located
Calcinosis cutis + nail-fold capillary changes	Scleroderma
	Location of calcinosis cutis is mostly periungual
Poikiloderma atrophicans vasculare + scaling + pruritus	Cutaneous T cell lymphoma; other features of dermatomyositis are absent
Violaceous hue of skin lesions + Wickham's striae-like appearance on the surface of older lesions + pruritus	Lichen planus
Scaling of scalp and scaly patch over elbows, knees, etc.	Psoriasis
Scaly, pruritic skin lesions	Atopic dermatitis (especially in juvenile dermatomyositis)
Muscle pain + periorbital edema	Trichinosis
	In endemic areas, trichinosis may present with these features but other features of dermatomyositis are absent.

MANAGEMENT

Assessment of Disease Severity[11]

Initial and thereafter follow up assessment of disease severity is helpful in monitoring therapeutic dosages. Various cutaneous disease assessment tools are available. These are Dermatomyositis Skin Severity Index and Cutaneous Dermatomyositis Disease Area and Severity Index (CDASH); the latter can be used for both adult and juvenile patients. The CDASI assesses the parameters like erythema, thickness, scaling, excoriation, and ulceration over 16 body areas in addition to Gottron's lesions, periungual lesions, and alopecia. The muscle involvement can be assessed clinically by MMT using 5-point or 10-point scale.

Supportive Measures[15]

Patients with DM must adopt photoprotection by physical methods and regular use of broad-spectrum sunscreens. During acute stage, bed rest and relatively sedentary lifestyle is suggested as these patients are unable to carry out daily activities due to muscle pain and weakness. Strenuous exercise may damage the compromised muscles further and affected patients are counseled to avoid such activities even during remission. Children with JDM are prone for joint contracture, and active and passive physiotherapy must be performed routinely. In case of malignancy-associated DM, underlying condition must be treated. If there is history of any drug intake, which may precipitate DM, it must be stopped. Psychological support of the patient and family is important as the disease course is long-term and may be relapsing.

The primary aims of treating a case of DM is to reduce morbidity and prevention of disfiguring cutaneous (calcinosis cutis and ulceration) and life-threatening systemic complications.[23] Moreover, early institution of therapy prevents acute muscle damage, muscle atrophy, and contracture in the long run and disease relapse. Various therapeutic modalities used in DM have been discussed below:

- Topical therapy: Topical steroid and calcineurin inhibitors are useful in treating localized, pruritic skin lesions in children and adults
- Systemic therapy
  - Corticosteroids: The first line of therapeutic intervention used for any form of DM is systemic corticosteroid. Oral prednisolone is started at a dose of 1–2 mg/kg body weight (initially as high as 60 mg/day), and this dose is maintained till serum CPK level is normalized. Thereafter, it is tapered slowly over several months or 1–2 years. During this maintenance period, a dose of 5–15 mg/day is used and the tapering must be done very slowly. In case, there is return of symptoms while tapering prednisolone, the previous effective dose should be resumed promptly.

    The clinician must take care of such long-term corticosteroid therapy-related side effects and morbidity. Dosage monitoring for systemic steroids should be guided by clinical improvement and reduction of initially raised muscle enzymes.

    Intravenous pulse of methyl prednisolone (1 g for 3 consecutive days) may be used with or without immunosuppressive drugs in severe cases or during acute flare-up.[16] The clinician may decide to switch over to intravenous methyl prednisolone pulse from oral prednisolone, if the patient's CPK level does not come down satisfactorily over time. In patients with JDM, judicious corticosteroid therapy decreases the risk of calcinosis.[17] Oral steroid is the treatment of choice for pregnant women.

    Systemic corticosteroids are considered ineffective if after 3 months of treatment, the patient continues to have muscle weakness or there is disease flare-up with reduction of dosage.
  - Immunosuppressive therapy: Inability to achieve adequate response with appropriate dose of systemic steroid over sufficient period of time or presence of any complications even earlier, or appearance of significant corticosteroid-related side effects are the indications for addition of immunosuppressive therapy.

    Various immunosuppressive drugs used in DM are methotrexate, cyclophosphamide[18] and azathioprine. These drugs are used as adjunct to corticosteroid therapy. Of these, methotrexate and cyclophosphamide are the most widely used drugs. These drugs are almost always used in conjunction with systemic steroid. Various regimens of combination therapy of corticosteroids and immunosuppressive drugs in adults and JDM are available.[18]

- Other adjunctive therapies: Cyclosporine, oral tacrolimus, mycophenolate mofetil, and hydroxychloroquine have been used in patients not responding to the combination of corticosteroid and immunosuppressive drug.

Key points about the use of various adjunctive therapies in patients with DM have been presented in table 13.

- Plasmapheresis: Before the advent of immunosuppressive drugs, plasmapheresis was a therapeutic modality for severe JDM with evidence of improvement; but this is ineffective in adult disease
- Intravenous immunoglobulin (IVIg): Severe disease refractory to treatment with corticosteroid and immunosuppressive drugs may respond to IVIg. The dosage is 1 mg/kg/day for consecutive 2 days/month for 4-6 months. Treatment with IVIg improves skin lesions as well as myositis. It can also be used at the onset of the disease.[17,19] and is associated with less side effects
- Biological therapy: Anti-TNF agent etanercept, infliximab, and the B cell

Table 13: Use of adjunctive therapy in patients with dermatomyositis[7,15,19]				
Drugs	Dosage	Immediate effect	Long-term effect	Comments
Methotrexate (MTX)	• Low dose: 7.5-15 mg, divided dosage/week • High dosage therapy (0.5-1 mg/kg/week), oral/subcutaneous dose	Rapid control of active disease	Prevention of calcinosis	• More effective in patients with predominant cutaneous involvement • Addition of MTX early during disease allows faster tapering of corticosteroids
Cyclophosphamide	• 1-2 mg/kg/day, orally • Pulse dosage (500-1,000 mg/m²/dose) 6-7 monthly pulses, followed by quarterly pulses till disease is stabilized[18]	Improvement of ulceration, severe muscle weakness, interstitial pneumonitis, gastrointestinal hemorrhage	Help in achieving disease stability	• Good therapeutic agent for severe and complicated cases
Azathioprine	• Oral, 1.5-3 mg/kg/day	–	–	–
Mycophenolate mofetil	• 1-3 g/day	–	–	• Effective in recalcitrant disease and pulmonary complications
Cyclosporine	• Oral, 5 mg/kg/day	–	–	• Useful for treating severe pulmonary complications • Easy to use-drug in juvenile dermatomyositis
Hydroxychloroquine	• Oral, 5-6 mg/kg/day, two divided doses	Both skin lesions and muscle disease may respond	–	• Good steroid-sparing agent for milder disease and juvenile dermatomyositis • Rarely exacerbation of skin lesions may occur

targeted therapy rituximab are the newer addition in the list of therapeutic agents for both adult DM and JDM. Of these, infliximab and rituximab have been proved to be successful in the management of cases refractory to conventional treatment.[8] Biological therapies are useful in ameliorating both cutaneous and muscle symptoms, reduce disease activity and help to achieve remission. However, relapse rate is similar to other therapeutic modalities. At present, there are no definite guidelines for treating DM with biologicals as most of the information regarding their effectiveness is based on observations from small series of patients[20]

- Other therapies: Autologous stem cell therapy has been tried in children and adults with DM (and other IIMs), who failed to respond to even rituximab therapy; it has been found to be effective in reducing disease activity and requirements for corticosteroid and immunosuppressive therapy.[21]

Antihistamines are to be prescribed in patients with significant pruritus.

Calcium and vitamin D supplementation is necessary as patients with DM are prone to develop osteopenia resulting from the disease process (related to restricted mobility), as well as due to prolonged corticosteroid use.

Calcinosis, a complication of especially JDM, has been treated with various agents like diltiazem, aluminum hydroxide, bisphosphonates, colchicine, etc.[17] Individual lesion of calcinosis cutis may be incised and drained when painful or restricts mobility.[22]

MONITORING A PATIENT WITH DERMATOMYOSITIS WHILE ON TREATMENT

While on treatment, patients with DM should regularly be assessed by physical examination of skin and muscles at regular intervals. Though nonspecific, CPK level is estimated as its fluctuations correlate with disease course and indicates treatment failure or disease flare.

> **Box 2: Distinguishing features between steroid myopathy and worsening dermatomyositis**
>
> **Clinical**
> Neck-flexor strength is preserved in steroid-induced myopathy, worsens with disease progression
>
> **Laboratory parameter**
> Serum creatine phosphokinase level is normal in steroid myopathy but increased in progressive disease (24 hours urinary creatine excretion is elevated in both the situations)
>
> **Muscle biopsy**
> Histopathology: Lack of interstitial inflammatory cells in steroid myopathy
>
> **Immunohistochemistry**
> Stained with myosin adenosine triphosphatase (mATPase): Selective involvement of type II muscle fibers in steroid myopathy, whereas in dermatomyositis both type I and type II fibers are involved
>
> **Electromyography**
> Insertional irritability, seen in dermatomyositis is lacking in steroid myopathy. Myopathic motor unit potentials are seen in steroid myopathy
>
> *Note:* Steroid-induced myopathy is reversible with tapering of dosage, but it may take about 4 months and is not a practical way to differentiate the two conditions.

If initial CPK level was normal, disease activity is detected by rise in GOT and LDH.

Some patients on long-term systemic corticosteroid therapy may experience sudden worsening of proximal muscle weakness. This may be due to disease relapse or manifestation of corticosteroid-induced proximal myopathy. The distinguishing features between these two conditions have been listed in box 2.

When MSA titer has been assessed at the disease onset, it may be repeated while the patient is on therapy, as the titers correlate with disease activity and disappear during complete remission.

CONCLUSION

Dermatomyositis is a unique disorder with distinct clinical features. Yet it may be difficult to diagnose at first visit unless skin lesions are evident and the patient presents with vague symptoms like fatigue, related to underlying myopathy. The disease course is chronic and often relapsing causing great morbidity to affected patients in terms of daily activities and quality of life. Systemic corticosteroids are the mainstay of therapy. Various adjuvant therapies are in use, but definite therapeutic regimens are not available. Supportive care plays an important role in the management of this debilitating disorder. Underlying malignancy must always be ruled out in elderly patients with DM.

REFERENCES

1. Kovacs SO, Kovacs SC. Dermatomyositis. J Am Acad Dermatol. 1998;39:899-920.
2. Bitsori M, Galanakis E. Modigliani's "fillette en bleu": a case of juvenile dermatomyositis? Int J Dermatol. 2003;42:327-9.
3. Bohan A, Peter JB. Polymyositis and dermatomyositis (first of two parts). N Eng J Med. 1975;292:344-7.
4. Sontheimer RD. Would a new name hasten the acceptance of amyopathic dermatomyositis (dermatomyositis sine myositis) as a distinctive subset within the idiopathic inflammatory dermatomyopathies spectrum of clinical illness? J Am Acad Dermatol. 2002;46:626-36.
5. Sontheimer RD, Hansen CB, Costner MI. Dermatomyositis. In: Goldsmith LA, Katz SI, Gilchrest BA, et al., editors. Fitzpatrick's dermatology in general medicine. Vol. 2. 8th ed. New York: McGraw Hill; 2012. pp. 1926-1942.
6. Jorizzo JL, Vleugels RA. Dermatomyositis. In: Bolognia JL, Jorizzo JL, Schaffer JV, editors. Dermatology. Vol. 1. 3rd ed. New York: Elsevier Saunders; 2012. pp. 631-41.
7. Goodfield MJ, Jones SK, Veale DJ. The 'Connective Tissue Diseases'. In: Burns T, Breathnach S, Cox N, et al., editors. Rook's textbook of dermatology. Vol. 3. 8th ed. Oxford: Wiley-Blackwell; 2010. pp. 51.1-51.138.
8. Chiu YE, Co DO. Juvenile Dermatomyositis: Immunopathogenesis, role of myositis-specific autoantibodies, and review of rituximab use. Pediatr Dermatol. 2011;28:357-67.
9. Shelley WB, Shelley ED. Dermatomyositis. In: Shelley WB, Shelley ED, editor. Advanced dermatologic diagnosis. Philadelphia: W.B.Saunders Company; 1992. pp. 454-56.
10. Habif TP. Connective tissue diseases. In: Habif TP, editor. Clinical dermatology. A color guide to diagnosis and therapy. 5th ed. New Delhi: Mosby Elsevier; 2010. pp. 671-709.
11. Huber AM. Juvenile dermatomyositis: Advances in pathogenesis, evaluation, and treatment. Paediatr Drugs. 2009; 11:361-74.
12. Constantin T, Ponyi A, Orbán I, et al. National registry of patients with juvenile idiopathic inflammatory myopathies in Hungary—Clinical characteristics and disease course of 44 patients with juvenile dermatomyositis. Autoimmunity. 2006;39:223-32.
13. Feldman BM, Rider LG, Reed AM, et al. Juvenile dermatomyositis and other idiopathic inflammatory myopathies of childhood. Lancet. 2008;371:2201-12.
14. Euwer RL, Sontheimer RD. Amyopathic dermatomyositis (dermatomyositis sine myositis). Presentation of six new cases and review of the literature. J Am Acad Dermatol. 1991:24:959-66.
15. Palit A, Inamadar AC. Current treatment strategies: collagen vascular diseases in children. Indian J Dermatol. 2012;57: 449-58.
16. Halbert AR. Juvenile dermatomyositis. Australas J Dermatol. 1996;37:106-8.
17. Reed AM, Lopez M. Juvenile dermatomyositis. Recognition and treatment. Paediatr Drugs 2002;4:315-321.
18. Riley P, Maillard SM, Wedderburn LR, et al. Intravenous cyclophosphamide pulse therapy in juvenile dermatomyositis: a review of efficacy and safety. Rheumatology (Oxford). 2004;43:491-6.
19. Cordeiro AC, Isenberg DA. Treatment of inflammatory myopathies. Postgrad Med J. 2006;82:417-24.
20. Levine TD. Rituximab in the treatment of dermatomyositis: an open-label pilot study. Arthritis Rheum. 2005;52:601-7.
21. Holzer U, van Royen-Kerkhof A, van der Torre P, et al. Successful autologous stem cell transplantation in two patients with juvenile dermatomyositis. Scand J Rheumatol. 2010;39:88-92.
22. Wu JJ, Metz BJ. Calcinosis cutis of juvenile dermatomyositis treated with incision and drainage. Dermatol Surg. 2008; 35:575-7.

CHAPTER 8

Systemic Sclerosis

Savita Yadav, Neetu Bhari

INTRODUCTION

The word scleroderma refers to the characteristic hardening and thickening of the skin. It is the most important characteristic feature in the patients of systemic sclerosis (SSc). The clinical manifestations of SSc range from primarily skin involvement to significant systemic involvement in which multiple organ systems can be affected. This disorder causes significant morbidity as well as mortality, and so far there is no cure for it though many new treatment options have recently evolved.

The management is symptom directed and organ specific, along with monitoring and timely intervention for the complications. With the better understanding of the disease, advent of many new drugs, and treatment modalities, the survival and quality of life of the patients has improved dramatically over last decade. In this chapter, we will review pathogenesis, clinical features, diagnostic techniques, and treatment of SSc.

EPIDEMIOLOGY

Prevalence of SSc is estimated at 266/1,000,000 in the United States, while countries like the United Kingdom (88/1,000,000) and Japan (38/1,000,000) report lower figures of the incidence.[1-3] There is a striking female predominance (sex ratio ranging between 4 and 14:1) and more common in the fourth and fifth decades of life.[4] Parameters predicting worse prognosis are male sex, black race, older age at diagnosis, internal organ involvement and elevated erythrocyte sedimentation rate.

PATHOGENESIS

The pathogenesis of SSc is complex and multifactorial and can be described as a characteristic triad of severe and progressive cutaneous and visceral fibrosis; proliferative vasculopathy; and humoral and cellular immunologic abnormalities. Three types of cells, which are thought to be responsible for the development of the clinical and pathologic manifestations of the disease, include:
1. Fbroblasts
2. Endothelial cells
3. Cells of the immune system, particularly T and B lymphocytes.

Genetic factors contribute in the disease development but environmental factors also play a significant role.

Environmental Factors

Infectious agents play a crucial part in pathogenesis of SSc. Herpes viruses, retroviruses, and human cytomegalovirus infections have been suggested as possible causative agents. Production of specific autoantibodies in SSc is said to be the result of an antigen-driven response caused by "molecular mimicry". However, there is no definitive evidence to conclude that SSc has an infectious origin.[5,6]

Organic solvent like vinyl chloride exposure increases the risk for skin thickening, the Raynaud's phenomenon, and digital ulcers. Exposure to several other environmental chemicals like pesticides, hair dyes, industrial fumes, and silica and metal dust have been associated with the development of SSc.[7]

Genetic Factors

Role of genetic factors is supported by occurrence of familial clustering of disease and the high frequency of autoimmune disorders and autoantibodies in family members of patients with SSc.

Disease expression appears to differ among different ethnic groups. African-American persons have more anti-topoisomerase I antibodies positivity and more severe visceral manifestations such as pulmonary fibrosis. In contrast, in white persons, anti-centromere antibodies and limited disease with less severe systemic manifestations are more common.[8]

Protein tyrosine phosphatase nonreceptor type 22 and signal transducers and activators of transcription-4 mutation, single nucleotide polymorphisms at codon 10 of the transforming growth factor (TGF)-β, and fibrillin are found to be associated with SSc. Anti-topoisomerase 1 antibody is most commonly associated with DPB1*1301, while anti-centromere antibody is associated with DQB1*0501 and DQB1*26 epi alleles.[9,10]

Humoral Immune System Alterations

Most of the SSc patients exhibit specific autoantibodies. Antinuclear antibodies can be seen in more than 90% of patients with SSc. Anti-Scl-70 antibodies react with deoxyribonucleic acid topoisomerase I and are seen in 30–40% of patients with the diffuse form of SSc. Anti-centromere antibodies are present in 80–90% of patients with the limited form of SSc but these antibodies are also seen in less than 10% of patients with diffuse SSc.

Other auto-antibodies include anti-ribonucleic acid polymerases I and III antibodies in patients with rapidly progressive disease and severe internal organ involvement, anti-fibrillarin antibodies in diffuse SSc patient, and anti-PM-Scl antibodies in patients with SSc who develop an inflammatory myopathy.[11]

Autoantibodies are helpful in establishing the diagnosis and predicting a probable pattern of organ involvement, severity, and disease progression but are not directly involved in the clinical manifestations of the disease.

Cellular Immune System Alteration

Chronic and persistent inflammation may be the initiating step in the pathogenesis of SSc, as cytokines and growth factors released by these inflammatory cells precipitate endothelial alteration as well as fibrosis. Systemic sclerosis patients have elevated levels of interleukin-2 in serum and abnormalities in numerous other cytokines have also been described.[12]

Transforming growth factor-β is one of the most crucial growth factor as it stimulates extracellular matrix synthesis by stimulating production of matrix protein as fibronectin. This growth factor is also known to inhibit production of protease and metalloproteinase, involved in the breakdown of extracellular matrix. Transforming growth factor-β also injures the endothelial cells by upregulating expression of major histocompatibility complex class I and II antigens and intercellular adhesion molecule-1. This growth factor induces transdifferentiation of vessel wall fibroblast into myofibroblast, resulting in vessel wall thickening and fibrosis.[13] Connective tissue growth factor is an another important growth factor involved in the process of fibrosis.[14]

Other cytokines released by inflammatory cells damage endothelial wall which exposes subendothelium to circulating platelets. These platelets adhere to subendothelium, initiate fibrin deposit and intravascular thrombus formation. Vasodilator deficiency and presence of vasoconstrictor like endothelin-1 induces vascular ischemia and maintain this vicious cycle of endothelial cell injury and fibrosis.[15]

CLASSIFICATION

On the basis of the extent of skin fibrosis, SSc is classified into limited cutaneous or diffuse cutaneous SSc (Table 1). Limited cutaneous SSc involves skin of the face, hands, and feet distal to the elbows and the knees, respectively, while diffuse form also affects the trunk.[16] Limited cutaneous SSc is also known as CREST (Calcinosis Cutis, Raynaud's Phenomenon, Esophageal Dysfunction, Sclerodactyly and Telangiectasia)

Table 1: Key features of localized and diffuse cutaneous systemic sclerosis		
Features	Localized cutaneous systemic sclerosis	Diffuse cutaneous systemic sclerosis
Skin	• Skin thickening occurs late; limited to distal part of upper and lower extremities, face, neck and upper chest. Telangiectasias and calcinosis are common	• Skin thickening occurs early; moves up to proximal part of extremities and trunk • Telangiectasias and calcinosis cutis may occur
Gastro-intestinal tract	• Esophageal dysmotility is more common than small and large intestine involvement	• Esophageal dysmotility can occur. Small and large intestinal involvement is more common
Pulmonary	• Pulmonary fibrosis is less frequent and less severe • Severe pulmonary hypertension is more common	• Pulmonary fibrosis is more common and severe • Pulmonary hypertension is less frequent
Kidney	• Renal crisis is uncommon	• Renal crisis is more frequent
Autoantibody association	• Anticentromere antibodies are predominant	• Anti-Scl-70 antibody is predominant • Anti-ribonucleic acid polymerase antibody is more common

syndrome.[17] A third, less common form "SSc *sine scleroderma*" is also recognized, in which there is primarily internal organ involvement with occasional fibrosis of distal digits.[18]

Diagnostic Criteria

One major or two or more minor criteria are required for the diagnosis of SSc.[19]

Major Criteria

Proximal scleroderma: Symmetric thickening, tightening, and induration of skin of the fingers and also skin proximal to the metacarpophalangeal or metatarsophalangeal joints (Figs 1 and 2).

Minor Criteria

1. Sclerodactyly: The above-mentioned skin changes occurring on the fingers (Fig. 3)
2. Digital pitted scars or loss of substance from the finger pad: Depressed areas at tips of fingers or loss of digital pad tissue as a result of ischemia (Figs 4 and 5)
3. Basilar pulmonary fibrosis: Bilateral reticular pattern of linear or linear-nodular densities most pronounced in basilar portions of the lungs on standard chest roentgenogram, not attributable to primary lung disease (Fig. 6).

The American College of Rheumatology or European League Against Rheumatism criteria for the classification of SSc have been described recently (Table 2).[20] Patients with a total score of

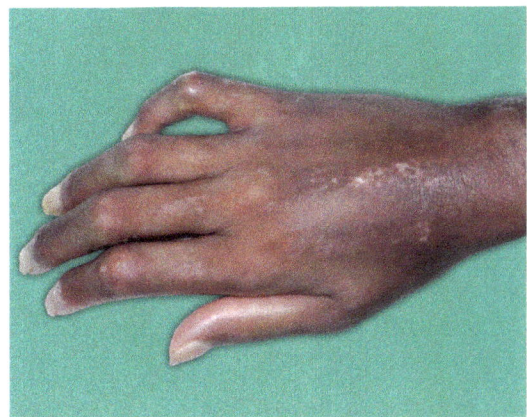

FIGURE 1: Shiny bound down skin extending beyond the metacarpophalangeal joints.

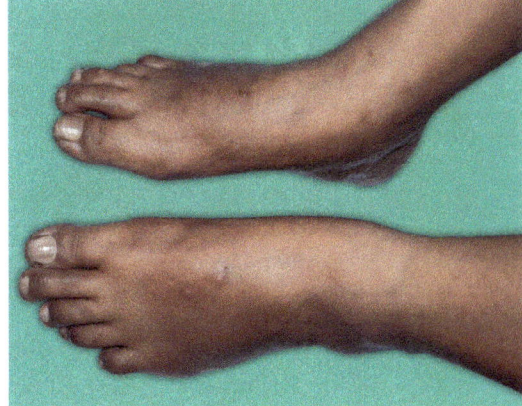

FIGURE 2: Shiny edematous bound down skin over toes and dorsum of feet extending to lower legs.

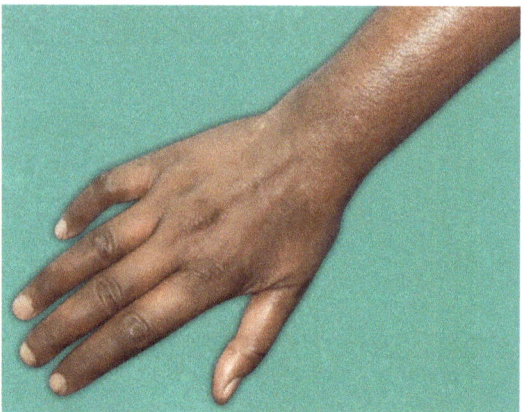

FIGURE 3: Sclerodactyly.

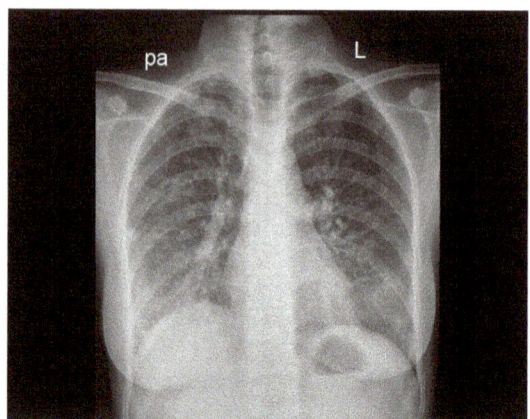

FIGURE 6: Chest X-ray showing basilar pulmonary fibrosis.

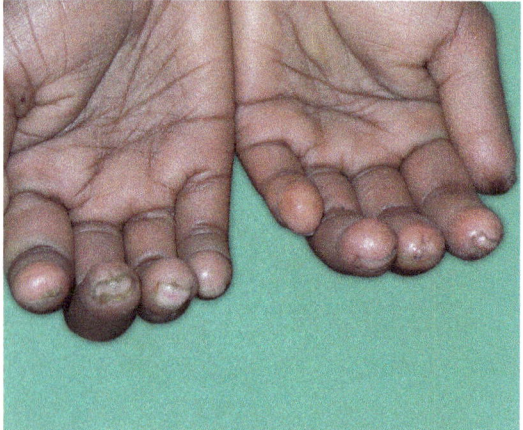

FIGURE 4: Digital pitted scars over the tips of the fingers in a systemic sclerosis patient.

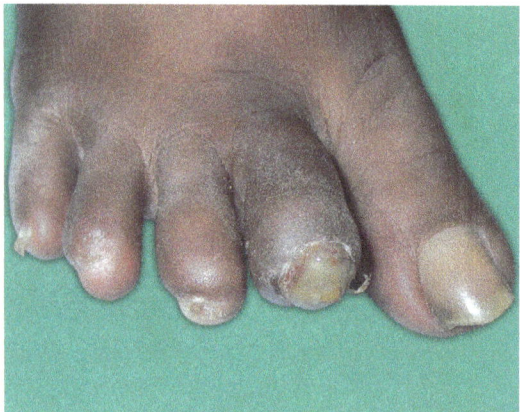

FIGURE 5: Ischemic scars with secondary infection over tips of the toes in a patient with systemic sclerosis.

Table 2: American College of Rheumatology or European League Against Rheumatism criteria for systemic sclerosis

Item	Subitem(s)	Weight or score
Skin thickening of the fingers of both hands extending proximal to the metacarpophalangeal joints (sufficient criterion)	–	9
Skin thickening of the fingers (only count the higher score)	• Puffy fingers	2
	• Sclerodactyly of the fingers (distal to the metacarpophalangeal joints but proximal to the proximal interphalangeal joints)	4
Fingertip lesions (only count the higher score)	• Digital tip ulcers	2
	• Fingertip pitting scars	3
Telangiectasia	–	2
Abnormal nailfold capillaries	–	2
Pulmonary arterial hypertension and/or interstitial lung disease (maximum score is 2)	• Pulmonary arterial hypertension	2
	• Interstitial lung disease	2

Continued

Systemic Sclerosis

Continued

Table 2: American College of Rheumatology or European League Against Rheumatism criteria for systemic sclerosis

Item	Subitem(s)	Weight or score
Raynaud's phenomenon	–	3
SSc-related autoantibodies (anticentromere, anti-topoisomerase I [anti-Scl-70], anti-RNA polymerase III) (maximum score is 3)	• Anticentromere • Antitopoisomerase I • Anti-RNA polymerase III	3

9 or more are classified as having definite SSc. The sensitivity and specificity of the new SSc criteria are 91% and 92%, respectively.

CLINICAL FEATURES

Skin

Skin changes evolve through three sequential stages. The earliest phase is edematous phase, which is characterized by puffiness, swelling, and decreased flexibility of the face, fingers, and hands (Figs 7 and 8). Subsequently in next indurated phase there is gradual diffuse sclerosis. The affected skin appears shiny, taut, thickened, and bound down leading to pinched nose, loss of wrinkles over forehead, and bird-like or mask-like facies (Figs 9 to 11). The mouth opening gets restricted (Fig. 12) and radial furrows appear in perioral area, giving a purse-string or pursed-lip appearance (Fig. 13). Lower eyelid retraction becomes difficult (Fig. 14). The severity of binding down of skin can be assessed by modified Rodnan skin scoring which includes assessment of skin thickening at 17 sites. Skin thickness is assessed by palpation and rated on a scale of 0 (normal), 1 (mild), 2 (moderate), or 3 (severe). The total skin score is the sum of the individual skin assessments in the 17 body areas, giving a possible range of 0–51. Finally, in the end stage, the skin becomes thin, atrophic, and often tightly tethered to the underlying tissue.

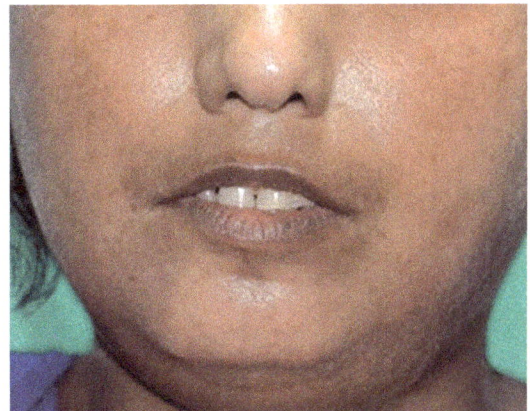

FIGURE 7: Initial edematous phase: Swelling, edema and tightening of the skin over face.

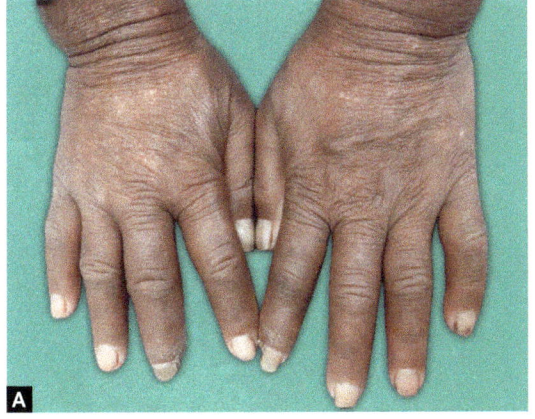
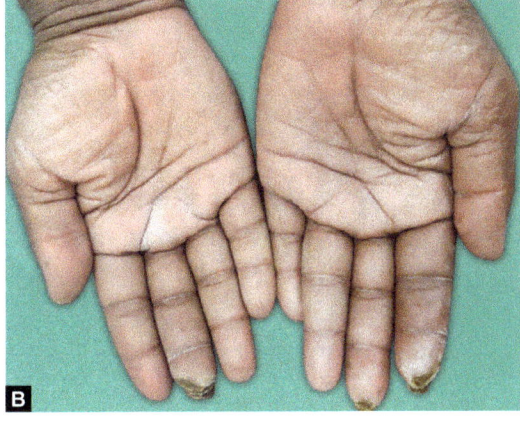

FIGURE 8: Initial edematous phase: Swelling and edema over the fingers and hand. Also visible are the ischemic ulcers over the tips of the fingers.

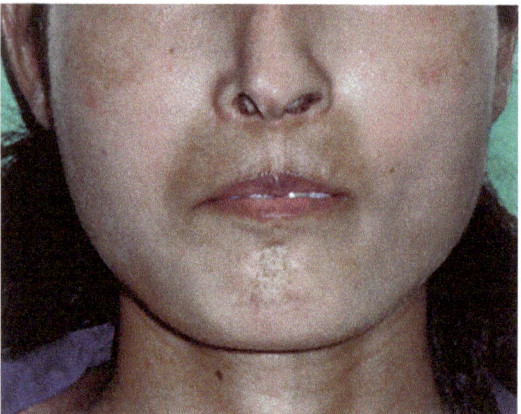

FIGURE 9: Mask like face, pinched nose, thinned out lips in an adult female systemic sclerosis patient.

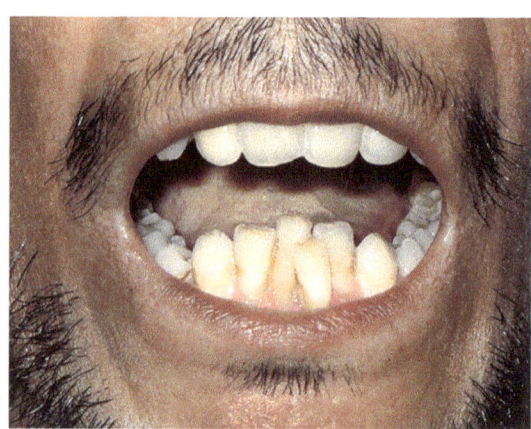

FIGURE 12: Reduced mouth opening in systemic sclerosis patient.

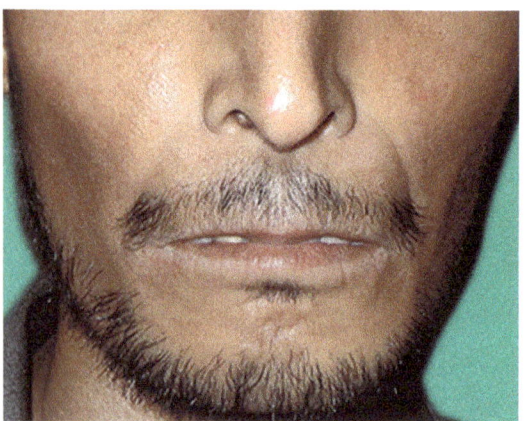

FIGURE 10: Adult male systemic sclerosis patient with loss of facial expressions, pinched nose, and thinned out lips.

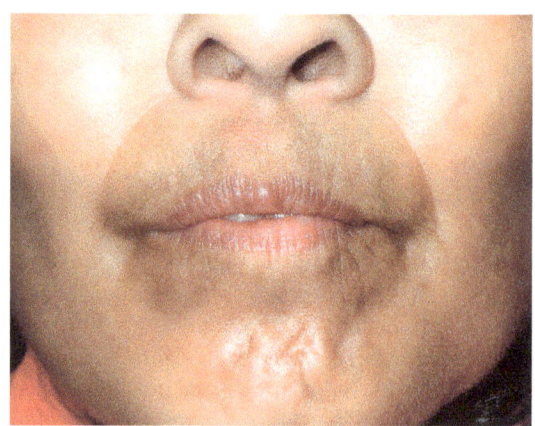

FIGURE 13: Pursed lip appearance in an adult female patient.

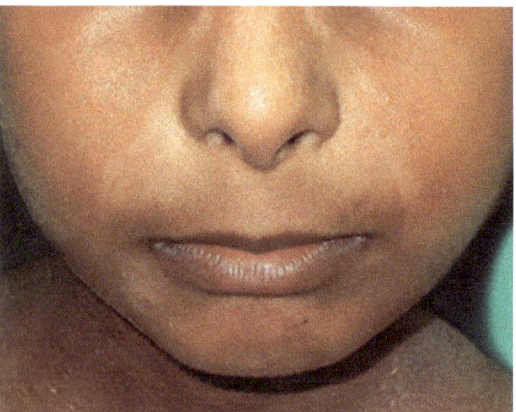

FIGURE 11: A 14-year-old female patient of systemic sclerosis with tightening of skin over face and pigmentary anomalies over face and neck.

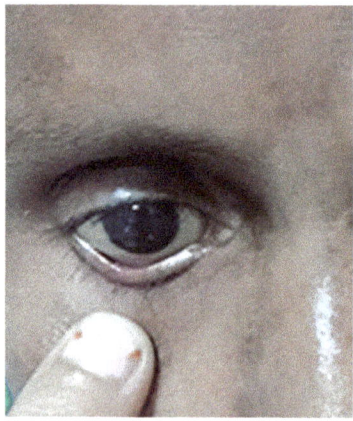

FIGURE 14: Difficulty in lower eyelid retraction.

Skin thickening in SSc patients is frequently accompanied by pigmentary changes. Different patterns of pigmentary anomalies seen in these patients include diffuse hyperpigmentation, salt and pepper pigmentation, and localized hyper/hypopigmentation. Variable incidences of hyperpigmentation ranging from 73.1 to 91% have been noted in previous studies. Diffuse pigmentation is the most common pattern. It usually starts from the fingers and extends proximally and face is also often involved (Fig. 15). Salt and pepper pattern of pigmentation is seen commonly on forehead, neck, upper chest, and back (Figs 16 and 17). This peculiar pattern arises due to perifollicular sparing in diffuse depigmented patches. Third pattern is localized hyperpigmentation or hypopigmentation seen in less number of cases (Figs 18 and 19). Often patients have combination of different patterns of pigmentary anomalies (Fig. 20). These changes can be quite severe and bothersome in some patients especially in the Indian skin type. Mat-like telangiectasia measuring 2-20 mm are commonly observed over face, and lips (Fig. 21) but can also be seen over neck, upper trunk, and hands (Fig. 22).

Extremities especially the finger tips are worst affected in SSc patients. Damage done depends upon the duration and severity of Raynaud's phenomenon. In the early stage, patient develops binding down of skin over fingers and small painful ischemic ulcers appear over the tips of fingers which heal leaving pitted scars (Fig. 4). These pitted scars can also be seen over the sides of the fingers as well as dorsa of fingers over the joints (Figs 23 and 24). Gradually, over a period of time the fingers appear smooth shiny and tapered (Fig. 25) and those with longstanding severe disease can have significant loss of tissue volume from the digital pulp along with acroosteolysis (Figs 26 and 27).

Nails become small, shiny, pale; have ragged cuticles; may curve over the atrophic phalanges; and can be lost completely in severe cases (Figs 5, 28, and 29). Nail fold capillary abnormality can be seen with dermatoscope (Figs 30 to 32) and the findings correlate with severity of Raynaud's phenomenon and occurrence of digital pitted scars. In early stage there is a uniform capillary dilatation alone, and later there is capillary drop out along with more dilated capillaries and hemorrhages. In advanced stage, we see avascular areas, arborising vessels, and irregularly enlarged giant capillaries.

Some patients with severe bound down skin develop flexion contractures of fingers (Figs 33 and 34), sometimes limbs and have functional disability (Fig. 35). Also, cutaneous atrophy and ulceration is seen in late stage, especially over the bony prominences (Fig. 36) and extensor surfaces of the interphalangeal joints (Fig. 37).[21]

Gangrene of the fingers and toes is not uncommon and is usually a dry gangrene (Fig. 38).

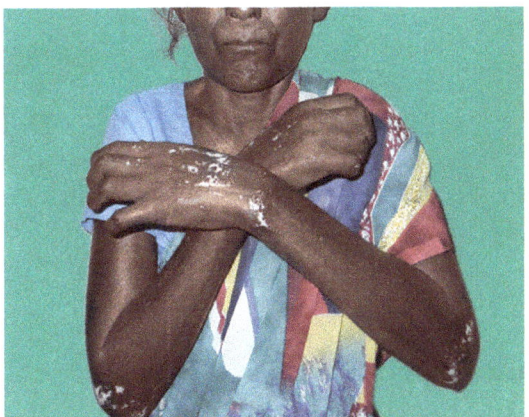

FIGURE 15: Diffuse hyperpigmentation over face, neck, and upper limbs in systemic sclerosis patient. Also visible is patchy depigmentation over trauma-prone sites.

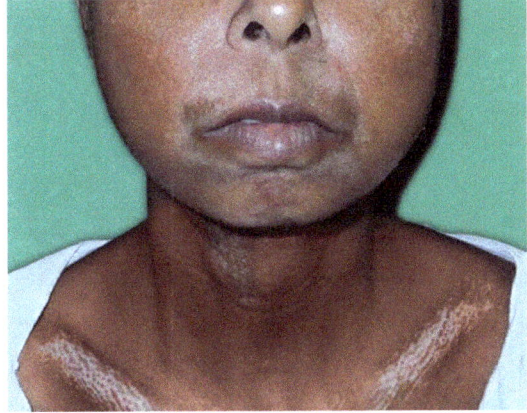

FIGURE 16: Salt and pepper pigmentary anomaly seen over face.

… Skin in Rheumatologic Diseases

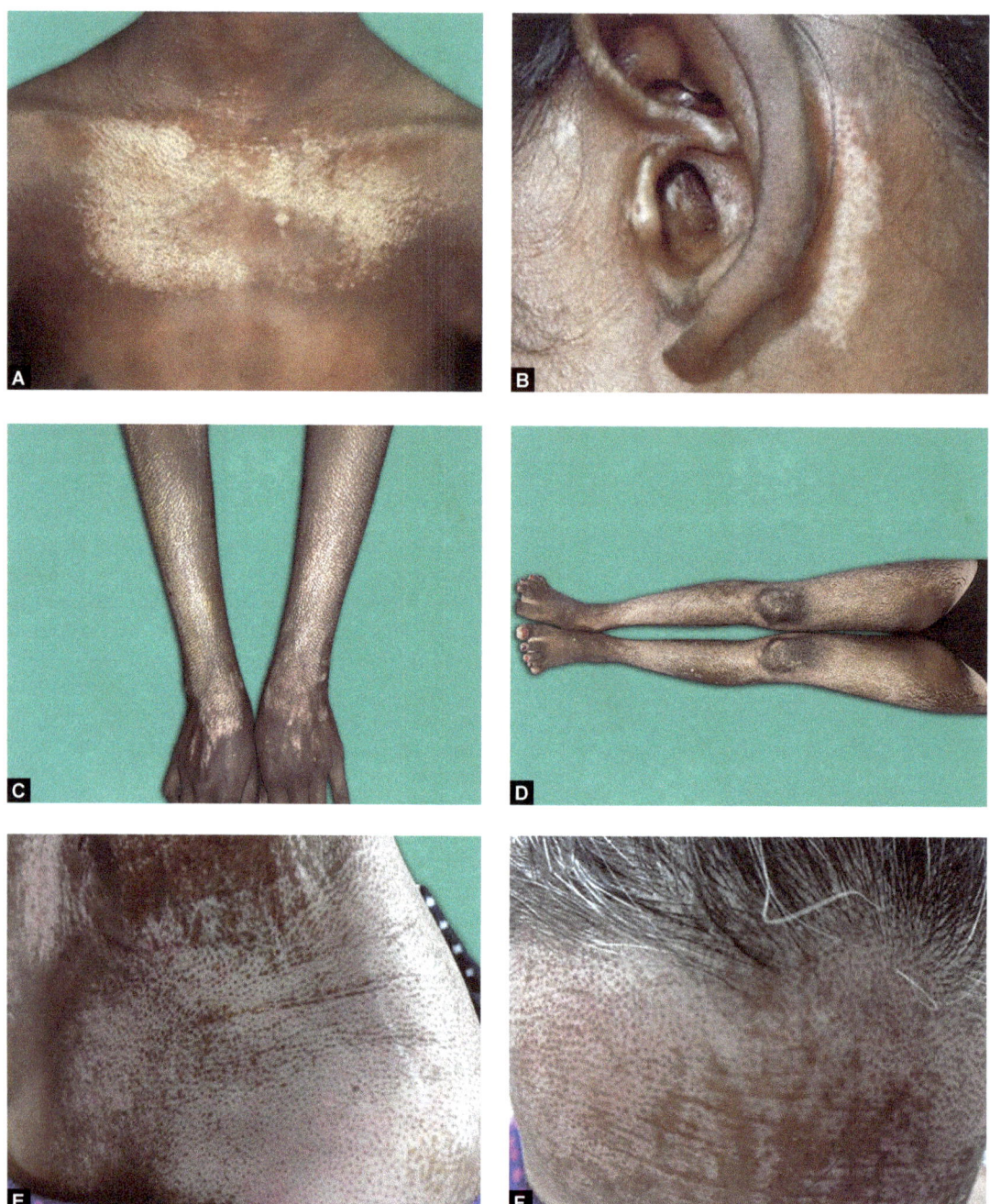

FIGURE 17: Salt and pepper pigmentary anomaly seen over: **A,** Upper anterior chest; **B,** Retroauricular area; **C,** Forearm; **D,** Thigh and leg; **E,** Shoulder; **F,** Forehead.

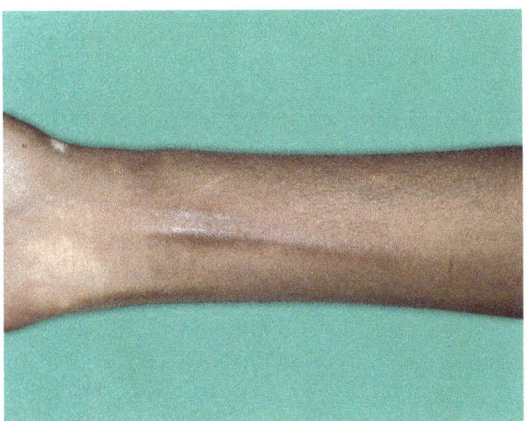

FIGURE 18: Localized hyperpigmentation of the skin overlying the flexor tendons of the wrist.

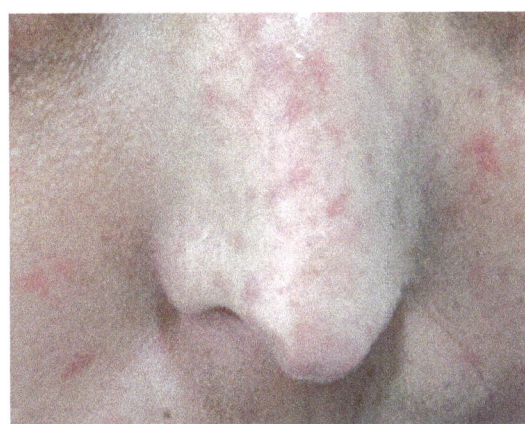

FIGURE 21: Matt-like telangiectasias over face in female adult systemic sclerosis patient.

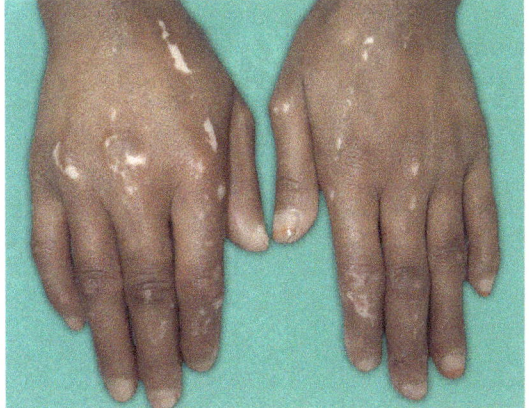

FIGURE 19: Patchy depigmentation over dorsum of both hands in a systemic sclerosis patient.

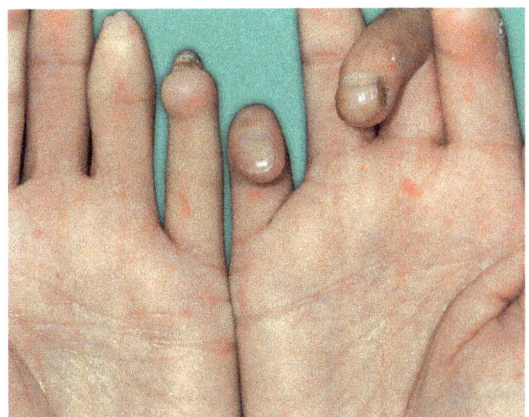

FIGURE 22: Matt-like telangiectasias over palms.

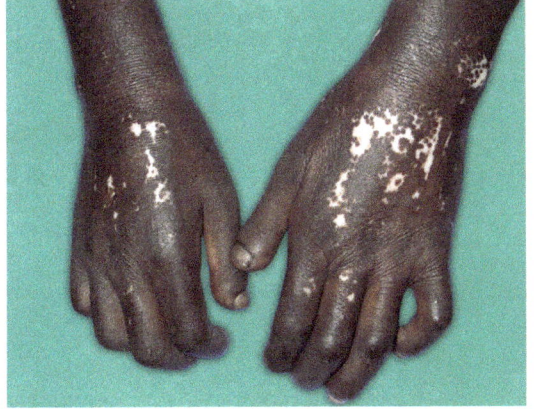

FIGURE 20: Salt and pepper depigmentation with background diffuse hyperpigmentation seen over dorsum of hands in a systemic sclerosis patient.

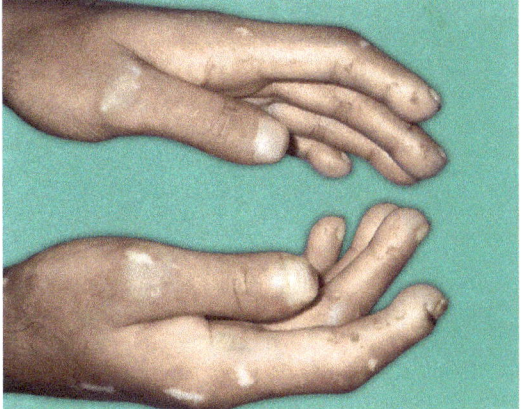

FIGURE 23: Digital pitted scars over the sides of the fingers.

Skin in Rheumatologic Diseases

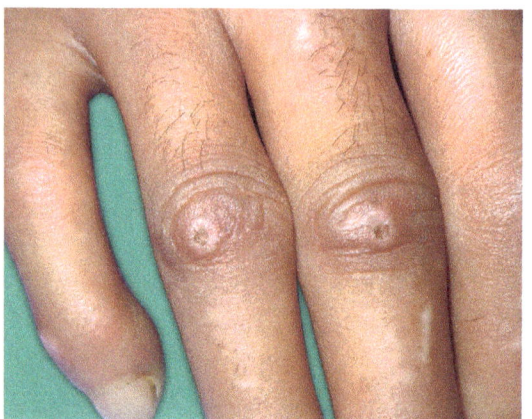

FIGURE 24: Pitted scars over the interphalangeal joints.

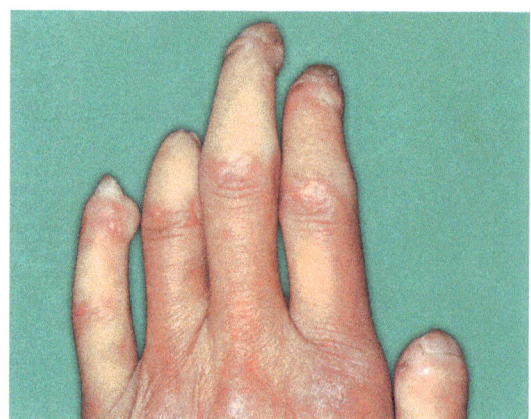

FIGURE 25: Tapering of fingers and acroosteolysis in a patient of systemic sclerosis with severe Raynaud's phenomenon.

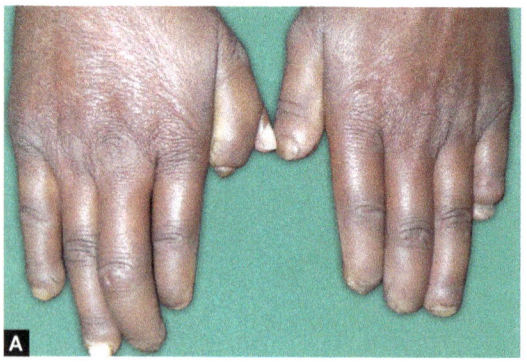

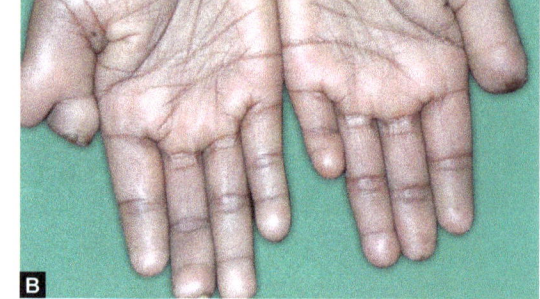

FIGURE 26: Acroosteolysis in a systemic sclerosis patient.

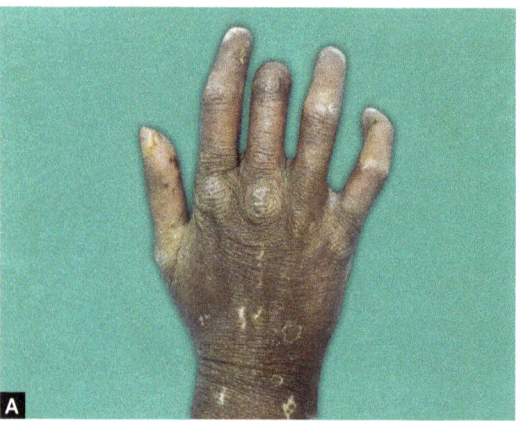

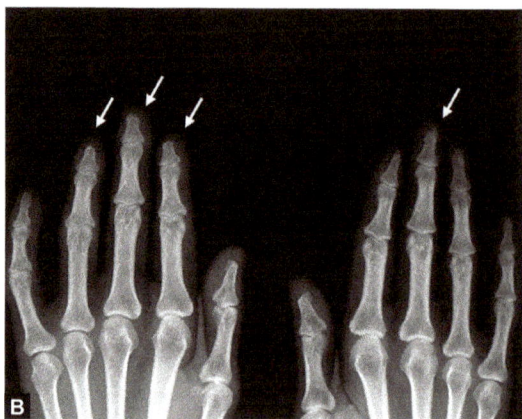

FIGURE 27: **A,** Acroosteolysis in middle finger of right hand along with loss of pulp tissue in other fingers; **B,** X-ray of hand showing bony resorption (white arrows) in multiple terminal phalanx of both hands in a systemic sclerosis patient.

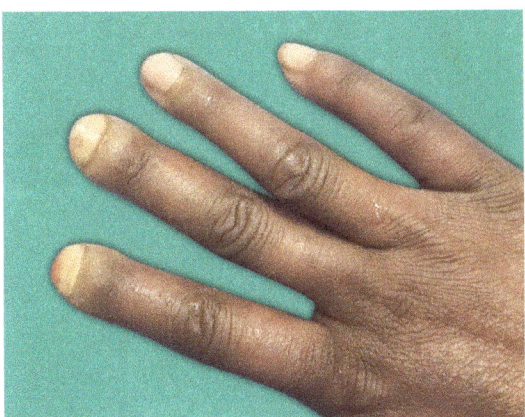

FIGURE 28: Pale and shortened nails of second and third finger of right hand.

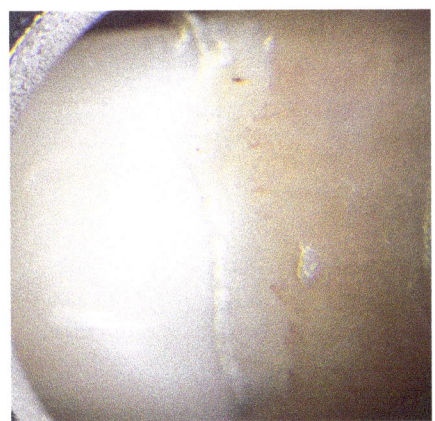

FIGURE 31: Capillaroscopy: During active established disease stage, capillary drop outs, irregularly more dilated capillary loops can be seen.

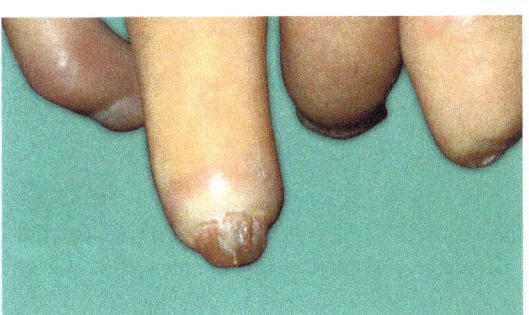

FIGURE 29: Curved dystrophic nail with severe pallor of the proximal nail fold in systemic sclerosis patient.

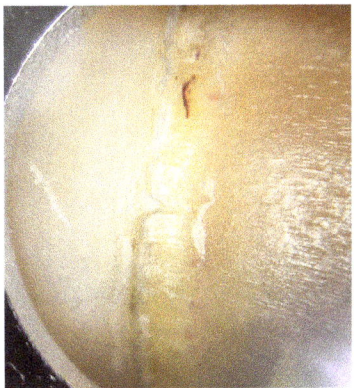

FIGURE 32: Capillaroscopy: In advanced stage of the disease, large ischemic areas along with scant dilated capillary loops can be seen.

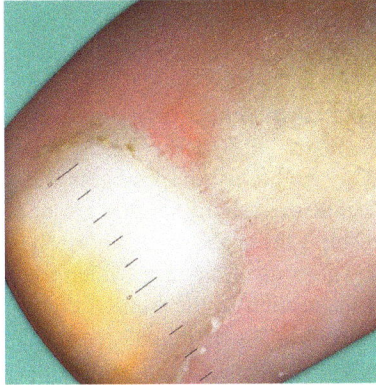

FIGURE 30: Capillaroscopy: Multiple dilated capillary loops in proximal nail fold seen in early stage of the disease.

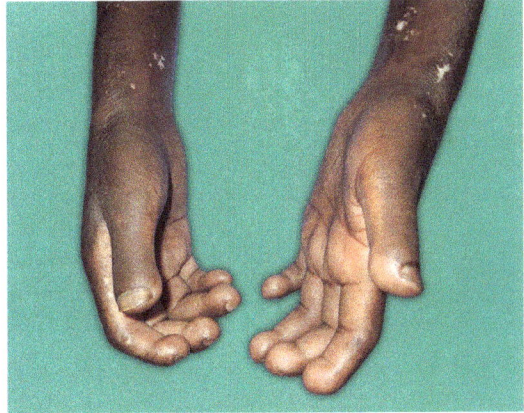

FIGURE 33: Flexion contractures of fingers due to severely bound down skin of the fingers and palm.

Skin in Rheumatologic Diseases

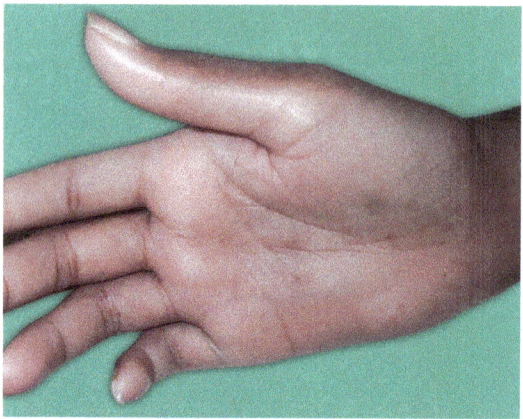

FIGURE 34: Flexion contractures and scalerodactyly due to systemic sclerosis.

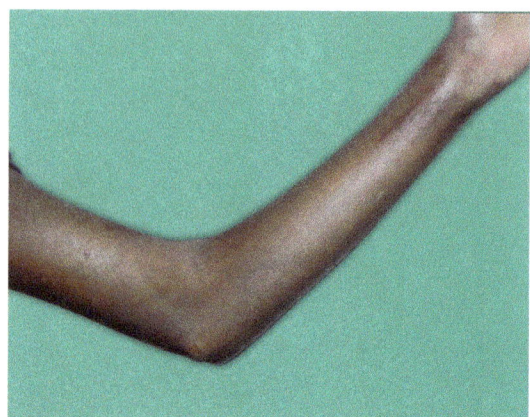

FIGURE 35: Flexion contracture at the left elbow joint due to severely bound down and contracted skin.

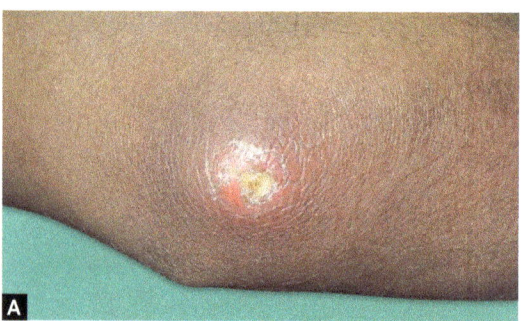

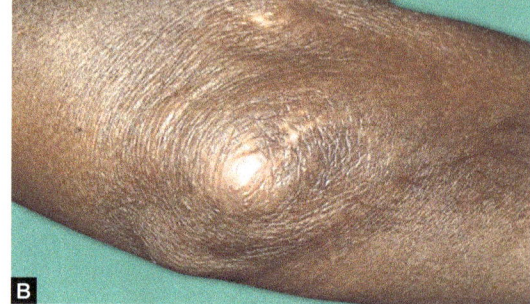

FIGURE 36: A, Ischemic ulcer over the extensor aspect of right elbow; **B,** Ulcer healed completely in 3 months with dressing and conservative management.

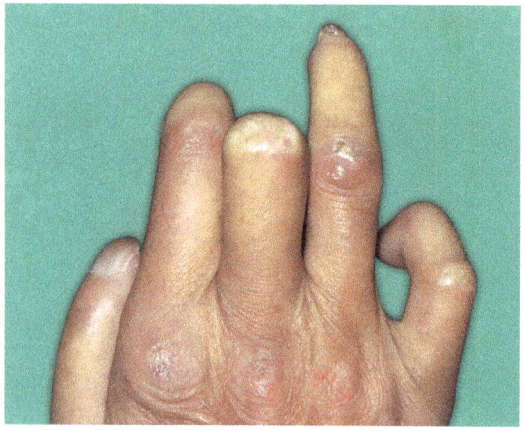

FIGURE 37: Fingers of systemic sclerosis patients with severe sclerodactyly, and ischemic ulcers and scars can be seen over knuckles and interphalangeal joints.

It affects the tips of the digits and then can extend more proximally. Severe pain in the tip of digit is the harbinger of impending gangrene and should alert the treating physician to make the treatment more aggressive. Early identification and initiation of treatment can prevent its progression to some extent.

Bilateral mandibular condylosis and apertognathia (open bite) have been reported as presenting symptoms in progressive SSc. It is believed that these bony lesions are of ischemic origin, resulting from obstruction of small muscular arteries. Tightness of the skin, which may lead to pressure resorption of the bone, can be another factor contributing to mandibular resorption.[22,23]

Subcutaneous calcifications composed of amorphous calcium hydroxyapatite occur mainly

Systemic Sclerosis

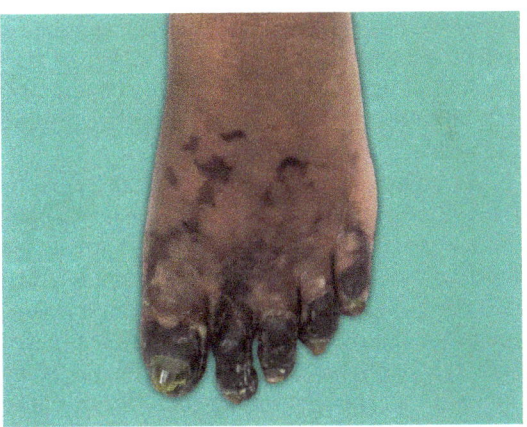

FIGURE 38: Dry gangrene of the toes of left foot in systemic sclerosis patient.

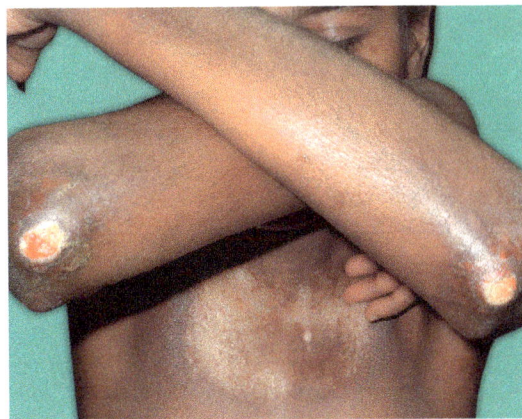

FIGURE 40: Cutaneous ulcers due to secondary calcinosis cutis over extensors of the elbow joint.

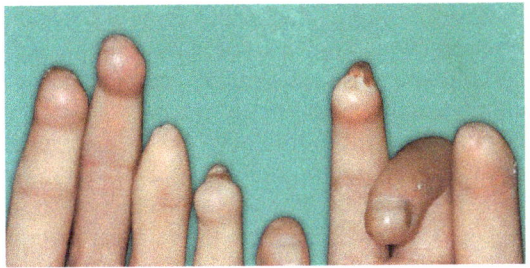

FIGURE 39: Dystrophic calcium deposits over the tip of many fingers.

in periarticular tissues. Dystrophic calcification of acral distribution (volar aspect of finger tips, extensor aspect of metacarpophalangeal, interphalangeal, elbows, and knee joint) is the most common type of calcinosis (Fig. 39). It occurs in approximately 25% of patients with SSc causing pain, local inflammation, ulceration, secondary infection (Fig. 40), and joint contractures. Radiographs show the radiopaque deposits in the subcutaneous plane.

In a prospective study of 46 patients of SSc by Ghosh et al., Raynaud's phenomenon was present in 84.8% patients, dyspigmentation in 86.9%, sclerodactyly in 82.6%, inability to open the mouth in 82.6%, mat-like telangiectasia in 23.1%, fingertip ulceration and scarring in 63%, cutaneous calcinosis in 2.2%, digital gangrene in 4.3%, generalized pruritus in 8.7%, cutaneous small vessel vasculitis in 4.3%, chronic urticaria in 4.3%, flexion contractures of the fingers in 28.3%, and amputation of the digits in 6.5%. Mucosal changes were seen in 21.7% patients and nail changes in 28.2% patients.[24]

Raynaud's Phenomenon

Raynaud's phenomenon is seen in almost all patients of SSc and manifests as classical triad of pallor followed by cyanosis, and then hyperemia accompanied by numbness and pain. The three stages reflect the underlying pathomechanisms of vasoconstriction, ischemia, and reperfusion. Raynaud's phenomenon often predates skin sclerosis by many years in the limited subtype and often occurs concurrently with skin sclerosis in those with diffuse cutaneous SSc.

Raynaud's phenomenon can be seen in 4–5% of the general population; however, presence of capillary nail fold microscopic abnormalities seen in association with Raynaud's phenomenon can be considered as a predictor of future development of connective tissue disease. In addition, capillary nail fold microscopic findings can help in assessment and subclassification of SSc as diffuse cutaneous or limited cutaneous SSc. Presence of capillary drop-out in nail folds is more suggestive of diffuse form of SSc, while presence of capillary dilatation is more in favor of limited form of disease. Presence of the antinuclear antibody in a patient with Raynaud's phenomenon is also considered as a predictor of future development of SSc.[21]

Pulmonary

Pulmonary manifestations of SSc include interstitial lung disease (ILD), pulmonary hypertension (PHT), and sometimes pleuritis, pleural effusion, and aspiration pneumonia. Dyspnea on exertion and nonproductive cough are the most common clinical symptoms. Interstitial fibrosis is more likely to occur among persons with diffuse scleroderma than in those with limited scleroderma, while PHT is more common in limited form of the disease.

Interstitial lung disease is the foremost cause of morbidity and mortality in SSc patients and associated with anti-Scl-70 antibody positivity. On chest auscultation, end-inspiratory rales are heard, and chest radiograph shows reticular interstitial thickening in a linear or nodular pattern more evident in the lower lung bases (Fig. 6). However, chest radiograph is a less sensitive mean for detecting lung involvement rather more useful for evaluation of any chest infections in these patients.

Pulmonary function testing (PFT) is a sensitive method for detecting and monitoring ILD (Tables 3 and 4). Pulmonary function abnormalities can reveal a restrictive ventilatory defect, suggested by a reduction in forced vital capacity (FVC) and decreased lung compliance and diffusing capacity of the lung for carbon monoxide.

A high-resolution computed tomography (HRCT) scan is more sensitive and can detect early disease when chest radiographs are normal. The most common pattern is nonspecific interstitial pneumonia (Fig. 41), which carries a better prognosis than the usual interstitial pneumonia (Fig. 42). High-resolution computed tomography shows intra- and interlobular reticular opacities in a predominantly subpleural and basilar distribution. Ground-glass opacification, alone or in combination with a reticular pattern, is seen in 50% of patients. Other findings include mediastinal lymphadenopathy, nodules, traction bronchiectasis, and in some cases, honeycomb cystic changes. High-resolution computed tomography grading of the thorax includes: (i) parenchymal opacification alone; (ii) parenchymal opacification more extensive than a reticular pattern; (iii) parenchymal opacification equal in extent to a reticular pattern; (iv) reticular pattern

Table 3: Pulmonary function test report of a patient with severe restrictive chest abnormality due to interstitial lung disease: Forced vital capacity is markedly reduced						
Parameter	UM	Description	Pred.	LLN	BEST#5	%Pred.
Best FVC	L (btps)	Best forced vital capacity	4.23	3.38	1.00	24
FVC	L (btps)	Forced vital capacity	4.23	3.38	1.00	24
FEV1	L (btps)	Forced expiratory volume in 1 sec	3.58	2.86	0.90	25
PEF	L/s	Peak expiratory flow	9.34	7.47	3.46	37
PIF	L/s	Peak inspiratory flow	–	–	1.02	–
FEV1/FVC%	%	FEV1 as % of FVC	82.0	65.6	89.9	110
FEF 25–75%	L/s	Forced mid-expiratory flow	4.75	3.80	1.88	40
MEF 75%	L/s	Max expiratory flow @ 25% FVC	7.97	6.38	3.46	43
MEF 50%	L/s	Max expiratory flow @ 50% FVC	5.19	4.16	2.64	51
MEF 25%	L/s	Max expiratory flow @ 75% FVC	2.34	1.87	0.71	30
FET 100%	s	Forced expiratory time	–	–	3.6	–
IC	L (btps)	Inspiratory capacity	–	–	0.58	–

Diagnosis:
Suspected restrictive abnormality: Restrictive abnormality: Very severe
UM: unit of measure; Pred.: predicted; LLN: lower limit of normal; BEST: best obtained value out of 5 times ; %pred.: percent predicted.

Table 4: Report showing reduced diffusing capacity of the lungs for carbon monoxide in a systemic sclerosis patient

Parameter	UM	Description	Pred.	LLN	BEST#6	%Pred.
Vt	L (btps)	Total volume	–	–	0.24	–
FiO$_2$	%	Inspiratory O$_2$ concentration	–	–	21.00	–
DLCO	mL/min/mm Hg	CO diffusing capacity	32.70	26.16	13.09	40
DLCO (corr)	mL/min/mm Hg	DLCO corrected for Hb, CHb and PB	32.70	26.16	13.51	41
DLCO/VA	mL/min/mm Hg/L	DLCO per unit of alveolar volume	5.03	4.02	4.80	96
FiCO	%	Inspired CO concentration	–	–	0.300	–
FiCH4	%	Inspired CH4 concentration	–	–	0.294	–
FaCO	%	Alveolar CO concentration	–	–	0.037	–
FaCH4	%	Alveolar CH4 concentration	–	–	0.067	–
Breathold	s	Breathold time	–	–	9.21	–
VA	L (btps)	Alveolar volume	–	–	2.81	–
Hb	g/dL	Hemoglobin concentration	–	–	13.10	–
Sample vol	mL	Sample collection volume	–	–	300	–
Washot vol	mL	Washout volume	–	–	461	–
IVC (DLCO)	L	Inspiratory vital capacity during DLCO	4.91	3.93	0.79	16
TLC (DLCO)	L	Total lung capacity during DLCO	6.50	5.20	2.88	44
RV (DLCO)	L	Residual volume during DLCO	1.64	1.31	2.09	128
RV/TLC (DLCO)	%	RV (DLCO)/TLC (DLCO)	25.3	20.2	72.5	287
FetCH4	%	End tidal CH4 concentration	–	–	0.003	–
DLCO3eq	mL/min/mm Hg	CO diffusing capacity (3 equations)	32.70	26.16	6.99	21
DLCOmean	mL/min/mm Hg	CO diffusing capacity (mean)	32.70	26.16	13.09	40
DLCO/VAmean	mL/min/mm Hg/L	DLCO per unit of alv. (mean)	5.03	4.02	4.80	96
VAmean	L (btps)	Alveolar volume (mean)	–	–	2.81	–
DLCO	mmol/min/mm Hg	CO diffusing capacity (mmol)	97.64	78.11	39.08	40

Diagnosis:
Suspected restrictive abnormality: Restrictive abnormality: Very severe
UM: unit of measure; Pred.: predicted; LLN: lower limit of normal; BEST: best obtained value out of 6 ; %pred.: percent predicted.

more extensive than parenchymal opacification; and (v) reticular pattern alone.

A "ground-glass" appearance is a feature of pneumonitis.

Pulmonary hypertension (mean pulmonary arterial pressure more than 25 mm Hg and with pulmonary capillary wedge pressure less than 15 mm Hg) is more frequently seen with limited SSc than with diffuse disease and often occurs late in the disease course. Early pulmonary arterial hypertension is asymptomatic, afterwards patient present with dyspnea on exertion and late stages symptoms of right-side heart failure (angina, exertional near syncope, pedal edema) ensue. Physical examination may reveal accentuation of the S2 and later patient may develop signs of right-sided heart failure. An echocardiogram or right-sided cardiac catheterization can be done to confirm the diagnosis.[21]

Cardiovascular

The major cardiac complications are pericarditis, constrictive pericardium, arrhythmias, and con-

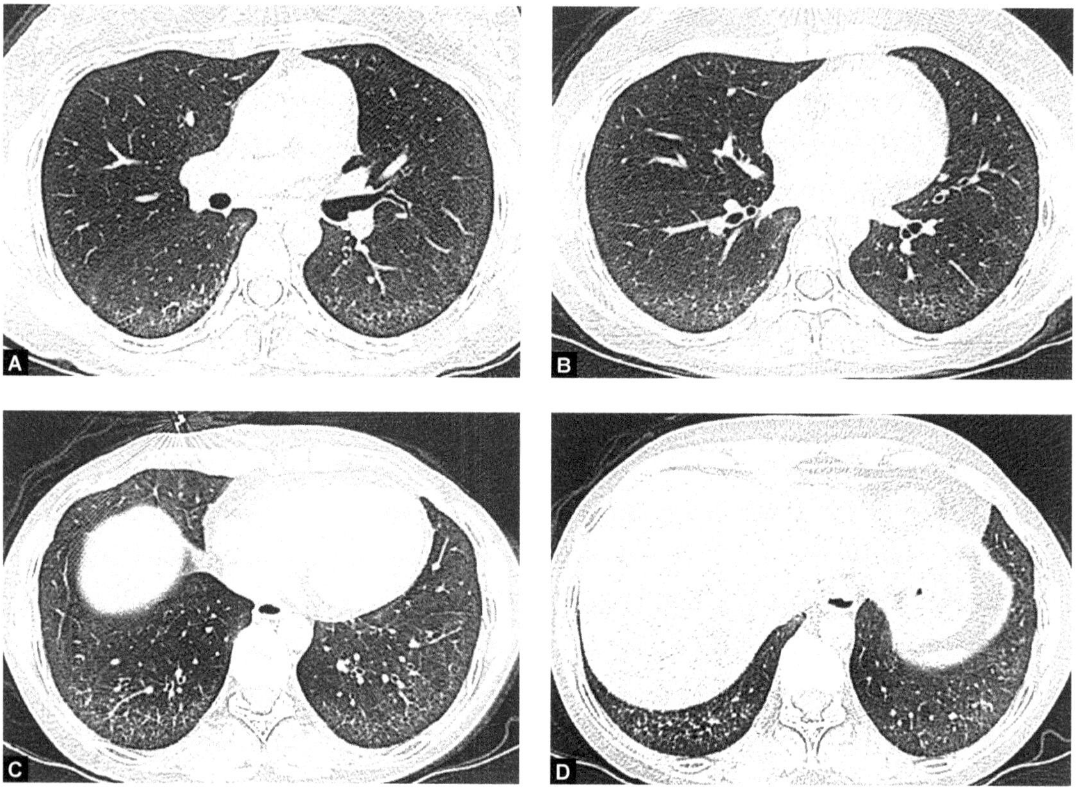

Skin in Rheumatologic Diseases

FIGURE 41: Nonspecific interstitial pattern in cranial to caudal high-resolution computed tomography (HRCT) sections: A 32-year-old female systemic sclerosis patient in HRCT sections showing ground-glass opacities with septal thickening and microcystic changes. The changes show a peripheral and basal predominance.

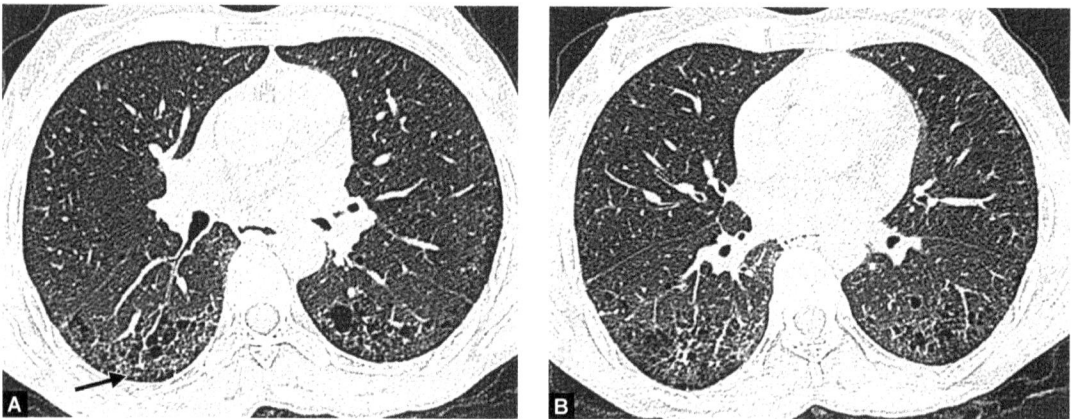

FIGURE 42: Usual interstitial pattern in high-resolution computed tomography (HRCT) sections: A 35-year-old male systemic sclerosis patient HRCT showing changes of honeycombing (arrow) seen in peripheral and subpleural distribution.

gestive heart failure; degeneration of myocardial fibers with replacement by fibrosis has been seen in autopsies.[21]

Renal

Scleroderma renal crisis (SRC) occurs in 5% of patients with SSc and used to be the most common cause of mortality before the advent of angiotensin converting enzyme (ACE) inhibitors. The risk factors include diffuse form of the disease, use of corticosteroids and cyclosporine A, and the presence of anti-RNA polymerase III antibodies. It is sometimes triggered by nephrotoxic drugs and/or intravascular volume depletion.

Scleroderma renal crisis is defined as the new onset of accelerated arterial hypertension and/or rapidly progressive oliguric renal failure during the course of SSc. Nonmalignant hypertension alone, without azotemia, is not renal crisis. There is a abrupt rise in blood pressure over days to weeks and rapidly progressive renal failure if untreated, usually within the first 5 years of the disease. It also results in hypertensive encephalopathy, congestive heart failure, and arrythmia.[25] Normotensive SRC occurs in 10% patients and is associated with poorer outcome.

Gastrointestinal

Systemic sclerosis can affect the entire gastrointestinal tract from esophagus to rectum. There is atrophy and replacement of smooth muscles by the collagen bundles, and small vessel obliterative vasculopathy in affected area. Esophagus is most commonly involved and up to 96% of patients can have esophageal complications, including esophageal motility abnormalities, lower esophageal sphincter abnormalities, esophageal dilatation (Fig. 43), gastroesophageal reflux disease, and Barrett's esophagus. It is found to be more common in patients with positive anticentromere antibodies.

Stomach involvement occurs in 10–75% of SSc patients and includes gastric dysmotility (gastroparesis) and gastric antral vascular ectasia (watermelon stomach). Patients present with symptoms of early satiety, bloating, dyspepsia, gastric bleeding, nausea, and vomiting. Peristaltic abnormalities (hypomobility) of small and large intestine result in constipation in initial stages and later lead to overgrowth of intestinal microorganisms, malabsorption, diarrhea, and cachexia.[26]

The most common liver disease usually associated to scleroderma is primary biliary cirrhosis.

Musculoskeletal

Joint pain, arthritis (Fig. 44), tendonitis, muscle weakness, and joint contractures can be seen in SSc. Flexion contractures usually occurring in the fingers, wrists, elbows and ankles are due to tendon and periarticular fibrosis and shortening

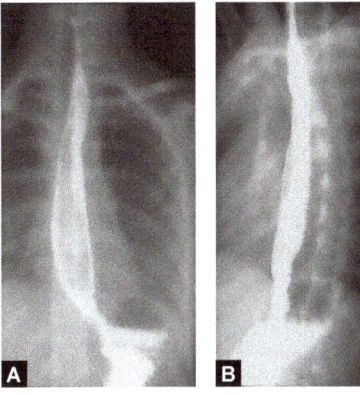

FIGURE 43: Barium swallow (**A,** anteroposterior and **B,** oblique) showing impaired motility of thoracic esophagus with delayed passage of barium and mid dilatation of thoracic esophagus.

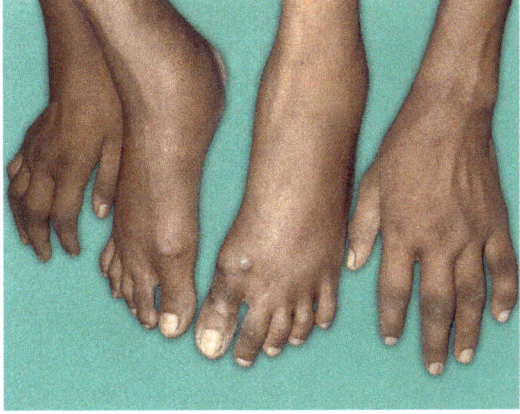

FIGURE 44: Systemic sclerosis patient with arthritis of many proximal interphalangeal joints and bilateral ankle joints.

along with severe bound down skin. Myopathy with mild muscle weakness and slight elevation of creatinine kinase can occur.[21]

Other

Disorders of the nervous system include depression, neuropathy from carpal tunnel syndrome, trigeminal neuralgia, or other compressive phenomenon. In patients with SSc and Sjögren's syndrome, vasculitis involving the skin and peripheral nervous system (sensory neuropathy) involvement may occur. Urogenital symptoms are rare. Vaginal symptoms such as tightness, dryness, and dyspareunia can occur and in men, erectile dysfunction due to reduced penile blood flow has been observed.[27] Ocular involvement presents as swelling and hardening of eyelids, decreased lacrimation, keratoconjunctivitis sicca, and endophthalmitis.

In a cohort of 1,000 patients, Hudson et al. found that common clinical features included Raynaud's phenomenon (98%), sclerodactyly (92%), clinically visible mat-like telangiectasias (78%), skin involvement above the fingers (58%), lung fibrosis (35%), PHT (15%), and gastrointestinal tract involvement. Almost 90% of patients had at least one SSc-related autoantibody, including 34% with anticentromere, and 16% with anti-topoisomerase I. The sensitivity of Raynaud and proximal finger skin thickening for the diagnosis of SSc was only 57%. Addition of clinically visible mat-like telangiectasias and SSc-related antibodies improved the sensitivity to 97%.[28]

MANAGEMENT OF SYSTEMIC SCLEROSIS

The management includes early diagnosis and evaluation, prompt and appropriate treatment, and regular follow-up. Routine investigations including complete hemogram, liver function test, kidney function test, and urine examination have to be done in all the patients. Relevant investigations for systemic involvement have been detailed in table 5.

Table 5: Assessment of various organ involvements in systemic sclerosis patients[29]			
Organ system	Diagnostic technique	Follow-up	Remarks
Skin	Modified Rodnan score	Every 6 months	Skin USG proposed as noninvasive and reproducible method
Renal	Glomerular filteration rate: Creatinine clearance, urinary protein excretion	Every 6 months	–
	Renal blood flow and vascular resistance: Renal Doppler	Every 12 months	
Gastrointestinal	Esophageal manometry	Every 12 months	Follow-up with manometry and pH studies reserved for patients with severe GI involvement
	Barium studies		
	24 h pH studies		
Pulmonary	PFT/DLCO (Table 3)	Every 6 months	BAL not recommended routinely. Role of proBNP levels
ILD	HRCT	Every 12 months	
PAH	2D echo, 6 min walk test (Appendix 1)	Every 6 months	
Cardiac	Standard ECG	Every 6 months	Holter monitoring can detect arrhythmias and conduction defects not seen in standard ECG. It should be done in case of clinical suspicion of arrhythmias.
	24 h Holter		
	2D echo		
Vascular	Nail fold capillaroscopy	Every 6 months	–

USG, ultrasound sonography; ILD, interstitial lung disease; PAH, pulmonary arterial hypertension; PFT, pulmonary function test; DLCO, diffusing capacity of the lungs for carbon monoxide; GI, gastrointestinal; 2D echo, two-dimensional echocardiography; ECG, electrocardiogram.

Skin biopsy is indicated when the diagnosis is not clear especially in milder disease or early stage of the disease or in long standing ulcers over bony prominences where calcinosis cutis or malignant transformation need to be ruled out.

Serological test are not routinely indicated except when the diagnosis is not clear. There role is more in predicting prognosis and as marker of particular organ involvement.

TREATMENT OF SYSTEMIC SCLEROSIS

Treatment of SSc is primarily organ directed and there is no diseases modifying therapy with good efficacy. In the absence of good treatment options, there has been no consensus on choice of therapy, at what stage to start treatment and what is the endpoint. Recently, European League Against Rheumatism (EULAR) and the EULAR Scleroderma Trials and Research group (EUSTAR) have formulated a set of recommendations for the treatment of SSc (Box 1).

> **Box 1: Treatment summary**
> - Early assessment of all potentially involved organs is mandatory
> - At present, no treatment is available that can change the course of systemic sclerosis. Currently, treatment is directed at specific organ involvement
> - Digital vasculopathy: Calcium channel blockers regarded as first-line agents followed by prostacyclins (mainly for improvement of existing ulcers) and endothelin anatagonists (for prevention of new ulcers formation)
> - Interstitial lung disease: Cyclophosphamide should be considered in the management as induction agent. Role of azathioprine and mycophenolate mofetil needs to be evaluated as maintenance agents
> - Pulmonary arterial hypertension: Endothelin antagonists as first-line agents followed by phosphodiesterase type 5 inhibitors and prostacyclins
> - Skin involvement: Methotrexate may be considered in the management
> - Renal involvement: Angiotensin converting enzyme inhibitors should be used in the treatment of scleroderma renal crisis
> - Gastrointestinal disease: Proton pump inhibitors for gastroesophageal reflux disease, prokinetic drugs for motility disorders and rotating antibiotics for malabsorption caused by bacterial overgrowth

For the purpose of better understanding, the treatment of SSc is categorized as described in table 6.

Therapies with Disease Modifying Potential

There is no single medication for the constellation of manifestations. The best "disease modifying therapy" at present seems to be immunosuppression.

Dexamethasone Cyclophosphamide Pulse Therapy or Dexamethasone Pulse Therapy

In 1990, Pasricha et al. used dexamethasone pulses to treat SSc.[30] Binding down of skin, dysphagia, and respiratory complaints usually improve within 3–6 months of treatment. Sameem et al. treated 47 patients of SSc with 100 mg intravenous dexamethasone in 500 mL 5% dextrose for 3 consecutive days. There was significant improvement in skin scoring, Raynaud's phenomenon, and digital ulcers; however, 13 patients developed tuberculosis and 1 patient developed steroid psychosis and avascular necrosis of femur.[31]

Majority reports of steroid pulse therapy for SSc are from India. There is no consensus on the number of pulses to be given and when to give

Table 6: Classification of the management guidelines for systemic sclerosis

Disease modifying therapy	Organ-targeted therapy for	Treatment of complications
Pulse therapy (DCP/DP)	Raynaud's phenomenon or digital ulceration	Gangrene or critical digital ischemia
Stem cell transplantation	Skin binding	Calcinosis
	Interstitial lung disease	Pulmonary artery hypertension
	Renal involvement	Scleroderma renal crisis
	GIT involvement	–

DCP, dexamethasone-cyclophosphamide pulse; DP, dexamethasone pulse; GIT, gastrointestinal tract up the treatment. Response to treatment is more satisfying in case the pulse treatment is started early during the course of the disease. High dose steroids are considered to increase the risk of renal crisis but same has not been observed in the studies on corticosteroid pulse therapy for SSc. Other limitation is the recurrence or deterioration of the symptoms in some patients usually 3–6 months after stopping the pulse therapy. Thus, pulse therapy halts the disease progression and results in clinical improvement in a good number of patients, and, therefore, can be considered a treatment option with some disease modifying potential, but side effects are common requiring close monitoring, precautions, and appropriate treatment. There are no randomized controlled trials of pulse therapy.

Stem Cell Transplantation

Recently few large multicenter studies have been conducted to establish the safety and efficacy of autologous hematopoietic stem cell transplantation (HSCT) as a disease modifying therapy for SSc. Hematopoietic stem cell transplantation consists of an initial phase of peripheral blood stem cell mobilization by administering either granulocyte colony stimulating factor (G-CSF) or a combination of cyclophosphamide with G-CSF. The patient is then subjected to a conditioning regimen that in most cases consists of cyclophosphamide and anti-thymocyte globulin (ATG), with or without total body irradiation (800 cGy, with lung and renal shielding only in recent years). This is followed by reinfusion of stem cells. The rationale behind its use in scleroderma and other autoimmune diseases is that high dose immunosuppression used in the conditioning regimen depletes the dysregulated immune cells and the new stem cells infused can serve to reset the immune system homeostasis.

At present we have some data about role of HSCT in SSc from large multicenter randomized controlled trials:

- American Systemic Sclerosis Immune Suppression versus Transplant (ASSIST) trial:[32] It was a phase II open label randomized trial comparing the effects of autologous nonmyeloablative HSCT versus cyclophosphamide in 19 patients with SSc-ILD. Study demonstrated an improvement in the FVC and lung volumetric measurements of the patients in the HSCT group at the end of 2 years, whereas a decline in these parameters was noted in the cyclophosphamide group. The authors reported zero mortality at the end of 2 years attributing the low mortality rate to pretransplant screening for cardiac disease (exclusion criteria was total lymphocyte count <45%, left ventricular ejection fraction <40% symptomatic cardiac disease) and proposed that treatment in the form of HSCT early in the course of disease before the onset of cardiac dysfunction may lead to better outcomes
- Autologous Stem Cell Transplantation International Scleroderma (ASTIS) trial: It was a phase III RCT conducted in Europe under the auspices of the EULAR and the European Group for Blood and Bone Marrow Transplantation (EBMT). Study included 156 patients and compared high-dose immunosuppressive treatment (HDIT) and autologous HSCT with 12 monthly intravenous cyclophosphamide (750 mg/m^2) pulse treatment. Hematopoietic stem cell transplantation was found to be more effective than pulse cyclophosphamide and resulted in greater improvement in skin scores, functional ability, lung functions and quality of life. So HSCT resulted in significant long-term event free survival benefit but was associated with increased treatment-related mortality in the first year after treatment[33]
- Scleroderma: Cyclophosphamide or Transplantation (SCOT) trial: It is an ongoing phase II RCT in the United States funded by the National Institute of Health, comparing HSCT with high dose intravenous monthly cyclophosphamide.

The available data indicate that stem cell transplantation is a potential treatment modality which may result in significant and sustained clinical benefit, and the serious adverse events can be minimized by means of careful selection of patients.

Organ-targeted Therapies

Digital Vasculopathy: Raynaud's Phenomenon or Digital Ulcers

The management of Raynaud's phenomenon and digital ulcers depends on its severity and comprise of general measures along with pharmacologic therapy.

General Measures

All SSc patients need to take cold protective measures like avoiding cold temperature and cold water and should wear gloves, socks, and covered clothes. Patient is also advised to quit smoking or any other nicotine addiction, and protect hands and feet from trauma and vibration. In case of digital ulcers, proper wound care measures need to be taken and secondary infection if any treated as per the severity with topical and or oral antibiotics.

Calcium Channel Blockers

Calcium channel blockers (CCBs) are the mainstay therapy for Raynaud's phenomenon. Nifedipine, amlodipine and felodipine act on smooth muscle calcium channels, resulting in vasodilatation. Nifedipine is the most widely used and studied CCB used in secondary Raynaud's phenomenon.

Thompson et al. performed a metaanalysis of eight randomized, placebo-controlled, and double blind trials looking at the efficacy of CCBs for the treatment of secondary Raynaud's phenomenon due to SSc. They concluded that there is clinical improvement in the frequency and severity of ischemic attacks with a reduction in severity of symptoms by 35%. Hence, the efficacy of CCBs is modest at best. Potential side effects include headaches, lower extremity edema, and worsening of lower esophageal sphincter function.[34]

According to EULAR recommendations for the treatment of SSc, CCBs are the first-line therapy for Raynaud's phenomenon. These drugs have the potential to reduce the risk of developing new ulcers. However, there are limited data to support the use of CCBs in the treatment of digital ulcers once they have developed.[35]

Prostanoids or Prostacyclins

Prostacyclin is released by endothelial cells; its binding to platelet G protein-coupled receptors activates cyclic adenosine monophosphate and inhibits platelet activation and myosin light chain kinase causing smooth muscle relaxation and vasodilatation by activating protein kinase A. The prostacyclins currently available are iloprost and epoprostenol, both of which have been administered intravenously to promote primary healing of the ulcers.

A meta-analysis indicates that iloprost is also effective in reducing the frequency and severity of Raynaud's phenomenon in SSc patients. Iloprost, given intravenously (0.5-3 ng/kg per minute for 3-5 consecutive days sequentially) or orally (50-150 mg twice a day) significantly reduced the frequency of ischemic attacks. Oral prostanoids seem to be generally less effective than intravenous iloprost in the treatment of SSC and Raynaud's phenomenon, although some beneficial effects could be seen with higher doses.

Thus, prostaglandins should be considered first-line therapy in the treatment of digital ulcers as they reduce the ulcer healing time and prevent development of new ulcers as well.[36]

Prostanoids can be given for treatment of Raynaud's phenomenon in case the CCBs cannot be given or if there is poor control of symptoms with CCBs alone.

Endothelin Receptor Antagonists

Endothelin 1, a vasoconstrictive agent acts on both ETA and ETB receptors on endothelial cells. Bosentan, a dual endothelin receptor antagonist, has been used in the dose of 62.5 mg twice a day and has shown significant reduction in the development of new digital ulcers, although it does not hasten healing of existing ulcers.[37] It is also generally ineffective in the control of Raynaud's phenomenon.

The most common side effects include stomach upset, nausea, diarrhea, headache, anemia and peripheral edema. Teratogenicity and deranged liver enzymes are serious side effects. Monitoring of patient on Bosentan will include liver function test done at baseline and every month, thereafter, urine pregnancy test at baseline and every month, hemogram at baseline, 1 month and then every 3 months.

European League Against Rheumatism recommendation is to give Bosentan when CCBs and prostanoids have failed to prevent the formation of multiple new ischemic ulcers.

Phosphodiesterase Inhibitors

Sildenafil is a phosphodiesterase type 5 inhibitor that allows accumulation of cyclic guanosine monophosphate. Cyclic guanosine monophosphate causes a decrease in intracellular calcium, and the result is vascular smooth muscle relaxation and dilatation. Sildenafil has been shown to benefit patients with the Raynaud's phenomenon episodes, but data related to its effects on digital ulcers is very limited.[38] It is given in dosage of 50–100 mg/day. Tadalafil and verdinafil are other phosphodiesterase inhibitors which have been given for control of Raynaud's phenomenon. Cilostazol is a selective phosphodiesterase III inhibitor found to be effective in treatment of Raynaud's phenomenon in SSc patients in a recent open-label study.[39]

Surgical Options

Sympathectomy

Sympathectomy as cervical or thoracic sympathectomy or digital sympathectomy can be performed for persistent Raynaud's phenomenon or digital ischemia. This results in interruption of the sympathetic tone that is responsible for the exaggerated vasoconstriction in response to cold.[40]

Other treatment options described for Raynaud's phenomenon include pentoxyphylline, angiotensin II receptor blocker, prazosine, fluoxetine, topical nitroglycerine, and botulinum toxin.[40]

Binding Down of Skin

Binding down of skin is the most common manifestation of SSc and its extent of involvement is the basis of its classification into localized and diffuse forms. The modified Rodnan skin score, a measure of the extent of skin involvement, has been used as the primary outcome measure in clinical trials of SSc.

Methotrexate

Methotrexate has been shown to improve binding down of skin in approximately 80% of the SSc patients.[41] It is a safe, cost-effective, and EULAR recommends that it can be considered for treatment of skin manifestations of early diffuse SSc.

D-penicillamine

Penicillamine prevents collagen formation by blocking aldehyde groups involved in the inter- and intramolecular cross linkage of mature collagen. It also accelerates the turnover of insoluble collagen by cleaving intermolecular bonds that stabilize the fibrous structure. Derk et al. treated 84 patients with diffuse cutaneous SSc with D-penicillamine 750 mg/day and it showed statistically significant reduction in skin involvement as well as improvement of renal, cardiac and pulmonary involvement.[42]

Clements et al. reported that low dose (120 mg every other day) was as effective as high dose (750–1,000 mg/day) and the safety profile of low dose was significantly better. Barring few positive studies, majority literature does not support the role of penicillamine in the treatment of skin sclerosis.

Other drugs which have shown anecdotal role in reduction in skin binding down are detailed in table 7.[43,44]

Interstitial Lung Disease

Decision regarding the treatment of ILD is based on the symptoms of the patient and results of PFT and HRCT findings. Also we need to take into account weather the lung disease is still progressive or not as the currently available treatment options primarily halt the further progression of disease.

Goh et al. have suggested a useful prognostic algorithm based on HRCT findings and FVC. It classifies patients with SSc-related ILD into having "limited" (up to 20% lung involvement) and "extensive" (more than 20% lung involvement) disease based on HRCT findings. In indeterminate cases, an estimation of FVC helps to classify these patients with a FVC of 70%

Table 7: Various drugs for the management of binding down of skin in systemic sclerosis

References	Treatment modality	Dose	No. of patients	Remarks
Tashkin et al. (2006)[43]	Cyclophosphamide	50 mg once daily	158 (72 cyclophosphamide, 73 placebo)	Significant reduction in skin thickness at 12 months in patients with diffuse cutaneous systemic sclerosis
Le et al. (2011)[44]	Mycophenolate mofetil	500 mg twice daily for 2 week, if well tolerated dose was increased to 1,000 mg twice daily	98	Significant reduction was seen in modified Rodnan skin scores at 3, 6, and 12 months
Khanna et al. (2009)[45]	Relaxin	10 µg/kg/day and 25 µg/kg/day for 24 weeks	n = 42 (10 µg/kg/day), n = 95 (25 µg/kg/day for 24 weeks), and n = 94 (placebo)	No difference among the placebo, 10 µg/kg/day, and 25 µg/kg/day relaxin-treated patients for change in skin score
De souza et al. (2010)[46]	Pentoxiphylline/vitamin E	800 mg/800 IU QID	12	Significant reduction in TSS
Levy et al. (2004)[47]	Intravenous immunoglobulin	2 g/kg/course for 3–6 monthly courses	15	Significant reduction in the TSS
Bosello et al. (2010)[48]	Rituximab	1 gram 2 doses 2 weeks apart	9	May be effective for the treatment of SSc as studies showing significant improvement in skin scores and lung function
Khanna et al. (2011)[49]	Imatinib	600 mg/day for 1 year	20	Improvement not only in skin thickening, but also in Raynaud's phenomenon and pulmonary function test. However, further double blind, randomized, placebo-controlled trials are needed
Tamaki et al. (2012)[50]		100 mg/day for 6 months	3	
Pope et al. (2011)[51]		400 mg/day for 6 months	10	
Sakakibara et al. (2008)[52]	PUVA/UVA1	–	3	Histological improvement

PUVA, psoralen and ultraviolet A; UVA1, ultraviolet A1; TSS, total suspended solids.

or greater qualifying for limited disease. This algorithm correlates well with survival and also helps in making clinical treatment decisions.

Cyclophosphamide

In many clinical trials, cyclophosphamide has shown consistent improvement in ILD of SSc. Cyclophosphamide given orally at a dose of 1–2 mg/kg per day improved lung function tests, dyspnea score, and quality of life compared with placebo.[53,54] Thus, cyclophosphamide should be considered for treatment of ILD in SSc though the therapeutic benefits are modest and persist only for a short while after the drug is stopped.

In another trial, cyclophosphamide monthly pulses combined with low dose daily steroids lead to improvement in FVC.[54] Refer to table 8 for other studies on cyclophosphamide.

Mycophenolate Mofetil

Mycophenolate mofetil is a less toxic alternative to cyclophosphamide for treating SSc-related ILD. It has shown its efficacy in prospective studies and metaanalysis.[55]

Other useful drugs include azathioprine and rituximab.[56,57] Azathioprine (Table 8) is mainly useful as maintenance treatment after initial disease stabilization with intravenous or oral cyclophosphamide.

Lung transplant is an option in advanced cases of lung failure (Table 9).

Many other therapies have been tried in treatment of ILD (Table 10 and Appendix 1).

Renal Involvement

Previously, renal involvement was the most common cause of mortality but with advent of ACE inhibitors, prognosis of renal disease has

Table 8: Various drugs for the management of pulmonary involvement in systemic sclerosis				
References	Type of study	No. of patients	Dosing regimen	Remarks
Poormoghim et al. (2014)[18]	Retrospective study	36 patients: AZA (n = 15) Oral CYC (n = 21)	• AZA: 1.5–2 mg/kg/day • CYC: 2 mg/kg/day	Azathioprine can be effective in stabilizing lung function in selected SSc patients
Berezene et al. (2008)[58]	Retrospective study	27	• 6 monthly intravenous CYC followed by oral AZA 18 months	Stable improvement in PFT by 70% and 58% at 6 months and 2 years, respectively
Paone et al. (2007)[59]	Prospective	13	• 12 monthly pulses of CYC followed by AZA 100 mg/day	Initial improvement with CYC was maintained with AZA
Nadashkevich et al. (2006)[60]	RCT	60 CYC (n = 30) AZA (n = 30)	• CYC: 2 mg/kg/day 12 months maintained on 1 mg/kg/day • AZA: 2.5 mg/kg/day 12 months maintained on 2 mg/kg/day	A decline in the FVC and DLCO of the patients in the AZA group was noted at the end of 18 months whereas these parameters in the CYC group were reported to be stable
Dheda et al. (2004)[56]	Retrospective study	19	• Azathioprine and steroid given 12 months	Improvement in the mean percent predicted FVC and dyspnea score from a baseline value. Overall, five patients improved and three remained stable

AZA, azathioprine; CYC, cyclophosphamide; PFT, pulmonary function test; FVC, forced vital capacity; DLCO, diffusing capacity of the lungs for carbon monoxide.

Table 9: Various studies showing efficacy of lung transplantation in systemic sclerosis		
References	No. of patients	Remarks
Bernstein et al. (2015)[61]	229	A diagnosis of SSc may confer an increased risk of death 1 year following lung transplantation compared to a diagnosis of ILD but this risk is similar to that of PAH
Sottile et al. (2013)[62]	69 SSc-related ILD (23) ILD not SSc related (46)	Outcome of lung transplantation was similar whether it was done in SSc group or for non-SSc-related ILD
Saggar et al. (2010)[63]	52 SSc-ILD (14) IPF (38)	Comparable survival between IPF and SSc-ILD posttransplant patients (80% at 632 days). Analysis of post-transplant complications showed that acute graft rejection was significantly higher among patients with SSc-ILD while no difference was noted in pulmonary function and risk of infection
Shitrit et al. (2009)[64]	54	There was no difference in infection and rejection rates between the patients with scleroderma and other lung transplant recipients

SSc, systemic sclerosis; ILD, interstitial lung disease; IPF, idiopathic pulmonary fibrosis; PAH, pulmonary arterial hypertension.

Table 10: Other therapies used in the management of interstitial lung disease in systemic sclerosis

Treatment modality	References	Dose regimen	Number of patients	Remarks
Mesenchymal stem cells and induced pleuripotent stem cells	Andrade et al. (2009)[65]	–	–	Their potential to enhance epithelial cell repair is currently studied
Bosentan	Furaya et al. (2011)[66]	62.5 mg BD 24 months	9	Failed to show any beneficial effects
	Siebold et al. (2010)[67]	62.5 mg twice daily, increasing to 125 mg twice daily after 4 weeks	163 Bosentan (n = 77) Placebo (n = 86)	Failed to show any beneficial effects
Sildenafil	Zisman et al. (2010)[68]	–	180	Failed to show any beneficial effects
Rapamycin	Su et al. (2009)[69]	48 weeks	18 Mtx (n = 9) Rapamycin (n = 9)	There was decline in FVC in patient group treated with rapamycin. Significant improvement in MRSS was noted in both groups.
Cyclosporine	Clements et al. (2010)[70]	–	10	Effective in skin fibrosis but not in lung fibrosis
Antithymocyte globulin	Matteson et al. (1996)[71]	100 mg/kg over 4 h for 5 consecutive days	10	No improvement in PFT
Rituximab	Daoussis et al. (2010)[72]	4 weekly pulse	14	Higher improvement in PFT at 1 year follow-up in the rituximab group.
	Bosello et al. (2015)[48]	Two infusions 1 g 2 weeks apart	20	Increase in FVC, TLC at 12 month follow-up and improvement in mRSS
Imatinib	Fraticelli et al. (2011)[73]	200 mg/day 6 months	30	Lung function was stabilized. No improvement in skin binding
	Khanna et al. (2011)[49]	600 mg/day 1 year	20	Trend toward improvement in FVC and mRSS but higher rates of side effects
Tocilizumab	Shima et al.[74]	–	2	No change in lung parameters
Pirfenidone	Udwadia et al. (2015)[75]	200 mg TDS 20 months	Case report	Lung function showed trend toward improvement
	Nagai et al. (2002)[76]	40 mg/kg body weight 1 year	8	No change in lung parameters. No side effects reported.

PFT, pulmonary function tests; FVC, forced vital capacity; TLC, total lung capacity.

significantly improved.[25] All patients of SSc need to be monitored for SRC and more frequently in those who are at higher risk of SRC. Angiotensin converting enzyme inhibitors should not be given for prophylaxis against SRC rather started at the earliest stage of development of SRC.[77,78]

Gastrointestinal Involvement

Proton pump inhibitors have shown efficacy in reducing gastric reflux disease. Prokinetic drugs are used to reduce dysmotility-related symptoms like dysphagia, bloating, and pseudoobstruction. Mozapride is the most commonly used prokinetic drug.[79] Repeated courses of oral antibiotics need to be given when suspecting malabsorption due to bacterial overgrowth in gut.

CALCINOSIS CUTIS

Most of the treatment tried in calcinosis is not supported by enough evidence.[80]

Warfarin

Systemic warfarin therapy has been shown to be effective for small calcified deposits. Cukierman et al. reported that two of three patients with SSc and calcinosis cutis responded well to a 1-year treatment with low-dose warfarin (1 mg/day).[81]

Bisphosphonates

Bisphosphonates showed decrease in size and number of ulcers as well as reduction in pain in patients of calcinosis cutis as early as 3 months with no relapse.

Minocycline in the dose of 50–100 mg/day and diltiazem in a dose of 180 mg/day have also been found to be effective in calcinosis cutis.

Other treatment options include intralesional corticosteroid, extracorporeal shock wave therapy, surgical intervention, CO_2 laser, and rituximab.

CONCLUSION

Systemic sclerosis is a multifactorial autoimmune disease with complex pathogenesis. Its clinical features have been well characterized. Based on clinical findings patients classified into two subgroups—diffuse and localised cutaneous systemic sclerosis. Extent and severity of systemic involvement is varied. Every patient should be investigated in detail to find the extent of systemic disease as the therapy is mainly organ targeted. No therapy has definitive disease modifying effect but systemic corticosteroids and stem cell transplantation are two therapies with some disease modifying potential. Therapy is mainly directed towards treatment of raynauds phenomenon, skin thickening and hardening, lung, cardiac and renal disease. Besides emphasis should be laid on taking the general precautions as described before, good diet, and exercise. Patients should be followed up regularly in order to detect the complications at the earliest and manage accordingly. Mortality has reduced significantly with the current treatment options but the morbidity continues to be high.

REFERENCES

1. Maricq HR, Weinrich MC, Keil JE, et al. Prevalence of scleroderma spectrum disorders in the general population of South Carolina. Arthritis Rheum. 1989;32:998-1006.
2. Allcock RJ, Forrest I, Corris PA, et al. A study of the prevalence of systemic sclerosis in northeast England. Rheumatology (Oxford). 2004;43:596-602.
3. Tamaki T, Mori S, Takehara K. Epidemiological study of patients with systemic sclerosis in Tokyo. Arch Dermatol Res. 1991;283:366-71.
4. Chandran G, Smith M, Ahern MJ, et al. A study of scleroderma in South Australia: prevalence, subset characteristics and nailfold capillaroscopy. Aust NZ J Med. 1995;25:688-94.
5. Jimenez SA, Diaz A, Khalili K. Retroviruses and the pathogenesis of systemic sclerosis. Int Rev Immunol. 1995;12:159-75.
6. Pandey JP, LeRoy EC. Human cytomegalovirus and the vasculopathies of autoimmune diseases (especially scleroderma), allograft rejection, and coronary restenosis. Arthritis Rheum. 1998;41:10-5.
7. Diot E, Lesire V, Guilmot JL, et al. Systemic sclerosis and occupational risk factors: a case-control study. Occup Environ Med. 2002;59:545-9.
8. Reveille JD. Ethnicity and race and systemic sclerosis: how it affects susceptibility, severity, antibody genetics, and clinical manifestations. Curr Rheumatol Rep. 2003;5:160-7.
9. Crilly A, Hamilton J, Clark CJ, et al. Analysis of transforming growth factor beta1 gene polymorphisms in patients with systemic sclerosis. Ann Rheum Dis. 2002;61:678-81.
10. Tan FK, Wang N, Kuwana M, et al. Association of fibrillin 1 single-nucleotide polymorphism haplotypes with systemic sclerosis in Choctaw and Japanese populations. Arthritis Rheum. 2001;44:893-901.

11. Ho KT, Reveille JD. The clinical relevance of autoantibodies in scleroderma. Arthritis Res Ther. 2003;5:80-93.
12. Sakkas LI, Xu B, Artlett CM, et al. Oligoclonal T cell expansion in the skin of patients with systemic sclerosis. J Immunol. 2002;168:3649-59.
13. Attisano L, Wrana JL. Signal transduction by the TGF-beta superfamily. Science. 2002;296:1646-7.
14. Leask A, Holmes A, Abraham DJ. Connective tissue growth factor: a new and important player in the pathogenesis of fibrosis. Curr Rheumatol Rep. 2002;4:136-42.
15. Herrick AL. Vascular function in systemic sclerosis. Curr Opin Rheumatol. 2000;12:527-33.
16. LeRoy EC, Black C, Fleischmajer R, et al. Scleroderma (systemic sclerosis): classification, subsets and pathogenesis. J Rheumatol. 1988;15:202-5.
17. Barnett AJ, Miller M, Littlejohn GO. The diagnosis and classification of scleroderma (systemic sclerosis). Postgrad Med J. 1988;64:121-5.
18. Poormoghim H, Lucas M, Fertig N, et al. Systemic sclerosis sine scleroderma. Demographic, clinical, and serological features and survival in forty-eight patients. Arthritis Rheum. 2000;43:444-51.
19. Masy AT, Rodnan GP, Medsger TA Jr, et al. Preliminary criteria for the classification of systemic sclerosis (scleroderma). Arthritis Rheum. 1980;23:581-90.
20. Van den Hoogen F, Khanna D, Fransen J, et al. 2013 classification criteria for systemic sclerosis: an American College of Rheumatology/European League against Rheumatism Collaborative Initiative. Ann Rheum Dis. 2013;72:1747-55.
21. Silver RM. Clinical aspects of systemic sclerosis (scleroderma). Medicine (Baltimore). 2010;89:159-65.
22. Ramon Y, Samra H, Oberman M. Mandibular condylosis and apertognathia as presenting symptoms in progressive systemic sclerosis (scleroderma). Pattern of mandibular bony lesions and atrophy of masticatory muscles in PSS, presumably caused by affected muscular arteries. Oral Surg Oral Med Oral Pathol. 1987;63:269-74.
23. Pogrel MA. Unilateral osteolysis of the mandibular angle and coronoid process in scleroderma. Int J Oral Maxillofac Surg. 1988;17:155-6.
24. Ghosh SK, Bandyopadhyay D, Saha I, et al. Mucocutaneous and demographic features of systemic sclerosis: a profile of 46 patients from eastern India. Indian J Dermatol. 2012;57:201-5.
25. Mouthon L, Bérezné A, Bussone G, et al. Scleroderma renal crisis: a rare but severe complication of systemic sclerosis. Clin Rev Allergy Immunol. 2011;40:84-91.
26. Tian X-P, Zhang X. Gastrointestinal complications of systemic sclerosis. World J Gastroenterol. 2013;19:7062-8.
27. Vincent FM, Van Houzen RN. Trigeminal sensory neuropathy and bilateral carpal tunnel syndrome: the initial manifestation of mixed connective tissue disease. J Neurol Neurosurg Psychiatry. 1980;43:458-60.
28. Hudson M, Fritzler MJ, Baron M; Canadian Scleroderma Research Group (CSRG). Systemic sclerosis: establishing diagnostic criteria. Medicine (Baltimore). 2010;89:159-65.
29. Kaloudi O, Matucci-Cerinic M. Organ involvement in systemic sclerosis from early detection and assessment to follow-up. Eur Musculoskel Rev. 2011;6:38-42.
30. Pasricha JS. Systemic sclerosis and dexamethasone cyclophosphamide pulse therapy. Indian J Dermatol Venereol Leprol. 2009;75:510-11.
31. Sameem F, Hassan I, Ahmad QM, et al. Dexamethasone pulse therapy in patients of systemic sclerosis: is it a viable proposition? A study from Kashmir. Indian J Dermatol. 2010;55:355-8.
32. Burt RK, Shah SJ, Dill K, et al. Autologous non-myeloablative haemopoietic stem-cell transplantation compared with pulse cyclophosphamide once per month for systemic sclerosis (ASSIST): an open-label, randomised phase 2 trial. Lancet. 2011;378:498-506.
33. van Laar JM, Farge D, Sont JK, (EBMT/EULAR Scleroderma Study Group) et al. Autologous hematopoietic stem cell transplantation vs intravenous pulse cyclophosphamide in diffuse cutaneous systemic sclerosis: a randomized clinical trial. JAMA. 2014;311:2490-8.
34. Thompson AE, Shea B, Welch V, et al. Calcium-channel blockers for Raynaud's phenomenon in systemic sclerosis. Arthritis Rheum. 2001;44:1841-7.
35. Kowal-Bielecka O, Landewé R, Avouac J, et al. EULAR recommendations for the treatment of systemic sclerosis: a report from the EULAR Scleroderma Trials and Research group (EUSTAR). Ann Rheum Dis. 2009;68:620-8.
36. Pope J, Fenlon D, Thompson A, et al. Iloprost and cisaprost for Raynaud's phenomenon in progressive systemic sclerosis. Cochrane Database Syst Rev. 1998;CD000953.
37. Matucci-Cerinic M, Denton CP, Furst DE, et al. Bosentan treatment of digital ulcers related to systemic sclerosis: results from the RAPIDS-2 randomised, double-blind, placebo-controlled trial. Ann Rheum Dis. 2011;70:32-38.
38. De LaVega AJ, Derk CT. Phosphodiesterase-5 inhibitors for the treatment of Raynaud's: a novel indication. Expert Opin Investig Drugs. 2009;18:23-29.
39. Negrini S, Spanò F, Penza E, Rollando D, Indiveri F, Filaci G, Puppo F. Efficacy of cilostazol for the treatment of Raynaud's phenomenon in systemic sclerosis patients. Clin Exp Med. 2016;16:407-12.
40. Levien TL. Advances in the treatment of Raynaud's phenomenon. Vasc Health Risk Manag. 2010;6:167-177.
41. Krishna Sumanth M, Sharma VK, Khaitan BK, et al. Evaluation of oral methotrexate in the treatment of systemic sclerosis. Int J Dermatol. 2007;46:218-23.
42. Derk CT, Huaman G, Jimenez SA. A retrospective randomly selected cohort study of D penicillamine treatment in rapidly progressive diffuse cutaneous systemic sclerosis of recent onset. Br J Dermatol. 2008;158:1063-8.
43. Tashkin DP, Elashoff R, Clements PJ, et al. Scleroderma Lung Study Research Group. Effects of 1-year treatment with cyclophosphamide on outcomes at 2 years in scleroderma lung disease. Am J Respir Crit Care Med. 2007;176:1026-34.
44. Le EN, Wigley FM, Shah AA, et al. Long-term experience of mycophenolate mofetil for treatment of diffuse cutaneous systemic sclerosis. Ann Rheum Dis. 2011;70:1104-7.

45. Khanna D, Clements PJ, Furst DE, et al. Recombinant human relaxin in the treatment of systemic sclerosis with diffuse cutaneous involvement: a randomized, double-blind, placebo-controlled trial. Arthritis Rheum. 2009;60:1102-11.
46. de Souza RB, Macedo AR, Kuruma KA, et al. Pentoxyphylline in association with vitamin E reduces cutaneous fibrosis in systemic sclerosis. Clin Rheumatol. 2009;28:1207-12.
47. Levy Y, Amital H, Langevitz P, et al. Intravenous immunoglobulin modulates cutaneous involvement and reduces skin fibrosis in systemic sclerosis: an open-label study. Arthritis Rheum. 2004;50:1005-7.
48. Bosello SL, De Luca G, Rucco M, et al. Long-term efficacy of B cell depletion therapy on lung and skin involvement in diffuse systemic sclerosis. Semin Arthritis Rheum. 2015;44:428-36.
49. Khanna D, Saggar R, Mayes MD, et al. A one-year, phase I/IIa, open-label pilot trial of imatinib mesylate in the treatment of systemic sclerosis-associated active interstitial lung disease. Arthritis Rheum. 2011;63:3540-6.
50. Tamaki Z, Asano Y, Hatano M, et al. Efficacy of low-dose imatinib mesylate for cutaneous involvement in systemic sclerosis: a preliminary report of three cases. Mod Rheumatol. 2012;22:94-9.
51. Pope J, McBain D, Petrlich L, et al. Imatinib in active diffuse cutaneous systemic sclerosis: results of a six-month, randomized, double-blind, placebo-controlled, proof-of-concept pilot study at a single center. Arthritis Rheum. 2011;63:3547-51.
52. Sakakibara N, Sugano S, Morita A. Ultrastructural changes induced in cutaneous collagen by ultraviolet-A1 and psoralen plus ultraviolet A therapy in systemic sclerosis. J Dermatol. 2008;35:63-9.
53. Tashkin DP, Elashoff R, Clements PJ, et al. Cyclophosphamide versus placebo in scleroderma lung disease. N Engl J Med. 2006,354:2655-66.
54. Hoyles RK, Ellis RW, Wellsbury J, et al. A multicenter, prospective, randomized, double-blind, placebo-controlled trial of corticosteroids and intravenous cyclophosphamide followed by oral azathioprine for the treatment of pulmonary fibrosis in scleroderma. Arthritis Rheum. 2006,54:3962-70.
55. Simeon-Aznar CP, Fonollosa-Pla V, Tolosa-Vilella C, et al. Effect of mycophenolate sodium in scleroderma-related interstitial lung disease. Clin Rheumatol. 2011;30:1393-8.
56. Dheda K, Lalloo UG, Cassim B, Mody GM. Experience with azathioprine in systemic sclerosis associated with interstitial lung disease. Clin Rheumatol. 2004;23:306-9.
57. Yoo WH. Successful treatment of steroid and cyclophosphamide-resistant diffuse scleroderma-associated interstitial lung disease with rituximab. Rheumatol Int. 2012;32:795-8.
58. Bérezné A, Ranque B, Valeyre D, et al. Therapeutic strategy combining intravenous cyclophosphamide followed by oral azathioprine to treat worsening interstitial lung disease associated with systemic sclerosis: a retrospective multicenter open-label study. J Rheumatol. 2008;35:1064-72.
59. Paone C, Chiarolanza I, Cuomo G, et al. Twelve-month azathioprine as maintenance therapy in early diffuse systemic sclerosis patients treated for 1-year with low dose cyclophosphamide pulse therapy. Clin Exp Rheumatol. 2007;25(4):613-6.
60. Nadashkevich O, Davis P, Fritzler M, et al. A randomized unblinded trial of cyclophosphamide versus azathioprine in the treatment of systemic sclerosis. Clin Rheumatol. 2006;25:205-12.
61. Bernstein EJ, Peterson ER, Sell JL, et al. Survival of adults with systemic sclerosis following lung transplantation: a nationwide cohort study. Arthritis Rheumatol. 2015;67:1314-22.
62. Sottile PD, Iturbe D, Katsumoto TR, et al. Outcomes in systemic sclerosis-related lung disease after lung transplantation. Transplantation. 2013;95:975-80.
63. Saggar R, Khanna D, Furst DE, et al. Systemic sclerosis and bilateral lung transplantation: a single centre experience. Eur Respir J. 2010;36:893-900.
64. Shitrit D, Amital A, Peled N, et al. Lung transplantation in patients with scleroderma: case series, review of the literature, and criteria for transplantation. Clin Transplant. 2009;23:178-83.
65. de Andrade JA, Thannickal VJ. Innovative approaches to the therapy of fibrosis. Curr Opin Rheumatol. 2009;21:649-55.
66. Furuya Y, Kuwana M. Effect of Bosentan on systemic sclerosis-associated interstitial lung disease ineligible for cyclophosphamide therapy: a prospective open-label study. J Rheumatol. 2011;38:2186-92.
67. Seibold JR, Denton CP, Furst DE, et al. Randomized, prospective, placebo-controlled trial of bosentan in interstitial lung disease secondary to systemic sclerosis. Arthritis Rheum. 2010;62:2101-8.
68. Zisman DA, Schwarz M, Anstrom KJ, et al. A controlled trial of sildenafil in advanced idiopathic pulmonary fibrosis. N Engl J Med. 2010;363:620-8.
69. Su T-IK, Khanna D, Furst DE, et al. Rapamycin versus methotrexate in early diffuse systemic sclerosis: results from a randomized, single-blind pilot study. Arthritis Rheum. 2009;60:3821-30.
70. Clements PJ, Lachenbruch PA, Sterz M, et al. Cyclosporine in systemic sclerosis. Results of a forty-eight-week open safety study in ten patients. Arthritis Rheum. 1993;36:75-83.
71. Matteson EL, Shbeeb MI, McCarthy TG, et al. Pilot study of antithymocyte globulin in systemic sclerosis. Arthritis Rheum. 1996;39:1132-7.
72. Daoussis D, Liossis SN, Tsamandas AC, et al. Experience with rituximab in scleroderma: results from a 1-year, proof-of-principle study. Rheumatology (Oxford). 2010;49:271-80.
73. Fraticelli P, Gabrielli B, Pomponio G, et al. Low-dose oral imatinib in the treatment of systemic sclerosis interstitial lung disease unresponsive to cyclophosphamide: a phase II pilot study. Arthritis Res Ther. 2014;16:R144.
74. Shima Y, Kuwahara Y, Murota H, et al. The skin of patients with systemic sclerosis softened during the treatment with anti-IL-6 receptor antibody tocilizumab. Rheumatology (Oxford). 2010;49:2408-12.
75. Udwadia ZF, Mullerpattan JB, Balakrishnan C, et al. Improved pulmonary function following pirfenidone

treatment in a patient with progressive interstitial lung disease associated with systemic sclerosis. Lung India. 2015;32:50-2.
76. Nagai S, Hamada K, Shigematsu M, et al. Open-label compassionate use one year-treatment with pirfenidone to patients with chronic pulmonary fibrosis. Intern Med. 2002;41:1118-23.
77. Steen VD, Costantino JP, Shapiro AP, et al. Outcome of renal crisis in systemic sclerosis: relation to availability of angiotensin converting enzyme (ACE) inhibitors. Ann Intern Med. 1990;113:352-7.
78. Steen VD, Medsger TA Jr. Long-term outcomes of scleroderma renal crisis. Ann Intern Med. 2000;133:600-3.
79. Sallam H, McNearney TA, Chen JD. Systematic review: pathophysiology and management of gastrointestinal dysmotility in systemic sclerosis (scleroderma). Aliment Pharmacol Ther. 2006;23:691-712.
80. Bienvenu B. Treatment of subcutaneous calcinosis in systemic disorders. Rev Med Interne. 2014;35:444-52.
81. Cukierman T, Elinav E, Korem M, et al. Low dose warfarin treatment for calcinosis in patients with systemic sclerosis. Ann Rheum Dis. 2004;63:1341-3.

9

CHAPTER

Morphea and Morpheaform Disorders

CR Srinivas, Pradeep Balasubramanian

INTRODUCTION

The word morphea is derived from Greek which means form or structure.[1] It is characterized by circumscribed area(s) of skin induration due to sclerosis of dermis and subcutaneous tissue which in some cases can extend to involve fascia, muscle, and underlying bone.

Clinically, morphea is characterized by an asymmetric distribution confined to localized area(s), thus called localized scleroderma. It is differentiated from systemic sclerosis (SSc) which has the following features in addition:
- Symmetric skin involvement
- Involvement of acral areas (sclerodactyly)
- Diffuse involvement of face
- Internal organ involvement (commonly lungs and gastrointestinal tract)
- Presence of Raynaud's phenomenon
- Nail-fold capillary abnormalities.

INCIDENCE

Though all ages are affected, the peak incidence is between 20 to 40 years. Female to male ratio is 3:1. Linear morphea is more common in children whereas circumscribed and generalized morphea are more common in adults.[2]

ETIOPATHOGENESIS

The exact etiology is unknown. The possible triggers mentioned are trauma, radiation, drugs (penicillamine, bromocriptine, and bleomycin), vaccines (Bacillus Calmette–Guérin, diphtheria, pertussis, and tetanus, measles, mumps, and rubella, and tetanus), vitamin B12 and vitamin K injections, and following varicella and herpes zoster. The role of *Borrelia* as a cause is controversial.[3]

The autoimmune nature of the disease can be explained by the presence of the following antibodies:
- Antinuclear antibodies (ANA) are positive in approximately 50% patients
- Antihistone antibodies
- Anti-single-stranded deoxyribonucleic acid (ssDNA) antibodies.

These antibodies are more frequently detected in generalized scleroderma followed by linear scleroderma and with lesser frequency in localized scleroderma.

The trigger factors and autoantibodies incite endothelial changes characterized by swelling and expression of adhesion molecules. This leads to the recruitment of T lymphocytes which produce transforming growth factor-β and other inflammatory mediators. These mediators stimulate the fibroblast thus resulting in the synthesis of type-1 collagen, glycosaminoglycans and fibronectin.

CLINICAL FEATURES

The various clinical types of morphea are as follows:

Morphea and Morpheaform Disorders

- Circumscribed plaque morphea (morphea en plaque)
- Morphea profundus or subcutaneous (deep) morphea
- Linear morphea
- En coup de sabre (frontoparietal morphea)
- Generalized morphea
- Superficial morphea
- Bullous morphea
- Guttate morphea
- Nodular (keloidal) morphea
- Zosteriform morphea
- Mixed morphea.

Commonly Involved Sites

- Circumscribed and generalized morphea commonly involves the trunk
- Linear scleroderma commonly involves extremities
- Except for en coup de sabre and progressive facial hemiatrophy, face and acral areas are typically spared; these areas are characteristically involved in systemic sclerosis.

Stages of Cutaneous Lesions

Following are the three stages of evolution of morphea cutaneous lesions:

1. There is marked inflammation (inflammatory stage) at the beginning of the disease which kindles the fibroblasts resulting in collagen synthesis. This stage is not clinically apparent in all the patients
2. As the disease progress, the inflammation wanes whereas the sclerosis progresses (sclerotic stage)
3. Over months to years, the indurated plaque softens resulting in an atrophic plaque with hypo- or hyperpigmentation (atrophic stage).

Patients usually present in stage 2 or 3 to the dermatologist and it is important to identify the stage as the plan of treatment differs for different stages.

Table 1 depicts the pathological changes correlated with the clinical features during the course of disease progression.

Circumscribed Plaque Lesions (Morphea En Plaque)

It presents as single or multiple round to oval patch or plaque which is erythematous or dusky red initially (Fig. 1) then progresses in size to

Table 1: Co-relation of clinical findings and pathological changes in the skin

Pathologic changes	Clinical features
Inflammation	Erythematous patch or thin plaque
Inflammation and early sclerosis	Central sclerotic (indurated) plaque with peripheral erythema/lilac borders (Fig. 1)
Sclerosis and waning inflammation	Central sclerosis and peripheral hyperpigmented borders
Scarring and damage	Atrophy of dermis and subcutis, sometimes extending to involve fascia, muscle, or bone

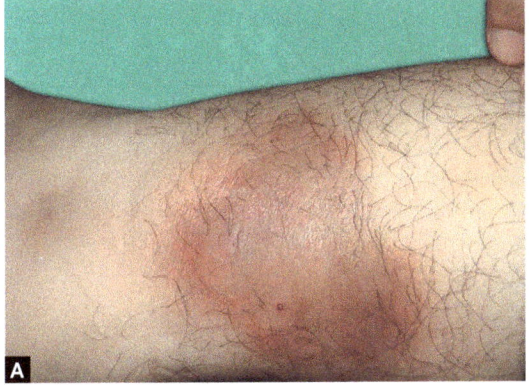 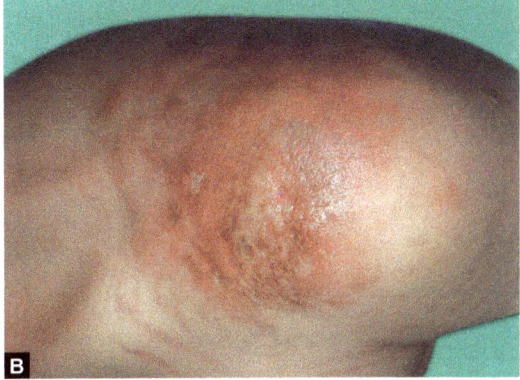

FIGURE 1: Recent onset Ill-defined morphea plaques showing prominent erythema at the margins. **A,** Leg; **B,** Shoulder.

Skin in Rheumatologic Diseases

achieve a maximum dimension of 2-15 cm. When multiple, the lesions are asymmetrical. The central portion turns ivory colored and border becomes lilac colored which later on turns hyperpigmented (Fig. 2). In darker skin types, lilac colored annular border is less apparent and the whole lesion turns sclerotic and epidermis develops brownish hyperpigmentation which often dominates over the white sclerosis. The surface is smooth and shiny which can rarely be nodular. The lesions are devoid of hair and it fails to sweat. Some patients may complain of itching which is due to the xerosis as a consequence of impaired sweating.

The course of the lesion is usually variable. The disease resolves in 3-5 years without treatment during which the sclerosis resolves leaving hypo- or hyperpigmented atrophic patch. Patients with circumscribed morphea should be closely followed up as linear and segmental morphea can begin with initial plaque lesions.

The atrophic stage (Fig. 3) is characterized by:
- Cigarette paper wrinkling of the surface (papillary dermal atrophy)
- Cliff drop appearance (deep dermal atrophy)
- Deep indentations (subcutaneous atrophy).

Deep Morphea (Morphea Profundus)

This variant involves the deep dermis, subcutis, fascia, and muscle. The skin feels thick and is bound down to the underlying fascia and muscle. Groove sign (depression) can be present at the site of tendon and ligaments. Overlying skin can be hypo- or hyperpigmented. The surface may have cobblestone or pseudo-cellulite appearance. Osteoma cutis may develop within such lesions.[4]

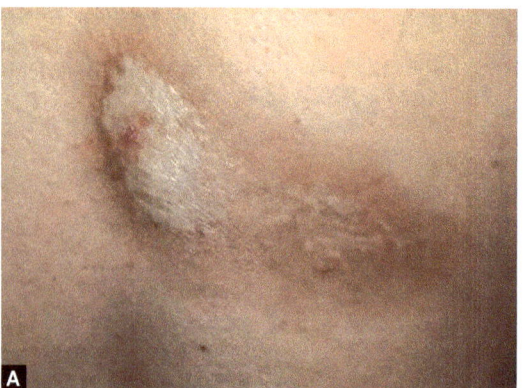 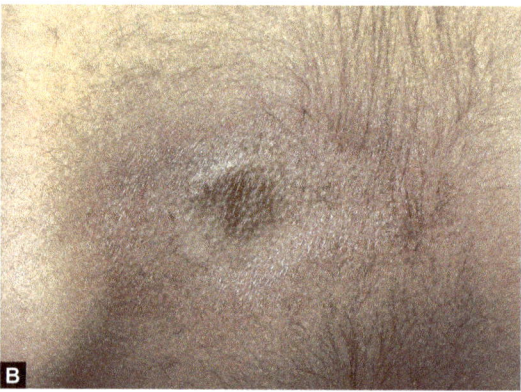

FIGURE 2: A, Morphea en plaque over back with prominent central ivory sclerosis; **B,** Morphea en plaque with central sclerosis and erythematous margins suggesting activity.

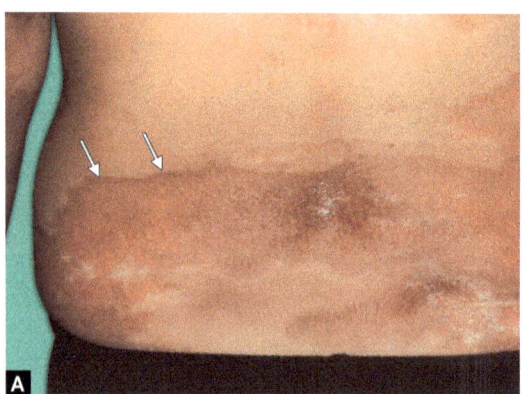 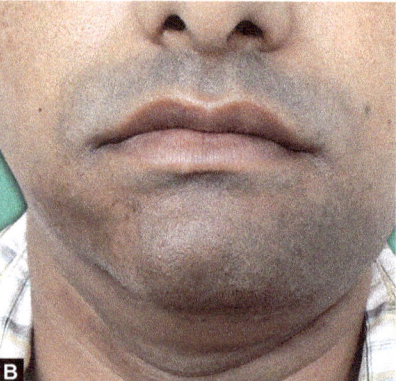

FIGURE 3: A, Cliff drop appearance at the margins of morphea plaque in a subsiding stage; **B,** Deep indentation at atrophic stage in morphea plaque over chin.

Linear Morphea

It involves limbs or face causing functional disability and severe aesthetic sequelae. It is more common in children. Limbs are affected twice as often as face. Three subtypes exist namely:

1. Linear Limb Morphea: It more commonly involves the lower limb (legs) than the upper limb, and is usually unilateral but can be bilateral (Figs 4 and 5). Rarely thorax, abdomen, and buttocks can be involved by the linear lesions. The essential morphological features are similar to plaque morphea, but the lilac ring is inconspicuous or only present at the advancing border. The lesion can involve the deeper tissues similar to morphea profunda resulting in severe flexion deformity or growth disturbance. Sometimes the circumferential band surrounding the limb or finger can result in limb atrophy or ainhum. The tissue, distal to the band can develop edema. The linear lesions can have skip lesions in between. Linear morphea may follow lines of Blaschko (Fig. 6)[5]

2. En Coup De Sabre: It means scar of a sabre-wound. It presents as an atrophic linear plaque (groove) on the forehead (fronto-parietal region) extending to the scalp where it causes cicatricial alopecia and it may extend to involve eye brow, nose, and lips (Fig. 7). It commences either as linear streak or row of small plaques (Fig. 8) that coalesce. Paramedian aspect is more common than the median aspect (Fig. 9). It can sometimes involve the underlying muscle and bone (Fig. 10). Neurological manifestations such as seizures, focal neurological deficit, and headache can be associated.[6] It may involve the jaw and gum on the corresponding side causing alteration in spacing and direction. Corresponding side of tongue and salivary glands can also become atrophic. A variety of ocular lesions of the corresponding side can result such as enophthalmos, atrophy of eyelids, oculomotor muscles, iris, and fundus[7]

3. Parry-Romberg Syndrome or Progressive Hemifacial Atrophy: It is characterized by progressive unilateral facial atrophy involving the skin, subcutis, muscle, and bone. Though it can be accompanied by morphea elsewhere,

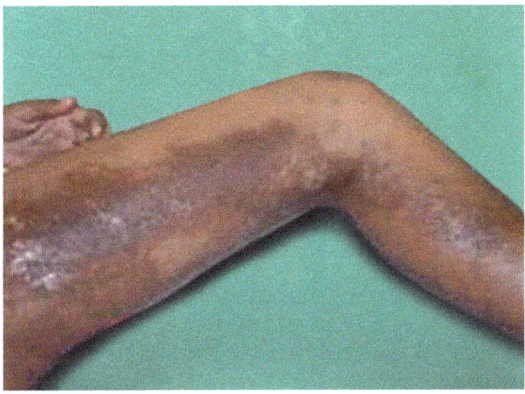

FIGURE 4: Linear morphea involving the left lower limb in a child.

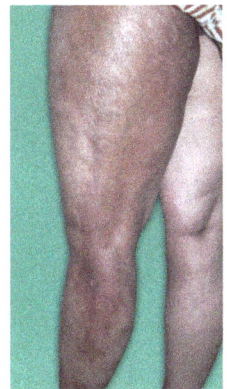

FIGURE 5: Wide linear plaque of morphea over left leg.

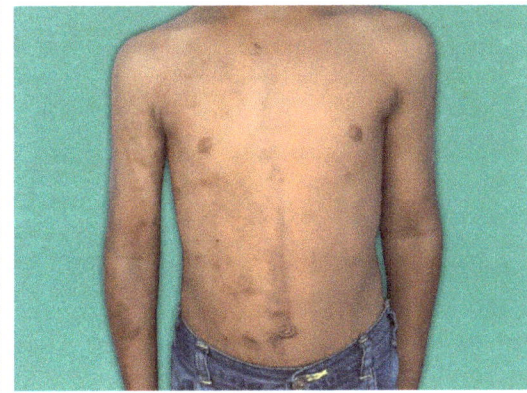

FIGURE 6: Blaschkoid morphea over the right hemi-thorax and the right upper limb.

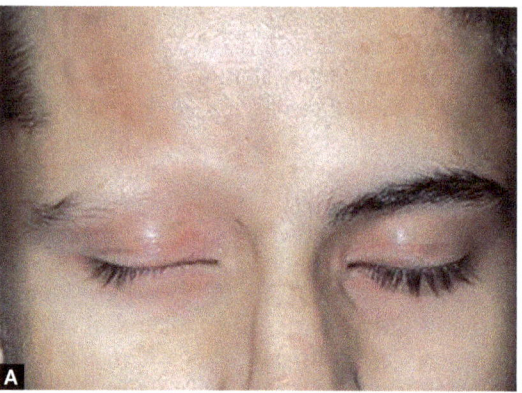
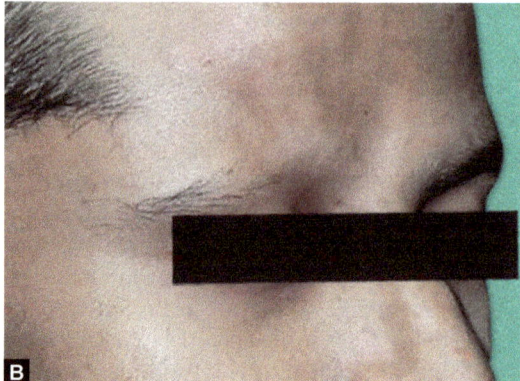

FIGURE 7: En coup de sabre over right frontoparietal region.

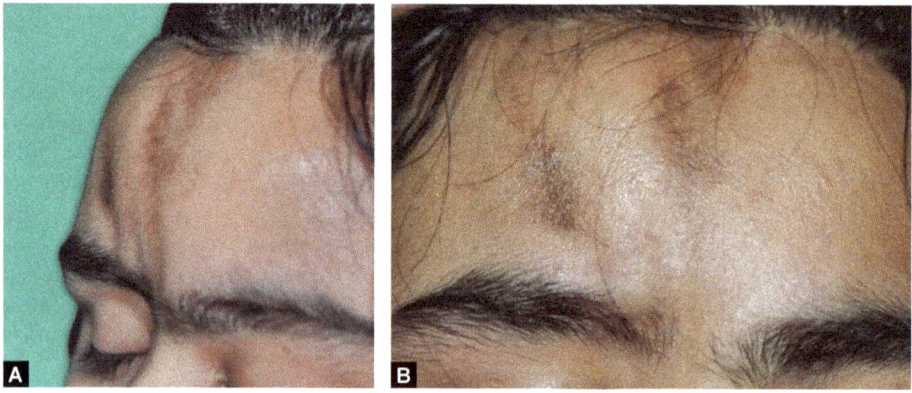

FIGURE 8: Multiple small plaques coalescing to form en coup de sabre.

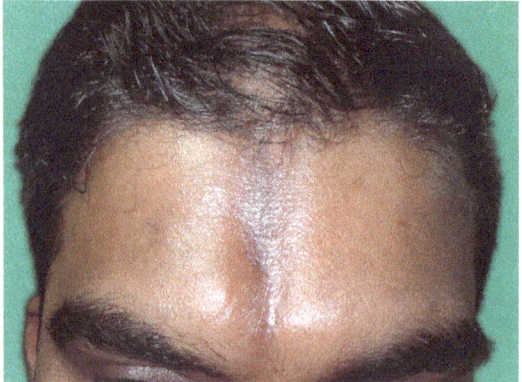

FIGURE 9: Liner morphea over centre of forehead with severe hyperpigmentation in overlying skin.

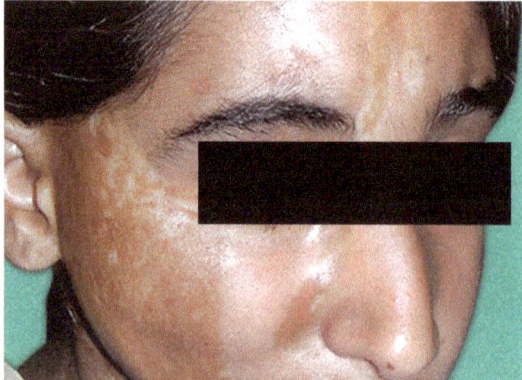

FIGURE 10: Extensive morphea over face affecting underlying muscles and bone.

the site involved by Parry-Romberg syndrome or progressive hemifacial atrophy will not be preceded by sclerotic lesion (Fig. 11).

Generalized Morphea (Fig. 12)

To be called so, the disease must satisfy the following criteria:
- Presence of four or more morphea lesions.

Involvement of two or more body areas out of seven areas, i.e., head and neck, right upper limb (UL), left UL, right lower limb (LL), left LL, anterior trunk and posterior trunk.8 The common sites involved are upper trunk, breast, abdomen, and upper thighs.

It can sometimes be symmetric, in which case it must be differentiated from systemic sclerosis by the features mentioned previously.

Superficial Morphea

It is characterized by hyperpigmented (sometimes hypopigmented) patches without induration as seen in morphea. There is mild to moderate dermal sclerosis limited to upper dermis. It is most frequent in females. Atrophoderma of Pasini and Pierini, characterized by cliff drop borders, bears a close resemblance to superficial morphea and some authors use these two terms interchangeably (Fig. 13).

Bullous Morphea

In some morphea lesions, the obstruction of the lymphatics by the sclerosing process might result in blister formation. It is more commonly seen in the lower limbs. O'Leary suggested eosinophilic major basic protein (MBP) could also be a cause,

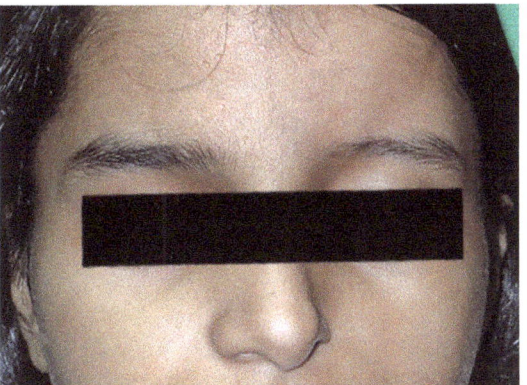

FIGURE 11: Parry-Romberg syndrome.

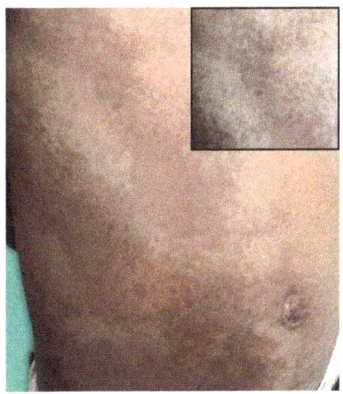

FIGURE 13: Superficial morphea and atrophoderma of Pasini and Pierini.

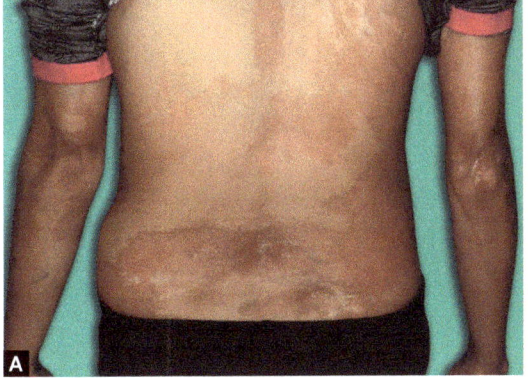

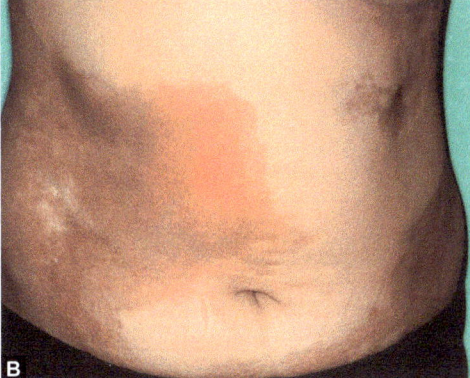

FIGURE 12: Multiple large morphea plaques present over the back, anterior abdomen and upper limbs in a case of generalized morphea.

since MBP from eosinophils was demonstrated in the base of the blister which would have caused tissue destruction resulting in the bulla formation.[9]

Guttate Morphea

It presents as multiple nummular plaques, which start as superficial lesions and later on may become deeper. It might closely resemble lichen sclerosus et atrophicus. These two disorders can have similar pathogenesis and sometimes can coexist.

Nodular (Keloidal) Morphea

It is characterized by development of keloidal nodules on the area of localized scleroderma, the histopathology of which is similar to keloid. Rarely, it may occur with systemic sclerosis too.

Zosteriform Morphea

It is characterized by distribution of the lesions along a dermatome, more commonly on the trunk (Fig. 14). There are reports of morphea arising as Wolf's isotopic response at the site of healed herpes zoster.[10]

Mixed Morphea

When two or more morphea subtypes exist in a same patient, then it is described as mixed morphea.[11]

LOCALIZED SCLERODERMA OF CHILDHOOD

Prevalence of morphea in children is similar to that of adults. Linear scleroderma is most common variant, followed by plaque type, generalized and sclerotic.[12]

Disabling Pansclerotic Morphea of Childhood

It is a rare variant characterized by involvement of skin, even extending further to involve muscle and bone in some patients (Figs 15 and 16). Severe joint contractures can result. It may cause claw hand and patients may walk on the tip of toes due to the involvement of Achilles tendon. Intense

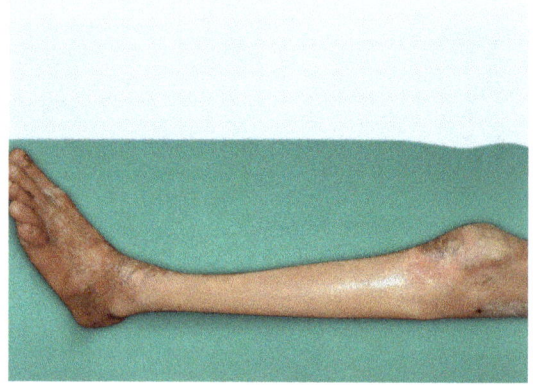

FIGURE 15: Pan sclerotic morphea over left leg.

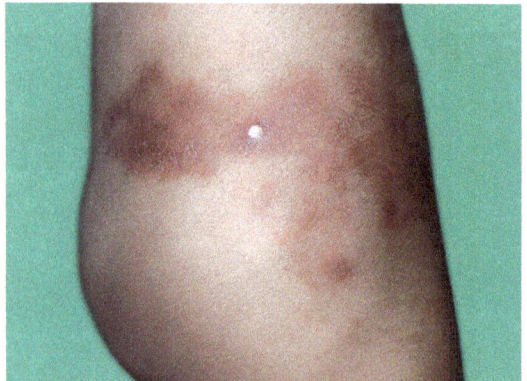

FIGURE 14: Linear morphea in segmental distribution over lower trunk in 10 year boy.

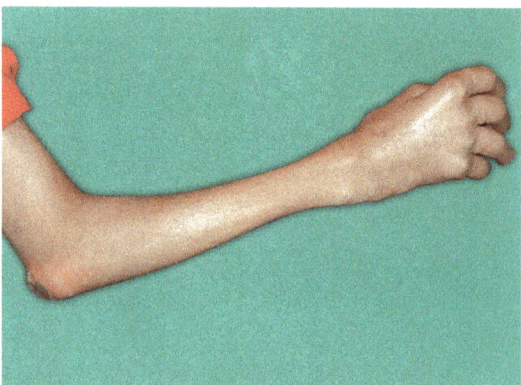

FIGURE 16: Pan sclerotic morphea resulting in contracture at elbow.

pain due to involvement of cutaneous nerves can happen. Osteoporosis and other bony changes may result. Few patients can have esophageal, pulmonary, and periodontal changes. Treatment is unsatisfactory many a times.[13]

Associated Disorders and Complications

Morphea can be associated with extracutaneous manifestations (ECMs) more commonly in the proximity of the morphea lesions. Extracutaneous manifestations involving the affected extremities include restricted joint mobility, limb length discrepancy, muscle weakness, carpel tunnel syndrome and peripheral neuropathy particularly in linear and deep morphea. En coup de sabre can be associated with neurological and ocular manifestations as mentioned earlier (refer Box 1).

ECMs unrelated to the proximity of the skin lesion include arthritis, myalgia, neuropathies, Raynaud's phenomenon and esophageal dysmotility. ECMs are more common in generalized and linear morphea. Circumferential sclerosis of limbs may cause compartment syndrome. Rarely, chronic ulcer (Fig. 17) secondary to Pansclerotic morphea can get transformed to squamous cell carcinoma (SCC). Autoimmune disorders associated with increased frequency in morphea include psoriasis, systemic lupus erythematosus (SLE), multiple sclerosis, vitiligo, thyroiditis, hepatitis, pernicious anemia and myasthenia gravis.

Histopathology

The biopsy must be of adequate depth so as to include the subcutis. The histopathology

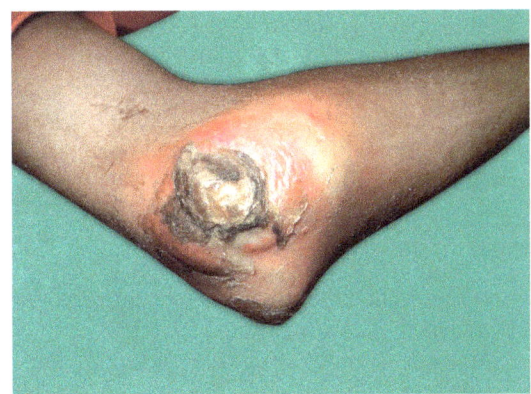

FIGURE 17: Ischemic ulcer over elbow in a morphea patient.

depends on the stage of morphea and the depth of involvement by the disease process. Biopsy taken from the early lesion depict infiltrates comprised of lymphocytes admixed with plasma cells and occasional eosinophils in the interstitial space of dermis (more in reticular dermis), perivascular area and the septa of the subcutis. The biopsy from the sclerotic lesion demonstrates vertically cut borders. There is increased collagenization of the dermis and subcutaneous tissue which is thickened, tightly packed, homogenous, and hypereosinophilic. The pilosebaceous unit appears to be pulled up (an illusion due to the collagenization of the subcutis). The epidermis is normal unto the sclerotic stage after when it becomes thinned out with loss of rete ridges. In morphea profunda and pansclerotic morphea, even the fascia and muscle show sclerosis (Also refer chapter 3: Dermatopathology of Rheumatologic Diseases).

Laboratory Abnormalities

As mentioned earlier, antibodies against ssDNA, anti-histone antibodies, and ANA are frequently detected in patients with generalized and linear morphea when compared to other morphea subtypes. Presence of these antibodies, eosinophilia, hypergammaglobulinemia, and elevated erythrocyte sedimentation rate or C-reactive protein indicates the disease activity. Carboxy terminal peptide of serum procollagen-1 signifying the disease activity needs detailed evaluation.[14]

Ultrasonography (USG) is a useful tool in assessing the extent and depth of the lesions

---

Box 1: Associations of morphea

- Morphea over extremities: Restricted joint mobility, limb length discrepancy, muscle weakness, carpal tunnel syndrome, peripheral neuropathy
- En Coup De Sabre: Neurological abnormalities and ocular abnormalities
- Autoimmune disorders: Systemic lupus erythematosus, psoriasis, vitiligo, thyroiditis, hepatitis, pernicious anemia, myasthenia gravis
- Others: Arthritis, myalgia, Raynaud's phenomenon, esophageal dysmotility

(involvement of subcutis, muscle, or bone). Disease activity correlates with the intensity of hyperemia and echogenicity. Magnetic resonance imaging (MRI) is also a useful tool, but USG is preferred over MRI because of the simplicity and cost-effectiveness.[15]

MANAGEMENT

From the therapeutic perspective, morphea can be conveniently classified into:
- Active (inflammatory and early sclerotic) stage
- Late sclerotic stage
- Atrophic stage.

The active stage must be treated aggressively with the aim of stabilizing the existing lesions and to prevent the eruption of newer lesions. Late sclerotic stage must be treated with efficacious but safer treatment options; thus, buying the chance even if there is a minimal scope for improvement. Atrophic stage does not improve with anti-inflammatory or immunomodulatory agents which are to be avoided in this phase of the disease.[16]

The patients must be succinctly explained that the initial view point in the management of morphea is to halt the progression of the disease. After putting the disease into halt, the measures to improve the cosmesis if possible may be performed.

The various therapeutic options directed towards controlling the disease activity are as follows:
- Topical medications
- Systemic medications
- Phototherapy
- Other modalities: Intralesional steroids, excimer laser.

Topical Medications

It is the treatment of choice in circumscribed plaque lesions. It can be combined with systemic medications or phototherapy in linear or generalized morphea.

Topical Tacrolimus 0.1% Ointment

It is the preferred topical agent since it is devoid of adverse effects of topical steroids namely atrophy, telangiectasia, and hypopigmentation. It is to be applied twice a day. The efficacy can be improved by applying it under occlusion.[17] Pimecrolimus 1% cream can also be used with similar efficacy.

Topical Steroid

Betamethasone dipropionate 0.05% ointment is the topical steroid molecule widely studied in morphea, even though other potent steroids can be used as well. To avoid its adverse effects, its use must be limited to around a month. It can also be given in combination with calcipotriol.

Topical Calcipotriene 0.005% Ointment

A vitamin D analogue is effective in morphea because in addition to its immunomodulatory action, it also inhibits the activity of fibroblasts thus decreasing the collagen synthesis. Its efficacy can be improved when applied under occlusion. Since there is a mild risk of hypercalcemia following its extensive application, the quantity to be applied should be limited to less than 100 g/week in adults and 50 g/week in children less than 12 years. It is prescribed in combination with steroids too. It can be combined with phototherapy and recent studies have shown that the clinical efficacy is not diminished when calcipotriol application is followed by phototherapy.[18] Topical tacalcitol ointment (4 µg/g) is an analogous molecule with similar efficacy.

Topical Imiquimod (5%) Cream

It is applied as a thin layer overnight on non-consecutive days and is found to be effective. Patients can encounter mild irritation as an adverse effect which can be decreased to certain extent by combining it with topical steroid in the day time.

Intralesional Steroid Injection

Intralesional triamcinolone acetonide 5 to 10 mg/mL can be injected into the advancing inflammatory border exercising caution so as to prevent the occurrence of atrophy.

Systemic Medications

It is administered in the following subtypes of morphea:
- Progressive plaque lesions

- Linear limb morphea
- En coup de sabre
- Generalized morphea.

The medications preferred in morphea are systemic steroids, methotrexate, and mycophenolate mofetil.

Systemic Steroids

It can be given as daily oral dose or intravenous pulse therapy to improve the initial inflammatory phase of the disease. The dose of daily oral steroids administered is 0.5-1 mg/kg of prednisolone for an average of 3 months. Methylprednisolone pulse therapy in a dose of 0.5-1 g in adults or 30 mg/kg in children is administered on 3 consecutive days a month for 3 months with a good therapeutic response. Betamethasone oral mini-pulse can also be administered which need further trials.[19,20]

Methotrexate

It is usually administered along with systemic steroids to control the active phase of the disease. For maintaining the remission and for less severe cases, it can be used as a stand-alone treatment. In a dose, 10-15 mg/week in adults or 0.3 mg/kg/week in children, it is given until the disease becomes quiescent and for 6-12 months further.[21]

Other Immunomodulatory Drugs

Mycophenolate mofetil is the preferred drug because of its safer adverse effect profile and its additional property of inhibiting the fibroblastic activity apart from its immunomodulatory action. It is administered in a dose of 1 g/day to 3 g/day in adults or 40 mg/kg in children in two divided doses. It is found to be effective in some patients who had failed to show remission with systemic steroids and methotrexate.[22]

There are few reports which describe response of severe morphea to cyclosporine. Other systemic treatment modalities namely cyclophosphamide, azathioprine, calcitriol, hydroxychloroquine, penicillamine, photodynamic therapy, and intravenous immunoglobulins were used with varying response.

Phototherapy

Ultraviolet A1 (UVA1) is the phototherapy of choice in morphea. It has a deeper penetration and it tackles the main pathomechanisms involved in morphea namely:
- Depletes T lymphocytes
- Down regulates the cytokines such as IL1, IL6, and IL8
- Upregulates matrix metalloproteinases
- Inhibits fibroblastic activity
- It can be administered in 3 dosage intensities namely low dose UVA1 (20 J/cm^2/treatment with a maximum dose of 600 J/cm^2), moderate dose UVA1 (70 J/cm^2/treatment with a maximum dose of 2100 J/cm^2), and high dose UVA1 (130 J/cm^2/treatment with a maximum dose of 3900 J/cm^2).[13]

Moderate dose UVA1 is preferred as it is significantly superior to mild dose UVA1 and has equal efficacy as that of the high dose UVA1.[23,24]

The efficacy of narrow band ultraviolet B (NB UVB) is comparable to that of mild dose UVA1.[25] Topical or systemic psoralen with UVA (PUVA) has also been studied with moderate response.[26] These phototherapeutic modalities can be combined with topical or systemic modalities of treatment for better and synergistic efficacy.

Excimer Laser

There are isolated case reports of morphea treated with excimer laser (308 nm). In one such report, excimer laser was combined with weekly methotrexate.[27]

Physiotherapy

It is of beneficial role in limb morphea with joint contracture for improving the range of movements. It also helps in preventing contracture to a certain extent.

Camouflage Cream

It helps in concealing the lesions or scars in the exposed areas, thus improving the self-esteem of the patient.

Fillers

Fillers are useful in patients with en coup de sabre or morphea lesion over exposed parts of body which have healed with atrophy and depression and patients demand a better cosmesis. Hyaluronic acid, poly L-lactic acid, autologous fat, and dermal grafts are used with improved cosmesis of the atrophic lesions.[28-30]

Surgical Correction

It may be necessary in patients with debilitating contractures and limb length discrepancies.

MORPHEAFORM SKIN DISORDERS

Cutaneous lesions resembling localized plaque morphea can be a varied presentation of other disorders as listed in box 2.

Lichen Sclerosus et Atrophicus

It is a chronic inflammatory disorder characterized by white sclerotic and atrophic lesions involving the genital and nongenital skin. Lichen sclerosus et atrophicus (LSA) commonly affects perineal skin in female and penile foreskin, prepuce in male. Genital and extragenital lesions can coexist in same patients. The disease is more predominant in female being 10 times more prevalent than male.[31] Patients with LSA have increased incidence of autoimmune disorders (Box 3).[32]

Clinical Features

Nongenital lesions: Though any site can be involved, it commonly involves the lower back, abdomen, buttocks, shoulder, axillae, inframammary area, flexor aspect of the wrist, and around the eyes. Lesions can occur at sites of pressure (underneath bra strap or belts) or show Koebner's (isomorphic) phenomenon.[33] The lesions begin as porcelain white papules that coalesce into plaques (Figs 18 and 19). It is

> **Box 2: Differential diagnosis of morpheaform skin lesions**
> - Chronic graft versus host disease
> - Eosinophilic fasciitis
> - Eosinophilia myalgia syndrome
> - Lichen sclerosus et atrophicus*
> - Lipodermatosclerosis*
> - Sclerosis at injection site*
> - Contact with chlorinated hydrocarbons*
> - Nephrogenic systemic fibrosis
> - Toxic oil syndrome
> - Radiation-induced morphea*
> - Porphyria cutanea tarda*
> - Muckle-Wells syndrome
> - Winchester syndrome
> - Linear melorheostosis*
> - Morpheaform sarcoidosis*
> - Morpheaform basal cell carcinoma*
>
> The disorders marked with (*) will be discussed in this chapter.

> **Box 3: Autoimmune disorders commonly associated with lichen sclerosus et atrophicus**
> - Morphea
> - Alopecia areata (in males)
> - Pernicious anemia (in females)
> - Systemic sclerosis
> - Systemic lupus erythematosus
> - Lichen planus

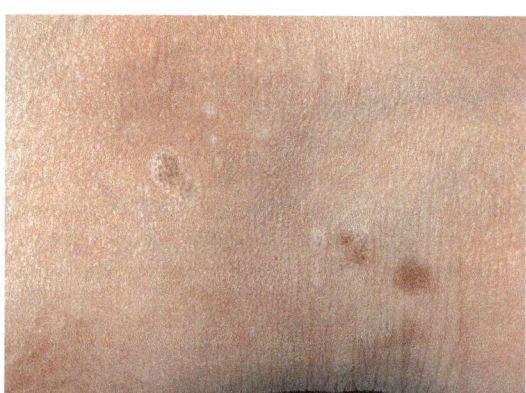

FIGURE 18: Small papules coalescing to form lichen sclerosus et atrophicus plaques and prominent follicular plugging.

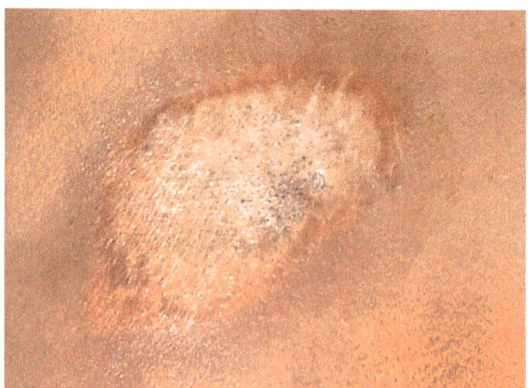

FIGURE 19: Large lichen sclerosus et atrophicus plaque.
Courtesy: Dr Neena Khanna, Professor, AIIMS, New Delhi.

usually asymptomatic. The size of the lesions can be variable. The evenly spaced dells or follicular plugs correspond to the appendiceal ostea which is succinctly demonstrated by dermascopy. This is not specific to LSA since it can also occur in chronic cutaneous lupus.

Sometimes patient continue to have small papular lesions only and are referred to be having guttate LSA (Fig. 20).

In later stages, atrophy occurs making the lesions to develop wrinkles, become depressed and pigmented (Fig. 21). Occasionally, the lesions can develop blister, telangiectasia, or purpura. Rarely, SCC transformation can occur.[34] Lichen sclerosus et atrophicus can be differentiated from morphea by the presence of multiple discrete papules around the coalesced plaque. Often LSA and morphea coexist and colocalize (Fig. 22).

Anogenital lesions in women: It commonly occurs in the prepubertal, peri and postmenopausal age groups. Vulval (Fig. 23) and perianal region are commonly involved (figure of 8 or hour glass configuration results when both are involved).[35] It may extend to involve the inner thigh. Patients often complain of pruritus, soreness, and dyspareunia. Atrophy of the vulva (kraurosis vulvae), stenosis of the introitus, burying of the clitoris and fusion of the labia can occur. Despite this, pregnancy and delivery are uninfluenced. Chances of SCC transformation are higher in genital LSA compared to extra-genital LSA (Fig. 24).

Penile lichen sclerosis (Balanitis xerotica obliterans): It presents as atrophic leukodermic (sclerotic) patches involving the glans penis or prepuce. It can result in phimosis, paraphimosis,

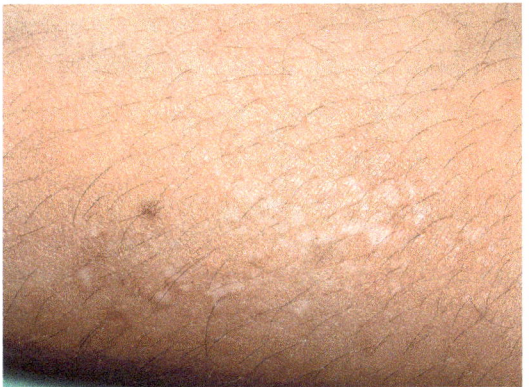

FIGURE 20: Guttate lichen sclerosus et atrophicus.
Courtesy: Dr Neena Khanna, Professor, AIIMS, New Delhi.

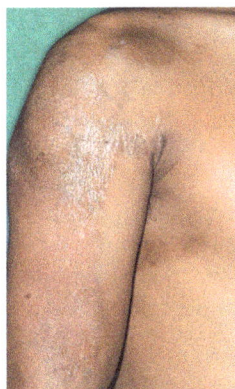

FIGURE 22: Lichen sclerosus et atrophicus and morphea overlap.

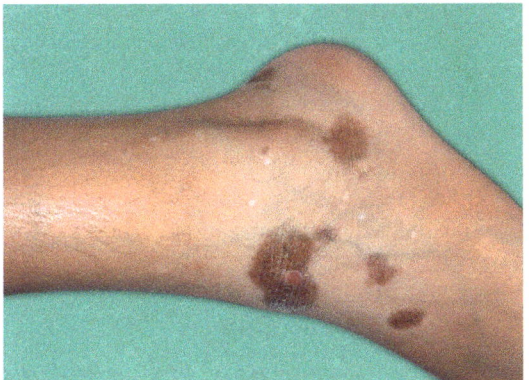

FIGURE 21: Old pigmented atrophic lichen sclerosus et atrophicus plaques with new small lesion in periphery.

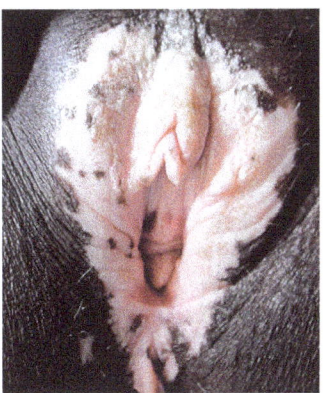

FIGURE 23: Female genital lichen sclerosus et atrophicus.

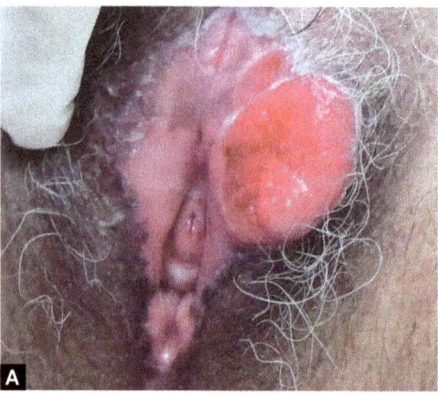
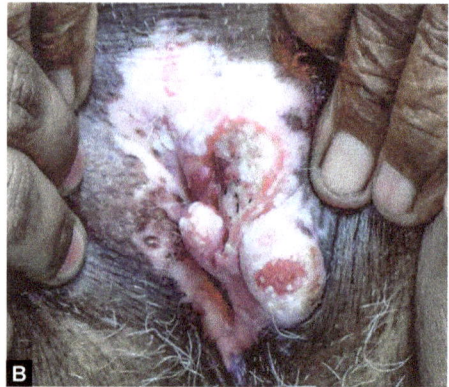

FIGURE 24: Lichen sclerosus et atrophicus with squamous cell carcinoma transformation.

narrowing of the meatus, (resulting in thin urinary stream) and urinary obstruction (Fig. 25). Involvement of perianal area is very rare in male.

Histopathology (Also refer chapter 3: Dermatopathology of Rheumatologic Diseases)

The classical histopathologic picture is called trilayered or striped appearance. It includes the following layers:
- The top most layer of hyperkeratosis and epidermal atrophy (dark pink layer)
- Upper dermis has pale hyalinized homogeneous collagen
- Inflammatory infiltrate predominantly composed of lymphocytes in the mid-dermis.

Treatment
- Topical steroid: Potent topical steroids (clobetasol or betamethasone) ointment or cream is to be used once daily. In circumcised penis, it is to be applied twice daily since it might get wiped off by the clothing. It is to be administered for 6–8 weeks following which the frequency of application is to be made to alternate day application until 12–16 weeks after which less potent steroid (mometasone) can be substituted
- Topical calcineurin inhibitors: Though topical tacrolimus or pimecrolimus are used, they are not first-line since the safety of long-term usage is not established
- Systemic medications such as steroids, acitretin, methotrexate or MMF can be given for extensive lesions

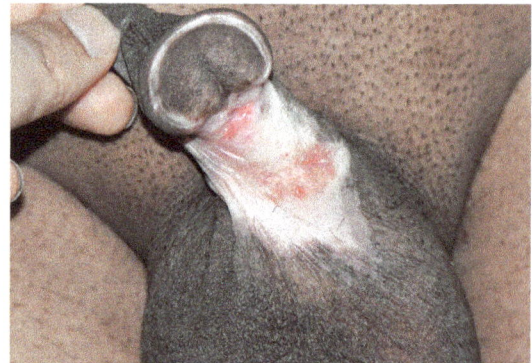

FIGURE 25: Male genital lichen sclerosus et atrophicus.

- Narrow band ultraviolet B or low dose UVA1 therapy can be done as an adjuvant
- Circumcision: It is to be performed if the topical medications are ineffective after 6 months of usage, or there is associated phimosis, paraphimosis
- For meatal stenosis: Meatotomy, meatoplasty, or urethroplasty is to be performed
- For vulvar lichen sclerosis, vulvectomy must not be done unless an associated malignancy is present.

Other topical medications of doubtful benefit include topical testosterone and topical estrogen.

Lipodermatosclerosis (Sclerosing Panniculitis)

It is a type of panniculitis, can be acute or chronic. It is frequently associated with venous insufficiency or obesity. It commonly involves the lower one-third of leg above the medial malleolus (Fig. 26). Acute lipodermatosclerosis is featured by erythematous, indurated and painful plaque with ill-defined borders. Chronic lipodermatosclerosis is characterized by marked sclerosis with well-defined borders and hyperpigmentation due to hemosiderin deposition. The affected leg resembles an inverted champagne bottle. The first-line treatment is limb elevation and elastic compression stockings. Surgical correction of incompetent veins/perforators or endovenous ablation is also useful. Anabolic steroids: Stanozolol 2 mg BD or Danazol 200 mg BD for 2–3 months is useful in acute lipodermatosclerosis because of its antifibrinolytic action (acts against the fibrin cuff).[36,37]

Sclerosis at Injection Site

This can be associated with following injections: Oil-soluble vitamin K_1 (Texier's disease), silicone or paraffin implant, interferon-β, bleomycin, glatiramer, enfuvirtide, opioids (e.g., pentazocine, methadone).[38]

Contact with Chlorinated Hydrocarbons

Morphea-like lesions can result from the contact with benzene or toluene.[39]

Radiation-induced Morphea

It is characterized by erythema, sclerosis, and pigmentary changes at the site of radiation exposure or even beyond it. It is more commonly seen in patients irradiated for breast carcinoma.[40] The disease onset can occur months or years after radiation therapy. Therapeutic options include topical or systemic steroids, methotrexate, and PUVA therapy. The response to therapy is unpredictable.[41]

Porphyria Cutanea Tarda

In porphyria cutanea tarda, UV-induced morphea like sclerosis can result in the sun exposed areas such as hairless scalp, face, dorsum of hands, and upper trunk.[42] Histopathologically, it resembles morphea except for the presence of periodic acid-Schiff positive deposits around the dermal blood vessels.

Linear Melorheostosis

It is rare disorder featured by linear hyperostosis of the bone more commonly involving the lower limb with a characteristic dripping candle wax appearance in the X-ray. It can be associated with induration (fibrosis) of the overlying soft tissue and skin. Pain is often present. It is a progressively debilitating disorder. The treatment consists of surgical correction of deformities.[43]

Morpheaform Sarcoidosis

Sarcoidosis is an idiopathic multisystem disease with protean manifestation. There are few reports of morphea-like lesions which on histopathology showed noncaseating granuloma. These patients had restrictive lung disease on pulmonary function test and had elevated angiotensin converting enzyme levels, thus diagnosed to have sarcoidosis.[44] The treatment of this condition consists of hydroxychloroquine, intralesional or systemic steroids.

Morpheaform Basal Cell Carcinoma

It presents as a depressed scar-like plaque. It is commonly located on the head and neck. It tend to be aggressive sometimes infiltrating the subcutis or muscle. Mohs micrographic surgery is the treatment of choice to avoid recurrences.

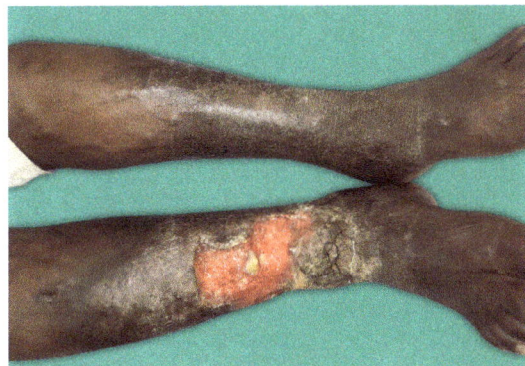

FIGURE 26: Lipodermatosclerosis over both legs, varicose vein and venous ulceration.

REFERENCES

1. National Institute of Musculoskeletal and Skin Diseases (NIAMS). (2006). Scleroderma. [online] Available from http://www.niams.nih.gov/Health_Info/Scleroderma/default.asp. [Accessed May 2017].
2. Zulian H, Athreya BH, Laxer R, Nelson AM, Feitosa de Oliveira SK, Punaro MG, et al. Juvenile localized scleroderma: clinical and epidemiological features in 750 children. An international study. Rheumatology (Oxford). 2006;45: 614-20.
3. Sartori-Valinotti JC, Tollefson MM, Reed AM. Updates on morphea: role of vascular injury and advances in treatment. Autoimmune Dis. 2013.
4. Julian CG, Bowers PW. Osteoma cutis in a lesion of solitary morphea profunda. Clin Exp Dermatol. 2003;28:673-4.
5. Soma Y, Kawakami T, Yamasaki E, Sasaki R, Mizoguchi M. Linear scleroderma along Blaschko's lines in a patient with systematized morphea. Acta Derm Venereol. 2003;83:362-4.
6. Amaral TN, Marques Neto JF, Lapa AT, Peres FA, Guirau CR, Appenzeller S. Neurologic Involvement in Scleroderma en coup de sabre. Autoimmune Dis. 2012;2012:719685.
7. Zannin ME, Martini G, Athreya BH, Russo R, Higgins G, Vittadello F, et al. Ocular involvement in children with localised scleroderma: a multi-centre study. Br J Ophthalmol. 2007;91(10):1311-4.
8. Dimitrova V, Yordanova I, Gospodinov D. Generalized morphea: A case report. J IMAB.2007;13:68-70.
9. O'Leary PA. In discussion on morphea. Arch Dermatol Syphilol 1954;70:387-8.
10. Ruiz-Villaverde R, Sánchez-Cano D, Galán-Gutiérrez M. Zosteriform morphea: Wolf's isotopic response in an immunocompetent patient. Dermatol Reports. 2011;3(2):e16.
11. Leitenberger JJ, Cayce RL, Haley RW, Adams-Huet B, Bergstresser PR, Jacobe HT. Distinct autoimmune syndromes in morphea: a review of 245 adult and pediatric cases. Arch Dermatol.2009;145(5):545-50.
12. Zulian F, Athreya BH, Laxer R, Nelson AM, Feitosa de Oliveira SK, Punaro MG, et al. Juvenile localized scleroderma: clinical and epidemiological features in 750 children. An international study. Rheumatology (Oxford). 2006;45:614-20.
13. Kura MM and Jindal SR. Disabling pansclerotic morphea of childhood with extracutaneous manifestations. Indian J Dermatol. 2013;58(2):159.
14. Kikuchi K, Sato S, Kadono T, Ihn H, Takehara K. Serum concentration of procollagen type I carboxyterminal propeptide in localized scleroderma. Arch Dermatol. 1994;130(10):1269-72.
15. Horger M, Fierlbeck G, Kuemmerle-Deschner J, Tzaribachev N, Wehrmann M, Claussen CD, et al. MRI findings in deep and generalized morphea (localized scleroderma). AJR Am J Roentgenol. 2008;190(1):32-9.
16. Fett NM. Morphea: Evidence based recommendations for treatment. Indian J Dermatol Venereol Leprol.2012;78:135-41.
17. Mancuso G, Berdondini RM. Localized scleroderma: response to occlusive treatment with tacrolimus ointment. Br J Dermatol.2005;152:180-2.
18. Adachi Y, Uchida N, Matsuo T, Horio T. Clinical effect of vitamin D3 analogues is not inactivated by subsequent UV exposure. Photodermatol Photoimmunol Photomed. 2008;24:16-18.
19. Kreuter A, Gambichler T, Breuckmann F, Rotterdam S, Freitag M, Stuecker M, et al. Pulsed high-dose corticosteroids combined with low-dose methotrexate in severe localized scleroderma. Arch Dermatol 2005;141:847-52.
20. Uziel Y, Feldman BM, Krafchik BR, Yeung RS, Laxer RM. Methotrexate and corticosteroid therapy for pediatric localized scleroderma. J Pediatr 2000;136:91-5.
21. Seyger MM, van den Hoogen FH, de Boo T, de Jong EM. Low-dose methotrexate in the treatment of widespread morphea. J Am Acad Dermatol 1998;39:220-5.
22. Martini G, Ramanan AV, Falcini F, Girschick H, Goldsmith DP, Zulian F. Successful treatment of severe or methotrexate-resistant juvenile localized scleroderma with mycophenolate mofetil. Rheumatology 2009;48:1410-3.
23. Stege H, Berneburg M, Humke S, Klammer M, Grewe M, Grether-Beck S, et al. High-dose UVA1 radiation therapy for localized scleroderma. J Am Acad Dermatol 1997;36:938-44.
24. Sator PG, Radakovic S, Schulmeister K, Honigsmann H, Tanew A. Medium-dose is more effective than low-dose ultraviolet A1 phototherapy for localized scleroderma as shown by 20-MHz ultrasound assessment. J Am Acad Dermatol 2009;60:786-91.
25. Kreuter A, Hyun J, Stucker M, Sommer A, Altmeyer P, Gambichler T. A randomized controlled study of low-dose UVA1, medium-dose UVA1, and narrowband UVB phototherapy in the treatment of localized scleroderma. J Am Acad Dermatol 2006;54:440-7.
26. Usmani N, Murphy A, Veale D, Goulden V, Goodfield M. Photochemotherapy for localized morphoea: effect on clinical and molecular markers. Clin Exp Dermatol. 2008;33:698-704.
27. Hanson AH, Fivenson DP, Schapiro B. Linear scleroderma in an adolescent woman treated with methotrexate and excimer laser. Dermatol Ther. 2014;27:203-5.
28. Arsiwala SZ. Persistence of Hyaluronic Acid filler for subcutaneous atrophy in a case of circumscribed scleroderma. J Cutan Aesthet Surg. 2015;8(1):69-71.
29. Zanelato TP, Marquesini G, Colpas PT, Magalhães RF, de Moraes AM. Implantation of autologous fat globules in localized scleroderma and idiopathic lipoatrophy - report of five patients. An Bras Dermatolol. 2013;88(6):120-3.
30. Onesti MG, Troccola A, Scuderi N. Volumetric correction using poly-L-lactic acid in facial asymmetry: Parry Romberg Syndrome and scleroderma. Dermatol Surg. 2009;35:1368-75.
31. Powell JJ, Wojnarowska F. Lichen sclerosus. Lancet. 1999; 353(9166):1777-83.
32. Kreuter A, Kryvosheyeva Y, Terras S, Moritz R, Möllenhoff K, Altmeyer P, et al. Association of autoimmune diseases with lichen sclerosus in 532 male and female patients. Acta Derm Venereol. 2013;93(2):238-41.

33. Pock L. Koebner phenomenon in lichen sclerosus et atrophicus. Dermatologica. 1990;181(1):76-7.
34. Carlson JA, Ambros R, Malfetano J, Ross J, Grabowski R, Lamb P, et al. Vulvar lichen sclerosus and squamous cell carcinoma: a cohort, case control, and investigational study with historical perspective; implications for chronic inflammation and sclerosis in the development of neoplasia. Hum Pathol. 1998;29(9):932-48.
35. Fistarol SK, Itin PH. Diagnosis and treatment of lichen sclerosus: am update Am J Clin Dermatol. 2013;14(1):27-47.
36. Vesić S1, Vuković J, Medenica LJ, Pavlović MD. Acute lipodermatosclerosis: an open clinical trial of stanozolol in patients unable to sustain compression therapy. Dermatol Online J. 2008;14(2):1.
37. Hafner C, Wimmershoff M, Landthaler M, Vogt T. Lipodermatosclerosis: successful treatment with danazol. Acta Derm Venereol. 2005;85(4):365-6.
38. Gettler SL, Fung MA. Off-center fold: indurated plaques on the arms of a 52-year-old man. Diagnosis: Cutaneous reaction to phytonadione injection. Arch Dermatol. 2001;137(7):957-62.
39. Haustein UF, Ziegler V. Environmentally Induced Systemic Sclerosis-like Disorders. Int J dermatol. 1985;24(3):147-151.
40. Alhathlool A, Hein R, Andres C, Ring J, Eberlein B. Post-Irradiation Morphea: Case report and review of the literature. J Dermatol Case Rep. 2012;6(3):73-77.
41. Spalek M, Jonska-Gmyrek J, Galecki J. Radiation-induced morphea-a literature review. J Eur Acad Dermatol Venereol. 2015;29(2):197-202.
42. Zemtsov R, Zemtsov A. Porphyria cutanea tarda presenting as scleroderma. Cutis. 2010 Apr;85(4):203-5.
43. Saghafi M, Sahebari M, Goshayeshi L. Linear scleroderma in association with melorheostosis. J Clin Rheumatol. 2010;16(2):99-100.
44. Choi SC, Kim HJ, Kim CR, Byun JY, Lee DY, Lee JH, et al. A case of morpheaform sarcoidosis. Ann Dermatol. 2010;22(3):316-8.

10

CHAPTER

Mixed Connective Tissue Disease

Varun Dhir

INTRODUCTION

Mixed connective tissue disease was first described by Sharp in 1972 and has continued to be a part of overlap syndromes in rheumatology despite the controversies and debates. It is characterized by overlapping features of rheumatoid arthritis (RA), systemic lupus erythematosus (SLE), scleroderma, and polymyositis. The major clinical features are Raynaud's phenomenon, puffy fingers, sclerodactyly, malar rash, arthritis, leukopenia, lymphadenopathy, pulmonary arterial hypertension, interstitial lung disease (ILD), and myositis. The criteria by Alarcon-Segovia is simple and has good accuracy; and thus most popular. The major serological characteristic of this disease is high titer antibody against uridine-rich U1 ribonucleoprotein (U1RNP), specifically the 70 Kda peptide attached to U1RNA. Treatment of this disease is as per its manifestations and consists of steroids for skin, joints, and myositis, immunosuppression for ILD and vasodilators for pulmonary arterial hypertension. Although initially considered benign, subsequently it has been shown to have a significantly higher risk of death.

HISTORICAL PERSPECTIVE

Sharp in 1972 from Stanford University and later from Missouri-Columbia in the USA described an apparently distinct rheumatic disease associated with a specific antibody to extractable nuclear antigen. He described a disease with overlapping features of SLE, scleroderma, and myositis.[1] This extractable nuclear antigen to which patients had high titer antibodies was ribonuclease and trypsin sensitive, i.e., contained both RNA and protein, thus was a ribonucleoprotein in contrast to the reactivity to DNA in SLE. Over the years, it has become clear that this nuclear antigen against which antibody in this disease is directed is part of the spliceosome complex and is specifically directed against U1RNP. Although, there may be some authorities who do not accept this as a distinct disease rather more as an overlap of diseases. There is no doubt that the clinical course in these patients is distinct.

DEFINITION

There have been four major criteria that have been published for mixed connective tissue disease (MCTD).[2-4] It is felt that the criteria by Alarcon-Segovia is the most simple as well as accurate for this disease. Commonly used criteria are given in table 1. It consists of serologic and clinical criteria. Another criteria that has been shown to perform well is the Japanese Ministry for health and welfare (JMHW).[5] Most studies have found a sensitivity of Alarcon-Segovia to be 100% and JMHW to be 87–99% and specificity of 99–100% and 87–94% respectively. Interestingly, it has been demonstrated that many of these patients would fulfill the criteria for RA as well as SLE.

Mixed Connective Tissue Disease

Table 1: Common criteria used to diagnose mixed connective tissue disease

Alarcon-Segovia criteria	Japanese Ministry for Health and Welfare (or Kasukawa criteria)

• Serologic criteria
  ○ Moderate to high titers of antibody against U1RNP (1:1600 or higher)
	• Common Symptoms
	  ○ Raynaud's phenomenon
	  ○ Swollen fingers and hands
	  ○ Anti-snRNP antibody positive

• Clinical criteria
  ○ Arthritis*
  ○ Raynaud's phenomenon
  ○ Acrosclerosis (sclerodactyly)
  ○ Myositis*
  ○ Finger edema
	• Mixed symptoms
	  ○ Systemic lupus erythematosus like findings
	    – Polyarthritis
	    – Lymphadenopathy
	    – Facial erythema
	    – Pericarditis or pleuritis
	    – Leuko or thrombocytopenia
	  ○ Scleroderma like findings
	    – Esophageal dysmotility or dilation of esophagus
	    – Pulmonary fibrosis, restrictive changes in lung or reduced diffusion capacity
	    – Sclerodactyly
	  ○ Polymyositis like findings
	    – Muscle weakness
	    – Myogenic pattern on electromyography
	    – Elevated muscle enzymes creatine phosphokinase

• Diagnosis requires serologic criteria and at least 3 of the following 5 clinical criteria and at least one of * must be present	• At least one of the two common symptoms plus positive snRNP plus one or more of mixed symptoms in at least 2 of the 3 disease categories.

PATHOGENESIS

Mixed connective tissue disease is closely associated with antibodies to U1RNP, specifically against the 70 Kda peptide attached to U1RNA. Although, the exact role of this antibody and whether it is pathogenic is not known, specific autoreactive T cell clones against this autoantigen have been demonstrated. This disease is associated with human leukocyte antigen (HLA)-DR4 in distinction with SLE that is associated with HLA-DR3.

DEMOGRAPHY

Sharp found that MCTD was less prevalent in the clinic than RA and SLE, but more common than polymyositis, dermatomyositis, or scleroderma. The gender ratio has been reported to vary from 4:1 to 16:1, being more prevalent in the female population.[6,7] The age of onset is usually in the thirties, although juvenile onset is well recognized.

SEROLOGIC TESTS

This disease is characterized by high titer antibodies directed against the U1RNP complex (Box 1). This was initially tested using hemagglutination, after coating RBCs with extractable nuclear antigen and then treating them with ribonuclease. The U1RNP complex consists of a U1RNA and associated noncovalently attached peptides that include 70 Kda and proteins A and C. The autoantibody has been specifically found to be directed against the 70 Kda peptide attached to the U1RNA.[8-10] This can be tested using immunoblot or enzyme-linked immunosorbent assay. Antibody to U1RNP and specifically the 70 Kda peptide may be found in around one-third of patients with SLE, however, are of a lower titer. On a fluorescent antinuclear antibody assay using human epithelial type 2 cells, this appears as a bright speckled nuclear fluorescence. In addition, MCTD is associated with rheumatoid factor (RF)

Skin in Rheumatologic Diseases

> **Box 1: Antibodies in mixed connective tissue disease**
>
> - High titers against uridine-rich U1 ribonucleoprotein
> - Antibody directed against 70 Kda protein attached to U1RNA
> - Detected using enzyme-linked immunosorbent assay or immunoblot
> - Not specific; seen in one-third systemic lupus erythematosus patients
> - Speckled nuclear fluorescence on IF

present in 50–75% of patients, anti-Ro in 33% and beta-2-glycoprotein I in 15% of the patients. It has been stated that patients of MCTD rarely have autoantibodies to Sm antigen.[11-13]

CLINICAL FEATURES

Common manifestations of MCTD are a combination of features of scleroderma, RA, SLE, and polymyositis (Box 2).[1,6,14-17]

Skin and Mucosal Manifestations (Box 3)

Raynaud's phenomenon is the most common manifestation of the skin (and vessels) occurring in 95% of patients. It is usually not associated with digital ulcers, but in few cases digital ulcers can occur. In some cases, digital gangrene occurs that has been ascribed to the obliterative vasculopathy occurring in this disease. Swollen fingers are very common at the onset of the disease (Fig. 1). Acrosclerosis (better known as sclerodactyly) occurs in many patients. Systemic lupus erythematosus like cutaneous manifestations like photosensitivity, malar rash (Fig. 2), subacute cutaneous lupus erythematosus rash, livedo reticularis, and livedoid vasculitis are known to occur in more than half the patients, however, discoid rash is uncommon. In a study on skin biopsies, two of the eight skin biopsies had a positive lupus band test. Features of dermatomyositis, like Gottron's papules can also occur in this disease. Telangiectasias over face and hands along with calcinosis can also occur in MCTD. Periungual dilated capillaries and a pattern of capillary dropouts and dilatation like

> **Box 3: Common mucocutaneous manifestations of mixed connective tissue disease**
>
> - Lupus like mucocutaneous manifestations
>   - Photosensitivity
>   - Malar rash
>   - Subacute cutaneous rash (papulosquamous)
>   - Livedo reticularis
>   - Discoid lupus erythematosis
>   - Leucocytoclastic vasculitis
> - Scleroderma like mucocutaneous manifestations
>   - Raynaud's disease
>   - Sclerodactyly
>   - Calcifications
>   - Telangiectasias
>   - Sjögrens syndrome
>   - Sicca syndrome

> **Box 2: Common clinical features of mixed connective tissue disease**
>
> Common clinical manifestations of mixed connective tissue disease[1,6,15,20-22]
>
> - Arthritis
> - Raynaud's disease
> - Sclerodactyly (or acrosclerosis)
> - Swollen fingers
> - Myositis
> - Esophageal dysmotility
> - Interstitial lung diseases
> - Pulmonary arterial hypertension
> - Skin rash
> - Hematological

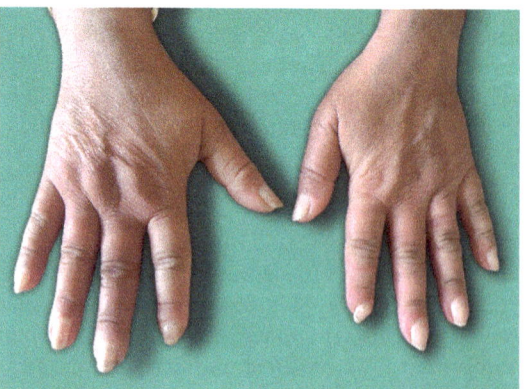

FIGURE 1: Finger edema or puffy fingers in a patient with mixed connective tissue disease.

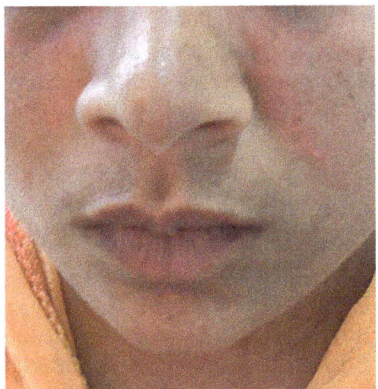

FIGURE 2: Malar rash in a patient.

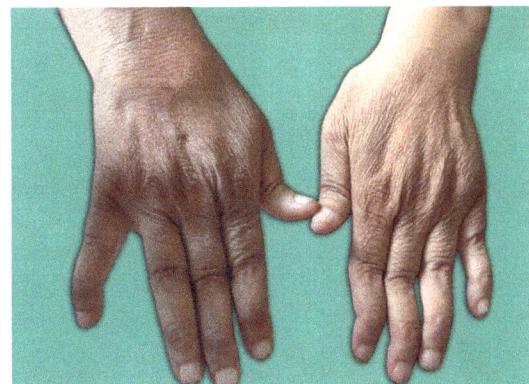

FIGURE 3: Rheumatoid like deformity (swan neck) in a patient with mixed connective tissue disease.

in scleroderma occurs in MCTD. Sicca symptoms are present in one-fourth to half the patients of MCTD.[12,18]

Arthritis

Arthralgias have been found to occur in most of the patients of MCTD and may be the presenting manifestation in half. Arthritis is a prominent feature of this disease occurring in more than half the patients, with some suggesting that RA is an important part of the overlapping diseases. Indeed, MCTD may fulfill the American college of Rheumatology classification criteria for RA. Common joints involved like RA are the small joints of the hands—the metacarpophalangeal and the proximal interphalangeal joints. Small marginal erosions may be found on radiographs of the hands that may be asymmetrical. However, additional features like terminal tuft erosions and periarticular calcifications may help to differentiate this disease radiographically from RA. Occasionally, patients also develop RA like deformities like swan neck etc. (Fig. 3). Correctable deformities like Jaccoud's arthritis have also been reported in MCTD. In one study, one-third of patients had deformities and a half had limited range of motion.

Myositis

This disease is characterized by inflammation of the muscles that is usually mild to moderate and associated with mild weakness apart from modest rise in the muscle enzymes like creatine phosphokinase. Many patients may be completely asymptomatic although biochemically show some elevation of muscle enzymes.

Pulmonary

This disease is associated with involvement of the pulmonary system in the form of interstitial lung disease, pleuropericardial effusion, and pulmonary arterial hypertension. Symptoms include cough, dyspnoea, or pleuritic chest pain. An important association of this disease is pulmonary arterial hypertension, which has also been ascribed to obliterative vasculopathy. It has been reported to occur in a fourth of the patients.[14] At autopsy, findings include interstitial fibrosis, obliterative vasculopathy of the pulmonary vessels with intimal proliferation, and medial hypertrophy of the pulmonary arteries and arterioles. In the heart, pericardial involvement occurs in one-third of the patients, with clinically apparent pericardial effusion in smaller numbers. Autonomic neuropathy can occasionally occur.

Gastrointestinal System

Esophageal dysmotility, including symptomatic reflux, is common in MCTD. Less commonly mesenteric vasculitis and pancreatitis have also been described. There are also reports of chronic autoimmune hepatitis and biliary cirrhosis in these patients. Some studies have found that although the esophageal manifestations are similar to that in scleroderma, the mean lower esophageal sphincter pressure is higher in MCTD than scleroderma.

Hematologic System

Mild lymphadenopathy occurs in 25–50% of the patients. Anemia, leucopenia, and lymphopenia are all common in this disease. Thrombocytopenia is less commonly found. There is significant hypergammaglobulinemia associated with MCTD, much more than in scleroderma.

Miscellaneous

Pericarditis occurs in up to one-third of the patients, myocardial involvement is uncommon. Trigeminal neuralgia is an important complication that occurs in this disease and has been reported to be a presenting feature as well.[19,20] A peripheral sensorimotor neuropathy can occur in this disease. Although considered rare, central nervous system involvement has been reported in the form of cerebellar dysfunction, psychosis, and seizures.[21,22] Renal disease is present in 25% patients. Membranous glomerulonephritis and membranoproliferative nephritis are more common rather than diffuse glomerulonephritis. Also, autopsy series show arterial intimal thickening like that seen in scleroderma. Malaise and low grade fever can occur in MCTD and rarely this can present as fever of unknown cause.

COURSE AND TREATMENT

Long term studies have shown that arthritis, swollen fingers, serositis and myositis, skin rash, Raynaud's phenomenon diminishes over time with treatment.[6] However, pulmonary hypertension, interstitial fibrosis, sclerodactyly, and nervous system involvement are less responsive and tend to persist or increase with time. There are no large controlled clinical trials to guide treatment. In general, the treatment is directed towards the specific clinical manifestation of the disease, taking a clue from the systemic autoimmune disease in which it is commonly found. Arthritis is often treated with steroids and if needed disease-modifying antirheumatic drugs like methotrexate. Raynaud's phenomenon can be treated as in scleroderma with vasodilators—calcium channel blockers, angiotensin converting enzyme inhibitors, and phosphodiesterase inhibitors. Interstitial lung disease is often treated with immunosuppressives like cyclophosphamide. Pulmonary arterial hypertension is treated with anticoagulation, phosphodiesterase inhibitors or endothelin receptor antagonists and may also respond to immunosuppression. Esophageal reflux symptoms are controlled using proton pump inhibitors and local measures like small frequent meals. Myositis, if clinically significant, is often treated with corticosteroids and if the patient is steroid dependent then with the addition of steroid sparing agents. Hematological involvement like leucopenia responds to steroids. Renal involvement in MCTD in the form of nephrotic syndrome has been shown to be steroid responsive, with resolution in three-fourths of the cases.

PROGNOSIS

Although, initially described by Sharp as a disease lacking serious renal or central nervous system involvement (in distinction with SLE), later studies, including a follow-up of the initial patients that were described by Sharp found a relatively high mortality rate. Indeed, currently MCTD is not considered to have a benign prognosis. The main predictors of poor long-term outcome are pulmonary arterial hypertension and lung involvement, apart from renal or nervous system involvement.[12,14]

CONCLUSION

Mixed connective tissue disease is an overlap disease characterized by specific criteria and high titer of U1RNP. Raynaud's phenomenon, puffy fingers and sclerodactly are commonly seen clinical features. In the skin, there can be SLE like manifestations such as malar rash and photosensitivity or scleroderma like features such as sclerodactly and telangiectasisas. Its treatment is dependant on clinical manifestations and includes steroids and immunosuppressants. Unlike in the past, it is not currently thought to have a benign prognosis.

REFERENCES

1. Sharp GC, Irvin WS, Tan EM, Gould RG, Holman HR. Mixed connective tissue disease--an apparently distinct rheumatic disease syndrome associated with a specific antibody to an extractable nuclear antigen (ENA). Am J Med. 1972;52(2):148-59.
2. Alarcon-Segovia D, Cardiel MH. Comparison between 3 diagnostic criteria for mixed connective tissue disease. Study of 593 patients. J Rheumatol. 1989;16(3):328-34.
3. Doria A, Ghirardello A, de Zambiasi P, Ruffatti A, Gambari PF. Japanese diagnostic criteria for mixed connective tissue disease in Caucasian patients. J Rheumatol. 1992;19(2):259-64.
4. Porter JF, Kingsland LC 3rd, Lindberg DA, Shah I, Benge JM, Hazelwood SE, et al. The AI/RHEUM knowledge-based computer consultant system in rheumatology. Performance in the diagnosis of 59 connective tissue disease patients from Japan. Arthritis Rheum. 1988;31(2):219-26.
5. Kasukawa Rm Sharp GC. Mixed connective tissue disease and anti-nuclear antibodies. Proceedings of the International Symposium on Mixed Connective Tissue Disease and Antinuclear Antibodies. New York, NY: Excerpta Medica; 1987.
6. Burdt MA, Hoffman RW, Deutscher SL, Wang GS, Johnson JC, Sharp GC. Long-term outcome in mixed connective tissue disease: longitudinal clinical and serologic findings. Arthritis Rheum. 1999;42(5):899-909.
7. Kotajima L, Aotsuka S, Sumiya M, Yokohari R, Tojo T, Kasukawa R. Clinical features of patients with juvenile onset mixed connective tissue disease: analysis of data collected in a nationwide collaborative study in Japan. J Rheumatol. 1996;23(6):1088-94.
8. Lerner MR, Boyle JA, Hardin JA, Steitz JA. Two novel classes of small ribonucleoproteins detected by antibodies associated with lupus erythematosus. Science. 1981;211(4480):400-2.
9. Takano M. [Clinical significance of antibodies to nuclear ribonucleoprotein in collagen diseases (author's transl)]. Ryumachi. 1978;18(4):256-66.
10. Holyst MM, Hill DL, Hoch SO, Hoffman RW. Analysis of human T cell and B cell responses against U small nuclear ribonucleoprotein 70-kd, B, and D polypeptides among patients with systemic lupus erythematosus and mixed connective tissue disease. Arthritis Rheum. 1997;40(8):1493-503.
11. Hoffman RW, Sharp GC, Deutscher SL. Analysis of anti-U1 RNA antibodies in patients with connective tissue disease. Association with HLA and clinical manifestations of disease. Arthritis Rheum. 1995;38(12):1837-44.
12. Setty YN, Pittman CB, Mahale AS, Greidinger EL, Hoffman RW. Sicca symptoms and anti-SSA/Ro antibodies are common in mixed connective tissue disease. J Rheumatol. 2002;29(3):487-9.
13. Mendonca LL, Amengual O, Atsumi T, Khamashta MA, Hughes GR. Most anticardiolipin antibodies in mixed connective tissue disease are beta2-glycoprotein independent. J Rheumatol. 1998;25(1):189-90.
14. Sullivan WD, Hurst DJ, Harmon CE, Esther JH, Agia GA, Maltby JD, et al. A prospective evaluation emphasizing pulmonary involvement in patients with mixed connective tissue disease. Medicine (Baltimore). 1984;63(2):92-107
15. Sharp GC, Irvin WS, May CM, Holman HR, McDuffie FC, Hess EV, et al. Association of antibodies to ribonucleoprotein and Sm antigens with mixed connective-tissue disease, systematic lupus erythematosus and other rheumatic diseases. N Engl J Med. 1976;295(21):1149-54.
16. Lundberg I, Hedfors E. Clinical course of patients with anti-RNP antibodies. A prospective study of 32 patients. J Rheumatol. 1991;18(10):1511-9.
17. Grant KD, Adams LE, Hess EV. Mixed connective tissue disease - a subset with sequential clinical and laboratory features. J Rheumatol. 1981;8(4):587-98.
18. Fraga A, Gudino J, Ramos-Niembro F, Aiarcon-Segovia D. Mixed connective tissue disease in childhood. Relationship Sjogren's syndrome. Am J Dis Child. 1978;132(3):263-5.
19. Searles RP, Mladinich EK, Messner RP. Isolated trigeminal sensory neuropathy: early manifestation of mixed connective tissue disease. Neurology. 1978;28(12):1286-9.
20. Vincent FM, Van Houzen RN. Trigeminal sensory neuropathy and bilateral carpal tunnel syndrome: the initial manifestation of mixed connective tissue disease. J Neurol Neurosurg Psychiatry. 1980;43(5):458-60.
21. Bennett RM, Bong DM, Spargo BH. Neuropsychiatric problems in mixed connective tissue disease. Am J Med. 1978;65(6):955-62.
22. Bennett RM, O'Connell DJ. Mixed connective tisssue disease: a clinicopathologic study of 20 cases. Semin Arthritis Rheum. 1980;10(1):25-51.

CHAPTER 11

Scleredema and Scleromyxedema

Biju Vasudevan, Ankan Gupta

INTRODUCTION

Sclerosis or sclerosus literally means hardening of the tissue. In dermatology, it refers to the increased fibroblast growth leading to thickening of skin and is the hallmark of systemic sclerosis. Pseudoscleroderma constitutes a heterogenous group of disorders other than morphea and systemic sclerosis, characterized by sclerosis of skin (Table 1).[1,2] Scleredema and scleromyxedema are cutaneous mucinoses where increased fibroblast growth produces increased mucin accumulation in the dermis.[3] Mucin, a jelly-like material, is a normal component of dermis containing acid GAGs (glycosaminoglycans), mainly hyaluronic acid and functions as the cushion in the skin, essentially helping in salt and water concentration in dermis.

MUCINOSES

The cutaneous mucinoses can be divided into primary cutaneous mucinoses where mucin deposition is the primary disorder and secondary cutaneous mucinoses where mucin deposition is only an additive finding in otherwise non-related dermatoses. Box 1 gives an elaborative classification of various mucinoses.

Pathogenesis

The exact cause of increased mucin deposition is unclear but the association with paraproteinemias, autoimmune disorders and endocrinal disorders

Table 1: Causes of pseudoscleroderma

Hereditary	• Phenylketonuria
	• Premature ageing syndromes
	   ◦ Werner's Syndrome
	   ◦ Hutchinson Gilford syndrome
	   ◦ Acrogeria
	• Stiff skin syndrome
	• Winchester syndrome
	• Huriez syndrome
	• Porphyria cutanea tarda

Infections	• Acrodermatitis chronica atrophicans (borrelia afzelii) • Scleredema of buschke (postinfectious)
Endocrinal	• Scleredema of Buschke (diabetes mellitus) • Hypothyroidism • Porphyria cutanea tarda
Malignancy	• Scleromyxedema • Carcinoid syndrome • POEMS syndrome • Primary systemic amyloidosis • Carcinoma en cuirasse
Iatrogenic	• Drugs: Bleomycin, vinca alkaloids, cisplatin, carboplatin, docetaxel, bromocriptine, carbidopa, methysergide, etc. • Chemicals: Vinyl chloride, silica dust, epoxy resins, etc. • Eosinophilia myalgia syndrome • Toxic oil syndrome

Continued

Continued

Table 1: Causes of pseudoscleroderma	
Immunologic	• Chronic GVHD • Eosinophilic fasciitis • Fibroblastic rheumatism
Miscellaneous	• Nephrogenic fibrosing dermopathy • Vibration disease • Radiodermatitis • Sudeck's dystrophy • Lipodermatosclerosis

POEMS, Polyneuropathy, organomegaly, endocrinopathy, monoclonal gammopathy, and skin changes; GVHD, graft versus host disease.

Box 1: Classification of cutaneous mucinoses

Primary
- Diffuse
  - Generalized myxedema
  - Pretibial myxedema
  - Lichen myxedematosus or papular mucinosis (scleromyxedema)
  - Scleredema
  - Hereditary progressive mucinous histiocytosis
  - Reticular erythematous mucinosis
- Follicular
  - Follicular mucinoses of Pinkus
  - Urticaria-like follicular mucinosis
- Focal
  - Cutaneous focal mucinosis or angiomyxoma
  - Mucinous cyst
  - Mucinous nevus

Secondary
- Lupus erythematosus, dermatomyositis
- Tumors
  - Basal cell carcinoma
  - Mesenchymal tumors: Myxosarcoma, dermatofibrosarcoma protuberans
  - Neural tumors: Neuromyxoma, neurofibroma
  - Cutaneous metastasis
  - Mucinous carcinoma of the eyelid
  - Cutaneous T-cell lymphoma
- Miscellaneous
  - L-tryptophan-induced eosinophilia-myalgia syndrome
  - Toxic oil syndrome
  - Degos' disease
  - Chronic GVHD
  - Granuloma annulare

GVHD, graft versus host disease.

suggest that there is an upregulation of mucin synthesis by autoantibodies or immunoglobulins. However, even after removal of antibodies or immunoglobulins by plasmapheresis, there seems to be no effect on the pathogenesis. Also, the amount of autoantibodies or paraproteins does not correlate with the severity of the disease. Presence of increased amount of Th1 cytokines like tumor necrosis factor-α, interleukin-1 suggest an immune-mediated pathway and they have proven to be responsible for increasing the production of GAGs *in vitro*.

SCLEREDEMA

INTRODUCTION

Scleredema is a primarily self-limiting cutaneous mucinoses characterized by thickened plaques due to deposition of mucin (especially acid mucopolysaccharides) in the dermis seen in association with diabetes mellitus or after a streptococcal infection.[4] Abraham Buschke described the first classical features in an adult patient in 1902 and named it scleredema adultorum of Buschke. However, it is now known that the name is erroneous as more than one-third of the cases are seen in children and about 50% of the cases occur before the third decade of life.[5] As the name suggests, the term was given by Buschke although it was originally described by Piffard.

CLASSIFICATION

There are three types of scleredema based on the Graff classification of 1968, namely:

Type I: It is the most common form including more than 55% cases and is especially found in the pediatric population and middle-aged women.[6] It typically follows a febrile illness, usually streptococcal throat infection or viral illnesses and is found in all races. It is characterized by thickening of the skin in the cervicofacial region with contiguous extension to the trunk and proximal upper limbs. There may be loss of facial expression lines and trismus in advanced cases. The mobility of the joints may be reduced. There is absence of Raynaud's phenomenon which is typically present in systemic sclerosis. There is usually no systemic organ involvement. The disease is generally self-limiting with active phase being 6-8 weeks and complete resolution within 6 months to 2 years. Occasionally, the disease may be progressive and fatalities have been noted.

Type II: It is a chronic, progressive variant with an insidious onset, clinically identical to type I and is associated with a monoclonal gammopathy, typically IgG kappa type. It constitutes around 25% of all cases.

Type III: Scleredema diutinum or scleredema diabeticorum constitutes around 20% of cases and is a known, rare complication of uncontrolled insulin-dependent diabetes mellitus.[7] The skin lesions are similar to type I but the patient may or may not have diabetic cheiroarthropathy, Huntley's papules, and acanthosis nigricans.[8]

EPIDEMIOLOGY

It is a very rare disease and association with diabetes mellitus is unquestionable. Type III is more common in men whereas other types are more commonly seen in women. There is a history of an infectious episode, from a few days to 6 weeks prior to onset, in 65-90% of cases.

PATHOGENESIS

The exact cause of the disease is unknown. It is postulated that increased insulin and insulin-like growth factor 1 along with microvascular and neural damage stimulate the fibroblasts, resulting in increased mucin production and glycosylation of collagen.[9] The other hypotheses suggested include obstruction to lymphatic channels by inflammation, immune sensitization, resistance to collagen degradation by collagenases, and neurohormonal alteration due to streptococcus. Sera from patients with paraproteinemia (Type II) has been found to stimulate collagen production in dermal fibroblast cultures.[10] There has been an incidence of occurrence of disease after using infliximab which spontaneously healed on discontinuation of the drug but the exact pathogenesis could not be understood.[11]

CLINICAL FEATURES

The disease is characterized by ill-defined, nonpitting, hard indurated plaques involving the cervicofacial region and trunk symmetrically, particularly the sides and the back of neck, giving a Peau d'orange appearance, extending onto the shoulders and proximal upper limbs (Fig. 1).[12] Rarely, the abdomen and legs may also be affected.[13] The hands and feet are usually spared and there is no acrosclerosis.

The induration is nonpitting and hard, and usually there is no sharp demarcation between normal and abnormal skin (Fig. 2). There is a characteristic sparing of epidermis which is evident by wrinkling of the skin when it is pinched or compressed between the thumb and index finger (Fig. 3).

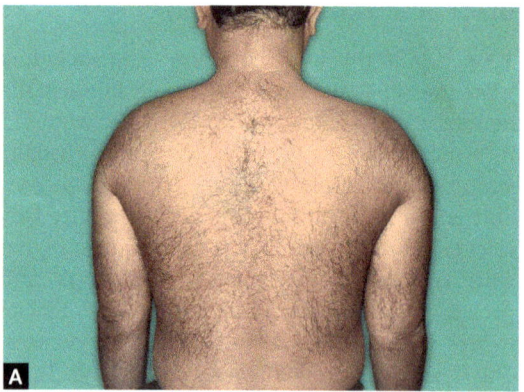 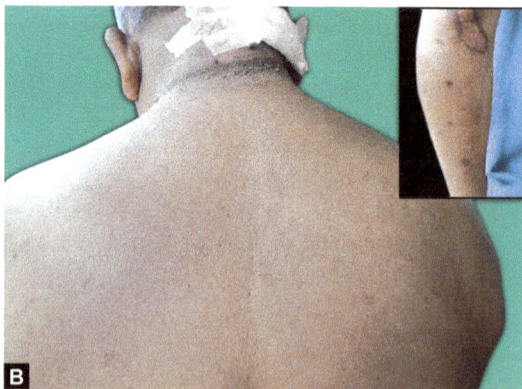

FIGURE 1: A, Scleredema affecting back and upper limbs in an adult; **B,** Scleredema in a diabetic patient with shin spots over the legs (inset).

Scleredema and Scleromyxedema

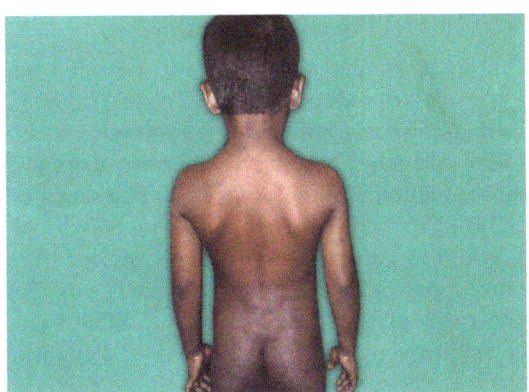

FIGURE 2: Scleredema affecting a child.

Facial involvement is characterized by loss of expression lines, difficulty in wrinkling the forehead and smiling, and sometimes there is trismus.[14] Mucosae are generally spared though there has been instances of involvement of eyes, tongue, and salivary glands.[15,16] The pharynx and esophagus may be involved, leading to difficulty in swallowing. Induration may lead to decrease in the respiratory capacity, presenting as sleep apnea syndrome.[17] In few cases, the induration may extend to involve joints, affecting normal joint movement.[18] More than two-thirds of the patients present with history of an infectious illness like influenza, upper respiratory tract infection, measles, mumps, or rubella prior to the onset of the disease process. So, prodromal symptoms of slight fever, malaise, muscle and joint pains are seen between the infectious episode and the onset of induration in such cases. Few give nonspecific history of a trivial triggering factor like trauma.

In type II and type III, patient may complain of systemic features like myositis, arthritis, dysphagia, hoarseness of voice, a myriad of ocular complaints, and congestive heart failure.[19] Rarely, pleural, pericardial, or peritoneal effusions can also occur. Complications of diabetes especially retinopathy, neuropathy, and peripheral vascular diseases may also be seen.

ASSOCIATIONS

All three forms may be associated with other auto-immune conditions like rheumatoid arthritis, hyperparathyroidism, hypothyroidism, Sjögren's syndrome, inflammatory bowel diseases, Waldenstrom's macroglobulinemia, anaphylactoid purpura, and malignant insulinomas.[20]

PATHOLOGY

In normal routine sections stained with Hematoxylin and Eosin, mucin is identified as an empty spaces between collagen bundles and it requires special stains to identify its presence.[21] The ground substance stains metachromatically with cresyl violet or toluidine blue. Metachromasia in scleroedema is caused by the presence of hyaluronic acid and is poorly seen in formalin fixed sections as the hyaluronic acid is removed by the fixative, and in tissues treated by hyaluronidase. So, specimen is best frozen

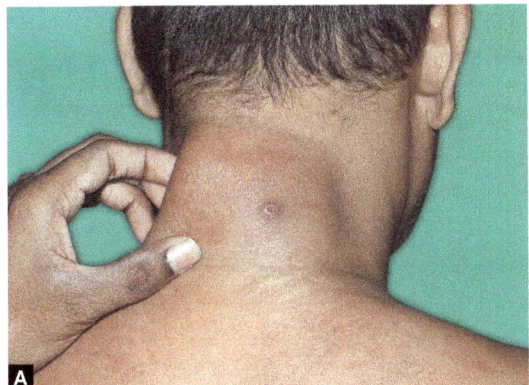
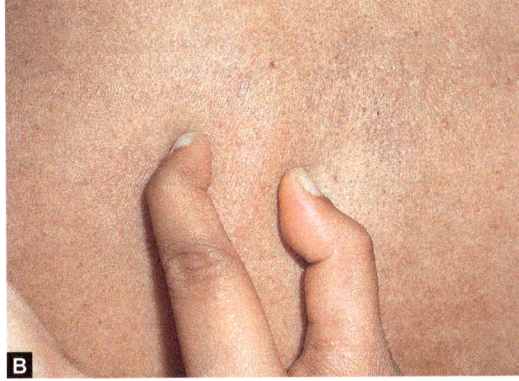

FIGURE 3: Scleredema patient with well-demarcated skin involvement over nape of neck and also surface wrinkling can be appreciated on pinching up of the skin.

Table 2: Special stains for mucin identification

For all GAGs	For sulfated GAGs only
Collodial iron	Alcian blue at pH 0.5
Alcian blue at pH 2.5	Toluidine blue at pH <2
Toluidine blue	-

GAG, glycosaminoglycans.

fixed if available or alcohol fixed. There is an excess of acid mucopolysaccharides, but neutral polysaccharides are normal. The various stains used are mentioned in table 2.

The epidermis is normal. There is a thickening of the reticular dermis along with large empty spaces filled with mucin, resulting in fenestration of the dermis. There is no increase in the number of fibroblasts, a sparse perivascular lymphocytic infiltrate is seen and the elastic fibers are reduced in number.[22,23] With progression of the disease, there is extension of the disease process into the subcutaneous tissue with replacement of fat by collagen bundles.[24]

INVESTIGATIONS

A rise in antistreptolysin O titre especially in children, erythrocyte sedimentation rate, C-reactive protein, and other acute phase reactants are seen. An estimation of immunoglobulin levels, particularly IgG kappa and IgA help in identification of monoclonal gammopathy. Serial monitoring by serum electrophoresis is advised for prognostification. Measuring blood sugar levels and glycated hemoglobin is also indicated.

DIFFERENTIAL DIAGNOSES

Other causes of sclerosis have to be ruled out especially scleroderma and morphea (Table 3). Dermatomyositis, Sjögren's syndrome, trichinosis, and other pseudosclerodermas also need differentiation. Scleromyxedema is differentiated clinically by presence of confluent papules in a grid-like pattern and insidious onset.[25] The other types of mucinosis are clinically different and easily differentiated clinically. Cellulitis and cutaneous amyloidosis may pose a diagnostic challenge at times.

In children, other causes of swelling of the body like renal, hepatic, cardiac, endocrinal, metabolic, anaphylactic, nutritional, connective tissue disorders, and even pulmonary conditions need to be ruled out.

TREATMENT

There is no treatment warranted for type I as it is self-limiting, though type II and III have shown some response to systemic (oral and pulse) steroid therapy and intralesional corticosteroids, immunesuppressants like colchicine,[26] cyclophosphamide, methotrexate,[27] chlorambucil, cyclosporine and azathioprine, phototherapy,[28,29] intravenous immunoglobulins (IVIg),[30] and electron beam therapy. Other reported therapeutic agents include radiotherapy, prostaglandin E1, factor XIII,[31] high-dose penicillin and d-penicillamine. Glycemic control does not seem to benefit patients with type III scleredema,[32] likewise an antibiotic course does

Table 3: Differential diagnosis of scleredema

	Systemic sclerosis	Morphea	Scleredema	Scleromyxedema
Clinical features				
Onset	Insidious	Insidious	Acute	Insidious
Raynaud's phenomenon	+	-	-	-
Acrosclerosis	+	-	-	-
Systemic involvement	+	-	-	±
Investigations				
Antinuclear antibodies	+	±	-	-
Monoclonal gammopathy	-	-	±	+

not decrease the duration of illness in the self-limiting type I scleredema.[33] In patients with raise in immunoglobulin levels, melphalan is the drug of choice and the only drug showing consistent benefits. In view of the self-limiting nature of the disease, ultraviolet A1 seems to be a good management option.

PROGNOSIS

The prognosis is variable with few cases showing self-remittance and few cases being associated with paraproteinemia showing high mortality too.[34] Some persistent cases are associated with moderate to severe diabetes mellitus, and both skin and diabetes are resistant to treatment. With detailed investigations, one can predict to great extent the outcome of the illness in any particular case.

CONCLUSION

Despite its rarity and relatively benign nature of scleredema and its diagnostic dilemma with similar conditions like scleroderma and scleromyxedema, with careful history, examination, and investigations, the diagnosis can be made and treated accordingly.

SCLEROMYXEDEMA

INTRODUCTION

Scleromyxedema is a primary cutaneous mucinoses characterized by numerous confluent papules later forming thickened plaques (Fig. 4). It is characterized by an increased fibroblast growth leading to mucin deposition along with increase in total collagen content of the dermis. It is also known as Arndt Gottron syndrome, lichen myxedematous, and papular mucinosis. It was identified by Montgomery and Underwood in 1953 but the term "scleromyxedema" was given by Gottron.[35,36]

CLASSIFICATION

Scleromyxedema can be classified into systemic or a generalized type which is often lethal and localized or cutaneous type (Box 2). The following criteria need to be fulfilled for diagnosis of systemic scleromyxedema:
- Generalized confluent papular eruptions
- Histopathology suggestive of scleromyxedema, using special stains
- Monoclonal gammopathy
- Normal thyroid profile.

EPIDEMIOLOGY

Scleromyxedema affects both sexes with most cases reported in middle age groups.[37] There are poor epidemiological data and cases are usually reported from specific regions.

CLINICAL FEATURES

Scleromyxedema is characterized by asymptomatic or mildly pruritic, multiple, linearly

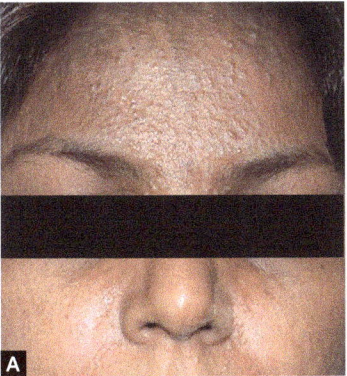
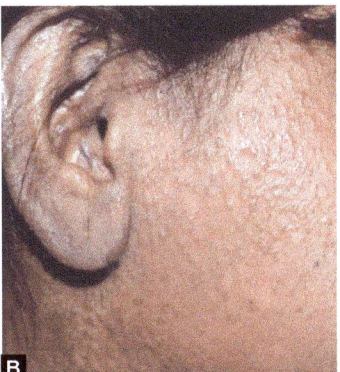
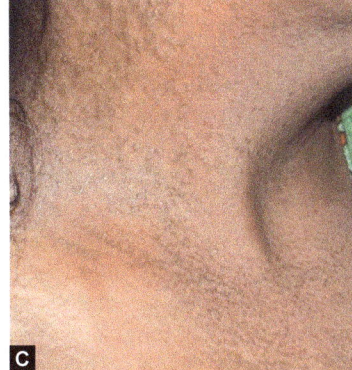

FIGURE 4: A female scleromyxedema patient having papular lesion present over face and neck with more dense lesions over forehead and side of the face.

Skin in Rheumatologic Diseases

> **Box 2: Classification of scleromyxedema**
> - Generalized scleromyxedema or generalized popular mucinosis or sclerodermoid lichen myxedematous
> - Localized scleromyxedema (seen in association with HIV and hepatitis C)
>   - Discrete papular form
>   - Randomly distributed over trunk usually, less number of papules and the face is spared with no systemic involvement
>   - Acral persistent popular mucinosis
>   - Present on the extensor aspects of the forearms and hands, have to be differentiated from Huntley's papules (seen in patients with insulin resistance)
>   - Papular mucinosis of infancy
>   - Self healing cutaneous mucinosis
>   - Juvenile form
>   - Adult form
>   - Nodular mucinosis
>   - Randomly distributed, simulate colloid milia
> - Atypical scleromyxedema
>   - Atypical localized form with systemic features
>   - Atypical generalized scleromyxedema without paraproteinemia

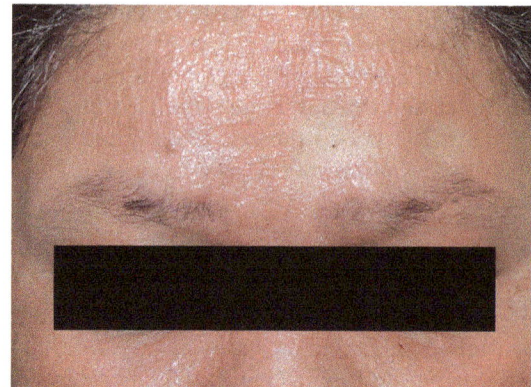

FIGURE 5: Linearly arranged papular lesion over forehead with background erythema and infiltration; also patient is having madrosis.

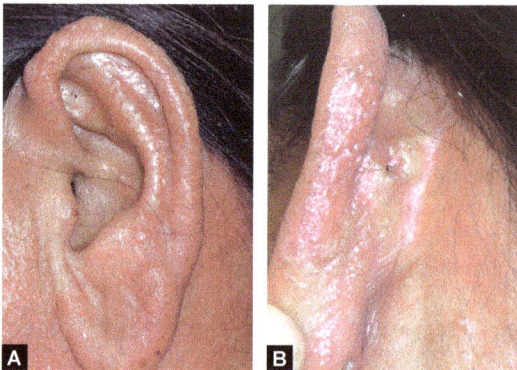

FIGURE 6: Erythema, infiltration and papular lesion over ear.

arranged, confluent waxy papules in a grid-like pattern (Figs 5 and 6), forming thickened plaques underneath, mostly involving the head and neck region (sparing the scalp), but may involve other parts of the body too (Fig. 7 to 9). The thickened plaques lead to loss of facial furrows and expression lines (Fig. 10) giving rise to leonine facies and trismus in some patients. Mucosa is characteristically spared but there may be presence of sclerodactyly in advanced cases. Absence of antinuclear antibodies, telengiectasias, Raynaud's phenomenon, and calcinosis cutis helps in differentiating it from scleroderma. Patient may or may not present with systemic features depending on the type of scleromyxedema. Systemic involvement includes myositis, arthritis, peripheral neuropathies, dermato-neuro syndrome (high fever, seizures, coma with a flu-like prodrome), and rarely visceral involvement including lungs and kidneys.[38]

Scleromyxedema is almost always associated with paraproteinemias.[39] The specific paraprotein

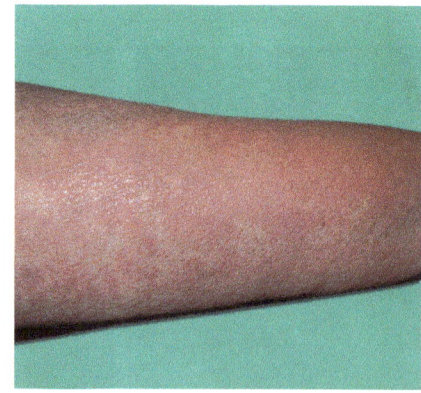

FIGURE 7: Papular lesion and erythema over forearm in a scleromyxedema patient.

Scleredema and Scleromyxedema

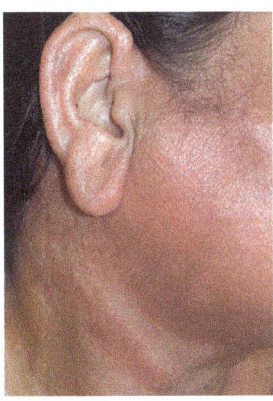

FIGURE 8: Sparing of neck folds in scleromyxedema patient.

Table 4: Types of paraprotein in various disorders	
Paraprotein	**Disease**
IgG kappa	• Scleredema • Necrobiotic xanthogranuloma • Primary systemic amyloidosis
IgG lambda	• Scleromyxedema
IgA	• Erythema elevatum diutinum • Pyoderma gangrenosum • Subcorneal pustular dermatosis • POEMS syndrome
IgM	• Schnitzler's syndrome

POEMS, Polyneuropathy, organomegaly, endocrinopathy, monoclonal gammopathy.

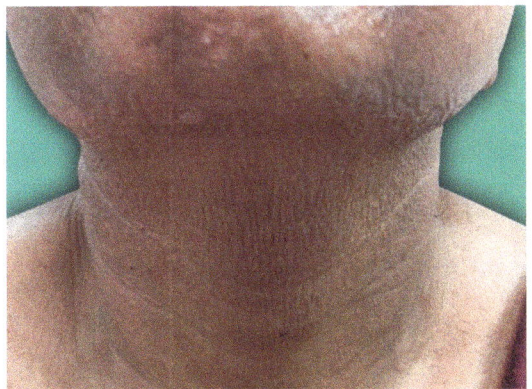

FIGURE 9: Linearly arranged papular lesion over neck.

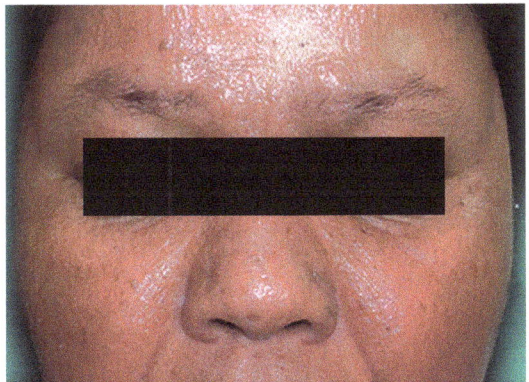

FIGURE 10: Diffuse erythema and infiltration with loss of wrinkles and furrows over face in scleromyxedema patient.

here is IgG lambda. The various skin disorders with their specific paraproteins are described in table 4.

PATHOLOGY

Scleromyxedema is characterized by a classical triad of
- Increased mucin deposition in upper and middle dermis
- Increased collagen deposition in upper and middle dermis
- Increased number of irregularly placed stellate fibroblasts.

The epidermis is normal or thinned out and there is loss of appendages. There is a presence of perivascular lymphocytes and plasma cells while the mucin is seen to cover the entire upper dermis between increased collagen fibers.

DIFFERENTIAL DIAGNOSIS

Other causes of sclerosis have to be ruled out especially scleroderma and morphea. The presence of paraproteinemia and characteristic papular lesions involving the head and neck suggest the diagnosis of scleromyxedema. A complete thyroid panel (to rule out generalized and pretibial myxedema), antinuclear antibody profile, blood sugar estimation (to rule out scleredema), renal function tests (to rule out nephrogenic fibrosing dermopathy) helps in reaching the diagnosis. In patients presenting in an advanced stage with leonine facies, other causes of leonine facies need to be ruled out, e.g., lepromatous Hansen's disease, lipoid proteinosis, primary systemic amyloidosis, actinic reticuloid, Paget's disease of the bone, neurofibromatosis 1, and multicentric reticulohistiocytosis.[40] The localized variant has a long list of differentials and histopathology is a must to confirm the diagnosis.

TREATMENT

The treatment in scleromyxedema is directed toward the plasma cell dyscrasias and melphalan is the drug of choice. Other anticancer agents including cyclophosphamide, chlorambucil and IVIg have been tried with mixed success. Corticosteroids,[41] calcineurin inhibitors,[42] oral retinoids,[43] thalidomide and its congeners,[44,45] have also been tried with some success. The advent of proteosome inhibitors like Bortezomib is reported to be helpful in a few cases but melphalan remains the preferred treatment of choice apart from autologous stem cell transplantation. The cutaneous manifestations respond to the systemic therapy with no or limited role of topical corticosteroids, retinoids and phototherapy as previously thought.

PROGNOSIS

Prognosis of patients with scleromyxedema is poor with no treatment option altering the disease process. The cause of death includes the monoclonal gammopathy per se, lower respiratory tract infections and cardiac complications.

CONCLUSION

Both conditions scleredema and scleromyxedema, are due to idiopathic accumulation of mucin. They are associated with paraproteinemia, connective tissue diseases, and endocrinal disorders. They are not always self-limiting and benign. They are usually not identified with normal histopathology and require special stains. Currently, there is no consensus on treatment protocols. There is a definite role for ultraviolet A1 phototherapy in treatment.

REFERENCES

1. Fracesco Z, James TC. The systemic sclerodermas and related disorders. In: James TC, Ross EP, Ronald ML, Carol BL (Eds). Textbook of Paediatric Rheumatology. Philadelphia: Saunders; 2011. p. 427.
2. Nashel J, Steen V. Scleroderma mimics. Curr Rheumatol Rep. 2012;14(1):39-46
3. Rongioletti F. Lichen myxedematosus (papular mucinosis): new concepts and perspectives for an old disease. Semin Cutan Med Surg. 2006;25:100-4.
4. Venencie PY, Powell FC, Su WP, Perry HO. Scleredema: a review of thirty-three cases. J Am Acad Dermatol. 1984;11:128-34.
5. Buschke A. Ueber Skleroedema. Berl Klin Wchnschr. 1902; 39:955.
6. Morais P, Almeida M, Santos P, Azevedo F. Scleredema of Buschke following Mycoplasma pneumonia respiratory infection. Int J Dermatol. 2011;50:454-7.
7. Murphy-Chutorian B, Han G, Cohen SR. Dermatologic manifestations of diabetes mellitus: a review. Endocrinol Metab Clin North Am. 2013;42(4):869-98.
8. Turchin I, Adams SP, Enta T. Dermacase. Scleredema adultorum, or Bushke disease. Can Fam Physician. 2003; 49:1089-93.
9. Ray V, Boisseau-Garsaud AM, Ray P, Pont F, Lin L, Hélénon R, et al. Obesity persistent scleredema: study of 49 cases. Ann Dermatol Venereol. 2002;129(3):281-5.
10. Varga J, Gotta S, Li L, Sollberg S, Di Leonardo M. Sceredema adultorum: case report and demonstration of abnormal expression of extracellular matrix genes in skin fibrobasts in vivo and in vitro. Br J Dermatol. 1995;132:992-9.
11. Ranganathan P. Infliximab-induced scleredema in a patient with rheumatoid arthritis. J Clin Rheumatol. 2005; 11(6):319-22.
12. Ioannidou DL, Krasagakis K, Stefaniclou MP, Karampekios S, Panayiotidis J, Tosca AD. Scleredema adultorum of Buschke presenting as periorbital oedema: diagnostic challenge. J Am Acad Dermatol. 2005;52:41-4.
13. Farrell AM, Branfoot AC, Moss J, Papadaki L, Woodrow DF, Bunker CB. Scleredema diabeticorum of Buschke confined to the thighs. Br J Dermatol. 1996;134:1113-5.
14. Rani JD, Patil SG, Murthy ST, Koshy AV, Nagpal D, Gupta S. Juvenile scleredema of Buschke. J Contemp Dent Pract. 2012;13(1):111-4.
15. Fernandez-Flores A, Gatica-Torres M, Ruelas-Villavicencio AL, Saeb-Lima M. Morphological clues in the diagnosis of sclerodermiform dermatitis. Am J Dermatopathol. 2014;36(6):449-64.
16. Basarab T, Burrows NP, Munn SE, Jones RR. Systemic involvement in scleredema of buschke associated with IgG-kappa paraproteinaemia. Br J Dermatol. 1997;136(6):939-42.
17. Miyares FJR, Kuriakose R, Deleu DT, El-Wahad NA, Al-Hail H. Scleredema diabeticorum with unusual presentation and fatal outcome. Ind J Dermatol. 2008;53(4):217-219.

18. Ray V, Boisseau-Garsaud AM, Ray P, Pont F, Lin L, Hélénon R, et al. Obesity persistent scleredema: study of 49 cases. Ann Dermatol Venereol. 2002;129(3):281-5.
19. Mohanasundaram K, Kumarasamy S, Kumar R, Rajendran CP. Scleredema adultorum of Buschke: with unusual manifestations in a young female. Indian J Dermatol Venereol Leprol. 2012;78:503-5.
20. Beers WH, Ince A, Moore TL. Scleredema adultorum of Buschke: a case report and review of the literature. Semin Arthritis Rheum. 2006;35(6):355-9.
21. Rongioletti F, Rebora A. Cutaneous mucinoses: microscopic criteria for diagnosis. Am J Dermatopathol. 2001;23(3):257-67.
22. Roupe G, Laurent TC, Malmstrom A, Suurküla M, Särnstrand B. Biochemical characterization and tissue distribution of the scleredema in a case of Buschke's disease. Acta Derm Venereol. 1987;67:193-8.
23. Varga J, Gotta S, Li L, Sollberg S, Di Leonardo M. Scleredema adultorum: case report and demonstration of abnormal expression of extracellular matrix genes in skin fibroblasts in vivo and in vitro. Br J Dermatol. 1995;132:992-9.
24. Tasanen K, Palatsi R, Oikarinen A. Demonstration of increased levels of type I collagen mRNA using quantitative polymerase chain reaction in fibrotic and granulomatous skin diseases. Br J Dermatol. 1998;139:23-6.
25. Conde Fernandes I, Sanches M, Velho G, Lobo I, Alves R, Selores M. Scleromyxedema vs scleredema: a diagnostic challenge. Eur J Dermatol. 2011;21(5):822-823.
26. Foti R, Leonardi R, Fichera G, Di Gangi M, Leonetti C, Gangemi P, et al. [Buschke Scleredema, case report]. Reumatismo. 2006;58(4):310-3.
27. Popadić S, Skiljević D, Antić D, Milenković B, Medenica L. Widespread scleredema associated with paraproteinemia and generalized osteoarthritis in an HLA-B39 positive patient. Acta Dermatovenerol Croat. 2011;19(3):191-4.
28. Yoshimura Y, Asano Y, Takahashi T, Uwajima Y, Kagami S, Honda H, et al. A case of scleredema adultorum successfully treated with narrow-band ultraviolet B phototherapy. Mod Rheumatol. 2014;15:3-5.
29. Kroft EBM, De Jong EMGJ. Scleredema diabeticorum case series: successful treatment with UV-A1. Arch Dermatol. 2008;144(7):947-8.
30. Aichelburg MC, Loewe R, Schicher N, Sator PG, Karlhofer FM, Stingl G, et al. Successful treatment of post streptococcal scleredema adultorum of Buschke with intravenous immunoglobulins. Arch Dermatol. 2012;148:1126-8.
31. Venturi C, Zendri E, Santini M, Grignaffini E, Ricci R, De Panfilis G. Scleredema of Buschke: remission with factor XIII treatment. Int J Tissue React. 2004;26(1-2):25-8.
32. Meguerditchian C, Jacquet P, Béliard S, Benderitter T, Valéro R, Carsuzza F, et al. Scleredema adultorum of Buschke: an under recognized skin complication of diabetes. Diabetes Metab. 2006;32(5):481-4.
33. Turchin I, Adams SP, Enta T. Scleredema adultorum or Buscke disease. Can Fam Phys. 2003;49:1089-93.
34. Sansom JE, Sheehan AL, Kennedy CT, Delaney TJ. A fatal case of scleredema of Buschke. Br J Dermatol. 1994;130(5):669-70.
35. Cokonis Georgakis CD, Falasca G, Georgakis A, Heymann WR. Scleromyxedema. Clin Dermatol. 2006;24:493-7.
36. Rongioletti F. Lichen myxedematosus (papular mucinosis): new concepts and perspectives for an old disease. Semin Cutan Med Surg. 2006;25:100-4.
37. Heymann WR. Scleromyxedema. J Am Acad Dermatol. 2007;57:890-1.
38. Marshall K, Klepeiss SA, Ioffreda MD, Helm KF. Scleromyxedema presenting with neurologic symptoms: a case report and review of the literature. Cutis. 2010;85(3):137-40.
39. Rongioletti F, Merlo G, Cinotti E, Fausti V, Cozzani E, Cribier B. Scleromyxedema: a multicenter study of characteristics, comorbidities, course, and therapy in 30 patients. J Am Acad Dermatol. 2013;69(1):66-72.
40. Montgomery H, Underwood LJ. Lichen myxedematosus; differentiation from cutaneous myxedemas or mucoid states. J Invest Dermatol. 1953;20(3):213-36.
41. Lun YC, Wang HC, Shen JL. Scleromyxedema: an experience using treatment with systemic corticosteroid and review of the published work. J Dermatol. 2006;3:207-10.
42. Rongioletti F, Zaccaria E, Cozzani E, Parodi A. Treatment of localized lichen myxedematosus of discrete type with tacrolimus ointment. J Am Acad Dermatol. 2008;58(3):530-2.
43. Hisler BM, Sovaj LB, Hashimoto K. Improvement of scleromyxedema associated with isotretinoin therapy. J Am Acad Dermatol. 1991;24:854-7.
44. Jacob SE, Fien S, Kerdel FA. Scleromyxedema, a positive effect with thalidomide. Dermatology. 2006;213(2):150-2.
45. Brunet-Possenti F, Hermine O, Marinho E, Crickx B, Descamps V. Combination of intravenous immunoglobulins and lenalidomide in the treatment of scleromyxedema. J Am Acad Dermatol. 2013;69(2):319-20.

CHAPTER 12

Sjögren's Syndrome

Sapan C Pandya, Avinash Jain

INTRODUCTION

The word "Sjögren" comes after the Swedish ophthalmologist Henrik Sjögren who in 1933 gave the first proper description of 19 patients with dry eyes and dry mouth, the combination of which he termed "keratoconjunctivitis sicca".[1] Mikulicz (Johann von Mikulicz Radecki) described a case of bilateral parotid and lacrimal enlargement with lymphocytic infiltration (now included in the IgG4-related diseases) and later in 1960s autoantibody associations of Sjögren's syndrome (SS) came to be known.

Sjögren's syndrome is an autoimmune inflammatory disorder characterized by diminished lacrimal and salivary gland functions. The "spectrum" of SS can be divided into:
- Primary versus secondary Sjögren's syndrome (pSS vs. sSS)
- Extraglandular versus exocrine predominant Sjögren's syndrome.
- Isolated "dry eye syndrome" and
- SS in the elderly and children as a special category.

Primary Sjögren's syndrome is not associated with any other autoimmune diseases while sSS is associated with mainly rheumatoid arthritis (RA) and lupus but also other diseases like scleroderma and mixed connective-tissue disease (MCTD). There are also overlaps with primary biliary cirrhosis or Grave's disease or hypothyroidism.

Within the pSS, two subsets are recognized: (i) the predominant exocrinopathy variant, wherein the patients have mainly sicca symptoms with or without mild constitutional or musculoskeletal symptoms and low titer antibodies and (ii) the predominant severe extraglandular variant with recurrent parotitis, submandibular gland enlargement, purpura, high acute phase reactants, low complements, high titer anti-Ro and/or La antibodies, the variant likely to evolve into a lymphoma. A third variant has been suggested with extraglandular features, sometimes single organ like interstitial nephritis or purpura with high titer antibody positivity but very little sicca symptoms if at all.

Sjögren's syndrome prevalence is higher in elderly while the disease is rare in children—the smallest child reported was 3 years old.[2]

EPIDEMIOLOGY

Sjögren's syndrome is the second most common inflammatory rheumatologic disease after RA. There are few epidemiologic studies defining the incidence and prevalence of this disease but none from India. Traditionally believed to be a disease of middle age (most common in the fourth to fifth decade of life), the disease can occur at young age as well as the elderly. The female to male ratio in various series has ranged from 9:1 to 20:1.[3]

The highest incidence has been reported from Greece—5.3/100,000 population. The prevalence of the syndrome has ranged from 0.03% (Japan) to 2.7% (Sweden). Prevalence has been higher in the elderly (6–14%).

Prevalence of sSS has been in the range of 6.5-19% with lupus (younger patients) and 5-29% in RA. Out of 25 MCTD patients, about 12 reported sicca symptoms. In scleroderma, keratoconjunctivitis sicca was reported in about 80% of patients but lymphocytic infiltration on biopsies was seen in only about 4.4%. Among overlap diseases, primary biliary cirrhosis and autoimmune hepatitis was seen in 11.9% and 4%, respectively. Hypothyroidism (14%), Grave's opthalmopathy (3%), and sarcoidosis (1-2%) are other autoimmune disease overlaps seen with SS.

ETIOPATHOGENESIS

There are many similarities between lupus and pSS etiopathogenesis, chief among which is the interferon (IFN) signature in both. There is, however, mucosal tropism in pSS. Why and how does that happen?

Viral triggers (Epstein-Barr virus, hepatitis C virus, Coxsackie A virus, or endogenous retroviral elements) in conjunction with toll-like receptors (TLR 3, 7, 9) or other activators of the innate immune system such as dysregulated activation of nuclear factor κB (NFκB) signaling (decreased expression of A20, a regulator of NFκB) lead to IFN production (Fig. 1). Viral injury leads to the release of ribonucleoproteins Ro and La on the salivary epithelial tissue and chemokines that bring in dendritic cells and plasmacytoid dendritic cells.[4] In which individuals does this happen? The preliminary results of the genome-wide association study done on pSS patients has shown

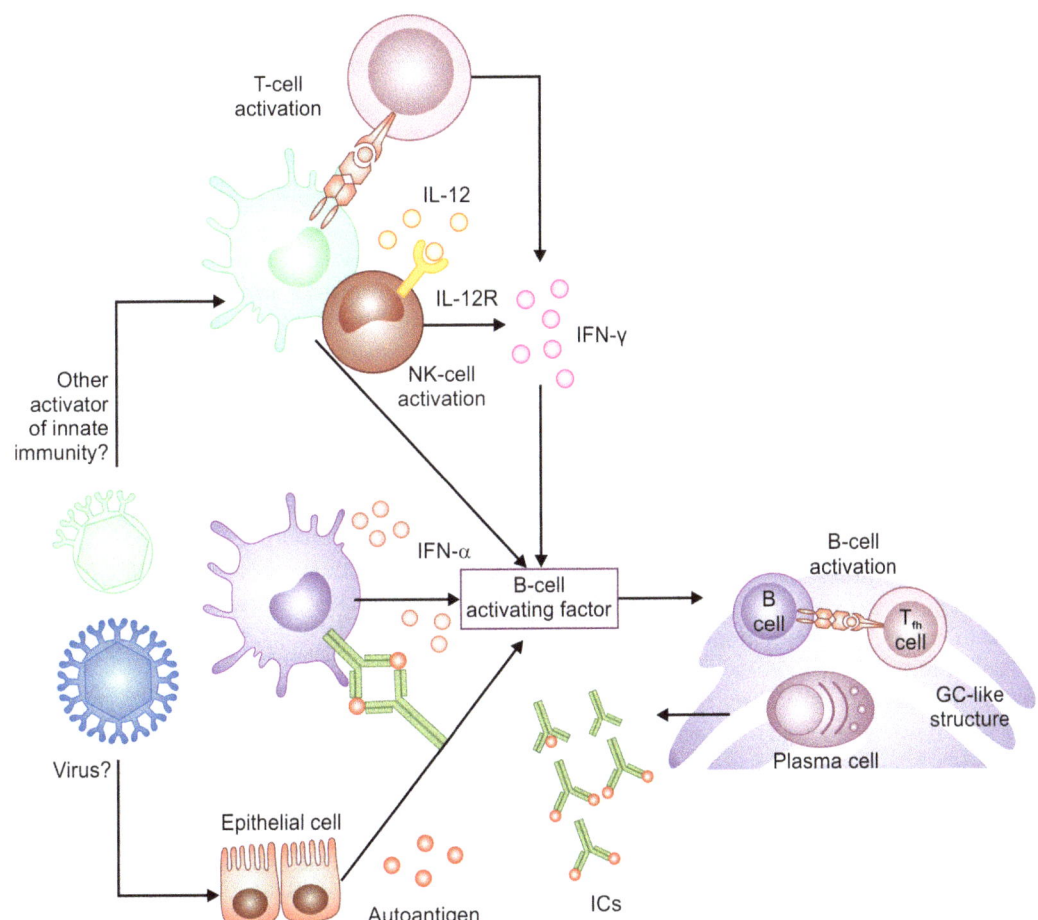

FIGURE 1: Pathogenesis of primary Sjogren's Syndrome.

associations with HLA-DQB1 and polymorphisms located in interferon regulatory factor 5, signal transducer and activator of transcription 4, B lymphocyte kinase, interleukin-12 subunit alpha, tumor necrosis factor-alpha induced protein 3 interacting protein 1, and C-X-C chemokine receptor type 5. Epigenetic mechanisms also might be involved. Epithelial activation in these individuals then leads to the secretion of type 1 IFN by the plasmacytoid dendritic cells and type 2 IFN by the dendritic cells through IL-12. The latter leads to tissue damage through activation of natural killer (NK) and Th1 cells. These events lead to lymphocyte migration to these areas which in turn leads to the secretion of B cell activating factor (BAFF). The B cell activation and BAFF promote autoantibody secretion anti-Ro and La—these bind to their respective antigens and these immune complexes in turn maintain IFN-α production thus leading to a vicious cycle. Interleukin-14 and IL-10 have been shown to be some of the other B cell activating cytokines in patients with pSS.

There has been a lot of work on "ectopic germinal centers" in patients with pSS. C-X-C chemokine receptor type 5 and its ligand CXCL13 are involved in the recruitment of B cells and follicular helper T cells to the B cell zone of these germinal blasts (GCs). Through IL-21, these follicular T cells provide T cell help to the B cells and regulate B cell differentiation to plasma cells and memory B cells. The GCs are an important marker for lymphoma development in these patients.

There have been some new developments on the role of NK cell subsets not dependent on IL-12 that express NK cell receptors, IL-7 (hematopoietic growth factor that promotes survival of mature naïve and memory T cells) and Th17 cells (found to be increased in pSS patients compared to normal). To date, no regulatory T cell defects have been found to be associated with pSS.

Why does this disease affect perimenopausal women predominantly? Estrogen deprivation leads to over-expression of retinoblastoma binding protein 4—the latter, in animal models, has been seen to lead to sicca symptoms. Dysfunction of hypothalamic-pituitary-gonadal axis and hypothalamic pituitary adrenal axis has been hypothesized in pSS.

Future research will tell us why pSS is "lupus of the mucosa"—the mechanisms of the mucosal tropism of the immune system activation in pSS.

CLASSIFICATION CRITERIA

There have been many a proposals for defining the classification criteria for pSS—at least 11 since 1965. Chief among them are the American European Consensus Group (Box 1) and the recently proposed American College of Rheumatology (ACR) criteria[5] (Box 2).

What are the main differences between these two criteria and why was there the need to bring about a new set of criteria? The problems with the American European Consensus Group criteria (2002) are:

- The subjective symptoms can be very nonspecific especially with aging

---

Box 1: The American European Consensus Group criteria

I. Ocular symptoms: a positive response to at least one of three validated questions
 1. Daily, persistent, troublesome dry eyes for more than 3 months?
 2. Recurrent sensation of sand or gravel in the eyes?
 3. Use of artificial tears >3 × per day?

II. Oral symptoms (at least one)
 1. Dry mouth >3 months?
 2. Recurrent or persistently swollen salivary glands as an adult?
 3. Need liquids to swallow dry foods?

III. Ocular signs: That is, objective evidence of ocular involvement defined as a positive result for at least one of the following two tests:
 1. Schirmer's test, without anesthesia (≤5 mm in 5 min)
 2. Rose Bengal score or other ocular dye score (≥4 according to van Bijsterveld's scoring system)

IV. Histopathology: Lip biopsy showing focal lymphocytic sialoadenitis (FLS) [focus score ≥1 per 4 mm². Focal lymphocytic sialoadenitis is number of lymphocytic foci (which are adjacent to normal-appearing mucous acini and contain more than 50 lymphocytes) per 4 mm² of glandular tissue]

V. Oral signs (at least one)
1. Unstimulated whole salivary flow (≤1.5 mL in 15 min)
2. Abnormal parotid sialography showing the presence of diffuse sialectasias
3. Abnormal salivary scintigraphy showing delayed uptake, reduced concentration, and/or delayed excretion of tracer

VI. Autoantibodies: Presence in the serum of the following autoantibodies:
1. Antibodies to Ro(SSA) or La(SSB) antigens, or both
   - For a primary Sjögren's diagnosis:
     a. Any 4 of the 6 criteria, must include either item IV (histopathology) or VI (autoantibodies)
     b. Any 3 of the 4 objective criteria (III, IV, V, VI)
   - For a secondary Sjögren's diagnosis:
     a. In patients with another well-defined major connective tissue disease, the presence of one symptom (I or II) plus 2 of the 3 objective criteria (III, IV, and V) is indicative of secondary Sjögren's syndrome

Exclusion criteria
- Past head and neck radiation treatment
- Hepatitis C infection
- Acquired immunodeficiency syndrome
- Preexisting lymphoma
- Sarcoidosis
- Graft-versus-host disease
- Use of anticholinergic drugs (since a time shorter than fourfold the half-life of the drug)

Source: Vitali C, Bombardieri S, Jonsson R, Moutsopoulos HM, Alexander EL, Carsons SE, et al. European Study Group on Classification Criteria for Sjögren's Syndrome. Classification criteria for Sjögren's syndrome: a revised version of the European criteria proposed by the American-European Consensus Group. Ann Rheum Dis. 2002;61(6):554-8.

Box 2: The American College of Rheumatology criteria

The classification of Sjögren's syndrome, which applies to individuals with signs or symptoms that may be suggestive of Sjögren's syndrome will be met in patients who have at least two of the following three objective features:

1. Positive serum anti-SSA/Ro and/or anti-SSB/La or (positive rheumatoid factor and antinuclear antibody titer 1:320)
2. Labial salivary gland biopsy exhibiting focal lymphocytic sialoadenitis with a focus score ≥1 focus/4 mm^2
3. Keratoconjunctivitis sicca with ocular staining score ≥3 (assuming that individual is not currently using daily eye drops for glaucoma and has not had corneal surgery or cosmetic eyelid surgery in the last 5 years)

Prior diagnosis of any of the following conditions needs to be excluded
- History of head and neck radiation treatment
- Hepatitis C infection
- Acquired immunodeficiency syndrome
- Sarcoidosis
- Amyloidosis
- Graft versus host disease
- Immunoglobulin G4-related disease

Source: American European Consensus Group. Shiboski SC, Shiboski CH, Criswell LA, Baer AN, Challacombe S, Lanfranchi H, et al. American College of Rheumatology Classification Criteria for Sjögren's Syndrome: a data-driven, expert consensus approach in the Sjögren's International Collaborative Clinical Alliance Cohort. Arthritis Care Res. 2012;64(4):475-87.

- While the Schirmer's test is an easy bedside test to screen for dry eyes, it lacks specificity for pSS and may not correlate with disease activity. The ocular staining tests are cumbersome and difficult to perform in day-to-day practice
- The histopathology is subject to pathologist interpretation which may differ—the sensitivity and specificity of this varies from 63% to 93% and 61% to 100%, respectively. Up to 22% of males and 36% of females on postmortem may show similar grades of lymphocytic infiltration
- Objective tests for oral dryness—does not specify the method of collection. Salivation may differ with age, sex, smoking, drugs, diurnal cycle, etc. Sialography and scintigraphy require referral to higher centers to perform and lack specificity for pSS
- Autoantibody tests are positive only about 60-65% of the times. They may be positive in other connective tissue diseases and hence are not specific.

The ACR criteria were proposed (2012) to overcome these limitations and to ensure high specificity so that they can be applied in clinical trials involving the use of biologic agents which are costly and not without side effects.

While the ACR criteria may be more specific because of the use of objective tests, they are not without problems, some of which are listed below:
- Autoantibody positivity as discussed above. Antinuclear antibody and rheumatoid facto positivity can be even more nonspecific
- Histopathology issues discussed above
- Corneal staining tests would need specialist ophthalmic referral and cannot be as easily done as bedside Schirmer's
- Those patients with subclinical immunologic disease which has not progressed to that much dryness so as to cause corneal scarring or focal lymphocytic score may be missed.

While both sets of criteria are being used in clinical trials and real life, outpatient departments both for classifying and diagnosing pSS, there is the need for more biomarkers, e.g., α Fodrin antibodies or magnetic resonance imaging salivary glands or sialography or easier bedside tools like the ultrasound of salivary glands to pick up those early patients who still have subclinical disease but a better chance of response to treatment.

CLINICAL FEATURES

The spectrum of clinical manifestations of pSS patients can be divided into glandular (exocrine function) and extraglandular (other parenchymal organs) (Table 1). The latter are also sometimes classified into the nonspecific (periepithelial infiltration by lymphocytes) and immune complex mediated (B cell hyperactivity).

Table 1: Clinical features of primary Sjögren's syndrome		
Symptoms/Organ involved	%	Glandular manifestations
Eye dryness (Fig. 2)	95	Foreign body sensation, grittiness, redness, itching, eye fatigue, thick mucus in inner canthus, absence of tear in conjunctival sac, devitalized tissue on slit lamp
Xerostomia (dry mouth) (Figs 3 and 4)	90	Difficulty chewing, swallowing, altered taste, dental caries, difficulty wearing dentures, dry sticky erythematous mucosa, loss of filiform papillae. Complications like fungal infection, angular cheilits
Parotid, submandibular gland swelling	30–40	Painless, chronic, unilateral to bilateral diffuse firm swelling. Acute presentation could be because of mucus inspissation. Rule out bacterial infection if there is associated fever. Rule out lymphoma in persistent, hard nodular swelling
Skin	10	Dry skin or itching (xerosis), eyelid dermatitis, donut-ring-like erythema, vitiligo
Other exocrine glands	–	Dyspareunia (vaginal), dry cough (xerotrachea), hoarseness (larynx)
Symptoms/Organ involved	%	Extraglandular symptoms*
Fatigue	75	Physical as well as mental fatigue, compounded by anxiety, depression, fibromyalgia, poor concentration, low stamina
Arthralgia	40–60	Nonerosive, asymmetrical or symmetrical, can be episodic
Raynaud	13–33	May precede glandular manifestations, digital ulcers rare
Lung	9–14	Dry cough, dyspnea, chest pain, bibasilar crackles; may precede glandular symptoms but typically occurs late; obstructive or restrictive pattern
Lymphadenopathy	14	Reactive or infection or lymphoma
Gastric or esophageal	33	Heartburn, dyspepsia, dysphagia
Liver	6	Obstructive jaundice, itching, fatigue

Continued

Continued

Table 1: Clinical features of primary Sjögren's syndrome		
Renal	2.5-9	Subclinical, distal renal tubular acidosis presenting as nephrocalcinosis, hypokalemic paralysis, very rarely hematuria, pedal edema hypertension (glomerulonephritis)
Bladder	4	Dysuria, urinary frequency, urgency, recurrent urinary tract infection
Peripheral nervous system	10	Paresthesia, ataxia, autonomic dysfunction, sensorimotor
Spinal cord	–	Myelopathy, myelitis
Central nervous systems and psychiatric	1-2	Stroke, multiple sclerosis like features, cognitive and mood disturbances, movement disorder, aseptic meningitis, neuromyelitis optica[9]
Cranial nerve	–	Commonly trigeminal neuralgia and optic neuritis, III, IV, VI, VII, cranial neuropathy. VIII coming with sensorineural hearing loss is often overlooked
Myositis	1	Mild inflammatory myopathy: severe cases rule out overlap
Vasculitis (Fig. 5)	Rare	Cutaneous vasculitis (10%) as purpura (palpable to nonpalpable), demyelinating polyneuropathy. CNS vasculitis rarely presenting as stroke or demyelinating lesion. Glomerulonephritis with or without cryoglobulinemia
Thyroid	10-70	Common associated disorder
Addison	17	Adrenal hyporesponsiveness
Cardiac	–	Rarely acute pericarditis, similar to general population
Pregnancy	–	Anti-Ro association with neonatal lupus, congenital; heart block

*Note: 75% patients experience it but only one-third have serious manifestations.

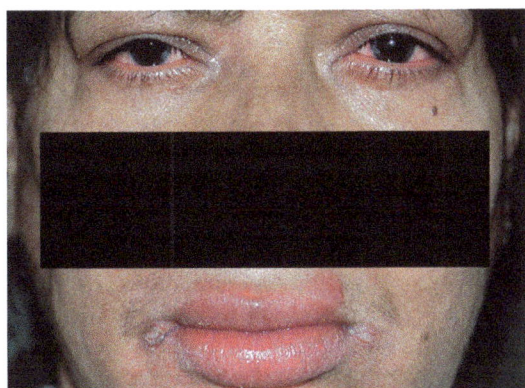

FIGURE 2: Dry eyes with angular cheilitis and dryness of mouth.

The earliest (1970s) extraglandular manifestations known were the respiratory (bronchitis sicca), renal (renal tubular acidosis—RTA), and lymphoma.[6] In the early 1980s, it was realized that while in the majority the disease is progressive and takes a 6-8 year span to develop into the full blown picture, in a few, it may start with nonspecific extraglandular manifestations like Raynaud's phenomenon (usually not leading to digital ulcer), arthralgias or arthritis (Jaccoud's), RTA, or purpura. Glomerulonephritis different from lupus (predominantly only immunoglobulin M in pSS) and vasculitis (skin, bowel, gangrene, gall bladder) were recognized in pSS around this time. Between the 80s and 90s, descriptions of gastrointestinal manifestations—esophageal dysfunction (does not correlate with grade of lymphocytic infiltration salivary glands or autoantibodies); subclinical pancreatitis, primary biliary cirrhosis (transaminitis in pSS patients), and myositis (vasculitis) were published. It is only in the last decade that the immunoglobulin G4-related disease came around as a close differential diagnosis of pSS.

An ataxic form of sensory neuropathy, which may take months or years to develop fully, may be seen in these patients due to dorsal ganglionitis and mononuclear cell infiltration. Not uncommonly,

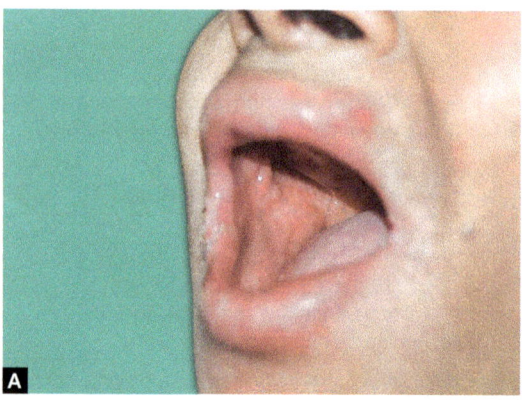
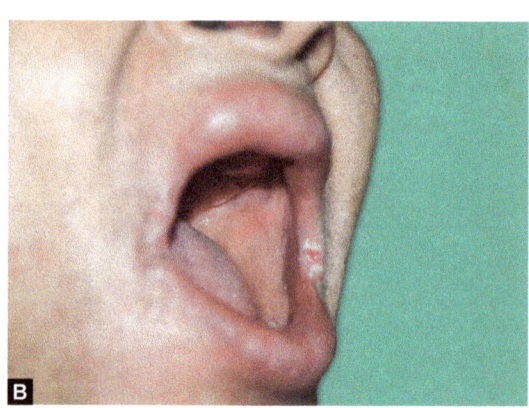

FIGURE 3: Angular cheilitis in Sjogren's Syndrome.

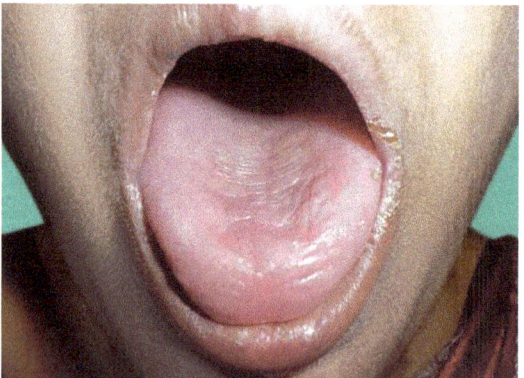

FIGURE 4: Severe tongue and lip dryness.

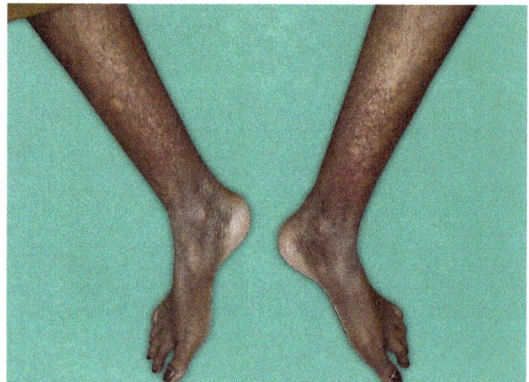

FIGURE 5: Dependent hypergammaglobulinemic purpura of Waldenstrom.

it is associated with pseudoathetosis. Trigeminal neuralgia with only sensory involvement and autonomic neuropathy which may manifest as diarrhea, syncope, abdominal pain, constipation, anhidrosis, orthostatic hypotension, or urinary symptoms are rarely seen. Central nervous system manifestations may include transient ischemic attacks, hemiparesis, and cognitive dysfunction. About 15% of patients of multiple sclerosis may fulfill criteria of pSS—cerebrospinal fluid (CSF) in such patients would show multiple bands instead of few in pSS. Magnetic resonance imaging white matter hyperintensities are also seen sometimes in patients of pSS. Low mood, depression, anxiety, and even dementia have been reported in these patients.

Patients of pSS with pulmonary involvement have fourfold rises in mortality compared to those without. Apart from the common manifestations described in the table, interstitial lung disease (ILD) is also reported in 11% of pSS patients clinically (histologically 75%). All types of ILDs—nonspecific interstitial pneumonitis (NSIP), lymphocytic interstitial pneumonitis (LIP, most common), usual interstitial pneumonitis, and organizing pneumonia have been reported.[7] Lymphocytic interstitial pneumonitis presents as cough, fever, night sweats, and dyspnea frequently mistreated as infection. High-resolution computed therapy will show ground glass opacities with thin walled cysts in up to 50% of patients. Histologically, one finds plasma cell and lymphocyte infiltration of interstitial septa and alveolar walls. Most commonly seen in the sixth decade of life, it may take up to 15 months for diagnosis from time of onset. Nonspecific interstitial pneumonitis is seen in various series ranging from 28 to 33% of patients. It also presents with cough and dyspnea with fever more commonly seen in NSIP than LIP. Pulmonary hypertension due to vasculitis or vasculopathy is uncommon but reported.

While arthralgias in pSS can be symmetric, arthritis is asymmetric in distribution. There are case reports of RA occurring in patients diagnosed with pSS after many years. These cases of RA overlapping with pSS had less of purpura, vasculitis, leucopenia, cryoglobulins, and Antinuclear antibodies compared to pSS alone. They also had less severe radiologic disease compared to RA alone. Fibromyalgia, (FMS) is reported in up to 20% of patients with pSS. Patients with primary FMS have lower threshold of pain compared to pSS with secondary FMS.

Vasculitis and vasculitic purpura in patients of pSS make them more vulnerable to lymphomas. Associations with low complements (especially C4), rheumatoid factor positivity, cryoglobulins, greater anti-Ro and La positivity, and lymphoma development have been reported by more than one investigator. All three types—flat hypergammaglobulinemic purpura, leukocytoclastic vasculitis, and medium vessel vasculitis (polyarteritis nodosa type but without aneurysms) have been reported.[8] Systemic vasculitis may present with neurologic deficits, cutaneous ulcerations, and even gall bladder perforation.

While there are scarce data published from India on pSS profile of patients, in those that have been published, the differences from the West were younger patients, less female to male ratio, and perhaps more extraglandular features in the form of arthritis and renal manifestations (particularly RTA—delay in diagnosis presenting both as hypokalemic palsy and less often pseudofractures).[9] There is also a report of an ultrasound study of the salivary glands correlating with the histopathology.

Skin in Primary Sjögren's Syndrome

Apart from the vasculitic purpura mentioned above, other cutaneous manifestations of pSS include xeroderma (dry skin), angular cheilits, eyelid dermatitis, and urticarial-like lesions

Box 3: Skin lesions in primary Sjögren's syndrome patient
- Xeroderma
- Vasculitis
- Annular erythema
- Angular cheilitis
- Eyelid dermatitis
- Urticarial rash
- Granulomatous panniculitis

(Box 3). Case reports of primary localized cutaneous nodular amyloid and granulomatous panniculitis also appear in literature.[10] Two cutaneous findings need special mention: (i) annular erythema and (ii) hypergammaglobulinemic purpura of Waldenstrom.

Annular erythema may precede the diagnosis of pSS. In a case series published, it was found to occur in 9% of pSS patients.[11] They were more often middle aged White females. The rash appeared on the face, neck, and upper extremities predominantly flared in the warmer months (photosensitive) and was strongly associated with anti-Ro antibodies. These may be difficult to differentiate from the lesions of subacute lupus erythematosus. Histopathology it shows dermal mucin deposition and features of lupus erythematosus tumidus.

Hypergammaglobulinemic purpura can be a presenting manifestation of pSS. Not infrequently these patients present with increasing eruption (in the lower limbs) in the dependent position which disappears or lessens in severity on elevating the legs. The rash has a strong association with globulin levels, anti-Ro and La and rheumatoid factor. A biopsy may show mononuclear or neutrophilic infiltration around blood vessels. Therapy is needed only if symptomatic and may be unrewarding at times.[12]

Lymphoma

Sjögren's syndrome holds the burden of being an autoimmune disease with the highest risk of lymphoma. Two Scandinavian studies and a recent data from a meta-analysis on the risk of lymphoma have been published.[13] The relative risk (RR) of development of non-Hodgkin's

> **Box 4: Prognostic markers for increased risk of lymphoma**
>
> - Persistent parotid enlargement
> - Purpura
> - Leucopenia
> - Low C4
> - Cyroglobulins
> - Anti-La antibodies
> - Gene polymorphism like TNFAIP3 serum cytokine FLT3-L
> - Ectopic germinal center' formation detected on HPE
>
> TNFAIP3, tumor necrosis factor α induced protein 3; FLT3L, FMS-related tyrosine kinase 3 ligand; HPE, holoprosencephaly.

lymphoma (NHL) in pSS patients was 6.1 as against 1.5 for RA and 4.5 for lupus. In the meta-analysis reported, the RR of developing lymphoma was 18.8 for pSS, 3.9 for RA, and 7.4 for lupus. These are mostly low-grade B cell NHL, mainly of marginal zone histological type and mucosal localization is predominant. Lymphomas often develop in organs where SS is active, such as salivary glands. Prognostic markers leading to increased risk of lymphoma are presented in box 4.[14] While most of these are low grade and indolent, survival is reduced in patients with B symptoms, lymph node more than or equal to 7 cm diameter and high or intermediate histological grade.

Overlap Diseases

Almost a third of patients with SS may have another autoimmune disease. The most common is hypothyroidism (14%). About 18–22% of patients with RA (especially with high titers of rheumatoid factor) have sSS. In a series of lupus patients, SS was reported in about 17%.[6] These patients were older, had arthritis and oral ulcers but less severe nephritis or central nervous system (CNS) involvement, had anti-Ro and La positivity and less of anti-Sm or cardiolipin antibodies. They generally had a more favorable prognosis. Some patients diagnosed as pSS may evolve into lupus or develop signs and symptoms of lupus after many years—in different series; this has been reported in 1.5–15% of patients. These patients were younger, had lower complement levels, higher globulins, and anti-La positivity. About 17–22% of scleroderma patients have sSS due to fibrosis of the salivary glands. They may have more of peripheral neuropathy and the overlap of SS in these seems to protect them against SSc-associated ILD.

The terms SS type 1 and 2 have been proposed for pSS and sSS.

DIAGNOSIS AND DIFFERENTIAL DIAGNOSIS

In addition to detailed clinical evaluation also including the questions mentioned in the classification criteria for pSS, the following tests should be offered to these patients for a complete work up: Schirmer's test using a filter paper strip (less than 5 mL in 5 minutes is positive—sensitivity of 77% and specificity ranging 4–72%) and the lissamine dye test for documenting corneal dryness and keratitis (sensitivity 64% and specificity 82%, the rose Bengal dye test is now considered obsolete, two scores are used—the van Bijsterveld score and the ocular staining score) for ocular dryness; unstimulated salivary flow rate using a graded tube (<1.5 mL over 15 minutes is positive for dryness—sensitivity 56% and specificity 81%) and minor salivary gland biopsy for focus score (defined as more than 50 lymphocyte clusters in an area of 4 mm² of surface in at least one of four lobules, sensitivity of 82% and specificity 86%) for oral dryness.[8]

It was around the 1980s that the antigens Ro and La were identified as ribonucleoproteins containing cytoplasmic ribonucleic acid (RNA) and proteins. The Ro 60 kD component is directly bound to the RNA in the complex and may have a role in deoxyribonucleic acid replication while the Ro 52 kD component is not RNA bound and may have a role in ubiquitation and modulation of innate immune system. While counter immunoelectrophoresis and immunoprecipitation assays are the gold standard for detecting antibodies against these, the western blot, enzyme-linked immunosorbent assay, and multiplex microbead immunoassays done commercially may show variable results especially with the Ro peptide. Specialized antibody tests like anti Ro and anti La (found in 70–100% and 35–70% patients respectively, latter more specific), and rheumatoid factor, hepatitis C, human T-cell lymphotropic virus type 1, human immunodeficiency virus (HIV), and serum electrophoresis are other tests that should be ordered as a part of work up. Complement levels, cryoglobulins, immunofixation, and other tests like the bone marrow biopsy or computed tomography scans may be done when lymphoma is a strong possibility complicating pSS. Flow cytometry using CD 38 and IgD is also used to identify subsets of B cells that can differentiate pSS from lupus and other autoimmune diseases. About 5–10% of pSS patients may have anticentromere antibody positivity—these patients have features of scleroderma like Raynaud's, dysphagia and telangiectasia—less severe pulmonary hypertension. Other antibody associations in overlap cases are anti-Ki SL (lupus pSS), anti-p80 coilin (primary biliary cirrhosis—pSS), and anti-Ku (SSc, myositis, cutaneous lupus with pSS). There is also some data on anti-α fodrin, anti-carbonic anhydrase, and antimuscarinic receptor antibodies in pSS patients but their diagnostic utility is still not clear.[15]

Salivary gland ultrasound is being used to diagnose pSS with a sensitivity of 63% and specificity of 95%. The Outcome Measures in Rheumatology group is working on validation of its use in pSS.[15]

Various conditions leading to sicca symptoms is shown in box 5.

Dysfunction of any component lacrimal functional unit (LFU) which comprises of lacrimal gland, meibomian glands, corneal and conjunctival epithelium, goblet cells and the tear film, and neural network that sends afferent signals to the CNS and efferents from there back to the glands of the LFU[16] can lead to dry eye. Hence, a thorough ophthalmic assessment including skin examination, blinking rate, eye and lid morphology, and slit lamp examination are a must apart from the ocular tests described before.

OUTCOME MEASURES

Since there are two components to the symptomatology of pSS—the subjective symptoms of dryness, fatigue, and pain (musculoskeletal), and the systemic complaints due to extraglandular manifestations, two validated indices have been developed to assess disease activity. For the former, the European League Against Rheumatism (EULAR) Sjögren's Syndrome Patient Reported Index (ESSPRI) is used to asses on a scale from 0 to 10 for dryness, fatigue, and pain over previous 2 weeks; mean of the three is the final score. For the latter (systemic extraglandular complaints predominantly), the EULAR Sjögren's Syndrome Disease Activity Index (ESSDAI) is use—a weighted 12 domain score (from 0 to maximum 123).[17] There are also some validated damage indices for pSS (e.g., SS damage index).

MANAGEMENT

The treatment of pSS aims at reducing the signs and symptoms of glandular and extraglandular manifestations. This often requires a multidisciplinary approach as the disease has a wide clinical spectrum. Mostly aimed at providing symptomatic relief, for the systemic manifestations, there is an important role for immunosuppressive therapy and even biologics in pSS.

Glandular Manifestations

Objective of treatment is not only to provide symptomatic relief but also limit the damaging effects of chronic sicca symptoms. General measures include:
- Maintenance of good hydration
- Avoidance of low humid climate, air conditioning, windy environment
- Avoidance of drugs with anticholinergic effects like tricyclic antidepressants, monoamine

> **Box 5: List of differential diagnosis**
> - Infections like tuberculosis, hepatitis C virus, HIV
> - Autoimmune and inflammatory diseases like autoimmune thyroiditis, sarcoid, amyloid; IgG4-related disease; metabolic diseases like diabetes or hyperlipoproteinemias (type 4 or 5);
> - Drug-induced dryness—diuretics, antipsychiatric and antianxiety agents, antihistaminics
> - Radiation
> - Graft-versus-host disease
> - Malignancies including lymphomas and parotid gland tumors

oxidase inhibitors, antihistaminics; diuretics, tramadol, neuroleptics, isotretinoin
- Avoidance of aerated drinks, coffee, tea, energy drinks, sugar-rich food, tobacco, cocaine
- Use of sugar-free chewing gums, fluorinated toothpastes
- Maintenance of open nasal passage
- Wearing appropriate sized glasses which cover the sides of the eyes too.

Dry Eyes

Mild Symptoms

For patients with mild symptoms like episodic discomfort or eye redness, apart from the general measures outlined above, following treatment options are available:
- Use of wraparound sunglasses
- Artificial tears like hypromellose 0.3% and carboxymethylcellulose 0.3% are easily available as over the counter drugs. Dosing frequency depends on the need; avoid preservative-containing solutions if the dosing is more than or equal to 4/day. Side effects include itching or irritation, blepharitis.

Moderate to Severe Symptoms

For patients with increased frequency of symptoms and signs occurring even in the absence of environmental stress, or having corneal erosions or filamentary keratitis, the following are recommended:
- More frequent instillation of artificial tears, use of long-acting lubricant ointment at night
- Topical cyclosporine 0.05%:[18] It can be applied twice daily to four times a day in severe cases. Effect would generally take 3 months and side effects like burning or stinging sensation, red eye, epiphora, and blurred vision are to be borne in mind and its use during active infection is to be avoided. A recent case series revealed that the local use of the tacrolimus 0.03% eye drops in eyes from eight patients for 3 months resulted in significant improvements in all objective measures
- Topical steroids (0.5% loteprednol, 0.1% fluorometholone, methylprednisolone drops): Find their role as an adjunct to topical cyclosporine to decrease associated burning sensation and also can be administered as pulse therapy with rapid tapering in 2 weeks if above treatment fails. Side effects like glaucoma, cataract, and fungal infection preclude long-term use
- Punctal occlusion: Temporary absorbable collagen plugs or subsequent permanent plugs often beginning with two inferior puncta first; laser and cautery is other modalities available for permanent occlusion. It is normally used as the last resort because of the skill needed in the procedure and side effects like discomfort, local infections, pyoderma granuloma
- Cholinergics: Patients often have associated severe dry eyes and use of pilocarpine,[19] cevimeline may provide some benefit
- Systemic anti-inflammatory and immunosuppressive therapy is reviewed under dry mouth.

In case of persistent dry eyes, make sure to check compliance, use of other over-the-counter drugs and look for complications such as blepharitis and fungal infection which can be mistaken as treatment failure.

Dry Mouth

Objective is to provide symptomatic relief and prevent complications such as dental caries and oral candidiasis. Apart from the general measures mentioned before, use of artificial saliva, composed of carboxymethylcellulose, polyethylene glycol, sorbitol, and electrolytes has shown benefit compared with placebo. Hydroxychloroquine (HCQ) may also help by inhibiting glandular cholinesterase. A recent study, JOQUER, did not find HCQ useful in improving dryness, fatigue or pain in patients with pSS (Table 2).[20]

Immunosuppressive Therapy

Use of immunosuppressants in severe sicca has been controversial.

Two small controlled studies confirmed rituximab's efficacy on fatigue and sicca symptoms, even if their primary endpoints were not met.[21] However, Tolerance and Efficacy of

Table 2: Sialogogues

Drugs	Mechanism of action	Dose Cevimeline	Side effects	Benefits
Pilocarpine	M1, M2, M3 agonist	Shorter half-life; 5 mg three to four times a day*	Flushing, diaphoresis, urinary frequency, diarrhea, hypotension	Some benefit also seen in dry eyes, nasal, vaginal, and skin dryness[7]
Cevimeline	M1, M2, M3 agonist	30 mg three times a day*	Lesser diaphoresis, flushing but more gastrointestinal side effects	

*Start at once a day dosing initially and take with food to minimize side effects.

Rituximab in pSS study reiterates that efficacy is not sufficient to allow its use in a large population of patients predominantly for glandular symptoms. Another study called TRACTISS[22] is ongoing, with reference to fatigue, oral and ocular dryness, quality of life, disease activity, and; damage once completed, a combined meta-analysis of the two studies is planned to determine which subgroup of pSS patients are more likely to benefit from this treatment.

Local IFN-α lozenges have been studied but overall efficacy was found to be low.

Treatment of Other Symptoms

Use of moisturizers, emollients, and mild cleansers for dry skin, vaginal moisturizers, lubricants, propionic acid gel and estrogen creams for vaginal dryness, and saline drops for nose is encouraged.

Focusing on complications such as secondary bacterial infections, blepharitis, oral candidiasis also forms an integral part of the management. Use of clotrimazole troche and nystatin oral suspension for 10-14 days is advised for oral candidiasis.

Parotid gland enlargement is managed with local wet heat, analgesics, and trial of prednisolone 0.25-0.5 mg/kg/day for 10-15 days; consider oral antibiotics for painful parotid associated with fever. Rule out lymphoma in persistent cases.

Extraglandular Manifestations

Treatment of extraglandular features of pSS has been largely empirical due to the lack of well-controlled randomized studies (Table 3). An algorithm for the same is represented in flowchart 1.

NEWER THERAPIES

With the use of outcome measures in pSS trials, especially ESSDAI, early and greater use of biologic therapies has been reported. Good number of studies have now shown significant effect of rituximab on fatigue, global health, and many clinical parameters.[23] Other B cell targeting molecules like epratuzumab (anti-CD22) and belimumab (BELISS trial) have also shown some promise.[24] Potential future therapies undergoing evaluation include alefacept, tocilizumab, abatacept, anakinra, and even infliximab.[25]

Intravenous gamma globulin therapy has been used for preventing anti-Ro mediated fetal congenital block in pregnant mothers. It has also been used in severe thrombocytopenia in such cases.

Other modalities under evaluation include mesenchymal stem cell therapy,[26] gene transfer involving interleukin-27, knockout of IFN-α receptor 1. Diquafosol eye drops, sphingolimod, salivary gland electrostimulation and rebapamide are some of the newer agents of treatment. The development of a molecular taxonomy of SS patients through the use of high-throughput molecular methods would be particularly interesting.

PROGNOSIS

Overall mortality is not increased in patients with pSS compared with the general population, although the subgroup of patients with extraglandular disease has an increased risk of morbidity and death. The latter include patients with severe life-threatening or organ-threatening manifestations such as vasculitis, CNS involvement,

Skin in Rheumatologic Diseases

Table 3: Treatment of systemic features	
Organ	**Management**
Pulmonary	
LIP, NSIP (in mild cases, monitoring PFT every 3–6 months and annual HRCT will help and guide the management. A fall in FVC by 10% warrants treatment. Some authors quote starting treatment even with FVC <83% from the previous cited 70%)	Prednisone 1 mg/kg/day, Reassess at 4–6 weeks and continue therapy at tapering dose for at least 6 months if response seen. Azathioprine (up to 2.5 mg/kg/day) and MMF 2–3 g/day have shown some benefit as steroid sparing agent[8,9]
Usual interstitial pneumonitis	No effective treatment, some follow NSIP management
Organizing pneumonia	Prednisone 1 mg/kg/day
Follicular bronchiolitis	Often associated with other ILD pattern
Pulmonary embolism	Anticoagulant. Rule out antiphospholipid antibody syndrome
CNS and PNS	–
Sensory neuropathy	Pregabalin, gabapentin, avoid TCAs
Sensory ataxic neuropathy, demyelinating, and axonal neuropathy	Prednisolone, cyclophosphamide (3–6 bolus), IvIg, plasma exchange, rituximab[21-24]
Trigeminal neuropathy	Pregabalin, gabapentin
Transverse myelitis, multiple sclerosis like disease, stroke	Pulse steroids, prednisolone, cyclophosphamide, azathioprine, rituximab
Vasculitis	Prednisolone, leflunomide, cyclophosphamide (3–6 boluses), plasma exchange, rituximab[21-24]
Kidney	
Renal tubular acidosis	See above, rule out associated thyroid disorders, oral or intravenous potassium in mannitol for hypokalemic paralysis
Tubular interstitial nephritis	Wait and watch (asymptomatic to mild), corticosteroids + MMF or CYC followed by AZA, rituximab
Glomerulonephritis (rule out cryoglobulinemia, amyloidosis, lymphoma)	Corticosteroids + MMF or CYC followed by AZA, rituximab
Gastrointestinal disorders	
Gastroesophageal reflux disease	PPIs, H2 blockers, antacid, prokinetic agent
Primary biliary cirrhosis (PBC)	Ursedeoxycholic acid 15–20 mg/kg/day
AIH, PBC AIH overlap	Prednisolone, azathioprine
Gastric antral vascular ectasia	Argon plasma coagulation, Nd:YAG laser
Endocrine	Rule out thyroid disorders, diabetes mellitus

LIP, lymphocytic interstitial pneumonitis; NSIP, nonspecific interstitial pneumonitis; PFT, pulmonary function tests; HRCT, high-resolution computed tomography; FVC, forced vital capacity; ILD, interstitial lung disease, CNS, central nervous system; PNS, peripheral nervous system; TCA, tricyclic antidepressants; IVIg, intravenous immunoglobulins; MMF, mycophenolate mofitil; CYC, cyclophosphamide; AZA, azathioprine; Nd:YAG, neodymium-doped yttrium aluminum garnet; AIH, autoimmune hepatitis.

or malignancy. Low C4, palpable purpura, hypergammaglobulinemia, and cryoglobulinemia have also been shown to be associated with increased risk of mortality. Judicious and early use of immunosuppressive agents, especially rituximab, in this subset of patients may improve survival.

CONCLUSION

The average time before diagnosis of primary Sjogren's syndrome is made in an individual patient used to be 4-5 years. This is now going down with increasing awareness of the disease amongst internists, ophthalmologists, dentists,

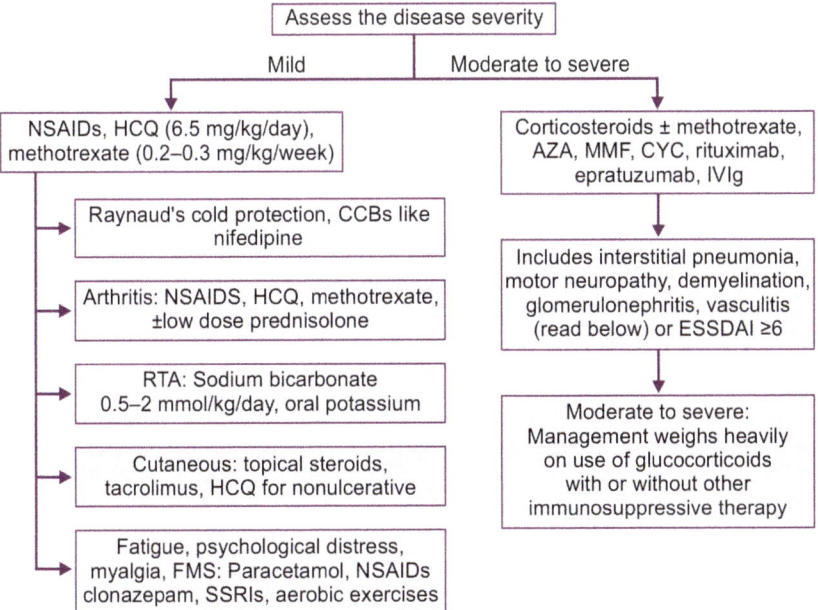

NSAIDs, nonsteroidal anti-inflammatory drugs; HCQ, hydroxychloroquine; CCBs, calcium channel blockers; RTA, renal tubular acidosis; FMS, fibromyalgia syndrome; SSRIs, selective serotonin reuptake inhibitor; AZA, azathioprine; MMF, Mmycophenolate mofetil; CYC, cyclophosphamide; IVIg, intravenous immunoglobulin; ESSDAI, EULAR Sjögren's syndrome disease activity index.

FLOWCHART 1: Treatment approach for extraglandular primary Sjogren's syndrome.

and rheumatologists. With the use of outcome measures like the ESSDAI which can gauge severity of the disease, treatment can be optimized for the patient. While the treatment for extraglandular features, which are not uncommonly a marker of aggressive disease, is getting better especially with the early use of biologics like rituximab, remedies for sicca symptoms, fatigue and noninflammatory pain in these patients is far from satisfactory. Much needs to be done to improve the quality of life of these patients. This is one disease where researchers from different disciplines need to collaborate to move from palliation to remission and then, if possible, cure.

REFERENCES

1. Sjögren H. Zur kenntnis der keratoconjunctivitis sicca. Acta Ophthalmol. 1933;11(suppl II):1-151.
2. Siamopoulou-Mavridou A, Drosos AA, Andonopoulos AP. Sjögren syndrome in childhood: report of two cases. Eur J Pediatr. 1989;148(6):523-4.
3. Tove R, Rekston, Mallin V Johnson. Sjögren's syndrome: an update on epidemiology and current insights on pathophysiology. Oral Maxillofacial Surg Clin North Am. 2014;26(1):1-12.
4. Nocturne G, Mariette X. Advances in understanding the pathogenesis of primary Sjögren's syndrome. Nat Rev Rheumatol. 2013;9(9):544-56.
5. Sankar V, Noll JL, Brennan MT. Diagnosis of Sjögren's syndrome. American-European and the American college of rheumatology classification criteria. Oral Maxillofacial Surg Clin North Am. 2014;26(1):13-22.
6. Moutsopoulos HM. Sjögren's syndrome: a forty-year scientific journey. J Autoimmun. 2014;51:1-9.
7. Lenopoli S, Carsons SE. Extraglandular manifestations of pimary Sjögren's syndrome. Oral Maxillofacial Surg Clin North Am. 2014;26:91-99.
8. Mavragani CP, Moutsopoulos H. Sjögren's syndrome. CMAJ. 2014;186(15):E579-86.
9. Misra R, Hissaria P, Tandon V, et al. Primary Sjögren's syndrome: rarity in India. J Assoc Physicians India. 2003;51:859-62.
10. Yoneyama K, Tochigi N, Oikawa A et al. Primary localized cutaneous nodular amyloidosis in a patient with Sjögren's syndrome: a review of the literature. J Dermatol. 2005;32(2):120-3.

11. Katayama I, Kotobuki Y, Kiyohara E, et al. Annular erythema associated with Sjögren's syndrome: review of the literature on the management and clinical analysis of skin lesions. Mod Rheumatol. 2010;20(2):123-9.
12. Finder KA, McCollough ML, Dixon SL, et al. Hypergammaglobulinemic purpura of Waldenstrom. J Am Acad Dermatol. 1990;23(4 Pt 1):669-76.
13. Liang Y, Yang Z, Qin B, et al. Primary Sjögren's syndrome and malignancy risk: a systematic review and meta-analysis. Ann Rheum Dis. 2014;73(6):1151-6.
14. Quartuccio L, Isola M, Baldini C, et al. Biomarkers of lymphoma in Sjögren's syndrome and evaluation of the lymphoma risk in prelymphomatous conditions: results of a multicenter study. J Autoimmun. 2014;51:75e80.
15. Cornec D, Jamin C, Pers JO. Sjögren's syndrome: where do we stand and where shall we go. J Autoimmun. 2014;51:109-14.
16. Tincani A, Andreoli L, Cavazzana I, et al. Novel aspects of Sjögren's syndrome in 2012. BMC Med. 2013;11:93.
17. Seror R, Theander E, Bootsma H, et al. Outcome measures for Sjögren's syndrome—a comprehensive review. J Autoimmun. 51(2014):51-56.
18. Sall K, Stevenson OD, Mundorf TK, et al. Two multicenter, randomized studies of the efficacy and safety of cyclosporine ophthalmic emulsion in moderate to severe dry eye disease. CsA Phase 3 Study Group. Ophthalmology. 2000;107:631.
19. Papas AS, Sherrer YS, Charney M, et al. Successful treatment of dry mouth and dry eye symptoms in Sjögren's Syndrome patients with oral pilocarpine: a randomized, placebo-controlled, dose-adjustment study. J Clin Rheumatol. 2004;10(4):169-77.
20. Gottenberg JE, Ravaud P, Puéchal X, et al. Effects of hydroxychloroquine on symptomatic improvement in primary Sjögren syndrome: the JOQUER randomized clinical trial. JAMA. 2014;312(3):249-58.
21. Meijer JM, Meiners PM, Vissink A, et al. Effectiveness of rituximab treatment in primary Sjögren's syndrome: a randomized, double-blind, placebo-controlled trial. Arthritis Rheum. 2010;62:960e8.
22. Brown S, Navarro Coy N, Pitzalis C, et al. The TRACTISS protocol: a randomised double blind placebo controlled clinical trial of anti-B-cell therapy in patients with primary Sjögren's syndrome. BMC Musculoskelet Disord. 2014;15:21.
23. Meiners PM, Arends S, Brouwer E, et al. Responsiveness of disease activity indices ESSPRI and ESSDAI in patients with primary Sjögren's syndrome treated with rituximab. Ann Rheum Dis. 2012;71:1297.
24. Mariette X, Seror R, Quartuccio L, et al. Efficacy and safety of belimumab in primary Sjögren's syndrome: results of the BELISS open-label phase II study. Ann Rheum Dis. 2015;74(3):526-31.
25. Sada PR, Isenberg D, Ciurtin C. Biologic treatment in Sjögren's syndrome. Rheumatology (Oxford). 2015;54:219-30.
26. Xu J, Wang D, Liu D, et al. Allogeneic mesenchymal stem cell treatment alleviates experimental and clinical Sjögren syndrome. Blood. 2012;120:3142e51.

13
CHAPTER

Sarcoidosis

Vikram K Mahajan, Devendra S Dadhwal

INTRODUCTION

Sarcoidosis is an immune-mediated multisystem granulomatous disease of unknown etiology. It is characterized by formation of noncaseating epithelioid cell granulomas in affected organs and tissues manifesting with a wide variety of clinical presentations. The consensus statement by the "American Thoracic Society" published in 1999 and subsequent results of ACCESS (A Case Control Etiologic Study of Sarcoidosis) have provided much insight into epidemiology, immunopathogenesis, and treatment of sarcoidosis.[1,2] Skin lesions of sarcoidosis are like tip of the iceberg, reflecting underlying disease in other organs. Ocular involvement and pulmonary changes are very common; therefore, all patients with skin lesions require detailed examination even in the absence of systemic features.

EPIDEMIOLOGY

Sarcoidosis occurs worldwide affecting individuals aged between 20 years and 40 years. Women are affected almost two times more often than men. Children constitute nearly 4% of sarcoidosis cases. It is less frequent in Central and South America, mainland China, and Africa but the prevalence is high in Scandinavian countries, Japan, England, Ireland, and North America. The reported prevalence in the United States is 40 cases/100,000 populations and estimated cumulative lifetime risk for sarcoidosis is 0.85% for whites and 2.4% for Blacks.[1,3] African Americans are affected eight times more than Whites and have severe, chronic, and disabling disease.[3] It is reported rarely from Spain, Portugal, Saudi Arabia, and South America. Its exact prevalence in India is not known for lack of population-based studies. This is perhaps due to lack of clinical suspicion and overwhelming prevalence of tuberculosis, which presents with very similar clinical, radiological, and histological findings. It has been variably estimated as 60 and 150 cases per 0.1 million outdoor patients in Delhi and Kolkata hospitals, respectively, in the past.[4] However, it is now being recognized more frequently with the availability of newer diagnostic modalities.[5,6]

ETIOPATHOGENESIS

The cause of sarcoidosis remains elusive despite plethora of investigations. Occupation, personal habits, pets, and use of drugs are not contributory. Environmental factors, both infectious, and noninfectious (Table 1) are believed to trigger an immune mediated inflammatory reaction in susceptible host.[7,8] The higher presence of *Propionibacterium acnes* from sarcoidal lymph nodes and its ability to induce granulomatous response akin to sarcoidosis in mice models suggests its possible pathogenetic role. Similarly, *Mycobacterium tuberculosis* DNA or mycobacterial protein, *Mycobacterium tuberculosis*-catalase-peroxidase (mKatG), demonstrated in sarcoidal granulomas is speculated to represent persistent antigen in sarcoidosis.[9,10] However, the evidence implicating mycobacteria is controversial at best and the identity of the antigen remains poorly elucidated. The role of atypical mycobacteria, *Borrelia burgdorferi*, viruses, and noninfectious environmental agents like insecticides, molds, and beryllium also needs authentication. Interaction between environmental and genetic factors remains the major key factor in determining pattern, presentation, progression, and prognosis in sarcoidosis.

Familial sarcoidosis without any consistent mode of inheritance is well recognized in at least 5% of sarcoidosis patients, especially among Irish or African Americans. Several non-human leukocyte antigen (HLA) genes are speculated to influence susceptibility or severity of sarcoidosis (Table 2).[11] In addition, different HLA haplotypes appear to influence clinical outcomes and pattern of sarcoidosis rather than its occurrence (Table 3).[11,12] The butyrophilin-like 2 (*BTNL2*) gene in class II major histocompatibility complex

Table 1: Etiologic agents implicated in sarcoidosis		
Infectious agents	Inorganic agents	Organic agents
Herpes virus, Epstein-Barr virus, Retrovirus, *Coxsackie B virus*, *Cytomegalovirus*, hepatitis C virus, human immunodeficiency virus	Aluminum	Pine pollens
Borrelia burgdorferi	Zirconium	Peanut dust
Propionibacterium acnes	Talc,	
Mycobacterium tuberculosis, M. avium complex, other atypical mycobacteria (cell-wall deficient mycobacteria)	Clay	
Rickettsia helvetica, Mycoplasma		

Table 2: Non-human leukocyte antigen candidate gene that may affect antigen processing, presentation, macrophage and T-cell activation, recruitment, and injury repair in sarcoidosis[11]	
Non-human leukocyte antigen candidate genes	Chromosomal Location
Angiotensin-converting enzyme	*17q23*
CC-chemokine receptor 2	*3p21.3*
CC-chemokine receptor 5	*3p21.3*
CD80, CD86	*3q21*
Clara cell 10 kD protein	*11q12-13*
Complement receptor 1	*1q32*
Cystic fibrosis transmembrane regulator	*7q31.2*
Heat shock protein A1L/HSP70-hom	*6p21.3*
Inhibitor κB-α	*14q13*
Interleukin-1α	*2q14*
Interleukin-4 receptor	*16p11.2*
Interleukin-18	*11q22*
Interferon-γ	*9p22*
Natural resistance associated macrophage protein	*2q35*
Toll-like receptor	*9q32*
Transforming growth factor	*19q13.2*
Tumor necrosis factor-α	*6p21.3*
Vascular endothelial growth factor	*6p12*
Vitamin D receptor	*12q12-14*

Table 3: Human leukocyte antigen haplotypes affecting clinical outcomes and pattern of sarcoidosis[11,12]

HLA gene	Effect on sarcoidosis
HLA-B8/DR3	Inherited as a sarcoid risk haplotype in patients with acute sarcoidosis
HLA-DRB1	Associated with sarcoidosis susceptibility and prognosis
HLA-DQB1*0201	Associated with mild disease, Löfgren's syndrome, decreased risk, and lack of progression
HLA-DQB1*0602	Associated with persistent disease
HLA-DQB1*0602-DRB1*150101	Associated with severe pulmonary disease
HLA-DRB3*1501	Associated with Löfgren's syndrome
HLA-DRB1*1101	Imparts genetic predisposition for sarcoidosis in Blacks and Whites

HLA, human leukocyte antigen.

Box 1: Immunologic abnormalities observed in sarcoidosis[1]

Immunologic abnormalities

- Intracellular and interstitial accumulation of CD4+ cells with helper-inducer activity and IL-2 release
- Expansion of T-cell bearing a restricted T-cell receptor repertoire in involved tissue
- Increased in situ production of Th1 cell derived IL-2 and IFN-γ during granuloma formation
- Increased expression of TNF-ligand and TNF-receptor super families by sarcoid T-cells
- B-cell hypersensitivity and spontaneous *in situ* production of immunoglobulins
- Increased spontaneous rate of proliferation of lung immunocompetent cells
- Accumulation of monocyte-macrophages with antigen-presenting cell capacity and increased expression of HLA-DR, HLA-DQ, CD71, and adhesion molecules CD49a, Cd54, CD102
- Increased release of macrophage-derived cytokines IL-1, IL-6, IL-8, IL-15, TNF-α, IFN-γ, GM-CSF and chemokines (RANTES, MIP-1α, IL-16). Most of these favor granuloma formation and lung damage
- Increased production of macrophage-derived fibrogenic cytokines (TGF-β and related cytokines, platelet-derived growth factor, insulin-like growth factor-1) favoring evolution of fibrosis

IL, interleukin; IFN-γ, interferon gamma; TNF-α, tumor necrosis factor alpha; GM-CSF, granulocyte-macrophage colony-stimulating factor; RANTES, regulation on activation, normal T-cell expression, and secretion; MIP-1α, macrophage inflammatory protein 1-alpha; TGF-β, transforming growth factor beta.

(MHC) region of chromosome 6p, a member of immunoglobulin superfamily with costimulatory action in T-cell activation, is suggested to predispose individuals of African American and German origins for developing sarcoidosis.[13]

IMMUNOPATHOPHYSIOLOGY

Granuloma formation in sarcoidosis requires complex interplay between antigen, antigen presenting cells, and T-cells in a genetically susceptible individual. The disease outcome will depend on disease modifying HLA and non-HLA genes. Immunologic abnormalities observed in sarcoidosis patients are listed in box 1.[1] Granuloma formation (Fig. 1) in sarcoidosis is a complex interplay between antigen and host immune responses.[14-17] The stage of granuloma formation is also marked by peripheral CD4+ T-cell lymphopenia and depressed cutaneous delayed hypersensitivity reactions to tetanus, candida, and tuberculin antigens. This immune paradox in sarcoidosis patients has been linked to a global T regulatory cell subset amplification whose activity is insufficient to control local inflammation. At the same time, peripheral T regulatory cells exert powerful antiproliferative activity that accounts for this anergy.[18]

Whether granulomatous inflammation will persist, resolve, or lead to fibrosis will depend upon balance of inflammatory cells, regulatory cells, apoptosis and Th1/Th2 cytokine responses. However, despite poor understanding the pathophysiology of fibrosis possibly involves a shift from Th1 to Th2 cell response.[15]

CLINICAL PRESENTATION

The onset of sarcoidosis is usually insidious in most cases and nonspecific constitutional symptoms like lethargy, weight loss, night sweats, and general malaise may occur in almost one-third of the patients. Nearly 70–80% patients also experience fatigue. Moderate to high fever and polyarthritis symptoms are common in

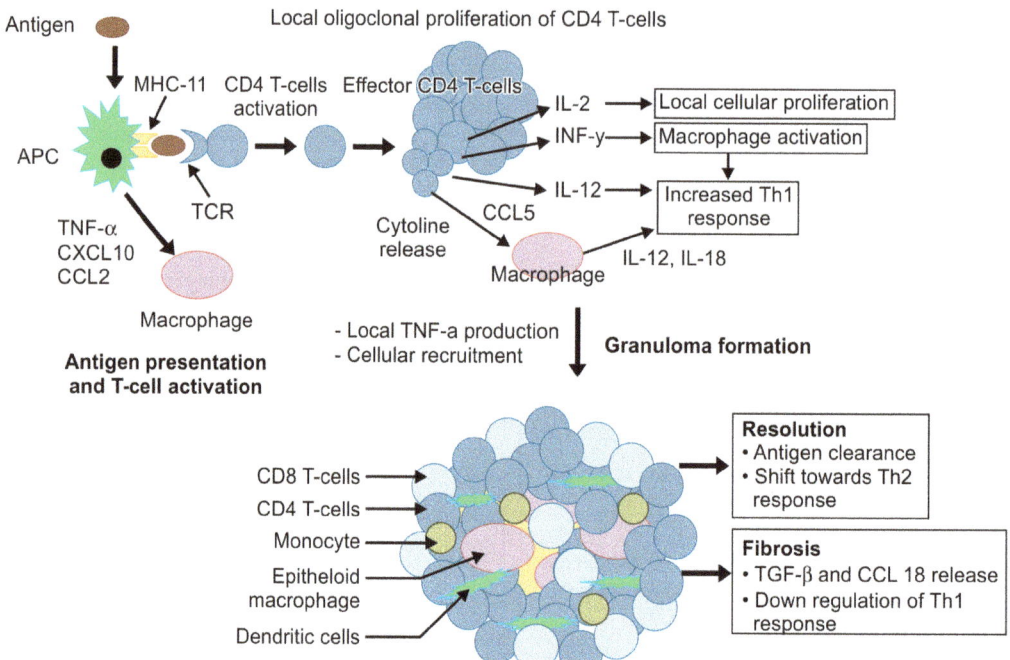

FIGURE 1: Schematic representation of immunopathophysiology of sarcoidosis. Unknown antigen (Ag) is taken up by the antigen-presenting cell (APC) via major histocompatibility complex (MHC) class-II peptide. The Ag-MHC complex binds to variable region of T-cell receptor (TCR). The MHC-Ag-TCR complex initiates activation of effector CD4+ T-cells and release of various cytokines. The Th1 predominant response leads to increased release of interferon-γ (INF-γ) interleukin-2 (IL-2) leading to granulomatous inflammation. The sarcoid granuloma consists of epithelioid cells, macrophages, few monocytes and predominantly CD4+ T-cells and small number of CD8+ T-cells characteristically at its periphery. Few dendritic cells may be present interspersed in the extracellular collagenous matrix. Fibroblasts will usually be present. Depending upon persistence or absence of the antigenic stimulation a shift to Th2 response or downregulation of Th1 response will lead to resolution/fibrosis.[17]

Source: Amin EN, Closser DR, Crouser ED. Current best practice in the management of pulmonary and systemic sarcoidosis. Ther Adv Resp Dis. 2014;8:111-32.

sarcoidosis patients presenting with erythema nodosum. Lymph nodes are involved in 50% patients. Bilateral pedal edema is rare and is due to iliac or para-aortic lymph node involvement. Sarcoidosis can affect almost all organ systems with varying frequency (Table 4). Sarcoidosis can be distinguished in acute/subacute or chronic forms based on presentation and clinical course (Table 5).

Cutaneous Sarcoidosis

Skin involvement in sarcoidosis occurs in 20–35% cases and nearly 73% patients had cutaneous lesions at the onset.[5,19] About 70% patients have systemic manifestations appearing concomitantly with skin lesions and other 30% develop the disease within 6 months to 3 years after the development of cutaneous lesions. Skin lesions of sarcoidosis are mostly asymptomatic, polymorphic, and exhibit mixed pattern and distribution (Figs 2 to 23). They have been classified classically as specific and nonspecific (Table 6). Specific lesions reveal noncaseating granulomas on histopathology and are indicative of more progressive disease. The nonspecific lesions lack classic noncaseating granulomas and represent a reactive process.

Among the specific lesions, the more common morphological types are the papular, maculopapular, plaque, and annular type. Papular/papulomacular (Figs 2 to 4) sarcoid lesions often involve face and trunk. Lesions appear as crops, are nonscaly, have orange-yellow-brownish red to violaceous color, and are associated with favorable prognosis. Maculopapular sarcoidosis (Fig. 5) is especially associated with acute other organ involvement like sudden lymphadenopathy, acute arthritis, and parotid gland enlargement. Plaque sarcoidosis (Fig. 6) lesions are one or multiple, often present on limbs, brownish-red, variable size, and shape with deeper granulomatous inflammation. These lesions are more persistent, may gradually enlarge to form diffuse large plaques, are associated with more chronic systemic disease, and often heal with macular atrophic scarring (Fig. 7). However, unlike lupus pernio which is another chronic cutaneous sarcoidosis, associated bone cysts are not seen. Annular plaques (Figs 8 and 9) result from peripheral evolution and central clearing with hypopigmentation, atrophy, or scarring in chronic disease of more than 2 years.

Other relatively less frequent types are lupus pernio, subcutaneous sarcoidosis, and scar sarcoidosis. In lupus pernio, the lesions are chronic, indolent, violaceous indurated papulo-plaques, involving cold sensitive areas (earlobes, nose, lips, cheeks, chin, forehead), and are cosmetically very disfiguring (Figs 10 and 11). However, it is not considered to be associated with cold exposure. It affects more commonly the African Americans women than Whites. It is usually associated with pharyngeal and laryngeal mucosal involvement, chronic fibrotic disease of lungs, and osteolytic lesions of digital bones especially in the presence of overlying skin lesions

Table 4: Frequency of common organ involvement in sarcoidosis

Organ system involved	Frequency of involvement (%)
Lungs	90–95
Intrathoracic and peripheral lymph nodes	75–90
Skin	24
Eye	12
Extrathoracic lymph nodes	15
Liver	12
Spleen	7
Neurologic	5
Cardiac	2
Rheumatological	1–15 (4–38)
Reproductive organs (breast, uterus, fallopian tubes, ovaries, prostate, epididymis, testis)	–

Table 5: Features of acute and chronic sarcoidosis

Features	Acute sarcoidosis	Chronic sarcoidosis
Age	<30 years	>40 years
Onset	Abrupt	Insidious
Duration	<2 years	>2 years
Histology	Epithelioid and giant cells	Hyaline fibrosis, interstitial pneumonitis
Chest X-ray	Hilar lymphadenopathy	Parenchymal infiltration, fibrosis
Eyes	Acute iritis, conjunctivitis, conjunctival nodule	Keratoconjunctivitis, chronic uveitis, glaucoma, cataract
Parotitis, lymphadenopathy, splenomegaly, Bell's palsy	Usually transient	Rarely permanent
Bone cysts	Not seen	Present
Calcium metabolism	Hypercalcemia, hypercalciuria	Nephrocalcinosis
Tuberculin test	Negative	May be negative
Kveim-Sultzbach test	Positive	May be negative
Acid phosphatase, leucine amino-peptidase, urinary hydroxyproline	Increased	Normal

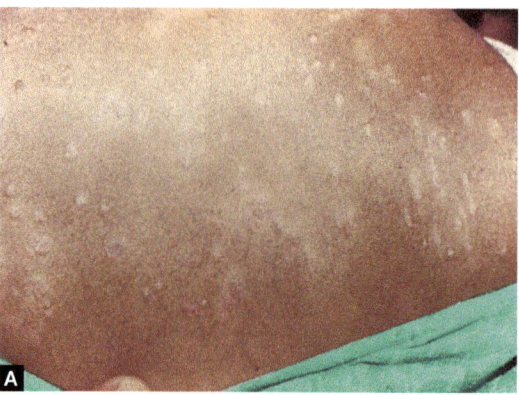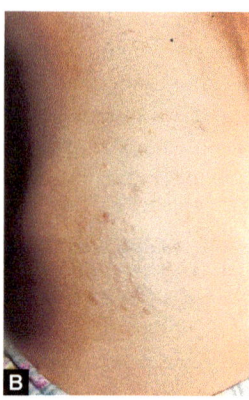

FIGURE 2: Multiple small 1–5 mm sized, flesh colored, papular lesions over left flank and back. They usually involute into papulomacular lesions.

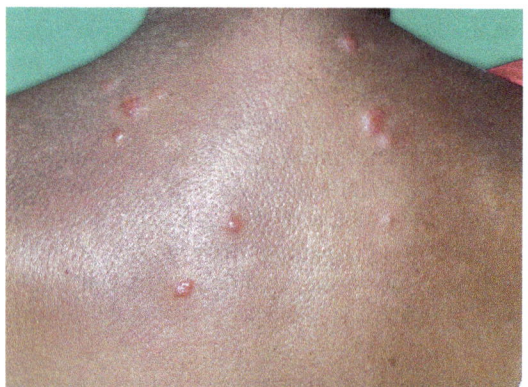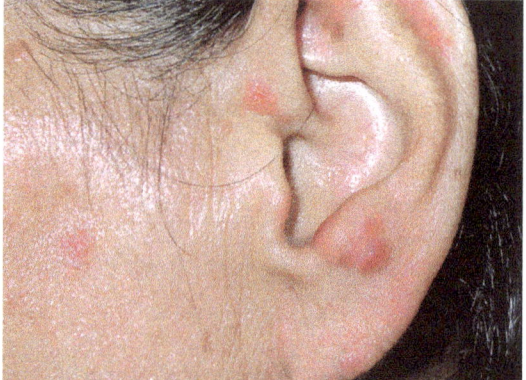

FIGURE 3: Reddish brown papular sarcoidosis lesions over upper back.

FIGURE 5: Papular and papulomacular sarcoidosis lesions over the left ear.

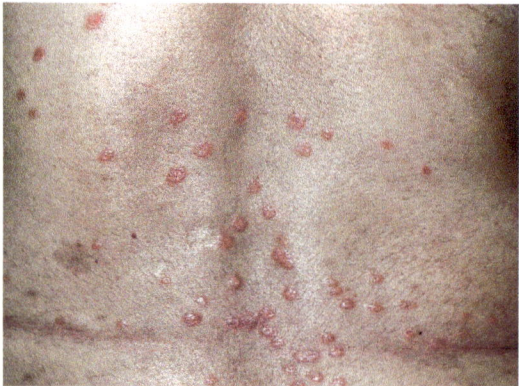

FIGURE 4: Papular sarcoidosis lesions over the lower back.

(Fig. 12). Nasal mucosa, septum, and adjacent bones may also be affected when the lesions are present around nostrils. This form of sarcoidosis is especially recalcitrant to treatment. Subcutaneous sarcoid lesions (Darier-Roussy sarcoid) occur in less than 5% patients, need biopsy for diagnosis, and have no predictive value. Nodules vary in number, arise in deep dermis and subcutaneous tissue of the extremities, are nontender, mobile, firm, and size ranges from 0.5 to 2 cm. Overlying skin may be normal or mildly erythematous and when lesions clear, overlying skin may develop depressions (Figs 13 and 14). Scar sarcoid, i.e., infiltration of previously silent scars (Fig. 15) is uncommon manifestation and represents

Sarcoidosis

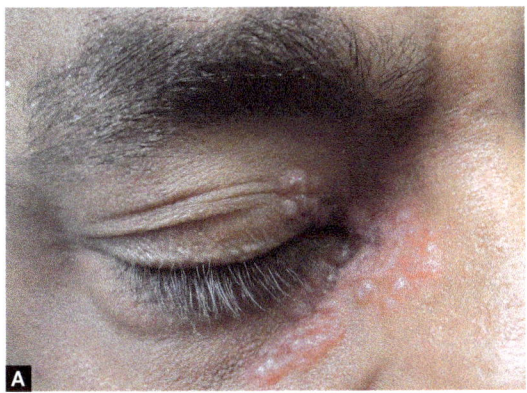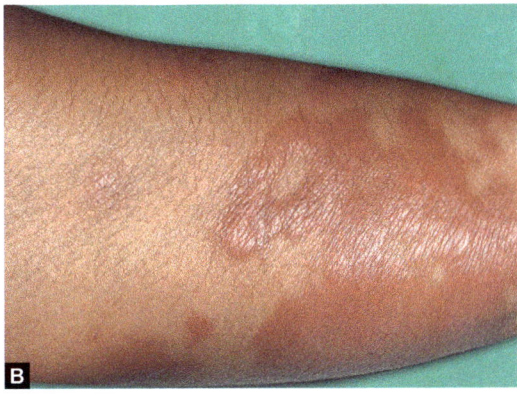

FIGURE 6: A, Plaque sarcoidosis as a result of coalescing papular lesions near right eye; **B,** Plaque sarcoidosis over left forearm. Other common sites of involvement are back, buttocks, cheeks.

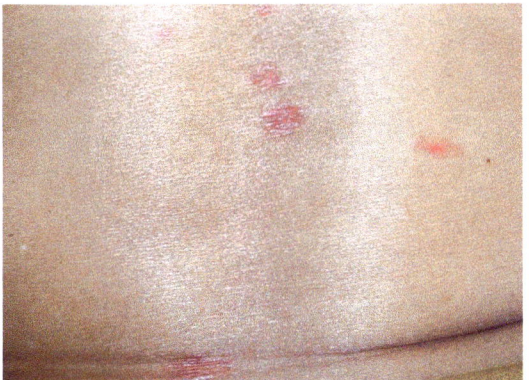

FIGURE 7: Atrophic lesion of cutaneous sarcoidosis over back.

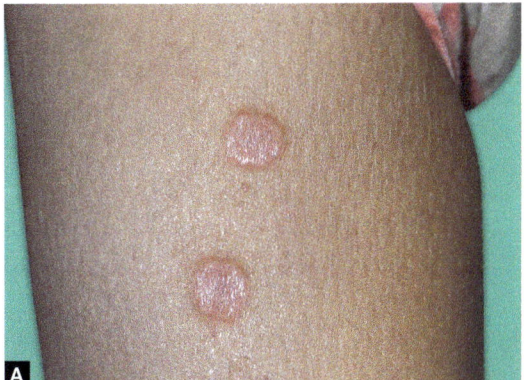

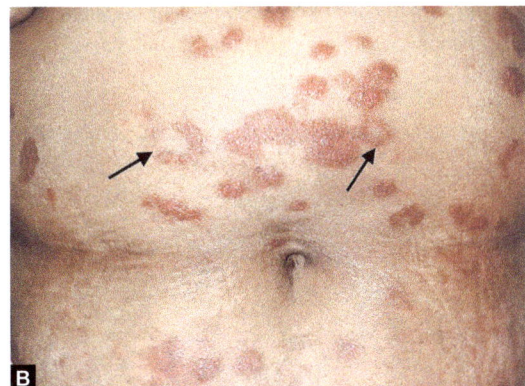

FIGURE 8: A, Annular sarcoidosis plaque over thigh. Center of plaque showing mild erythema, atrophy, and wrinkling; **B,** Annular sarcoidosis lesion (black arrows) over trunk in a patient with polymorphous sarcoidosis lesion.

benign disease. Similarly, sarcoidosis also occurs preferentially within the previously traumatized skin and around imbedded foreign material such as silica and tattoos (Fig. 16).

Sarcoidosis sometimes surprises with very atypical presentations and has, therefore, been called a great imitator and clinical chameleon. Uncommon morphological types include angiolupoid, hypopigmented, lichenoid, psoriasiform, ulcerative, verrucous, ichthyosiform (Fig. 17), erythrodermic, morpheaform, necrobiosis lipoidica like (Fig. 18), and tumoral sarcoidosis. Angiolupoid sarcoid (Fig. 19) lesions are rare, soft, reddish-brown nodules, or annular plaques with

Skin in Rheumatologic Diseases

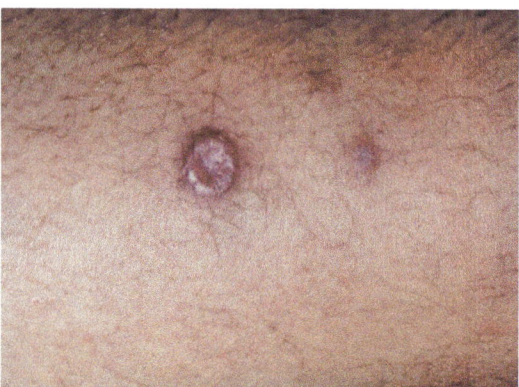

FIGURE 9: An umblicated lesion of cutaneous sarcoidosis over thigh in a patient of pulmonary sarcoidosis.

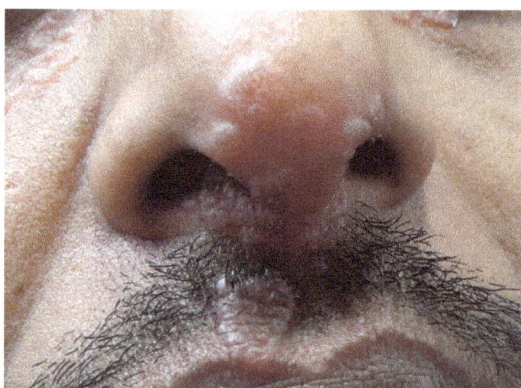

FIGURE 11: Lupus pernio. Erythematous to violaceous papular sarcoidosis lesions over nose tip, nasal philtrum, and extending into the nasal cavity.

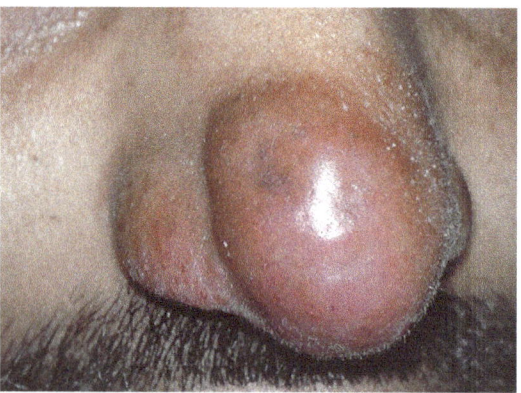

FIGURE 10: Lupus pernio. Violaceous erythematous granulomatous swelling over nose tip and ala nasi.

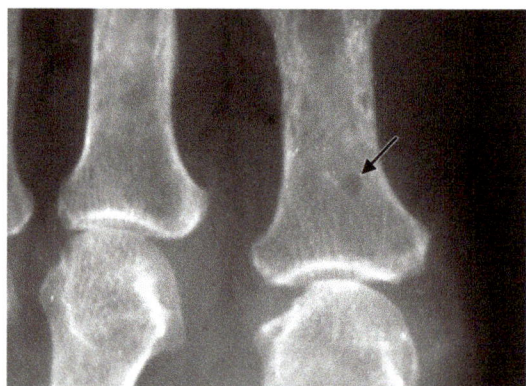

FIGURE 12: X-ray of hand showing lucent areas (lytic lesions) in left hand digital bones in a patient with pulmonary sarcoidosis (stage 1).

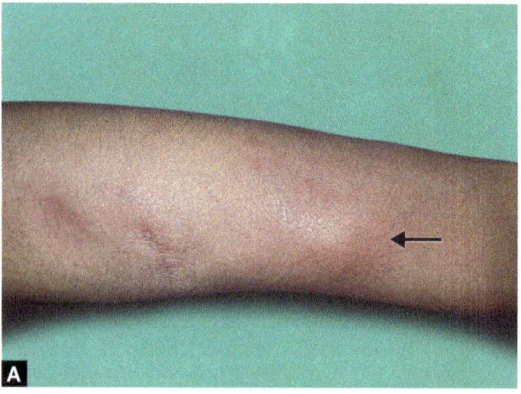
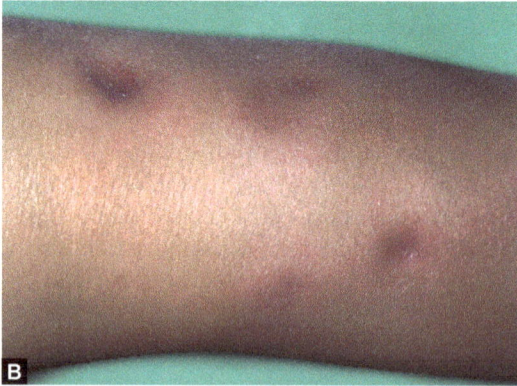

FIGURE 13: A, Subcutaneous sarcoidosis in a known pulmonary sarcoidosis patient. Note the skin colored swelling (black arrow) present over forearm; **B,** Subcutaneous sarcoidosis lesions over the arm with overlying skin showing erythema and depressions.

Sarcoidosis

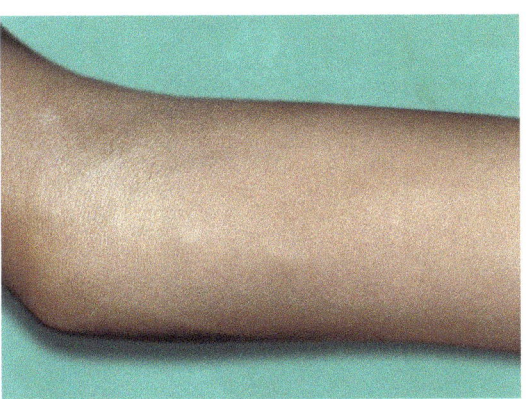

FIGURE 14: Skin colored deep seated swellings over the forearm in a sarcoidosis patient.

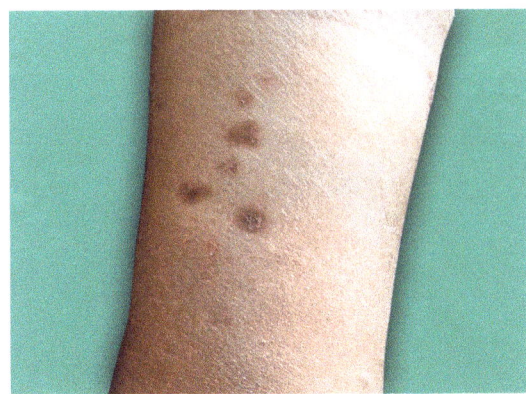

FIGURE 17: Ichthyosiform cutaneous sarcoidosis over leg.

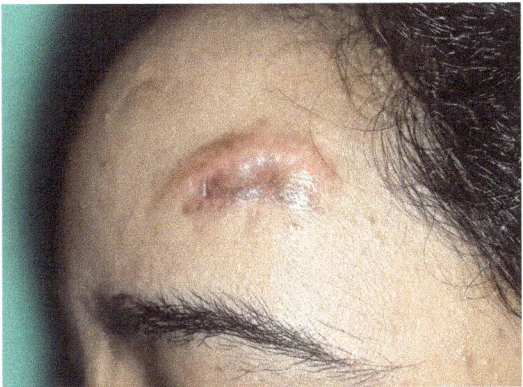

FIGURE 15: Scar sarcoidosis in 25-year-old post-traumatic scar.

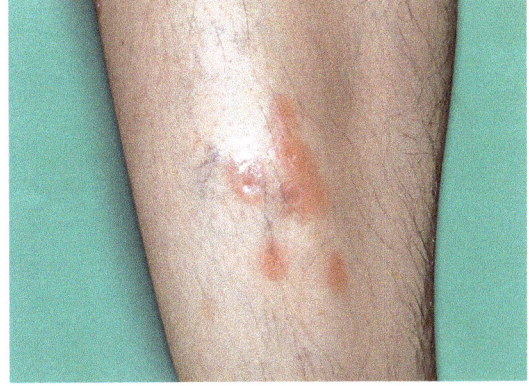

FIGURE 18: Necrobiosis lipoidica like lesions of cutaneous sarcoidosis over right shin.

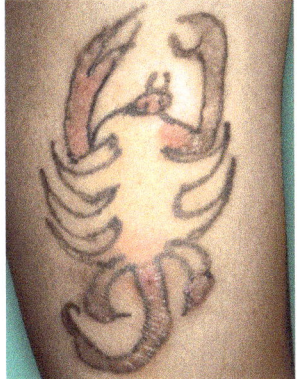

FIGURE 16: Sarcoidal granuloma in tattoo. Red pigment (cadmium or mercury salts) used for tattooing is a common cause for such granulomatous inflammatory reaction.

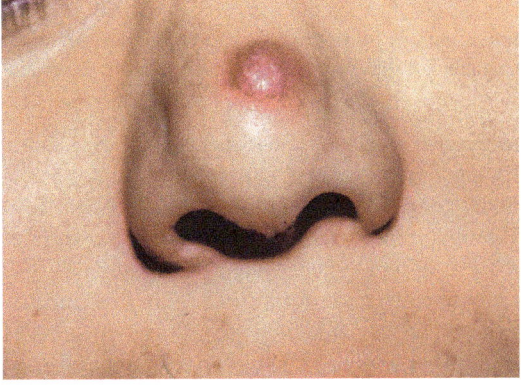

FIGURE 19: Angiolupoid sarcoidosis over nose. A soft, hemispherical lesion having reddish color due to telangectatic component.

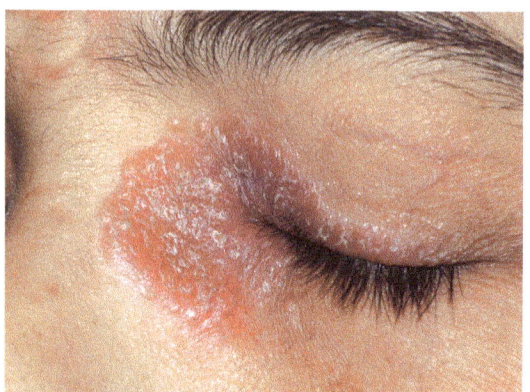
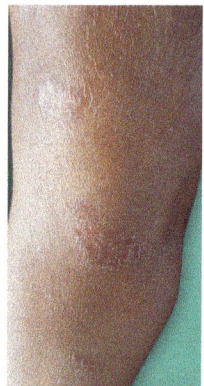

FIGURE 20: Psoriasiform plaque of cutaneous sarcoidosis over root of nose near medial canthus of left eye and extending to upper eyelid.

Courtesy: Dr Ramam, Professor, Department of Dermatology, All India Institute of Medical Sciences, New Delhi.

FIGURE 21: Psoriasiform lesion of cutaneous sarcoidosis over leg.

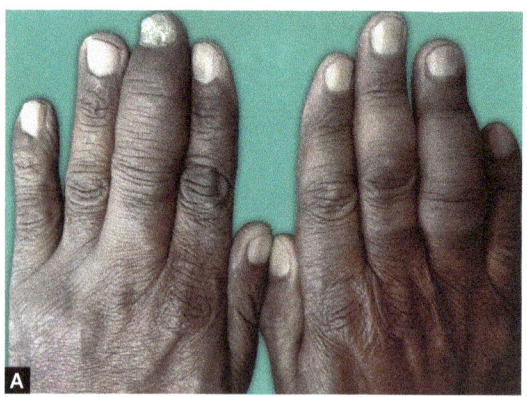
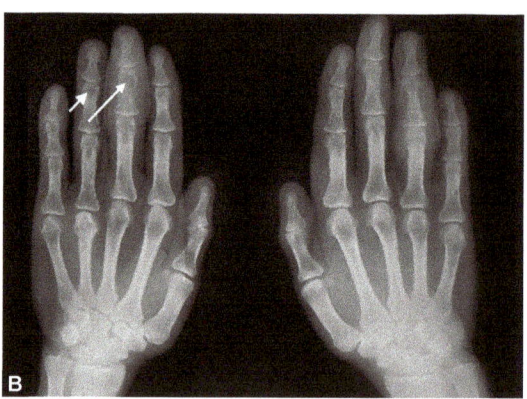

FIGURE 22: A, Dactylitis in a patient with pulmonary sarcoidosis. Note asymptomatic diffuse swelling of left middle and right middle and ring fingers. Left middle fingernail is also involved and has become dystrophic and brittle; **B,** X-ray of both hands shows lytic lesions (arrow) involving digital bones. Note soft tissue swelling of right ring and left middle fingers corresponding to dactylitis.

marked telangiectatic component preferentially located on nose and central face and have a little tendency for spontaneous resolution. Hypopigmented sarcoidosis is seen in people of African descent exclusively and presents as well demarcated hypopigmented patches mainly over the limbs. Lichenoid sarcoidosis presents as multiple 1–3 mm size maculopapules distributed extensively over the body. Psoriasiform sarcoidosis (Figs 20 and 21) lesion is different from classical psoriasis plaque which is redder in color, scales are thick and larger, and lesions heal without scarring.

Oral lesions are infrequent in sarcoidosis. Nail involvement is a marker of chronic disease and can present with all type of nail changes. It is often accompanied by phalangeal bone disease, sometimes dactylitis and intrathoracic sarcoidosis (Fig. 22).

Erythema nodosum classically presents as dusky erythematous, tender subcutaneous nodules over shins with constitutional symptoms (Fig. 23) in around one-fourth of the sarcoidosis patients. It is considered a hallmark nonspecific skin lesion reflecting acute benign disease. It is more common in patients of northern European countries, Ireland, and Spain but affects African Americans and Japanese less often.[20] It indicates good prognosis with spontaneous resolution of sarcoidosis in less than 2 years.

Other nonspecific cutaneous findings which may sometimes occur in sarcoidosis patients include sweet syndrome, pyoderma gangrenosum, vasculitis, and erythema multiforme (Fig. 24).

Other Systemic Manifestations

Systemic sarcoidosis such as cutaneous sarcoidosis has very protean manifestations and poses diagnostic challenge in many patients. Around one-third patients manifest with vague constitutional symptoms. Pulmonary involvement is the most common and important systemic affliction occurring in more than 90% patients, followed by sarcoidosis of intrathoracic, and peripheral lymph node in 75–90% cases. It remains asymptomatic in 20–30% cases and changes are observed only in routine chest X-ray films. Dyspnea, wheezing, cough, and chest pain are common symptoms and may occur with or without constitutional symptoms. Bilateral hilar

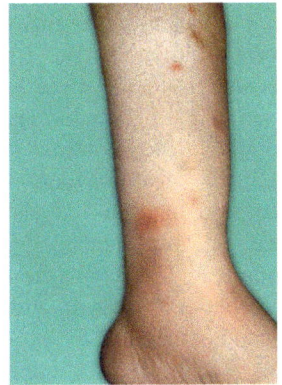

FIGURE 23: Erythema nodosum classically seen as dusky erythematous, tender subcutaneous nodules over shins with constitutional symptoms in a patient with stage-1 pulmonary sarcoidosis.

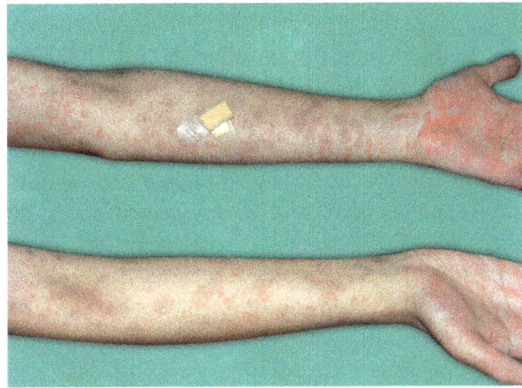

FIGURE 24: Erythema multiforme.

Table 6: Cutaneous sarcoidosis—morphologic variants		
Specific lesions	**Nonspecific inflammatory lesion (immune mediated)**	**Uncommon forms**
• Maculopapules • Papules • Nodules • Annular • Plaques • Scar sarcoidosis • Subcutaneous sarcoidosis (Darier-Roussy sacrcoid) • Lupus pernio • Angiolupoid sarcoid	• Erythema nodosum • Iritis, iridocyclitis • Arthritis	• Nail dystrophy, clubbing, onycholysis, subungual hyperkeratosis • Ulcerative, atrophic • Ichthyosiform sarcoid • Psoriasiform/verrucous form • Lichenoid • Erythrodermic • Hypopigmented/hyperpigmented • Alopecia • Calcinosis cutis with subcutaneous plaque • Faint erythema • Morphea like • Perforating lesions • Umbilicated lesions

(occasionally unilateral), mediastinal lymphadenopathy, and parenchymal involvement are frequent. Peribronchial thickening, random nodules (subpleural, septal and centrilobular), ground-glass opacities and interstitial lung disease are more characteristic. In sarcoidosis patients, decreased diffusion of carbon monoxide (DLCO) indicates involvement of lung parenchyma while improvement of DLCO indicates therapeutic response. Lung volumes may remain within normal range in about one-third cases with abnormal chest X-rays. Features of obstructive lung disease occur in nearly 50% cases manifesting as reduced ratio of forced vital capacity expired in time interval t (FEV t/FVC). Pleural effusion, pleural thickening, pneumothorax, and cavitation are observed less frequently. Hemoptysis is rare and is usually indicative of cavitation/aspergilloma. Nearly 10–30% patients have chronic progressive disease, while irreversible lung changes and severe respiratory disability occur in 10–20% patients because of end-stage lung fibrosis. Sarcoidosis-associated pulmonary hypertension is reported in 5–6% cases perhaps from direct pulmonary vascular involvement and in 70% patients with end stage lung fibrosis.[21]

Ophthalmic involvement varies between 30% in the United States and more than 70% among Japanese patients (Table 7). Anterior or posterior uveitis (acute, chronic), conjunctival nodule, and lacrimal gland, and duct lesions occur in order of frequency. Sicca and dry eye follows lacrimal gland disease. Ophthalmic involvement from active inflammation may remain asymptomatic or manifest with photophobia, blurred vision, retinitis, pars planitis, and smarting or sometimes blindness. Ophthalmic involvement is highly correlated with systemic disease activity. Hence, a complete ophthalmic examination is imperative in all patients even in the absence of symptoms.

Abdominal viscera are frequently involved in sarcoidosis, although this involvement usually does not produce symptoms. Anorexia, vague abdominal pain, hepatomegaly, splenomegaly, multiple intra-abdominal lymph node involvement, and features of Crohn's-like disease are some of the reported gastrointestinal manifestations. Hypersplenism may cause thrombocytopenia. Liver involvement often occurs as biochemical abnormality in 20–30% patients but can be identified in nearly 50% cases using biopsies. An elevated alkaline phosphatase

Table 7: Ocular sarcoidosis	
Sites of involvement	Features
Lacrimal glands	Keratoconjunctivitis sicca from decreased tears
Eyelid margins	"Millet seed" nodules
Orbit	Proptosis
Conjunctivae	Conjunctivitis with opaque, slate grey nodules
Iris	Granulomatous nodules of iris. Anterior or posterior uveitis—acute or chronic granulomatous iridocyclitis with mutton fat precipitates, or its complications (glaucoma, cataract, iris synechiae)
Retina/choroid	Retinochoroiditis from chronic uveitis
Optic nerve involvement from wide spread central nervous system involvement	Papilledema, retrobulbar disease, optic neuritis/atrophy
Syndromes of sarcoidosis and ocular involvement	
Löfgren's syndrome	Erythema nodosum, bilateral hilar lymphadenopathy, acute iridocyclitis, fever and polyarthritis
Heerfordt's-Waldenström syndrome	Fever, uveitis, parotid swelling, and facial nerve palsy
Mikulicz's syndrome	Keratoconjunctivitis sicca, bilateral swelling of lacrimal and parotid glands
	Chronic iridocyclitis, lupus pernio and bone cysts

levels is the most common abnormality of liver function and elevated bilirubin levels are seen with advanced disease. Elevated serum glutamine oxalate transaminase and serum glutamine pyruvate transaminase levels, extensive intrahepatic cholestasis, portal hypertension with esophageal varices, or ascites may occur in long standing cases.

Nearly less than 5% patients may have direct renal involvement from sarcoidal granulomas with increased calciuria with or without hypercalcemia being the most common. Hypercalcemia (in 2–10%) and hypercalciuria (in 6–30%) cases are more common in Whites than Blacks. This is attributed to increased intestinal absorption of calcium due to increased production of 1,25-dihydroxy vitaminosis D by granulomas and suppressed parathyroid hormone. Nephrocalcinosis, renal calculi, and acute renal failure may occur from hypercalcemia and hypercalciuria.

Sarcoidosis can involve central or peripheral nervous system in 5–10% cases. Cranial nerve involvement, basilar meningitis, myelopathy, anterior hypothalamic involvement with consequent neuroendocrine dysfunction (diabetes insipidus, hyperprolactinemia, or hypopituitarism), seizures, and cognitive changes are usual manifestations of neurosarcoidosis. Cranial nerves are involved either as part of more widespread leptomeningeal disease, or in isolation. Although any nerve can be involved, the facial and optic nerves get affected most commonly. Polyneuritis cranialis is considered pathognomonic. Small fiber neuropathy is a common complication of sarcoidosis and over 40% of patients with sarcoidosis have peripheral pain, paresthesias, or autonomic dysfunction attributable to it.[22]

The prevalence of cardiac involvement ranges from 5% based upon clinical criteria to more than or equal to 39% on the basis of latest imaging techniques.[23,24] Cardiac involvement has racial predilection and is a leading cause of sarcoidosis-related deaths in Japanese and the second most in sarcoid patients in the United States. Cardiac damage can be due to acute inflammation, fibrosis, or both causing pericarditis, papillary muscle dysfunction, or infiltrative cardiomyopathy. Cardiac manifestations are usually not apparent but may manifest as cardiac failure, arrhythmias, or sudden death. Clinically, chest pain, palpitation, and tachycardia are usual. Partial or complete cardiac blocks may occur from infiltration of sinoatrial or atrioventricular node, or Purkinje's system. Nonspecific ST segment depression and temporary T-wave inversion may be observed in routine electrocardiogram (ECG) and treadmill exercise. Doppler echocardiography (ECHO) may show cardiac dysfunction especially in diastolic dysfunction.

Bone and muscle involvement is documented in radio imaging studies, gallium scans, or biopsy in about 1–15% cases. Skeletal muscles weakness, chronic fatigue, and reduced exercise capacity occurs more often than perceived previously. Approximately 25% of patients with sarcoidosis have associated arthropathy. Monoarthritis or oligoarthritis, joint swelling and effusion, and tenosynovitis are more frequent in chronic sarcoidosis. Acute arthritis, polyarthralgia and myalgias also occur with acute sarcoidosis (Löfgren's syndrome) or as a part of chronic disease. Asymptomatic bone changes and lysis with bone cysts involving small digital bones are common and are more destructive in Black South Africans.

DIFFERENTIAL DIAGNOSIS AND DIAGNOSTIC PRINCIPLES

High index of clinical suspicion and compatible clinicopathologic findings are required to make a diagnosis of sarcoidosis in view of its varied clinical presentation. Formation of well-defined, compact, noncaseating, naked epithelioid cell granulomas with Langhans or foreign body type of giant cells in affected tissues is its hallmark feature (Fig. 25). Fibrinoid necrosis may occur in large granulomas. Asteroid, Schaumann's, or Hamasaki-Wesenberg inclusion bodies are not specific for sarcoidosis. Thus, the diagnosis of sarcoidosis remains by exclusion as a plethora of diseases share these histopathologic features (Table 8).

The diagnostic work-up[1,25] includes confirmation by histopathology, assessment for progression, extent and severity of organ involvement, and likelihood of therapeutic outcome (Table 9). The need of biopsy remains controversial in asymptomatic patients and when neoplasia or other granulomatous diseases have been excluded adequately. However, histological diagnosis is essential for patients requiring systemic corticosteroids. The patient should be examined for skin lesions as they are most accessible for biopsy and obviate the need of other invasive diagnostic procedures. Diagnosis of skin lesions or lymph node involvement by fine needle aspiration cytology appears possible with reasonable accuracy.

Bronchoscopy guided transbronchial lung biopsy and endobronchial biopsy are the direct ways to obtain tissue from lung parenchyma. Diagnostic yield of transbronchial lung biopsy is maximized when at least six good samples are obtained. Transbronchial needle aspiration (conventional or ultrasound guided) is less invasive method for sampling of the mediastinal lymph nodes. Endobronchial ultrasound-guided transbronchial needle aspiration has the highest diagnostic yield but need to be combined with transbronchial lung biopsy for the optimal results.[26] Other invasive procedures like mediastinoscopy for mediastinal lymph node sampling, video-assisted thoracoscopic lung biopsy, and open lung biopsy are needed when bronchoscopic procedures remain nondiagnostic. Video-assisted thoracoscopy permits biopsy of both lung and lymph nodes with precision and minimal trauma.

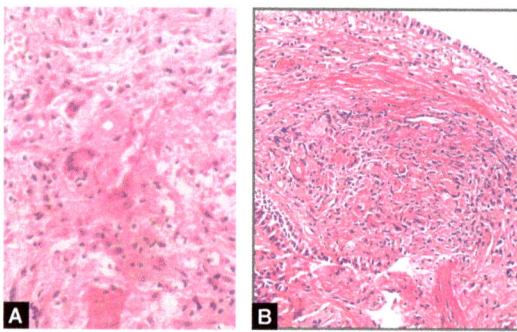

FIGURE 25: Histopathology. **A,** Noncaseating, epithelioid cell granuloma with giant cells in cutaneous lesion; **B,** Subepithelial endobronchial biopsy (H&E, ×40).

Radio Imaging Studies

Chest X-ray still remains the method of choice for detecting and monitoring the pulmonary sarcoidosis. High-resolution computed tomography scan is more sensitive method and has the advantage of diagnosing peribronchial thickening and reticular nodular lesions (parenchymal disease) even before it manifests in chest X-rays.

Table 8: Clinicopathological differential diagnosis of sarcoidosis			
Infective granulomatous diseases	**Noninfective granulomatous diseases**	**Neoplasia**	**Others**
• Tuberculosis, atypical mycobacteriosis • Cryptococcosis, aspergillosis, histoplasmosis, blastomycosis, coccidioidomycosis • *Pneumocystis jirovecii* (previously *P. carinii*) • Mycoplasma • Brucellosis • Toxoplasmosis • Cat-scratch disease • Schistosomiasis • Cytomegalovirus • Infectious mononucleosis • Cutaneous leishmaniasis • Donovanosis • All types of Leprosy lesions	• Pneumoconiosis • Hypersensitivity pneumonitis, chronic interstitial pneumonia • Foreign body impaction/aspiration with granulomatous inflammation, e.g., zirconium, tattooing • Granulomatous reaction in lymph nodes from carcinoma • Kikuchi's disease • Giant cell myocarditis • Rheumatoid nodules • Primary biliary cirrhosis • Drugs reactions • Granulomatous lesions of unknown significance (GLUS syndrome)	• Hodgkin's disease • Non-Hodgkin's lymphoma • Granulomatous mycosis fungoides • Lethal midline granuloma • Lymphomas with histiocytic infiltration (Lennert's disease)	• Granulomatous rosacea • Granuloma annulare and actinic granuloma • Necrobiosis lipoidica • Wegener's granulomatosis • Churg-Strauss disease • Crohn's disease

Table 9: Recommended investigative work-up in sarcoidosis patients		
For diagnosis in clinically suspected cases	To assess for vital organ involvement, extent and severity of sarcoidosis	To exclude other diseases
• Complete hemogram, serum biochemistry including hepatorenal function tests and serum calcium levels • Chest X-ray, pulmonary function tests (diffusion capacity and vital capacity are important parameters) • Urinalysis, 24 h urine calcium excretion, others based on history and clinical examination • Biopsy for histopathology, fine needle aspiration cytology of lymph nodes, tuberculin test, serum ACE	• Complete ophthalmic examination • Complete examination for cardiovascular system, ECG, echocardiogram, 24 h Holter monitoring • Complete neurological examination • HRCT, bronchoalveolar lavage, MRI brain, cardiac MRI, ^{67}Ga scans (when indicated)	• Detailed history and clinical examination (for pneumoconiosis or other pulmonary and cutaneous diseases, • Sputum examination (for *Mycobacterium tuberculosis*, fungal elements, abnormal cells) • Others as appropriate for the clinical diagnosis

ECG, electrocardiogram; ACE, angiotensin converting enzyme; HRCT, high-resolution computed tomography.

Table 10: Radiologic staging, features and mortality of lung sarcoidosis				
Radiologic Stage	Features on chest X-ray	Remarks	Spontaneous resolution rate	5-year mortality rate
0	Normal	5–10% patients have active disease	Low likelihood of progression	0%
1	Lymphadenopathy only	>50% patients have active disease	55–90%	Resolution within 1–2 years
2	Lymphadenopathy associated with pulmonary infiltrates	25–30% patients have active disease	40–70%	11%
3	Pulmonary infiltrate without lymphadenopathy	15% patients have active disease	10–20%	18%
4	Fibrosis and end-stage lung disease	Up to 20% patients progress to this stage	0%	50%

However, it is not considered a monitoring tool in pulmonary sarcoidosis. The Scadding radiologic staging system (Table 10) does not correspond to the chronologic progression of the disease but has prognostic value and helps assessing disease progression and therapeutic response. This is in spite of the fact that chest X-ray findings may not correlate sometimes with clinical presentation, pulmonary function/disease, parenchymal disease, or findings of CT or gallium (Ga) lung scans.

Chest X-rays show one of the three patterns—(i) bilateral hilar and mediastinal lymphadenopathy, (ii) diffuse parenchymal involvement with or without hilar, and (iii) mediastinal lymphadenopathy (Figs 26 to 29). Right paratracheal with bilateral hilar lymphadenopathy (Pawnbroker's sign, Garland's sign, 1-2-3 sign) is reliably diagnostic. Parenchymal infiltration in stage 3 and 4 is seen as reticular, acinar, and or large nodules. Pleural effusion in sarcoidosis is uncommon, and when occurs, is mostly unilateral, small, and more on right side. Deterioration in lung function (vanishing lung), bronchiectasis, and cavity formation signify progressive disease. The "fairy-ring" lesion (formation of rings by different sized granulomas) observed in posterior lung fields is characteristic. Punctate, amorphous, or eggshell calcification of hilar lymph nodes is observed in 5% patients with late stage sarcoidosis. Widespread small nodules in bronchovascular and subpleural distribution, thickened

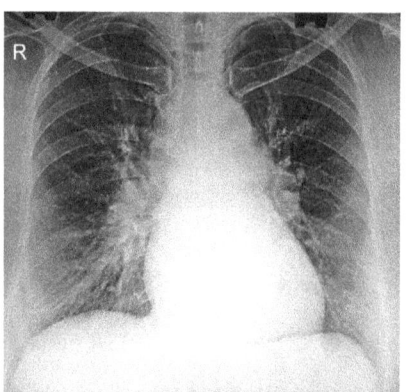

FIGURE 26: Chest radiograph in posteroanterior view with bilateral hilar lymphadenopathy (stage I pulmonary sarcoidosis).

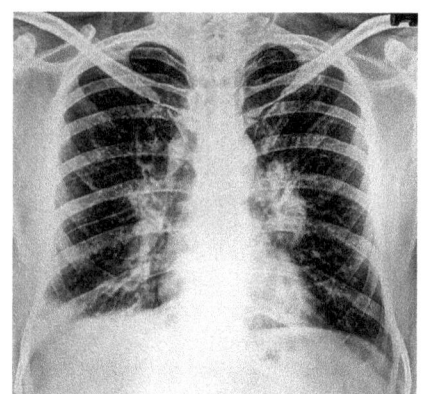

FIGURE 28: Chest radiograph in posteroanterior view with bilateral hilar lymphadenopathy, and patchy infiltrates right lower zone obscuring the costophrenic angle (stage II pulmonary sarcoidosis).

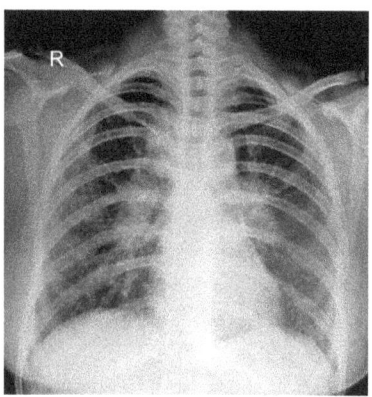

FIGURE 27: Chest radiograph in posteroanterior view with right paratracheal and bilateral hilar lymphadenopathy. Diffuse nodular opacities are present in both lung fields (stage II pulmonary sarcoidosis).

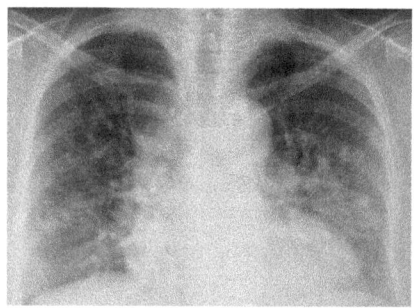

FIGURE 29: Chest radiograph in posteroanterior view with bilateral hilar lymphadenopathy and nodular opacities of variable size in both mid and lower zones (stage II pulmonary sarcoidosis).

interlobular septae, architecture distortion or conglomerate masses, and ground-glass opacity are more common findings in CT scan (Table 11, Figs 30 to 33). Honeycombing, apical fibrocystic disease, and giant bullous emphysema are less frequent. Pulmonary artery larger than 30 mm in diameter in contrast enhanced CT scan reflects the possibility of pulmonary hypertension.

The sensitivity of ^{67}Ga scintigraphy in detecting sarcoidosis is 60–90% and characteristic appearance of ^{67}Ga uptake in sarcoidosis has been described as "lambda" and "panda" patterns (Table 11). However, "panda" pattern alone is not considered specific for sarcoidosis and may be seen other conditions such as lymphoma. ^{67}Ga scintigraphy is useful in identifying extrathoracic sites of involvement, detecting active alveolitis, and in assessing response to treatment. Although CT and Ga lung scan obviate the need for invasive procedures, it may be abnormal in lymphoma, carcinoma, pneumonia, silicosis, or tuberculosis and radiation excess remains a limiting factor for routine use. However, magnetic resonance imaging (MRI) is seldom useful in evaluation of lung parenchyma and the role of technetium-99m labeled diethylene triamine penta-acetic acid (^{99m}Tc-DTPA) clearance test remains speculative.[25]

Sarcoidosis

Table 11: Classic features of pulmonary sarcoidosis in high-resolution computed tomography lung and ^{67}Ga scan

High-resolution computed tomography	^{67}Ga scan	Remarks
• Smooth or nodular peribronchial thickening. Predominant upper and midzone distribution • Small, well defined nodules along the interlobular septa, peribronchovascular bundles, and pleural surfaces • Patchy ground glass opacities • Fibrotic changes with lung distortion and traction bronchiectasis • Symmetric lymph node enlargement	• "Lambda" pattern-bilateral symmetrical uptake in parahilar and infrahilar lymph nodes, right paratraceal lymphnode (even with normal chest radiographs) • "Panda" pattern-symmetrical uptake in parotid, lacrimal, and salivary glands with normal nasopharyngeal capture producing facies resembling face of a panda	• "Lamba" plus "Panda" patterns together with bilateral hilar lymphadenopathy and parenchymal infiltration in chest radiographs is considered highly specific

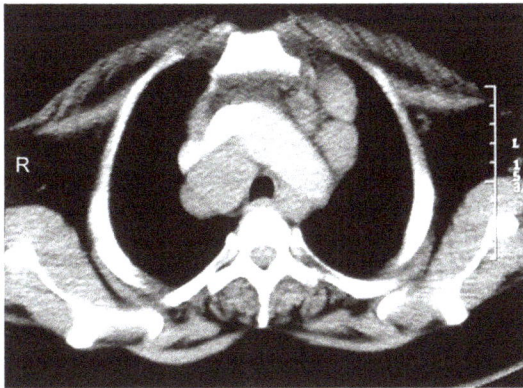

FIGURE 30: Contrast enhanced computed tomography scan chest shows enlarged right paratracheal (station 4R) and para-aortic (station 6) lymph nodes.

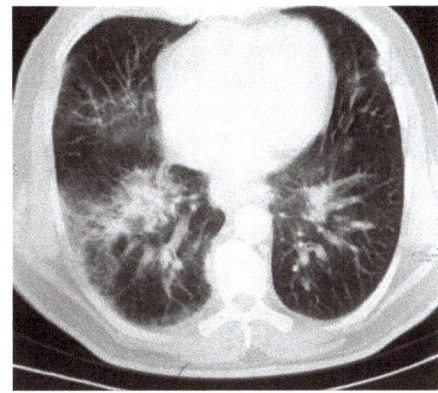

FIGURE 32: Computed tomography scan chest shows patchy infiltrates in posterior and lateral segments of right lower lobe.

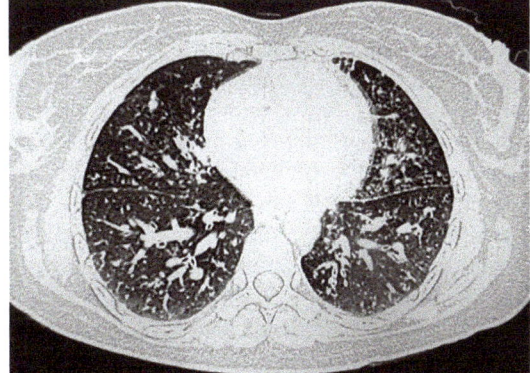

FIGURE 31: Computed tomography scan chest shows bilateral nodular opacities, ground glass opacities and irregular nodular thickening of major fissures.

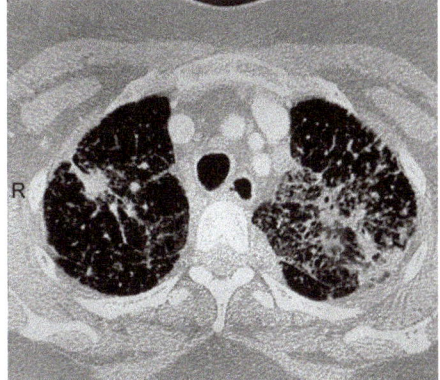

FIGURE 33: Computed tomography scan chest shows fibrotic mass right upper lobe, traction bronchiectasis and fibrosis in left upper lobe with bilateral parenchymal nodules (equivalent to stage IV of sarcoidosis).

The sensitivity and specificity of cardiac MRI remain uncertain in cardiac sarcoid but combined with myocardial T2 mapping is said to improve diagnostic outcome.[27,28] The sensitivity of F-fluorodeoxyglucose-positron emission tomography (FDG-PET) scans in cardiac sarcoidosis is higher than MRI but remains under evaluated (Fig. 34). Hydrocephalus, mass lesion(s), and leptomeningeal enhancement are common imaging findings in intracranial sarcoidosis. Gadolinium-enhanced MRI is preferred for evaluating neurosarcoid but findings are usually nonspecific.

Other Investigative Workup

Hematological abnormalities are frequent but not diagnostic. Anemia (hemoglobin <11 g/dL) occurs in 4–20% cases and nearly 40% patients have leukopenia. Elevated erythrocyte sedimentation rate is usual but hemolytic anemia, thrombocytopenia, and eosinophilia are rare. Abnormal serum biochemistry will suggest hepatorenal involvement. Suppression of tuberculin and other intradermal responses, elevated serum γ-globulins, calcium and angiotensin-converting enzyme (ACE) levels, and hypercalciuria support diagnosis in most cases. Serum ACE elevation (2 × normal) occurs in about 60% patients and the levels are higher in stage-2 pulmonary disease but not necessarily correlate with disease activity. It has limited diagnostic value due to false negative (40%) or false positive (10%) results. A poor correlation with disease severity also limits its use in monitoring of disease progression.

Baseline ECG, ECHO, urinary and serum calcium, pulmonary function tests, and ophthalmologic examination are indicated for all patients as these will help in deciding treatment with immunosuppressives. Bronchoalveolar lavage fluid analysis/culture helps rule out infective etiology. A high CD4/CD8 cell ratio in bronchoalveolar lavage is supportive of sarcoidosis rather than hypersensitivity pneumonitis. The presence of lymphocytes, elevated proteins, and ACE levels, increased CD4/CD8 ratio in CSF favors diagnosis of neurosarcoid and help exclude tuberculosis and fungal infections. Kveim-Siltzbach reaction is positive in patients with active disease but is neither approved by the Food and Drug Administration nor available for commercial use and has been given up due to high infective risk of injecting human tissue.

COMPLICATIONS AND PROGNOSIS

The skin lesions can be disfiguring, however, prognosis of cutaneous sarcoidosis is dictated by the involvement and severity of systemic disease. Sarcoidosis associated with erythema nodosum or acute/subacute inflammatory manifestations is self-limiting and resolves in 2–5 years. Blindness may occur even with asymptomatic ocular sarcoidosis. Glaucoma, cataract, and iris synechiae can complicate ocular sarcoidosis. It is also not uncommon to find these patients suffer significant psychosocial morbidity as it affects persons during most active years of life and the diagnosis is often delayed leading to increased financial burden, anxiety, and frustration.

The patients with other systemic manifestations suffer significant morbidity and relapses as the treatment is withdrawn. The risk of mortality is low in sarcoidosis except for patients presenting with

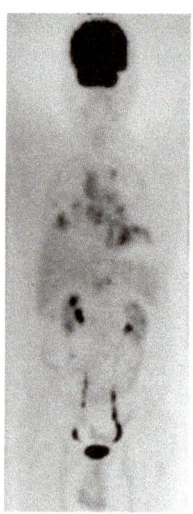

FIGURE 34: F-fluorodeoxyglucose-positron emission tomography scan shows uptake of radio contrast medium in fibronodular lesions in both lower lobe parenchyma. Physiological uptake is noted in liver, spleen and other organs.

advanced disease/pulmonary fibrosis, cardiac sarcoidosis, neurosarcoidosis, lupus pernio, renal failure/hypercalciuria/renal calculi, or bone cysts. Massive hemoptysis is usually from complications such as bronchiectasis or cystic lesions with aspergilloma in stage IV sarcoidosis. Pulmonary hypertension carries poor prognosis.

The most deaths are attributable to progressive lung disease (pneumonia, chronic obstructive lung disease, corpulmonale, ventilatory failure, lung fibrosis) or cardiac sarcoidosis (arrhythmias, sudden cardiac death) and happen in about 1–5% cases. However, mortality rates of patients with sarcoidosis are increasing in the United States by 3% per year over the past 2 decades where pulmonary complications account for greater mortality than deaths from cardiac complications in Japanese.[29]

Apart from racial predilection, old age, disease of more than 6 months, splenomegaly, and multiple organ involvement are other poor prognostic factors. However, pregnancy does not complicate sarcoidosis and the vice versa is true as well. There is also no specific risk to the fetus. However, elective pregnancy is discouraged because of treatment-associated toxicities.

TREATMENT AND FOLLOW-UP

Spontaneous remission provides an opportunity for conservative approach to treat sarcoidosis. Cutaneous lesions when present alone require a more conservative treatment approach unless they are very extensive or disfiguring. Intralesional triamcinolone or potent topical steroids (clobetasol propionate 0.05% cream) can be used for isolated limited skin involvement. Topical tacrolimus is a good alternative to steroids for lesions over face and flexures.

Systemic steroids are warranted when skin lesions are rapidly progressive, generalized and disfiguring. Once adequate clinical response has been achieved then taper steroid dose gradually to the lowest dose which prevents relapse. There is a long list of oral drugs that have been used as steroid sparing agents or as monotherapy when steroids cannot be given or when lesions not responding to steroids alone. Most commonly used agents include methotrexate, hydroxychloroquine, minocycline/tetracyclines, and mycophenolate mofetil. Other agents reported to be beneficial are allopurinol, low dose thalidomide, tumor necrosis factor-alpha inhibitors isotretinoin, pentoxifylline, chlorambucil, melatonin, fumaric acid esters, and PUVA. Laser treatment and surgery is reserved for very recalcitrant and disfiguring cutaneous sarcoidosis and results are variable with high chances of recurrences. Erythema nodosum generally reflects good prognosis and treatment with NSAIDs (indomethacin) and bed rest usually suffices. Associated acute iridocyclitis (Löfgren's syndrome) will respond to topical corticosteroids combined with mydriatic eye drops. However, more severe forms/failure of topical therapy will require periocular corticosteroid injections or systemic corticosteroids.

When managing systemic sarcoidosis there are specific indications for starting oral steroids (Box 2). In symptomatic and deteriorating pulmonary disease, the therapy is aimed at ameliorating symptoms, modifying disease activity, and to prevent fibrosis. Systemic corticosteroids are beneficial in all forms/stages of sarcoidosis: however, there is no consensus for the time of initiating therapy with systemic corticosteroids for lung sarcoidosis. A decline in the FVC of 10% or

---

Box 2: Common indications for systemic treatment in sarcoidosis

- Symptomatic pulmonary sarcoidosis, progressive or persistent parenchymal lung sarcoidosis
- Pathological changes in bronchoalveolar lavage
- A reduction of 10% functional vital capacity or 20% of diffusion capacity for carbon monoxide is considered significant for treatment
- Posterior ocular disease or anterior ocular disease not responding to topical steroids
- Liver involvement with significant dysfunction or hepatomegaly
- Cardiac sarcoidosis
- Renal involvement, persistent hypercalcemia/hypercalciuria
- Neurosarcoidosis
- Disfiguring, widespread, function-impairing skin lesions
- Myopathy or myositis
- Thrombocytopenia
- Persistent fever or weight loss

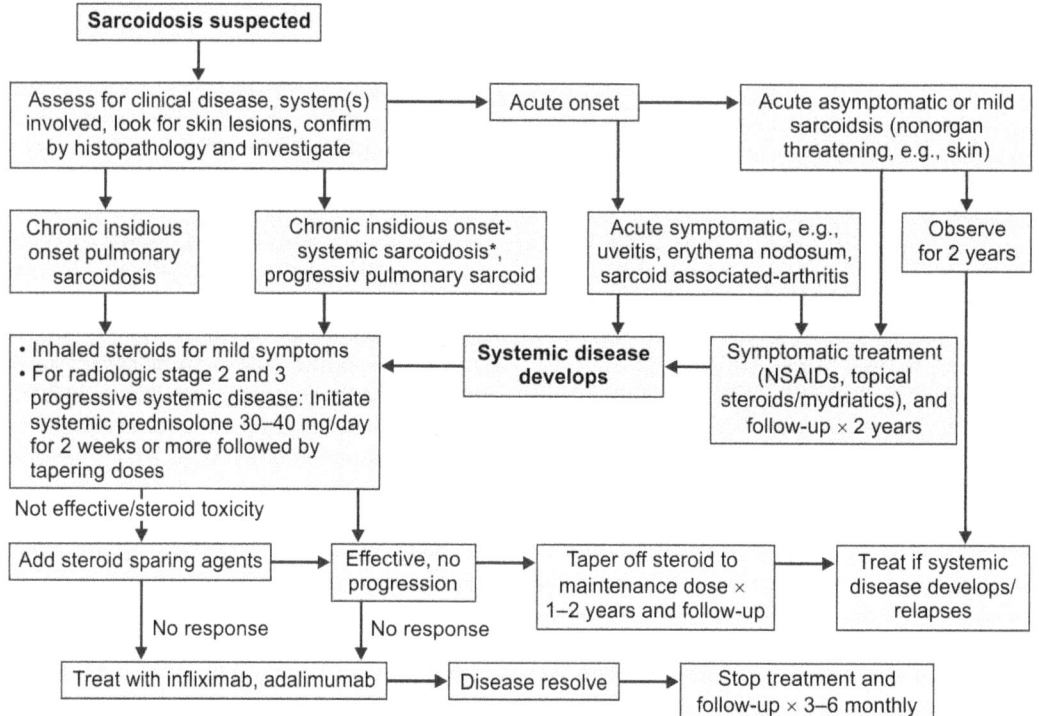

FLOWCHART 1: A suggested algorithm for management of suspected sarcoidosis

*Includes cardiac sarcoidosis, neurosarcoidosis, and complicated sarcoidosis that may need treatment for life.

DLCO of 20% is considered significant for initiating the treatment.[30,31] Flowchart 1 summarizes a suggested management approach for pulmonary sarcoidosis. American Thoracic Society consensus statement recommends prednisone 20-40 mg daily or on alternate days as a starting dose for 8-12 weeks.[1] Higher doses are needed for cardiac or neurosarcoidosis. The prednisone dose is tapered to 5-10 mg daily or on alternate days in patients who show clinicoradiological improvement. Then, a minimum maintenance dose which keeps the patient symptom free is continued for at least 1 year.

Steroid sparing agents are indicated in patients having intolerable corticosteroid side effects, progressive disease despite steroid therapy, or long-term corticosteroid need (Table 12).[32] Therapy with infliximab or adalimumab (for systemic and cutaneous sarcoidosis) is effective in steroid resistant cases but yet evolving.[33-35] Currently, infliximab appears more promising. Etanercept is least promising among biologic agents.[36,37]

High-dose inhaled corticosteroids (budesonide 800 μg twice daily) is said to improve pulmonary function and/or cough requiring systemic corticosteroids less frequently. Systemic antibiotics or antifungals (voriconazole, itraconazole, posaconazole) are indicated when bronchiectasis is complicated by bacterial infection or mycetoma/aspergilloma. Surgical lung resection may be needed in patients developing fatal hemoptysis. The patients with end stage disease will require lung transplantation. Therapeutic potential of perfenidon, an orally active drug having anti-inflammatory and antifibrotic effects in idiopathic pulmonary fibrosis, whether given alone or in combination with other drugs, in pulmonary fibrosis from sarcoidosis remains unevaluated.

Therapeutic potential of perfenidon, an orally active drug having anti-inflammatory and anti-fibrotic effects in idiopathic pulmonary fibrosis, whether given alone or in combination with other drugs, in pulmonary fibrosis from sarcoidosis remains unevaluated.

Sarcoidosis

Table 12: Nonsteroid therapies for the treatment of sarcoidosis

Drugs	Dose	Remarks
Cytotoxic drugs		
Methotrexate	10–15 mg/week	Pulmonary toxicity can complicate pulmonary sarcoidosis. Leflunamide is used in such cases. Also effective in cutaneous and musculoskeletal sarcoidosis. 70–80% response rate in cutaneous sarcoidosis. Takes 6 months to be effective. Add folic acid or folinic acid to minimize toxicity. Pregnancy category X drug
Azathioprine	2–3 mg/kg/day (50–200 mg/day)	Best used as steroid sparing drug. Also effective for extrapulmonary sarcoidosis. Pregnancy category X drug
Cyclophosphamide	50–100 mg/day or 500–2,000 mg intravenous every 2 weekly	Associated with higher efficacy and adverse effects. Pregnancy category X drug
Leflunomide	100 mg loading dose for 3 days, then 20 mg/kg/day	Can be combined with methotrexate for synergistic effect to reduce toxicity with enhanced therapeutic effect. Pregnancy category X drug
Mycophenolate mofetil	500–3,000 mg/day	Effective for extrapulmonary sarcoidosis like cutaneous, neuro, ocular, and cardiac sarcoidosis. Pregnancy category D drug
Antimicrobial agents		
Chloroquine	250–500 mg/day	Both are effective in cutaneous sarcoidosis, pulmonary sarcoidosis, steroid resistant neurosarcoidosis, and sarcoidosis-associated hypercalciuria, hypercalcemia. Hydroxychloroquine has better safety profile. Eye examination recommended at every 6-month interval. Pregnancy category C drug
Hydroxychloroquine	200–400 mg/day	
Minocycline	100–200 mg/day	Doxycycline (200 mg/day) or tetracycline 1,000 mg/day is also effective. Consider stopping tetracyclines if no response in 3 months. Pregnancy category D drug
Cytokine modulating drugs		
Pentoxifylline	400 mg thrice daily (25 mg/kg/day)	Best used as steroid sparing drug. Pregnancy category C drug
Thalidomide	50–200 mg/day	Best used as steroid sparing drug. Efficacy is not same in all patients. Absolute contraindication in women of childbearing age. Pregnancy category X drug
Infliximab	3–5 mg/kg, intravenously initially, then at every 4–8 weeks	Infliximab has been more promising but has risk of reactivation of tuberculosis or development of lymphoma, and hypersensitivity. It is a good choice for lupus pernio cases which are otherwise refractory to treatment. Pregnancy category B drug
Adalimumab	40 mg, subcutaneously, weekly or fortnightly	
Etanercept	25 mg subcutaneously, twice a week	Less effective in pulmonary sarcoidosis, and not effective in cutaneous or ocular sarcoidosis. Pregnancy category B drug
Ustekinumab, golimumab, rituximab		Emerging/evolving treatment modalities
Others		
Stem cell therapy		

Relapse may occur in 2–8% patients and regular follow-up is essential at 3–6 month intervals for patients with active disease, and at least once in 3 years when the disease is apparently inactive. Patients with persistent changes in X-rays require lifelong surveillance for recurrence of disease while those with new or worsening symptoms need monitoring of chest X-ray and pulmonary function tests. Patients with lung/heart transplant also require follow-up as sarcoidosis can develop in the transplant even when these were from donors without sarcoidosis.

CONCLUSION

Sarcoidosis, a systemic disease of unknown etiology, is characterized by granulomatous inflammation in affected organs and tissues. It can affect any organ system with a predilection for the lungs, skin, and eyes. It occurs worldwide but accurate epidemiological data are not available. It is considered a "rare disease" but the regional prevalence is much higher than previously estimated especially in Scandinavian countries, Japan, England, Ireland, and North America. African Americans are affected eight times more than Whites and have severe, chronic, and disabling disease. Granuloma formation in sarcoidosis requires complex interplay between antigen, antigen presenting cells, and T-cells in a genetically susceptible individual and the disease outcome will depend on disease modifying HLA and non-HLA genes. High index of clinical suspicion and compatible clinicopathological features are required to make its diagnosis.

All patients with skin lesions even in the absence of systemic features should be subjected to detailed clinical examination as ocular involvement is common and pulmonary changes dominate usually in the later stages. Skin biopsy also obviates the need of invasive diagnostic procedures. Routine chest X-ray is the method for detecting, staging and monitoring while high resolution computed tomography scan is sensitive diagnostic method for pulmonary sarcoidosis. The management of sarcoidosis requires a multidisciplinary approach. Systemic corticosteroids, with or without steroid sparing cytotoxic agents, remain mainstay of therapy for patients with progressive involvement of pulmonary, cardiovascular, nervous systems, and eyes. However, spontaneous remission provides an opportunity for conservative approach to treat sarcoidosis.

REFERENCES

1. Statement on sarcoidosis. Joint Statement of the American Thoracic Society (ATS), the European Respiratory Society (ERS) and the World Association of Sarcoidosis and Other Granulomatous Disorders (WASOG) adopted by the ATS Board of Directors and by the ERS Executive Committee, February 1999. Am J Respir Crit Care Med. 1999;160:736-55.
2. Rossman MD, Kreider ME. Lesson learned from ACCESS (A Case Control Etiologic Study of Sarcoidosis). Proc Am Thorac Soc. 2007;4:453-6.
3. Pierce TB, Margolis M, Razzuk MA. Sarcoidosis: still a mystery? BUMC Proceedings. 2001;14:8-12.
4. Gupta SK. Sarcoidosis: the Indian scene. Indian J Clin Prac. 1993;3:19-27.
5. Mahajan VK, Sharma NL, Sharma RC, et al. Cutaneous sarcoidosis: clinical profile of 23 Indain patients. Indian J Dermatol Venereol Leprol. 2007;73:16-21.
6. Joshi JM, Saxena S. Sarcoidosis in India. Med Update. 2012;22:408-12.
7. Ezzie ME, Crouser ED. Considering an infectious etiology of sarcoidosis. Clin Dermatol. 2007;25:259-66.
8. Newman LS, Rose CS, Bresnitz EA, et al. A case control etiological study of sarcoidosis: environ and occupational risk factors. Am J Respir Crit Care Med. 2004;170:1324-30.
9. Gupta D, Agarwal R, Agarwal AN, et al. Molecular evidence for the role of mycobacteria in sarcoidosis: a meta-analysis. Eur Respir J. 2007:30:508-16.
10. Song Z, Marzilli I, Greenlee BM, et al. Mycobacterial catalase-peroxidase is a tissue antigen and target of adaptive immune response in systemic sarcoidosis. J Exp Med. 2005;201:755-67.
11. Iannuzzi MC, Rybicki BA. Genetics of sarcoidosis: candidate genes and genome scans. Proc Am Thorac Soc. 2007;4:108-16.
12. Voorter CE, Drent M, van den Berg-Loonen EM. Severe pulmonary sarcoidosis is strongly associated with the haplotype HLA-DQB1*0602-DRB1*150101. Hum Immunol. 2005;66:826-35.
13. Rybicki BA, Walewski JL, Maliarik MJ, et al. The BTNL2 gene and sarcoidosis susceptibility in African American and Whites. Am J Hum Genet. 2005;77:491-9.
14. Noor A, Knox KS. Immunopathogenesis of sarcoidosis. Clin Dermatol. 2007;25:250-8.
15. Patterson K, Hogarth K, Husain A, et al. The clinical and immunologic features of pulmonary fibrosis in sarcoidosis. Transl Res. 2012;160:321-31.

16. Mahajan VK, Sharma NL, Kashyap S. Sarcoidosis (Lung). In: Lang F (Ed). Encyclopedia of Molecular Mechanisms of Disease, 1st edition. Berlin Heidelberg: Springer; 2009. pp. 1887-9.
17. Amin EN, Closser DR, Crouser ED. Current best practice in the management of pulmonary and systemic sarcoidosis. Ther Adv Resp Dis. 2014;8:111-32.
18. Miyara M, Amoura Z, Parizot C, et al. The immune paradox of sarcoidosis and regulatory T cells. J Exp Med. 2006;203:359-70.
19. Fernandez-Faith E, McDonnell J. Cutaneous sarcoidosis: differential diagnosis. Clin Dermatol. 2007;25:276-87.
20. Mana J, Marcoval J. Erythema nodosum. Clin Dermatol. 2007;25:288-94.
21. Nunes H, Humbert M, Capron F, et al. Pulmonary hypertension associated with sarcoidosis: mechanisms, haemodynamics and prognosis. Thorax. 2006;61:68-74.
22. Hoitsma E, Marziniak M, Faber C, et al. Small fibre neuropathy in sarcoidosis. Lancet. 2002;359:2085-6.
23. Bussinguer M, Danielian A, Sharma O. Cardiac sarcoidosis: diagnosis and management. Curr Treat Options Cardiovasc Med. 2012;14:652-64.
24. Crouser E, Ono C, Tran T, et al. Improved detection of cardiac sarcoidosis using magnetic resonance with myocardial T2 mapping. Am J Resp Crit Care Med. 2014;189:109-12.
25. Nunes H, Brillet PY, Valeyre D, et al. Imaging in sarcoidosis. Semin Resp Crit Care Med. 2007;28:102-20.
26. Gupta D, Dadhwal DS, Agarwal R, et al. Endobronchial ultrasound-guided transbronchial needle aspiration vs conventional transbronchial needle aspiration in the diagnosis of sarcoidosis. Chest. 2014;146:547-56.
27. Bussinguer M, Danielian A, Sharma O. Cardiac sarcoidosis: diagnosis and management. Curr Treat Options Cardiovasc Med. 2012;14:652-64.
28. Crouser E, Ono C, Tran T, et al. Improved detection of cardiac sarcoidosis using magnetic resonance with myocardial T2 mapping. Am J Resp Crit Care Med. 2014;189:109-12.
29. Swigris J, Olson A, Huie T, et al. Sarcoidosis-related mortality in the United States from 1988 to 2007. Am J Respir Crit Care Med. 2011;183:1524-30.
30. Lazar C, Culver D. Treatment of sarcoidosis. Semin Respir Crit Care Med. 2010;31:501-18.
31. Lynch J, Ma Y, Koss M, et al. Pulmonary sarcoidosis. Semin Respir Crit Care Med. 2007;28:53-74.
32. Baughman R, Nunes H, Sweiss N, et al. Established and experimental medical therapy of pulmonary sarcoidosis. Eur Respir J. 2013;41:1424-38.
33. Judson M, Baughman R, Costabel U, et al. Efficacy of infliximab in extrapulmonary sarcoidosis: results from a randomised trial. Eur Respir J. 2008;31:1189-96.
34. Kamphuis L, Lam-Tse W, Dik W, van Daele P, van Biezen P, Kwekkeboom D, et al. Efficacy of adalimumab in chronically active and symptomatic patients with sarcoidosis. Am J Respir Crit Care Med. 2011;184:1214-6.
35. Pariser R, Paul J, Hirano S, et al. A double-blind, randomized, placebo-controlled trial of adalimumab in the treatment of cutaneous sarcoidosis. J Am Acad Dermatol. 2013;68:765-73.
36. Utz JP, Limper AH, Kalra S, et al. Etanercept for the treatment of stage II and III progressive pulmonary sarcoidosis. Chest. 2003;124:177-85.
37. Baughman RP, Lower EE, Bradley DA, et al. Etanercept for refractory ocular sarcoidosis: results of a double-blind randomized trial. Chest. 2005;128:1062-7.

14

CHAPTER

Cryoglobulinemic Vasculitis

Liza Rajasekhar

DEFINITION

According to the Chapel Hill classification of vasculitis in 2012, cryoglobulinemic vasculitis (CV) is a disorder causing vasculitis of small vessels (predominantly capillaries, venules, or arterioles) due to deposition of cryoglobulin immune deposits.[1]

The disease is considered in the differential diagnosis of an illness which has a typical triad of purpura, weakness, and arthralgia with or without visceral involvement in the form of glomerulonephritis, liver involvement, or neuropathy.

NOMENCLATURE

The CV is called essential CV if the etiology is unknown. It is now recommended that if the etiology is known then it can be referred to in the nomenclature, e.g., Hepatitis C virus-related (HCV) CV. The other term often used in literature is essential mixed cryoglobulinemia. The evolution of these terms will be discussed here.

HISTORICAL LANDMARKS IN THE UNDERSTANDING OF CRYOGLOBULINEMIC VASCULITIS

In 1966, Metzler reported in the American Journal of Medicine, the nature of cryoglobulins in 29 patients.[2] They said that in 12 of them they found unusual rheumatoid factor activity. In 9 they found macroglobulins and in 8 they found immunoglobulins G (IgG) as seen in multiple myeloma and "idiopathic cryoglobulinemia". In a further report, they described clinical and laboratory studies in the 12 patients with rheumatoid factor activity.[3] In 11 of these 12 patients there was both IgM and IgG but the IgM was necessary for cryoprecipitation to occur. Seven of these 12 patients had low serum complement, 4 had antinuclear antibodies and in one the gamma globulin was deposited in the glomerular lesions.

In one female patient who had rheumatoid arthritis and died due to marked hyperviscosity they could isolate an IgG with rheumatoid factor activity. They described it as the first IgG rheumatoid factor.

In a landmark article in 1974 published in the American Journal of Medicine,[4] the authors established the nature of cryoglobulins from a sample of 86 patients using immunochemical methods. They then classified them into three types, naming them Type 1, Type 2, and Type 3.

The type I cryoglobulins were monoclonal immunoglobulins.

Type II cryoglobulins were also monoclonal immunoglobulins but directed against polyclonal immunoglobulin of only IgG isotypes. Most commonly they are IgMkRF. They are the cause of cryoglobulinemic syndrome seen in HCV and Sjogren's syndrome.

Type III cryoglobulins were polyclonal, mostly immunoglobulins and directed against polyclonal immunoglobulins. Some cryoglobulins in this class were not immunoglobulins but proteins like lipoproteins.

Type II and type III were called mixed cryoglobulins.

The authors then tried to draw an association between the chemical nature of these cryoglobulins and the diseases in which they were observed.

They observed that those with type I cryoglobulins had more severe Raynaud's phenomenon, while those with type II and type III cryoglobulins were more often associated with milder purpura, Raynaud's phenomenon, renal and neurologic involvement.

Immunoproliferative disorders were associated with type I or II cryoglobulins. The immunoproliferative disorders associated with type II cryoglobulins include non-Hodgkin's lymphoma, multiple myeloma, Waldenstrom's macroglobulinemia, chronic myeloid leukemia and angioimmunoblastic lymphadenopathy.

Autoimmune diseases such as Sjögren's syndrome, chronic infections, and lymphoproliferative disorders were associated with type II and III cryoglobulins.

They stated that in 30% of patients with cryoglobulinemia they could not find a disease despite 9 years of follow-up. These were referred to as essential cryoglobulinemia or essential mixed cryoglobulinemia depending on whether there was type I cryoglobulins or type II or III in serum, respectively.

We know now that most of cases in these two categories comprise HCV infected patients. This knowledge followed upon the discovery of HCV in 1989.

In 1991 Ferri et al.[5] reported that slightly more than half the patients with mixed cryoglobulins in their serum had antibodies to hepatitis C while almost none of the patients with other systemic autoimmune diseases had these antibodies. They further showed that in those subset of patients with mixed cryoglobulinemia and chronic liver disease or transaminitis the proportion testing positive for hepatitis C antibodies was higher than in those without. Using these results the authors comprehensively proved for all times to come that HCV has a role to play in the pathogenesis of disease associated with mixed cryoglobulinemia.

For some unknown reasons, very few, probably less than 5%, of patients with hepatitis B infection have associated CV.

PATHOGENESIS OF CRYOGLOBULINEMIC VASCULITIS

In the type I cryoglobulinemia the manifestations are due to hyperviscosity. In type 2 and 3 it is due to vasculitis. The cryoglobulins are deposited in the vessel wall as part of immune complex. These immune complexes activate complement. They are activators of classic and alternate pathway. This further leads to leukocyte migration to site and endothelial damage. The characteristic signature of very low levels of C4 and low levels of C1q and C2 suggests activation of the classical pathway.

Vasculitis occurs in only a variable proportion of patients with cryoglobulinemia and this is dependent on the rheological disturbance and endothelial cell activation arising out of immune complex formation by the cryoglobulins and subsequent complement activation. The variables which determine when a cryoglobulin results in a vasculitic syndrome are probably the isotype of the immunoglobulin, the tertiary configuration of the immune complex and the characteristics of the antigen, which is believed to be a constituent of the immune complex.

CLINICAL FEATURES OF CRYOGL OBULINEMIC VASCULITIS

The disease expression can vary from mild symptoms to severe life-threatening disease. Fatigue is the most common symptom noted in 80–90% individuals.

The paper best describing the clinical features of CV was published in 1980 again in the American Journal of Medicine by the group which had first published in 1966.

They described recurrent palpable purpura, polyarthralgias, and renal disease as the most common manifestations. If in the presence of vasculitic features, which are not usual for CV such as cerebral vasculitis or temporal arteritis one finds hypocomplementemia, rheumatoid factors in the serum and a histopathology suggestive of immune complex mediated vasculitis but cryoglobulin cannot be demonstrated then cryofibrinogen (CF) must be looked for. In a small report on 29 patients with CV,[6] 18 tested positive for CF. Of these 38% had cancer or hematologic disorders compared to none in the CF negative group.

The French CryoVas group which has a dataset of over 380 patients with CV, studied them retrospectively by dividing them into infectious and noninfectious related CV. In the group of noninfectious CV they showed that patients with type II cryoglobulins have a higher incidence of purpura, peripheral neuropathy, renal involvement, lower C4 levels, and lower glomerular filtration rate compared to patients with type III CV.

Cutaneous Manifestations

Skin lesions in CV result from hyperviscosity and thrombosis in type I while due to immune complex deposits in small vessels in type II and III CV.

Patients with type I CV can develop acrocyanosis, purpura, Raynauds, ischemic ulceration, gangrene, livedo reticularis, and arterial thrombosis in nondependent areas.

In patients with type II and III CV, palpable purpura represent the most common cutaneous manifestation occurring in 70-90% individuals starting over the lower limbs but can extend to involve the abdomen, and less frequently the trunk and upper limbs. These spots appear intermittently any time during the course of the disease and severity varies from isolated few lesions to florid vasculitic lesions. These lesions resolve leaving behind brownish pigmentation in 3-10 days (Fig. 1). In addition, patient may have Raynaud's phenomenon, acrocyanosis and disease course may be complicated by the cutaneous ulcers over lower limbs and less commonly the upper limbs and distal necrosis of the hands and feet (Fig. 2). Cutaneous ulcers are

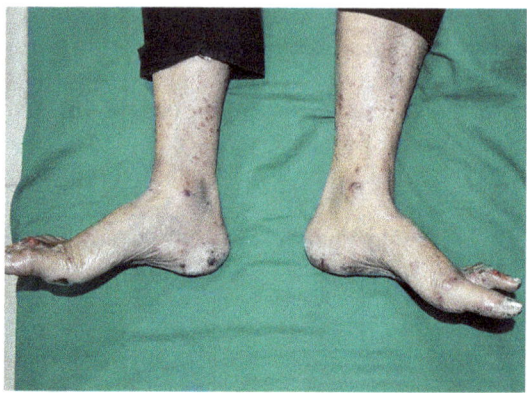

FIGURE 1: Palpable purpura, brownish spots over leg and feet and cutaneous ulcers over toes.

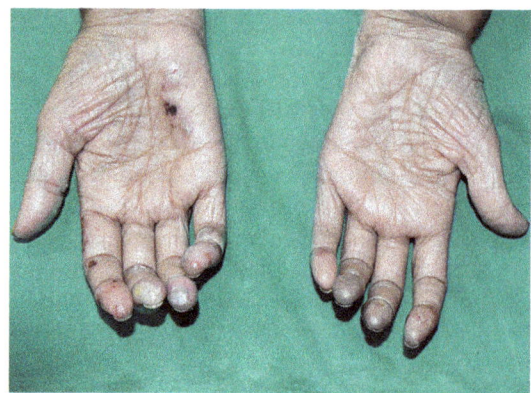

FIGURE 2: Acrocyanosis and vasculitic lesion over palms.

painful, nonhealing, and often develop secondary bacterial infection.

Arthralgia occurs in 40-60% patients and is bilateral, symmetric, nondeforming, involving the knees and hands. Frank arthritis is less common. Neurologic manifestation is present as distal sensory neuropathy or sensory motor polyneuropathy leading to painful paresthesias. Involvement of CNS is less frequent but can result in stroke, seizure and cognitive impairment.

Glomerulonephritis

Cryoglobulinemic glomerulonephritis is almost always found in association with the presence of type II CG in the serum. This means that the CGs are monoclonal Ig directed against polyclonal

IgG. The histology observed in decreasing order of frequency includes membranoproliferative and mesangioproliferative glomerulonephritis. Renal vasculitis of small and medium sized vessels is noted in one-third of patients and chronic renal failure may occur in up to half of the patients.

Hepatic Manifestations

The initial report which described the clinical findings in 40 patients seen over 2 decades reported hepatic involvement, though often subclinical, in around 70% of patients. On histopathology mild triaditis, chronic active hepatitis or cirrhosis was seen.

Peripheral Neuropathy

Sensory symptoms predominate in the peripheral neuropathy of CV. They are usually distal and very soon become symmetric. Motor symptoms are often delayed. Occasionally, mononeuritis multiplex may be seen.

Cardiac Involvement and Gastrointestinal Involvement

The clinical features of cardiac and gastrointestinal involvement do not correlate with the cryoprotein concentration.

LABORATORY FEATURES

Cryoglobulins are detected at the bedside by separating the serum at 37°C, i.e., core body temperature and then storing at 4°C to uncover the presence of these cryoglobulins. It is important that all processes till serum separation are done at 37°C. Once the serum is separated then presence of cryoglobulins is checked for by maintaining the serum at 4°C. If detected their cryoprecipitability is confirmed by rewarming the serum to 37°C for 24 hours. The cryocrit is measured at 7 days but does not correlate with the severity of symptoms.

The additional characteristic laboratory features of CV are normal or low level of C3 and very low level to absent C4.

On histopathology, some authors recommend that immune complex mediated vasculitis should be proven by immunohistochemistry or electron microscopy.

VALIDATION OF CLASSIFICATION CRITERIA FOR CRYOGLOBULINEMIC VASCULITIS

There have been efforts to bring the CV in to the same playing level as other vasculitis by developing and validating classification criteria.[7]

The multicenter European group developed a set of criteria over three domains which provide more than 90% sensitivity and more than 90% specificity for the diagnosis of CV. The three domains considered are questionnaire, clinical features, and laboratory features.

Using expert opinion questions relevant to the diagnosis of CV were formulated. These questions include five questions on purpura, four on neuropathy or muscle symptoms, and one related to HCV infection. After Delphi exercises, three questions were retained in the questionnaire domain, two of the three questions considered relate to the presence of purpura (past or current) and one to a history of viral hepatitis.

The clinical features considered include constitutional features, articular involvement, vascular involvement, and neurologic involvement.

- The constitutional symptoms include fatigue, fibromyalgia, low grade fever for more than 10 days or fever more than 38°C either without other obvious cause
- Arthralgia or arthritis constitutes the articular domain
- Vascular involvement is scored if any one of the five is present: (i) purpura, (ii) skin ulcers, (iii) necrotizing vasculitis, (iv) Raynaud's phenomenon, and (v) hyperviscosity syndrome
- Neuropathy is scored if peripheral neuropathy, cranial neuropathy, or CNS vasculitis is present.

Laboratory items considered are the presence of rheumatoid factor, low serum C4, and presence of monoclonal M spike in serum.

In a patient with cryoglobulins in serum, presence of more than 2 out of 3 of questionnaire criteria, more than 3 out of 4 of clinical criteria and more than 2 out of 3 of laboratory criteria provide the above-mentioned accuracy in diagnosis of CV.

It is important to note that none of these criteria score for the presence of cryoglobulins.

This is because these criteria have been developed for patients who have serum cryoglobulins. These criteria were tested in patients with other vasculitis (which could share some clinical features of CV except the presence of cryoglobulins), they were rarely found positive. This prompted the expert group to reinforce the message that if a patient without cryoglobulins in serum satisfied the criteria for diagnosis of CV the tests for cryoglobulins should be repeated using laboratory procedures of greater sensitivity.

THERAPY OF CRYOGLOBULINEMIC VASCULITIS

Therapy of Infection-related Cryoglobulinemic Vasculitis

Purpura of HCV related CV responds well to therapy but the glomerulonephritis and peripheral neuropathy respond poorly.

Antiviral Therapies

It is a fact that HCV related CV arises in patients with chronic hepatitis C infection and increases in frequency with the duration of the disease reaching a prevalence of around 70% in those with duration of infection of more than 20 years. Therapy therefore should logically include elimination of the virus.

Interferon-α is the agent most commonly employed to treat hepatitis C infection, the dose and duration being decided by the genotype which to some extent predicts clearance of the virus following interferon therapy. Relapse rates after 1 year of interferon therapy are high and maybe associated with relapses of the associated CV if present initially. Some experts prefer to add a proteasome inhibitor bortezomib in case of infection due to genotype I of hepatitis C.

If the associated CV is mild then antiviral therapy alone may be effective in removing the virus and resolving the vasculitis. Since hepatitis C infection as a cause of CV is so common experts recommend that both antibodies to HCV and HCV RNA estimation should be done in patients suspected to have a clinical course favoring CV. If they are repeatedly negative and serum cryoglobulins are present they even recommend separating the proteins of the immune complexes by acid treatment and then looking for the above markers of HCV infection. The strength of association between CV and hepatitis C infection is so high that it is recommended to look for infection even in a patient with normal transaminases.

Sometimes skin ulcers and peripheral neuropathy are worsened during interferon based antiviral therapy.

Since antiviral therapies are slow-acting, moderate to severe CV may require therapy to be initiated with both immunosuppression and antiviral therapy.[8]

Immunosuppressive Therapy

Though viral agents were accepted as an important etiologic agent in CV, the fact that vasculitis was widespread and that antiviral therapy did not reverse the vasculitic manifestations led to the sequential or concomitant use of immunosuppressives in the management of these conditions by experts.

Immunosuppressive Therapy in Cryoglobulinemic Vasculitis

Cyclophosphamide B-cell depleting therapies: Since most of MC or CV is associated with an IgMRF monoclonal Ig against polyclonal IgG, it stands to reason that there is an expanded B-cell pool producing them. Hence, the rationale of using B-cell depleting therapy in CV with type 2 MC.

In a randomized controlled trial (RCT) published in AR 2012 from a group I Italy,[9] it was demonstrated that in patients with hepatitis C associated severe mixed cryoglobulinemia and CV in whom antiviral therapy was ineffective, intolerant or not indicated as per the expert, rituximab infusions 1 g given twice 2 weeks apart and then given during relapse was significantly better (65%) compared to either steroids alone, or azathioprine or cyclophosphamide, or plasmapheresis (3.5%) in meeting the primary end point of patients continuing with the therapy they were initially randomized to. Rituximab was able to provide improvement in all the three disease manifestations of skin ulcers, worsening or refractory neuropathy, and active glomerulonephritis.

In the same year another group from Maryland, Bethesda[10] explored the role of rituximab in an open label RCT of four doses of weekly rituximab versus the best available therapy which could include maintenance therapy or an increase in immunosuppressive therapy in patients of HCV related CV who had failed to achieve remission with antiviral therapy. The primary endpoint of remission at 6 months was met in 83% of patients who received rituximab versus 8% in the other arm. In addition, viremia or transaminases did not deteriorate.

Therapy of Peripheral Neuropathy in Cryoglobulinemic Vasculitis

A recent Cochrane review in December 2014[11] analyzed studies on therapy of HCV related to peripheral neuropathy. They considered all studies which used any therapies such as interferon-α, ribavirin, corticosteroids, cyclophosphamide, plasmapheresis alone or in combination with a minimum follow-up of 6 months. They looked at primary outcome of improvement in sensory symptoms using any validated instrument. Secondary outcome of improvement in motor symptoms at 6 months was considered. Four studies were identified but none used the primary outcome measure. In one study which used pegylated interferon-α, ribavirin, and rituximab in one arm and pegylated interferon with ribavirin alone in the other did not show difference in efficacy.

Therapy in Noninfectious Mixed Cryoglobulinemic Vasculitis

In a large dataset of 242 patients with the CV syndrome[12] and no evidence of hepatitis C, B, or HIV infection, rituximab with steroids was more effective than steroids alone or steroids with alkylating agents in inducing remission and reducing the prednisolone dose to less than 10 mg at 6 months.

PROGNOSIS

In the series of 40 patients published in 1980[13] in which there was a 2-decade follow-up of patients, renal involvement was reported to be associated with poor prognosis. Autopsy in most patients revealed widespread vasculitis in addition to renal involvement.

Analyzing 150 hepatitis C RNA positive patients between 1993 and 2009 for clinical, biologic, and therapeutic factors associated with survival, the group from France[14] reported that severe liver fibrosis at baseline and severity of vasculitis as indicated by a high five factor score (FFS) of vasculitis as poor prognostic markers. The FFS of vasculitis includes one point each for proteinuria more than 1 g/day, serum creatinine more than 2 mg/dL, cardiomyopathy, and specific central nervous system involvement. Antiviral therapy had a positive impact while use of immunosuppressants had a negative effect.

Future reports on long-term change in prognosis after use of rituximab will be anticipated.

CONCLUSION

Cryoglobulinemic vasculitis involves small vessels due to deposition of cryoglobulin immune deposits and is classified into three types. The manifestations in type I cryoglobulinemia are due to hyperviscosity and due to vasculitis in type II and III. Vasculitis occurs in only a variable proportion of patients with cryoglobulinemia. The disease expression can vary from mild to severe with fatigue, purpura, polyarthralgia and renal disease as the most common manifestations. Apart from cryoglobulins additional characteristic laboratory features of CV are normal or low level of C3 and very low level of C4. A new set of criteria with three domains viz questionnaire, clinical features and laboratory features are about 90% sensitive and specific for the diagnosis of CV. Antiviral therapy is the mainstay of therapy in HCV CV. Rituximab has been proven to be effective in improving all manifestations of CV. Renal involvement, severe liver fibrosis at baseline and high five factor score of vasculitis are poor prognostic markers.

REFERENCES

1. Jennette JC, Falk RJ, Bacon PA, et al. 2012 revised International Chapel Hill Consensus Conference Nomenclature of Vasculitides. Arthritis Rheum. 2013;65(1):1-11.

2. Meltzer M, Franklin EC. Cryoglobulinemia—a study of twenty-nine patients. I. IgG and IgM cryoglobulins and factors affecting cryoprecipitability. Am. J. Med. 1966;40:828-36.
3. Meltzer M, Franklin EC, Elias K, et al. Cryoglobulinemia—a clinical and laboratory study. II. Cryoglobulins with rheumatoid factor activity. Am J Med. 1966;40:837-966.
4. Brouet JC, Clauvel JP, Danon F, et al. Biologic and clinical significance of cryoglobulins. A report of 86 cases. Am J Med. 1974;57:775-88.
5. Ferri C, Greco F, Longombardo G, et al. Antibodies to hepatitis C virus in patients with mixed cryoglobulinemia. Arthritis Rheum. 1991;34;1606-10.
6. Michaud M, Moulis G, Puissant B, et al. Cryofibrinogenemia: a marker of severity of cryoglobulinemic vasculitis. Am J Med. Am J Med. 2015;128(8):916-21.
7. De Vita S, Soldano F, Isola M, et al. Preliminary classification criteria for the cryoglobulinaemic vasculitis. Ann Rheum Dis. 2011;70:1183-90.
8. Cacoub P, Terrier B, Saadoun D. Hepatitis C virus-induced vasculitis: therapeutic options. Ann Rheum Dis. 2014;73:24-30.
9. De Vita S, Quartuccio L, Isola M, et al. A randomized controlled trial of rituximab for the treatment of severe cryoglobulinemic vasculitis. Arthritis Rheum. 2012;64:843-53.
10. Sneller MC, Hu Z, Langford CA. A randomized controlled trial of rituximab following failure of antiviral therapy for hepatitis C virus-associated cryoglobulinemic vasculitis. Arthritis Rheum. 2012;64:835-42.
11. Benstead TJ, Chalk CH, Parks NE. Treatment for cryoglobulinemic and non-cryoglobulinemic peripheral neuropathy associated with hepatitis C virus infection. Cochrane Database Syst Rev. 2014;12:CD010404.
12. Terrier B, Krastinova E, Marie I, et al. Management of noninfectious mixed cryoglobulinemia vasculitis: data from 242 cases included in the CryoVas survey. Blood. 2012;119:5996-6004.
13. Gorevic PD, Kassab HJ, Levo Y, et al. Mixed cryoglobulinemia: clinical aspects and long-term follow-up of 40 patients. Am J Med. 1980;69:287-308.
14. Terrier B, Semoun O, Saadoun D, et al. Prognostic factors in patients with hepatitis C virus infection and systemic vasculitis. Arthritis Rheum. 2011;63:1748-57.

CHAPTER 15

Psoriatic Arthritis

Sunil Dogra, Gitesh U Sawatkar

INTRODUCTION

Psoriatic arthritis (PsA) is one of the complex musculoskeletal chronic inflammatory disorders characterized by joint destruction in patients of psoriasis. Psoriatic arthritis was recognized as a specific entity by the American College of Rheumatology in 1964.[1] Psoriatic arthritis, even after being recognized as a separate entity, had been viewed as a benign counterpart of rheumatoid arthritis (RA), with fewer long-term sequel and unlikely progression to permanent joint damage. Patients of psoriasis with joint pains can be easily recognized early. However, still large numbers of psoriasis patients with the sole complaint of joint pain go unrecognized and are either undiagnosed/misdiagnosed and are deprived of appropriate treatment. The chapter highlights diagnosing PsA early and managing appropriately. Though a considerable amount of advancement has been made with regards to treatment, the ongoing research about the pathogenesis of the disease has enabled us to understand the disease more deeply. Likewise, many new drugs targeting the specific pathogenic pathways are in the way of evolution.

EPIDEMIOLOGY

Psoriatic arthritis is an inflammatory seronegative arthritis affecting a wide range of age group, the peak incidence is around 40–50 years of age.[2] Both the genders are affected equally, though reports quote a male-to-female ratio of 0.7:1 to 2.1:1.[2]

There is difference in prevalence based on study population. Clinic-based studies from European countries have shown PsA prevalence in psoriasis patients ranging from 6 to 42%, with recent estimates of 20–25%.[3] However, population-based studies in England and USA show prevalence of 11–13.8%.[4] The prevalence of psoriasis among Asians is reported to be about 0.1%, which is lower than the 2% reported among Westerners.[5]

A cross-sectional analysis of 2,009 patients with psoriasis from 13 dermatological hospitals and 129 dermatological private practices and outpatient clinics in Germany showed that 19% of the patients had PsA, including 14.8% previously confirmed and 4.2% newly diagnosed disease. Another 7.7% had intermittent joint symptoms that could not be clearly attributed to PsA.[6] In another study, among 1,511 psoriasis patients, 20.6% had PsA—85% of the PsA cases were newly diagnosed.[7] In a recent cross-sectional study from India, out of 1,149 of psoriasis screened patients, 8.7% had PsA with 83% of PsA cases were diagnosed for the first time.[8]

A multicentric, noninterventional, retrospective cross-sectional study from Japan revealed a pooled PsA prevalence of 14.3% among patients with psoriasis.[5] Another cross-sectional study from the Asian continent had 5.8% patients of PsA, of which 92% was newly diagnosed. The findings were consistent with a low prevalence of PsA among patients with psoriasis in Asia and confirmed a high percentage of undiagnosed cases with active arthritis among psoriasis patients in dermatologist's office.[9] Similar finding of undiagnosed PsA in psoriasis patients was reported by a multicentric study from the European/North American dermatology clinics.[10]

In a Singaporean study, ethnic Indians with psoriasis had twice the risk of developing PsA compared with ethnic Chinese and Malays, highlighting that ethnicity may affect the development of PsA.[11] This ethnic difference in the prevalence of PsA was demonstrated in a recent case-control study in a tertiary dermatology center in Singapore involving 400 patients with severe psoriasis.[12] The risk factors for development of PsA among psoriasis patients were family history of PsA, severe psoriasis by body surface area, and Indian ethnicity.

One of the reasons for the variable prevalence rate could be that diagnosis of PsA may be often missed by the dermatologist. Lack of awareness, less use of PsA screening tool in the dermatology community could be some factors. Often rheumatologists misdiagnose PsA when they fail to diagnose the presence of psoriasis in an individual presenting with joint pain.

ETIOLOGY AND PATHOGENESIS

Genetics

A complex array of genetic, immunological, and environmental factors contributes to the pathogenesis of PsA. Genetic associations in psoriasis are relevant to PsA as the two diseases are interrelated epidemiologically and share similar immunopathology.[13] Individuals with first degree relatives having PsA are more predisposed, which ranks second only behind ankylosing spondylitis.[14,15]

Within the major histocompatibility complex region, human leukocyte antigen (HLA)-Cw*0602 is the PSORS1 risk variant of psoriasis.[16] However, the magnitude of association with PsA is comparatively low and accounts for delayed onset of PsA in patients of psoriasis. Other HLA antigens associated with PsA include HLA-B13, HLA-B27, HLA-B38/39, HLA-B57, and HLA-DRB1*04.[17] Human leukocyte antigen alleles have also modest associations with disease expression and prognosis in PsA though with limited clinical utility (Table 1).[13]

Table 1: Human leukocyte antigen alleles associated with disease expression

Pattern of disease expression	HLA alleles
Peripheral polyarthritis	B38 and B39
Axial involvement	HLA-B27
Dactylitis	HLA-B27 allele
HLA alleles associated with a higher rate of disease progression	
HLA-B39 alone	
HLA-B27 only in the presence of HLA-DR7	
HLA-DQ3 only in the absence of HLA-DR7 and HLA-Cw*0602	

HLA, human leukocyte antigen.

Besides the PSORS1 locus located at chromosome 6p21.3, other prominent regions of linkage identified from all genome-wide linkage studies, are PSORS2-PSORS10.[16,18]

Genome-wide association study (GWAS) have identified genes in PsA that are commonly found in psoriasis consisting of *HLA-B/C, HLA-B, IL-12B, IL-23R, TNIP1, TRAF3IP2, FBXL19, and REL*. The results of these genetic studies have highlighted critical pathways in psoriatic disease including distinct signaling pathways comprising barrier integrity, innate immune response, and adaptive immune response, mediated primarily by Th-17 and Th-1 signaling.[13] Bowe et al., have reported GWAS of PsA loci to 10 including 4 that are PsA-specific: HLA-B, chromosome 5q31, PsA-specific variants within IL23R, and the rs2476601 variant in the *PTPN22* gene.[19]

Pathogenetic Mechanisms

The evidence suggests that in a genetically susceptible individual, trauma, drugs, infection, or emotional stress trigger PsA and that the initial inciting event probably occurs in the skin, which leads to activation of T lymphocytes.[20] Some studies suggest that streptococcal antigens may activate T cells. Type I keratin, particularly keratin 17 may act as autoantigens as they have structural similarities with streptococcal M protein.[21,22]

The infiltrating T lymphocytes enter deep layers, i.e., dermis and subsynovium, and promote hyperproliferation of cells native to the particular tissue, i.e., keratinocytes of skin and synovial lining cells in the joint.[20] In predisposed patients of psoriasis, local milieu in the joint promote angiogenesis followed by influx of T lymphocytes, increased expression of tumor necrosis factor-α (TNF-α) and interleukin (IL)-1β, and an elevated ratio of receptor activator of NF-κB ligand (RANKL) to natural antagonist osteoprotegerin. Circulating osteoclast precursors enter the joint after binding to activated endothelial cells and undergo osteoclastogenesis and resorb bone. Thus, leading to markedly altered bone remodeling which appears in the form of tuft resorption and large eccentric erosions.[23]

Periostitis and bony ankylosis, features suggestive of new bone formation are also seen. The events responsible for such new bone formation remain unknown although studies in animal models suggest that transforming growth factor-β and vascular endothelial growth factor may be important in this process.[24] In addition, metalloproteinases released by synovial lining cells degrade cartilage and foster blood vessel remodeling. Presumably, perpetual release of proinflammatory cytokines, particularly TNF, leads to persistent synovitis, enthesitis, and progressive matrix degradation. The events that drive the chronic release of these proinflammatory cytokines have not been elucidated.

CLINICAL FEATURES

Psoriatic arthritis, first reported by Louis Aliberti in 1818, is currently recognized as an inflammatory joint condition associated with skin psoriasis (Fig. 1) with negative rheumatoid factor (Box 1).[25] It is considered as part of the umbrella group of the seronegative spondyloarthritides (SpA) (ankylosing spondylitis, reactive arthritis, inflammatory bowel disease-related arthritis, and undifferentiated SpA) characterized by high prevalence of HLA-B27.[26]

Generally concomitant presence of skin psoriasis helps to differentiate PsA from other types of arthritis. Arthritis might precede, succeed, or be concomitant with the appearance of skin lesions. In approximately 75–80% of the cases, the skin condition precedes arthritis; in 15%, it appears after arthritis; and in 10%, the skin and articular involvements occur simultaneously.[25,27,28]

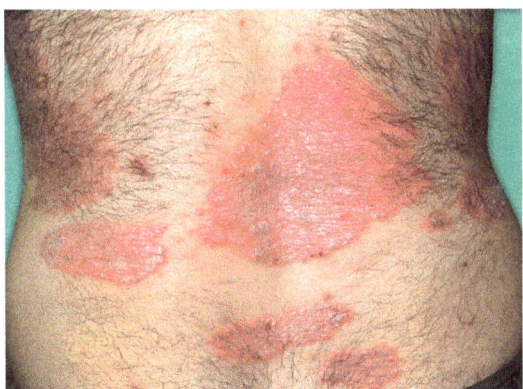

FIGURE 1: Severe chronic plaque psoriasis.

Box 1: Key points of psoriatic arthritis

- Seronegative spondyloarthritides with high prevalence of HLA-B27
- Both genders almost equally affected
- Common in 4th and 5th decade
- Usually occurs 5–12 years after skin disease onset
- Scalp lesions, nail dystrophy, perianal/intergluteal lesion, and extensive disease—higher risk for PsA
- Shows feature typical of any inflammatory arthritides
- Enthesitis, dactylitis, and distal interphalangeal joint involvement quite specific for PsA
- Severity of PsA does not correlate with extent of skin involvement

PsA, psoriatic arthritis.

The dermatologist plays an important role in identifying the joint involvement in psoriasis as majority of the psoriasis patients develop PsA usually 5–12 years after the onset of skin disease.[29] When skin lesions appear after joint involvement, it is called as "PsA sine psoriasis" and can be a diagnostic challenge to the treating physician. Presence of dactylitis and/or distal interphalangeal (DIP) arthritis, HLA-Cw6, and a family history of psoriasis are some of the soft pointer to clinch the diagnosis in such patients.[30]

Both the genders are equally affected, although males are more likely to have the spondylitic form (three to five times more).[25] Psoriatic arthritis typically begins in the fourth or fifth decade, however can occur at any age, in adults and children. Rouzaud et al., in their meta-analysis found mean age at onset of psoriasis to be similar among patients with skin disease alone and in those with PsA.[31]

The inflammatory nature of PsA is characterized by pain and stiffness that is typically aggravated by rest, associated with tenderness and swelling in the affected joints which tend to improve with activity. Long history of psoriasis probably leads to higher chances of PsA compared to patients having psoriasis of short duration, thus increasing the prevalence of PsA with the duration of psoriasis.[9,32,33]

Though a significant association between PsA and any specific psoriasis localization has not been characteristically demonstrated, literature review supports the belief that some psoriatic skin features, such as scalp lesions (Fig. 2), nail dystrophy, intergluteal/perianal lesions, and more extensive disease, are associated with a higher risk of PsA.[9,32,34,35] The notion that patients with extensive psoriasis have an increased risk of PsA has been suggested in most studies. However, the validity of this notion cannot be confirmed as mild cutaneous disease does not exclude the presence of PsA as also the severity of PsA does not reliably correlate with the extent of skin involvement.[31]

Nail alterations appear in up to 90% of patients with PsA but in only 45% of patients with psoriasis.[36] Nail involvement in psoriasis patients is commonly associated with PsA,[31] with DIP arthritis in particular as nail changes may be a part of enthesitis and could predict the onset of arthritis among patients with psoriasis.[37,38] Among the various types of nail changes, a significant association between onycholysis and PsA,[39,40] and also with nail bed hyperkeratosis[40] has been found though other type of nail involvement can also be present (Figs 3 and 4). Finger nails are likely to be more severely affected in PsA patients compared to psoriasis patients without articular lesion.[39] Psoriatic paronychia is also commonly seen in patients of PsA with nail involvement.[41]

Articular Manifestations

Psoriatic arthritis is characterized by swelling, warmth, stiffness, pain, limitation of movement, and tenderness of the joints along with the surrounding ligaments and tendons. Psoriatic arthritis often presents in an oligoarticular and sometimes monoarticular pattern, gradually becoming polyarticular and symmetric over time.

A systematic review revealed that peripheral PsA is the most frequent pattern, oligoarticular peripheral PsA was predominant in patients with shorter disease duration whereas polyarthritis is more frequent in long-standing disease. The data on axial PsA are controversial depending

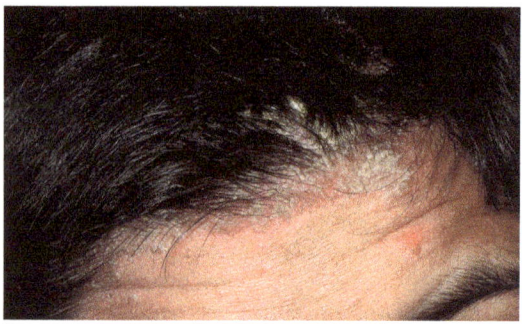

FIGURE 2: Scalp psoriasis.

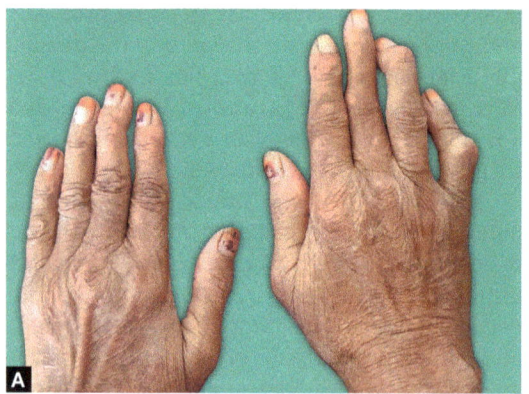
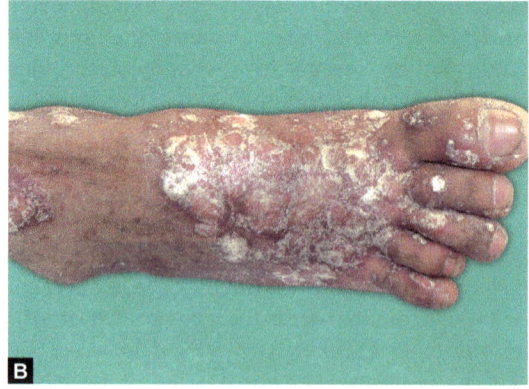

FIGURE 3: A, Involvement of the distal interphalangeal joint of both the hands and involvement of right little finger as well; **B,** Psoriatic arthritis deforming distal interphalangeal joint of fourth toe.

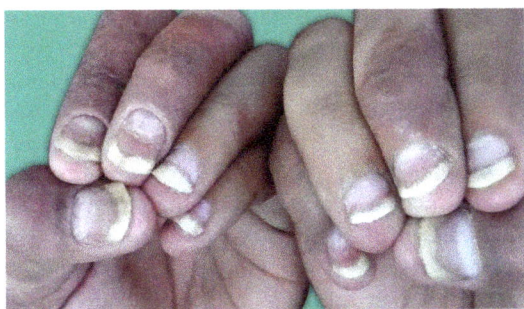

FIGURE 4: Fingernail showing Beau's line, distal subungual onycholysis, and subungual hemorrhage in few finger nails.

Distal Interphalangeal Joint Involvement

Classical PsA affects the DIP (Fig. 3A), and is usually accompanied by characteristic nail manifestations, such as pitting of nails, subungual hyperkeratosis, and Beau's line (Figs 4 and 5). Most of the patients will be having characteristic cutaneous lesions of psoriasis elsewhere on body. But at times, some patients in their course of disease can have lesions confined to flexural "hidden" sites, such as scalp, retroauricular area (Fig. 6), umbilicus, gluteal cleft making the lesions of psoriasis occult.

The prevalence of DIP joint involvement varies in different studies. Kumar et al. found predominant DIP arthritis in 3% of the patients on the method of classification based on axial symptoms or the demonstration of radiographic sacroiliitis.[42]

When considering the diagnosis of PsA, assessing the recurrent early morning stiffness, lasting longer than 30 minutes is a valuable question[29] to screen the patients for PsA. Physical examination should not be limited to just joint, but should also include skin, nail, enthesial, and spine disease, as well as dactylitis, which results from synovitis, tenosynovitis, and enthesitis. Also axial manifestations of PsA such as pain, stiffness and range of motion limitations in the neck or back should also be evaluated.

Joints are palpated for the purpose of determining if they are tender and/or swollen, the latter implying the presence of active synovitis, and both implying the presence of inflammation. The various joints assessed include DIP, proximal interphalangeal joints, and metacarpophalangeal joints of the hands; the wrist, elbow, shoulder, acromioclavicular, sternoclavicular, temporomandibular, hip, knee, ankle and midtarsal joints; and the metatarsophalangeal and PIP joints of the feet.

Assessment of joint with palpation is a critical step in the management of PsA as it acts as a marker for presence of inflammation in joints. The standard procedure for joint palpation involves applying approximately 4 kg/cm^2 of pressure (enough to blanch the tip of the examiner's fingernail) and ascertaining the presence/absence and in some indices, severity of tenderness.[43]

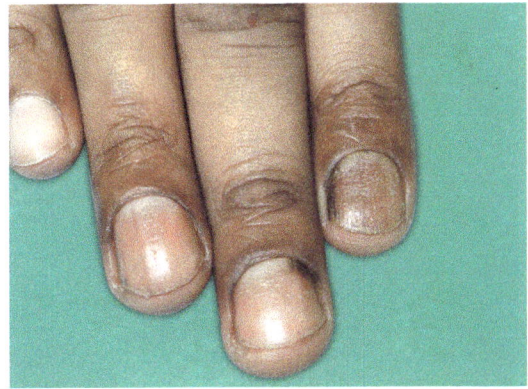

FIGURE 5: Finger nails showing prominent coarse pitting in nail plates.

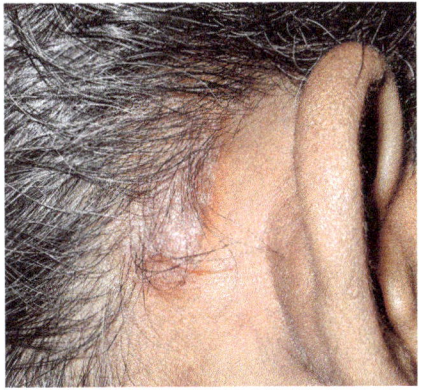

FIGURE 6: Psoriatic plaque over retroauricular area.

of PsA from north India.[8] A multicentric, non-interventional, retrospective cross-sectional study from Japan had DIP involvement in 8.9% of patients.[5] While a large cross-sectional observational study from China had 5.4% with DIP arthritis.[9] Studies from Turkey had 11.0% of DIP involvement.[44] In the largest clinical series, DIP arthritis has been reported in 1–59% of cases, with an increased frequency with disease duration.[42] DIP joint involvement is quite characteristic of PsA but some of these patients can also have additional PIP joint involvement (Fig. 7) or alone PIP joint involvement (Fig. 8).

Imaging studies can be helpful in differentiating PsA from other arthritis. The findings favoring PsA consist of concomitant presence of erosive and proliferative lesions, resorption of distal tuft, bony ankylosis, "pencil in cup" deformity, and minimum periarticular osteopenia (Figs 9 and 10).[25]

On imaging techniques such as magnetic resonance imaging (MRI), nail thickening has been the common finding along with the involvement of distal phalanx even when the clinical evidence of onychopathy is absent.[45] The Leeds group in their study found significantly more entheseal and ligament enhancement, extracapsular changes, and diffuse bone edema in PsA

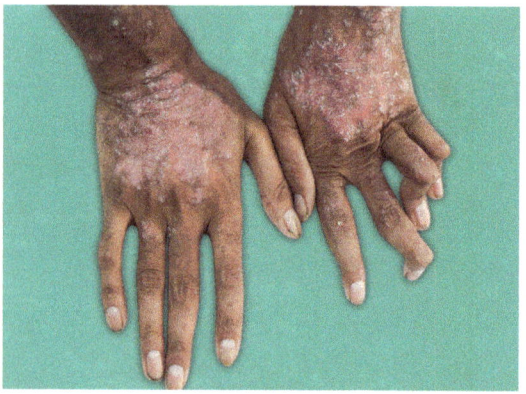

FIGURE 7: Psoriatic arthritis leading to deformities at distal interphalangeal and proximal interphalangeal joints in many fingers.

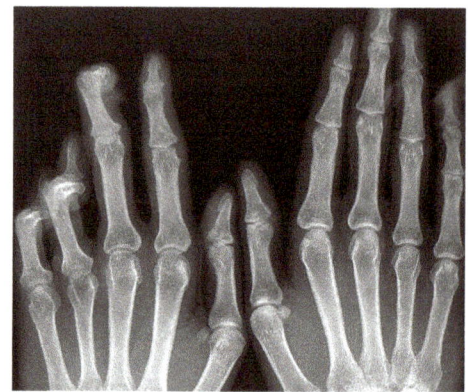

FIGURE 9: Radiological features of psoriatic arthritis of distal and proximal interphalangeal joint of fingers - periarticular erosions, bony ankylosis, deformities, soft tissue swelling and little osteopenia can be seen.

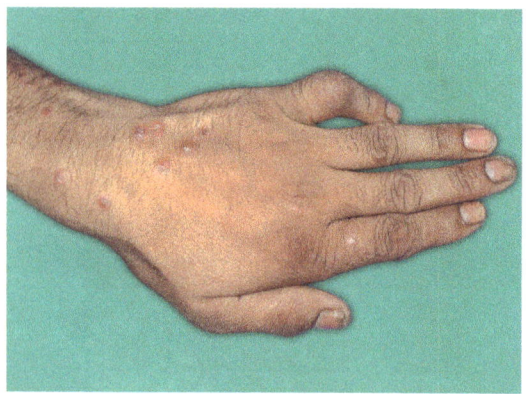

FIGURE 8: Psoriatic arthritis leading to deformity in left little finger proximal interphalangeal joint.

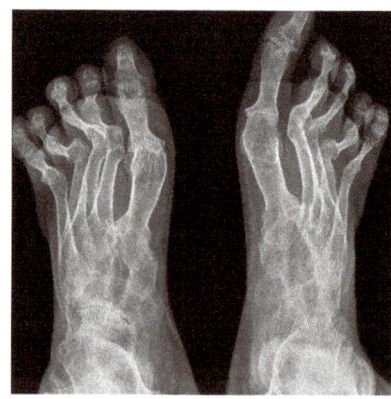

FIGURE 10: Radiological features of psoriatic arthritis of distal and proximal interphalangeal joint of toes- resorption of distal tuft, bony ankylosis, "pencil in cup" deformity, and minimum periarticular osteopenia can be seen.

patients compared to osteoarthritis patients.[46] Studies suggest that inflammation likely starts in the nail and spreads via the entheses proximally to the distal phalanx and then to the DIP joint.[45-47] This could be in accordance with the hypothesis generated by McGonagle et al., that the initial site of inflammation in peripheral PsA could be enthesitis of the extensor tendon of the fingers.[48,49]

Asymmetric Oligoarthritis

The most frequent initial presentation pattern is oligoarthritis.[20] Some authors suggest combination of enthesitis, dactylitis, and oligoarthritis almost characteristic of PsA.[50] One of the studies from Asia reports it as one of the most common patterns of PsA manifestation.[9] Asymmetric oligoarthritis has been observed in 78% of patients at disease onset, whereas asymmetric knee involvement has been reported in around 40% of cases at PsA onset.[42]

Spondylitis

The clinical features of the spondylitis include sacroiliitis, which is often asymmetric; and spinal disease similar to ankylosing spondylitis associated with pain and stiffness of the cervical, thoracic, and lumbar spine. It is one of the common symptoms in patients with PsA, usually starts unilaterally and becomes bilateral in the years to follow. Various studies report a prevalence of 22-78%.[2,9,44] Males are at threefold increased risk of developing sacroiliitis.[2]

Pain and stiffness of the affected spinal tract is one of the clinical manifestations or in case predominance of sacroiliac joint, alternating buttock pain can be the expression. Axial PsA has better prognosis and minor functional damage compared to ankylosing spondylitis as revealed by few studies.[42]

Dactylitis

Dactylitis is one of the hallmark clinical features of PsA. It manifests as a uniform swelling of a digit with inflammation causing a sausage digit (Fig. 11). Combination of flexor tenosynovitis and interphalangeal joint synovitis contributes to the swelling.[42] It has been reported to occur in 32-48% of reported cases and the morbidity increases with the prolonged duration of disease.[2] Dactylitis has been proposed as the expression of active disease in PsA which responds to anti-TNF therapy.[51]

It can be further characterized as acute/tender dactylitis where the digit is tender, often erythematous and warm, or as chronic/subacute/nontender dactylitis in which the digit is swollen but nontender.[52] Toe involvement is seen in around 75% of patients and multiple digits involved simultaneously can be seen in 50% of patients (Fig. 12).[53]

Dactylitis may occur in one or more digits concomitantly with presence of the typical signs of inflammation such as swelling, redness, pain, warmth, and limited range of motion. It is primarily diagnosed clinically and imaging studies such as ultrasound and MRI can be of help. The Leeds Dactylitis Instrument evaluates the median

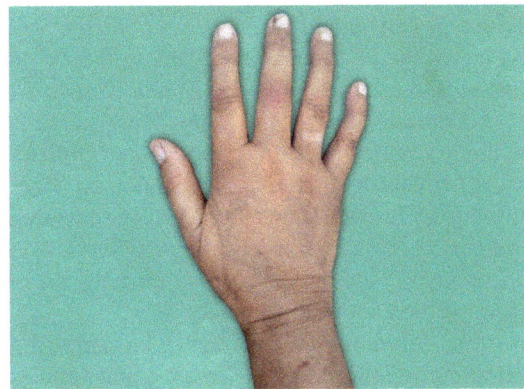

FIGURE 11: Dactylitis of the right third finger.

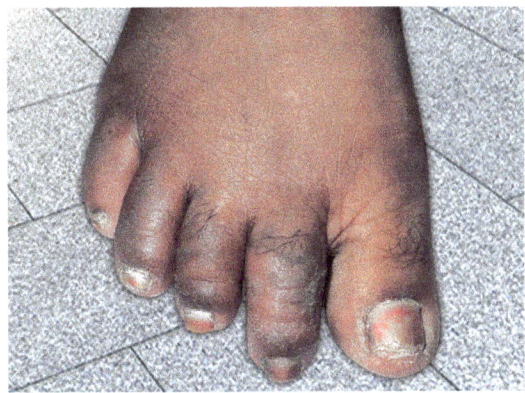

FIGURE 12: Dactylitis of second, third and fourth toes of the right foot.

difference in digital circumference between dactylitic and control digits, wherein dactylitis is defined as an increase in circumference of the digit of more than 10% compared to the contralateral nonaffected digit.[52]

Other conditions which could simulate dactylitis are tuberculosis, syphilis, sarcoidosis, soft tissue infections, sickle cell anemia, and gout.[42] Absence of tenderness on palpation along the flexor tendon course and the absence of fluid within the joints and tenosynovial sheath at ultrasound examination help to differentiate dactylitis of PsA from other conditions.

Enthesitis

Enthesitis is inflammation of the entheses, the site of attachment of ligament, tendon, and joint capsule fiber insertion into bone, and may present as tenderness and swelling at these sites (Fig. 13). Two types of enthesitis have been recognized based on the anatomical and MRI studies: (i) a purely fibrous insertion, and (ii) one containing fibrocartilage. The second type conceptualizes a unique functional unit, called as "enthesis organ" consisting of the insertional fibrocartilage together with an additional fibrocartilage covering the bone surface, periosteum, and synovial and bursa membranes. It assumes a crucial role in resisting the biomechanical stress.[42]

The common sites of enthesitis are the calcaneum (both at the attachment of the Achilles tendon and at the attachment of the plantar fascia), the muscular and tendon attachments around the pelvis, the inferior aspect of the patella, and the elbow. Among the PsA, enthesitis is found in around 25–53% of patients.[2] One study from Toronto revealed increased trend from 15% at the beginning of study to 36% during the course of disease.[54]

Variable pain depending on the location and severity of disease and loss of function are some of the clinical features of enthesopathy. Pain is usually more pronounced after a period of rest, with improvement with movement.[42]

Clinical examination consists of palpation and pressures application for the assessment of pain, tenderness, swelling at tendons, ligament, or capsule insertion sites. Achilles tendon enthesitis usually coexists with tenosynovitis and contributes to the "bombe-shaped" aspect of the tendon.[42]

Mander Enthesitis Index consisting of a measure of 66 entheseal sites graded on a semiquantitative score from 0 to 3 was the first enthesitis index developed.[52] Another index, the Maastricht Ankylosing Spondylitis Enthesitis Score, has not been validated for the PsA but has been found useful for the ankylosing spondylitis.[52] The Leeds Enthesitis Index which uses 6 most commonly involved entheseal sites has been tested in a randomized control trial and is the only measure developed specifically for PsA.[52] Ultrasound or MRI imaging studies can be of help for evaluation of entheses located in deeper sites.

Psoriatic Arthritis Mutilans

Psoriatic arthritis mutilans (PAM) is the most severe form of the disease leading to complete

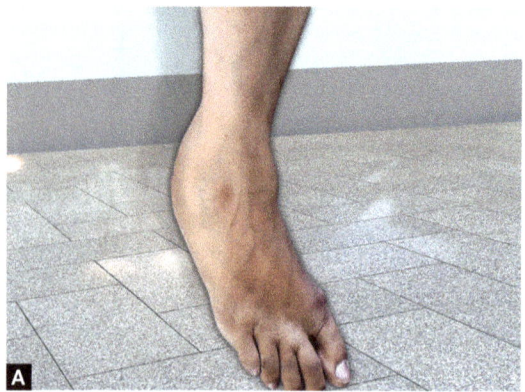
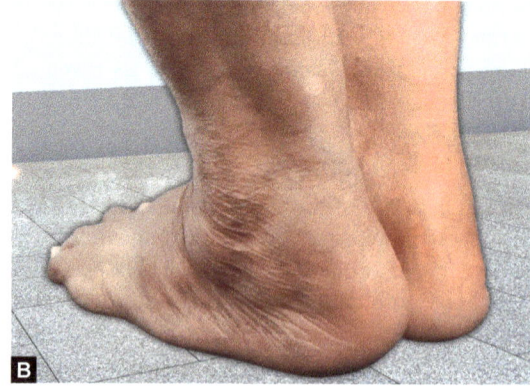

FIGURE 13: Heel enthesopathy.

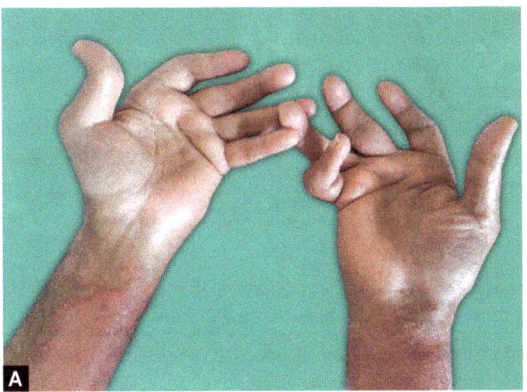
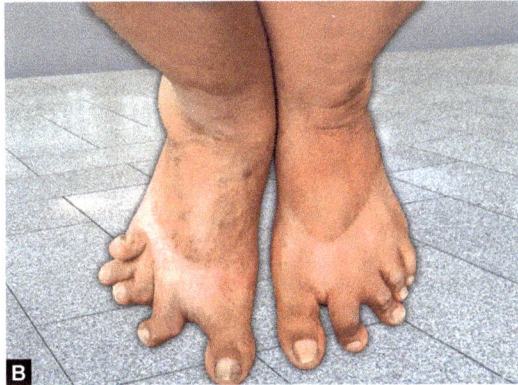

FIGURE 14: Psoriatic arthritis mutilans of the hands and feet leading to disfiguring disability.

resorption in entire phalanges and functional disability (Fig. 14). It is destructive and involves preferentially fingers and toes, as well as metacarpophalangeal and metatarsophalangeal joints. This finding, usually occurring in long-standing disease, has been observed in around 5% of cases,[55] but studies have reported a wide prevalence of 2–21%.[56]

It is believed that around 47% patients with PsA will eventually develop erosions within 2 years of symptoms onset and 20% of patients with polyarticular PsA are at risk of progressing to PAM.[57] PAM commonly affects the weight-bearing joints of the feet and hand joints involved in power/precision grip.[58]

It is associated with osteolysis of the phalanges involved, flail joints, causing a deformity clinically known as "opera glasses" or telescoping fingers due to collapse of the finger soft tissue as the bone support is lost,[25] and seems to be the most common clinical feature characterizing PAM.[56] As a result, fingers and toes can shorten, giving rise to thick transverse folds of skin, and digits that can be elongated with traction.[58] Features such as ankylosis and subluxation may be associated with PAM, but these may not be defining features.[56]

Radiographic features characteristic of PAM consist of severe osteolysis and bone resorption. Magnetic resonance imaging is considered as a potential radiological biomarker of progressing to PAM as MRI images demonstrates higher bone proliferation and edema scores in PAM compared with non-PAM cases.[59] A retrospective cohort study found PAM cases have earlier age at PsA diagnosis, poorer function, more prevalent nail dystrophy, and more radiographic axial disease/sacroiliitis compared with non-PAM cases.[58] Conditions associated with arthritis mutilans other than PAM are rheumatoid arthritis, chronic reactive arthritis, juvenile chronic arthritis, and mixed connective tissue disease.[58]

Distal Extremity Swelling with Pitting Edema

Distal extremity swelling with pitting edema described in 1985 by McCarty is often observed in PsA.[60] In a case-control study from the Prato Rheumatic Disease Unit, distal extremity swelling with pitting edema was recorded in 39/183 (21%) PsA patients, and in 18/366 (5%) controls, with a highly significant statistical difference ($p < 0.0001$). Furthermore, in 20% of patients, this feature represented the first manifestation of PsA.[61]

In PsA, the clinical picture of distal swelling with pitting edema may be related to lymphedema. The pain and pitting edema are more strictly localized along the tendon course and pitting is more easily induced and more defined in patients with tenosynovitis. Lymphoscintigraphy and MRI aids in its proper diagnosis.[42]

MEASURES TO ASSESS PSORIATIC ARTHRITIS

The outcome of any therapeutic measures is carried by clinical assessment and evaluated with the validated soring systems. These scoring

Table 2: Measures to assess psoriatic arthritis	
Composite psoriatic disease activity index[52]	It assesses five domains (joints, skin, entheseal, dactylitis, and spinal manifestations) with a measure of disease activity and impact on the patient for each domain
Psoriatic arthritis disease activity score[52]	It measures physician and patient visual analog scale, swollen and tender joint count, C-reactive protein, enthesitis, dactylitis count, and the physician component summary of the short-form 36
Disease activity in psoriatic arthritis[43]	It assess the swollen joint count, tender joint count, patient global, pain, and C-reactive protein level
Composite Psoriatic Disease Activity Index[43]	Disease involvement is assessed in up to 5 domains: peripheral joints, skin, enthesial, dactylitis, and spinal manifestations and the domains are scored from 0 to 3
Psoriatic arthritis response criteria[43]	Tender and swollen joint count and patient and physician global assessment are the four items which are assessed in this index

systems form an integral part of the various study design. The Group for Research and Assessment of Psoriasis and Psoriatic Arthritis and the Outcome Measures in Rheumatology clinical trials has identified a core set of domains for PsA to be assessed in clinical trials, including dactylitis and enthesitis (Table 2).[62]

CLASSIFICATION OF PSORIATIC ARTHRITIS

Many classification schemes for PsA have been proposed, among which the Moll and Wright diagnostic criteria was the first and most widely used. Five broad clinical groups were described in the original Moll and Wright description (Table 3).[15]

Subsequently, many other criteria have come along the way such as Bennett and McCarty, Gladman et al., Vasey and Espinoza, McGonagle et al., and Dougados et al.[63] A prospective, multicenter observational study of 588 consecutive clinic patients with PsA led to the formulations of classification of psoriatic arthritis (CASPAR) criteria (Table 4).[64] It is easier to use in epidemiologic studies and has a specificity and sensitivity of 98.7% and 91.4%, respectively.[2] The CASPAR criteria have been used in various epidemiological studies across populations of different ethnicity and have been validated and found to be superior to the previous criteria.[63-66]

Due to the variable nature of the disease, the current trend is to classify PsA into three major clinical presentations—polyarticular (≥5 involved joints), oligoarticular (≤4 involved joints), and axial with or without peripheral arthritis.[25,42]

Table 3: Moll and Wright criteria of classifying psoriatic arthritis		
S. No.	Pattern	Frequency (%)
1.	Monoarticular or asymmetrical oligoarticular with dactylitis	70
2.	Symmetrical polyarticular similar to rheumatoid arthritis	25
3.	Classical form, predominantly affecting the distal interphalangeal joints	5–10
4.	Arthritis mutilans	5
5.	Spondylitic	5–40

Extra-articular Manifestations

Ocular inflammation [conjunctivitis (20%), iritis, scleritis, and episcleritis, acute anterior uveitis (4–18%)], oral ulcerations, urethritis, gastrointestinal involvement in the form of inflammatory bowel disease, pulmonary fibrosis, and aortic insufficiency are some of the extra-articular manifestation which can occur with PsA.[2,25] Uveitis is more common in PsA patients with the spondylitis, with or without peripheral joint involvement.[2] Patients with PsA have a higher frequency of metabolic syndrome, cardiovascular morbidity and mortality, and a relative reduction in life expectancy as compared with that of the general population. Cardiovascular disease such as an increased prevalence of ischemic heart disease, cerebrovascular disease,

Table 4: Classification of psoriatic arthritis criteria for psoriatic arthritis

To meet the CASPAR criteria for PsA, patient needs to fulfill the three or more points from the following criteria along with the pre-requisite of having an inflammatory joint disease (peripheral, axial, or enthesitis)

1	Evidence of psoriasis	
	• Current	2 points
	• Personal history	1 point
	• Familial history	1 point
2	Psoriatic nail dystrophy	
	• Pitting, onycholysis, hyperkeratosis	1 point
3	Negative test result for rheumatoid factor	1 point
4	Dactylitis	
	• Current inflammation of an entire digit	1 point
	• History of dactylitis	1 point
5	Radiological evidence of juxta-articular new bone formation	
	• Well-defined ossification close to joint margins on plain radiographs of hands and feet	1 point

Box 2: Associations of psoriatic arthritis

- Ocular inflammation (conjunctivitis, iritis, scleritis, episcleritis, uveitis)
- Inflammatory bowel diseases
- Metabolic syndrome
- Pulmonary fibrosis
- Inflammatory noninfective urethritis
- Recurrent oral ulcerations
- Cardiovascular diseases
- Nonalcoholic fatty liver disease
- Reduced glomerular filtration rate
- Psychiatric morbidity—depression, anxiety

diastolic dysfunction, left ventricular dysfunction, abnormal carotid intimal thickness, and cardiovascular death represent a major source of morbidity for patients with PsA.[67] Psoriatic arthritis was found to be associated with a greater risk of arrhythmia, further indicating that inflammation may be an important link between arrhythmia and psoriasis.[68] Endothelial dysfunction has also been found in patients with PsA independent of risk factors for cardiovascular disease in a study from north India.[69] Type 2 diabetes mellitus, possibly related to insulin resistance driven by PsA inflammation, obesity and metabolic syndrome are also commonly seen in patients with PsA.[67] In a study from north India, around 58% patients of PsA had metabolic syndrome, especially in those with long-standing psoriasis and active joint disease.[70] A higher prevalence of osteoporosis in patients with PsA compared to that in patients with rheumatoid arthritis and AS has been observed (Box 2).[71]

Liver disease can result from the disease itself as well as the medications used to treat PsA.

Among patients with psoriasis, patients with PsA have the highest risk for nonalcoholic fatty liver disease.[72] Renal morbidity is also found in PsA patients, one study revealing reduced estimated glomerular filtration rate of 16% in patients with "seronegative arthritis" (patients with PsA and undifferentiated oligoarthritis), statistically similar to patients with RA (19%).[73] Depression and anxiety are very common among patients with PsA and can have a prevalence of 36.6% and 22.2%, respectively.[74]

DIAGNOSIS

The diagnosis of PsA is basically clinical. Presence of concomitant skin lesions of psoriasis assist in diagnosing the case. The real challenge is in those 15% of cases in which the onset of PsA is prior to the onset of cutaneous psoriasis lesions.

A number of questionnaires are available which aid as a screening tool for the physician. It possibly results in early referral for evaluation and treatment by rheumatologists and reduces the risk of joint destruction and disability.

These questionnaires include Psoriatic Arthritis Screening and Evaluation tool (PASE),[75] the Psoriasis Epidemiology Screening Tool (PEST),[4] Psoriasis and Arthritis Screening Questionnaire (PASQ),[76] the Toronto Psoriatic Arthritis Screen (ToPAS),[77] and a simpler recent questionnaire, Early Arthritis for Psoriasis Patients (EARP).[78] In a study from India, out of the four screening questionnaires for PsA, EARP was found to have most sensitivity while ToPAS II had highest specificity.[79]

INVESTIGATIONS

Laboratory assessment reveals elevation in acute phase proteins, such as erythrocyte sedimentation rate, C-reactive protein, and α-1-glycoprotein with polyclonal hypergammaglobulinemia. Other findings which are observed are anemia, hypoalbuminemia, mild hyperuricemia, and circulating immune complexes. Antinuclear antibodies are present in up to 10% of cases, but IgM rheumatoid factor is absent.[25]

Analysis of synovial fluid reveals an inflammatory pattern with reduced viscosity, increased number of leukocytes (>3,000/mm³), predominantly polymorphonucleates and protein concentration more than 3 g/dL.[42]

Imaging techniques such as radiography, ultrasonography, MRI, computed tomography (CT), and bone scintigraphy are of immense help for the diagnosis and at instance monitoring of PsA.[2]

Radiological imaging is one of the cheapest and easily available investigations. The characteristic findings observed are an asymmetrical distribution, DIP joints involvement, periostitis, bone density preservation, bone ankylosis, and pencil-in-cup deformity.[80] Resorption and erosion may be commonly seen in PsA, but more severe resorption or osteolysis and commonly bony proliferation are prominent features distinguishing PsA from RA.[57] Involvement of the axial skeleton shows features such as paravertebral ossification, syndesmophytes, interspinous or anterior ligament calcification, apophysis, sclerosis, and asymmetrical sacroiliitis. Cervical intervertebral disks may be narrowed, and ankylosis may be present with atlantoaxial fusion or subluxation.[2,81]

Ultrasound is being developed as an important tool in the evaluation of PsA. It helps in detecting subclinical enthesopathy in the Achilles tendon and to identify acute or degenerative tendinitis, rupture, peritendinitis, and retrocalcaneal or pre-Achilles bursitis.[82] Preliminary results demonstrate that peritenon extensor tendon inflammation pattern is a higher characteristic of PsA, helping to differentiate from rheumatoid arthritis. Power Doppler ultrasonography is helpful in monitoring the therapeutic efficacy and also to guide steroid injections at the level of inflamed sites.[83,84]

High-field MRI with contrast enhancement is arguably the "gold standard" for simultaneously imaging soft tissue and bony pathology in PsA.[47] Magnetic resonance imaging offers advantage of direct visualization of inflammation in the peripheral and axial joints along with peripheral and axial enthuses. It helps in differentiating PsA from rheumatoid arthritis, as PsA synovial inflammation usually secondary to extrasynovial involvement.[2] A "snapshot" of inflamed joint can be obtained by whole-body multijoint MRI. Computed tomography is useful in assessing the involvement of spine though it has limited role in the diagnosis of peripheral joints.

PROGNOSTIC MARKERS

Some particular clinical features and laboratory investigations at times can help in predicating the prognosis. Such clinical and laboratory parameters are summarized in table 5.

Table 5: Clinical parameters and biomarkers which suggest bad prognosis in psoriatic arthritis[20,25,42]

Clinical features	Laboratory features
Female gender	An increase in acute phase proteins both at the beginning and in the course of disease
Presence of familial history	Specific genetic markers (HLA-B27 in the presence of HLA-DR7; HLA-B39 and DQw3 in the absence of DR7)
Beginning of disease before the age of 20 years	Expression of gene polymorphism alleles TNF-α-308 and TNF-β-252
Extensive skin involvement	–
More than five swollen joints	–
Use of several different medications with persistence of polyarthritis	–
Accumulated joint damage between consultations	–

HLA, human leukocyte antigen TNF, tumor necrosis factor.

Objective molecules that indicate either normal or diseased processes in the body serve as biomarkers. Owing to the heterogeneous nature of rheumatoid arthritis and PsA, no single biomarker has so far emerged as a reliable predictor of joint damage; hence, a need for a panel of biomarkers. Some of the biomarkers that have been explored in PsA are summarized in table 6.[57]

Table 6: Biomarkers of joint damage in psoriatic arthritis

Biomarker*	Role in inflammatory arthritis
Calgranulin (S100A8/S100A9)	Ca^{2+} binding protein with pleiotropic effects. Regulates myeloid derived cells
IL-1	Promotes activation of keratocytes, endothelial cells, chondrocytes, and osteoclasts. Promotes the production of proinflammatory cytokines
IL-15	Induces T cell proliferation and B cell differentiation. Recruits memory T cells to the synovium and induces TNF-α production
CCL3	Lymphocyte, monocyte, basophil, eosinophil chemoattractant
CCL11	Eosinophil chemoattractant
Angiopoietin-2	Promotes angiogenesis
RANKL	Induces osteoclast bone destruction
M-CSF	Induces aggressive phenotype in macrophages

IL, interleukin; CCL, chemokine ligand; RANKL, receptor activator of nuclear factor kappa-B ligand M-CSF, macrophage colony-stimulating factor; TNF, tumor necrosis factor

*Besides these, the other biomarkers that have been evaluated in PsA patients MMP-3, DKK-1, M-CSF, CTX-1, and TRAIL.[85]

TREATMENT

The aim of PsA treatment is to alleviate the signs and symptoms of PsA, inhibit structural damage, and maximize quality of life. The treatment of psoriasis and PsA is long-standing, at times which can make the patient lose faith in therapy. As a rule, all PsA patients must be conversant with the characteristics of the disease, benefits, and risks of their treatments. A special psychological counseling and physiotherapy inputs are also recommended for such patients. Maintenance of a program of physical activity, postural orientation, stretching exercises, and muscle strengthening exercises should be encouraged. The patient needs to be into their treatment plan and should not discontinue treatment on their own (Table 7).

Nonsteroidal Anti-inflammatory Drugs

Nonsteroidal anti-inflammatory drugs (NSAIDs) are commonly used for the short time management of mild PsA. A trial period of 2–3 months is recommended before switching to another class of drugs such as methotrexate.[86] However, the evidence supporting the efficacy of NSAIDs is scarce.

Conventional Disease-modifying Antirheumatic Drugs

Disease-modifying antirheumatic drugs (DMARDs) consist of methotrexate, oral and parenteral gold, cyclosporine, leflunomide, azathioprine and 6-mercaptopurine, antimalarial agents, D-penicillamine, colchicines, retinoids, photo-chemotherapy, somatostatin, and sulfasalazine.[2]

Table 7: The group for research and assessment of psoriasis and psoriatic arthritis treatment guidelines for psoriatic arthritis categorized by disease characteristics and distinct organ involvement[51]

Peripheral arthritis	Skin and nail disease	Axial disease	Dactylitis	Enthesitis
NSAID	Topicals PUVA/UVB	NSAID	NSAID	NSAID
Intra-articular steroids	Systemics (MTX, CsA)	Physiotherapy	Steroid injection	Physiotherapy
DMARD (MTX, CsA, SSZ, LEF)	Biologics (anti-TNF, etc.)	Biologics (anti-TNF)	Biologics (anti-TNF)	Biologics (anti-TNF)
Biologics (anti-TNF)	–	–	–	–

NSAID, nonsteroidal anti-inflammatory drug; DMARD, disease-modifying antirheumatic drugs; TNF, tumor necrosis factor; LEF, leflunomide; SSZ, sulfasalazine; MTX, methotrexate; CsA, cyclosporine; PUVA, psoralen and ultraviolet A.

They are indicated for patients who have neither rapid nor satisfactory response to NSAIDs, or in the presence of radiological or functional progression.[25] Among the DMARDs, specifically methotrexate has been found to be potentially effective from two randomized controlled trials.[87] The efficacy of methotrexate, leflunomide, and cyclosporine in PsA is further supported by observational and open-label studies.[88] Careful monitoring is advised with the use of such drugs, as methotrexate and leflunomide are hepatotoxic. Combination of drugs such as methotrexate and cyclosporine can also be used for the treatment of PsA, as evident by a randomized, multicenter, double-blind, placebo-controlled trial combining oral cyclosporine with oral methotrexate in patients with PsA who had a prior incomplete response to methotrexate monotherapy.[89]

Methotrexate has been recommended as a first-line drug for the management of moderate-to-severe PsA. It reduces inflammation by increasing the release of adenosine, a potent anti-inflammatory autocoid. It reduces joint tenderness and swelling along with improvement in skin manifestations. In cases of minimal improvement in signs and symptoms, a waiting period of 12–16 weeks with methotrexate therapy with appropriate dose escalation [up to 25 mg per week (oral)] is advised before either adding or switching to a TNF-α inhibitor.[87] Combining methotrexate with biological drugs has a number of advantages such as it increases the serum concentration of infliximab and adalimumab, reduces the development of antibodies against anti-TNF agents, and significantly decreased risk of cardiovascular disease.[87]

Sulfasalazine has been examined in several PsA clinical studies. Clinical features such as morning stiffness, number of painful joints, articular score, and grip strength improve with the therapy of sulfasalazine for a period of 6 months. However, skin manifestations and radiographic progression of PsA are not altered with the use of sulfasalazine.[87] It is recommended for controlling moderate-to-severe peripheral arthritis according to studies with level of evidence A.[25] The benefit of sulfasalazine is usually confined to peripheral disease with no significant effect on axial disease. It is usually started at a low dose of 500 mg twice a day and the dose is increased weekly by 500 mg. The usual daily dose recommended is less than 4 g so as to avoid the adverse effects.

Leflunomide is a selective pyrimidine synthesis inhibitor that targets activated T cells unable to rely solely on a salvage pathway for expansion. A randomized double-blind placebo-controlled study of 6 months duration in 188 cases, 59% of leflunomide treated patients met the primary efficacy endpoint PsARC compared with 29.7% of placebo treated patients. The usual adult dose is 100 mg/day for 3 days, followed by 20 mg/day.[90] Leflunomide is a potential immunosuppressant, hepatotoxic, and is contraindicated in pregnant women. Women should not become pregnant for 2 years after the cessation of therapy or should undergo a rapid wash-out procedure with cholestyramine. Men wishing to father a child should discontinue leflunomide and should also undergo the wash-out procedure.[90]

Corticosteroids

In cases of pauciarticular joint involvement, intra-articular corticosteroids injection is one of the treatment options. It can also be considered in polyarticular disease with one or two active joints.[91] Risk of joint contamination, sepsis, and trauma are always associated with it. Systemic use of corticosteroids is generally not supported as withdrawal of it can lead to rebound flare of psoriasis.[92] Still corticosteroids are used systemically in low doses to treat patients who are poorly responsive to NSAIDs or DMARDs.[79]

Biological Agents

The discovery of TNF-α as one of the key molecules in the pathogenesis of psoriasis and PsA has led to the development of new array of anti-TNF-α drugs. On the same line many biological therapies are being developed for the treatment of moderate to severe psoriasis and PsA.

Patients with active PsA or skin disease that fulfills defined British Society for Rheumatology or British Association of Dermatologists guideline criteria, respectively, and who have failed or cannot use methotrexate may need to be considered for biologic treatment given the potential benefit of such treatment on both components of psoriatic disease.[91]

CONCLUSION

Psoriatic arthritis, a part of psoriatic disease, is a heterogeneous chronic inflammatory disease with a spectrum of manifestation and variable course. The incidence and prevalence of PsA vary worldwide. Research regarding the etiopathogenesis of this chronic disease has discovered many new potential molecules which can be targeted for treatment. Many patients of PsA remain underdiagnosed and/or under-treated due to the heterogenous clinical course. The distressing nature causes a significant physical and psychological morbidity causing a huge loss of manpower. The morbidity caused by deformities affects the patients individually, and the population is also affected as a result of work disability. Development of many screening questionnaire, attempts to classify and again to simplify the classification denotes the ongoing effort in this chronic arthropathy. Many new drugs have been developed targeting the specific pathomechanism. Such drugs are showing promising results to stop and even revert the disease process.

REFERENCES

1. Blumberg BS, Bunim JJ, Calkins E, et al. Ara nomenclature and classification of arthritis and rheumatism (Tentative). Arthritis Rheum. 1964;7:93-7.
2. Liu JT, Yeh HM, Liu SY, et al. Psoriatic arthritis: Epidemiology, diagnosis, and treatment. World J Orthop. 2014;5:537-43.
3. Chandran V, Raychaudhuri SP. Geoepidemiology and environmental factors of psoriasis and psoriatic arthritis. J Autoimmun. 2010;34:J314-21.
4. Ibrahim GH, Buch MH, Lawson C, et al. Evaluation of an existing screening tool for psoriatic arthritis in people with psoriasis and the development of a new instrument: the Psoriasis Epidemiology Screening Tool (PEST) questionnaire. Clin Exp Rheumatol. 2009;27:469-74.
5. Ohara Y, Kishimoto M, Takizawa N, et al. Prevalence and Clinical Characteristics of Psoriatic Arthritis in Japan. J Rheumatol. 2015;42(8):1439-42.
6. Radtke MA, Reich K, Blome C, et al. Prevalence and clinical features of psoriatic arthritis and joint complaints in 2009 patients with psoriasis: results of a German national survey. J Eur Acad Dermatol Venereol. 2009;23:683-91.
7. Reich K, Kruger K, Mossner R, et al. Epidemiology and clinical pattern of psoriatic arthritis in Germany: a prospective interdisciplinary epidemiological study of 1511 patients with plaque-type psoriasis. Br J Dermatol. 2009;160:1040-7.
8. Kumar R, Sharma A, Dogra S. Prevalence and clinical patterns of psoriatic arthritis in Indian patients with psoriasis. Indian J Dermatol Venereol Leprol. 2014;80:15-23.
9. Yang Q, Qu L, Tian H, et al. Prevalence and characteristics of psoriatic arthritis in Chinese patients with psoriasis. J Eur Acad Dermatol Venereol. 2011;25:1409-14.
10. Mease PJ, Gladman DD, Papp KA, et al. Prevalence of rheumatologist-diagnosed psoriatic arthritis in patients with psoriasis in European/North American dermatology clinics. J Am Acad Dermatol. 2013;69:729-35.
11. Thumboo J, Tham SN, Tay YK, et al. Patterns of psoriatic arthritis in Orientals. J Rheumatol. 1997;24:1949-53.
12. Tey HL, Ee HL, Tan AS, et al. Risk factors associated with having psoriatic arthritis in patients with cutaneous psoriasis. J Dermatol. 2010;37:426-30.
13. O'Rielly DD, Rahman P. Genetics of psoriatic arthritis. Best Pract Res Clin Rheumatol. 2014;28:673-85.
14. Chandran V, Schentag CT, Brockbank JE, et al. Familial aggregation of psoriatic arthritis. Ann Rheum Dis. 2009;68:664-7.
15. Moll JM, Wright V. Familial occurrence of psoriatic arthritis. Ann Rheum Dis. 1973;32:181-201.
16. Nair RP, Stuart PE, Nistor I, et al. Sequence and haplotype analysis supports HLA-C as the psoriasis susceptibility 1 gene. Am J Hum Genet. 2006;78:827-51.
17. Chandran V, Rahman P. Update on the genetics of spondyloarthritis—ankylosing spondylitis and psoriatic arthritis. Best Pract Res Clin Rheumatol. 2010;24:579-88.
18. Gladman DD, Ziouzina O, Thavaneswaran A, et al. Dactylitis in psoriatic arthritis: prevalence and response to therapy in the biologic era. J Rheumatol. 2013;40:1357-9.
19. Bowes J, Loehr S, Budu-Aggrey A, et al. PTPN22 is associated with susceptibility to psoriatic arthritis but not psoriasis: evidence for a further PsA-specific risk locus. Ann Rheum Dis. 2015.
20. Duarte GV, Faillace C, Freire de Carvalho J. Psoriatic arthritis. Best Pract Res Clin Rheumatol. 2012;26:147-56.
21. Lowes MA, Bowcock AM, Krueger JG. Pathogenesis and therapy of psoriasis. Nature. 2007;445:866-73.
22. Sabat R, Philipp S, Hoflich C, et al. Immunopathogenesis of psoriasis. Exp Dermatol. 2007;16:779-98.
23. Lacey DL, Timms E, Tan HL, et al. Osteoprotegerin ligand is a cytokine that regulates osteoclast differentiation and activation. Cell. 1998;93:165-76.
24. Braun J, Bollow M, Neure L, et al. Use of immunohistologic and in situ hybridization techniques in the examination of sacroiliac joint biopsy specimens from patients with ankylosing spondylitis. Arthritis Rheum. 1995;38:499-505.
25. Goldenstein-Schainberg C, Favarato MH, Ranza R. Current and relevant concepts in psoriatic arthritis. Rev Bras Reumatol. 2012;52:98-106.
26. Brewerton DA, Hart FD, Nicholls A, et al. Ankylosing spondylitis and HL-A 27. Lancet. 1973;1:904-7.
27. Gladman DD. Natural history of psoriatic arthritis. Baillieres Clin Rheumatol. 1994;8:379-94.

28. Fitzgerald O, Winchester R. Psoriatic arthritis: from pathogenesis to therapy. Arthritis Res Ther. 2009;11:214.
29. Menter A, Korman NJ, Elmets CA, et al. Guidelines of care for the management of psoriasis and psoriatic arthritis: section 4. Guidelines of care for the management and treatment of psoriasis with traditional systemic agents. J Am Acad Dermatol. 2009;61:451-85.
30. Olivieri I, Padula A, D'Angelo S, et al. Psoriatic arthritis sine psoriasis. J Rheumatol Suppl. 2009;83:28-9.
31. Rouzaud M, Sevrain M, Villani AP, et al. Is there a psoriasis skin phenotype associated with psoriatic arthritis? Systematic literature review. J Eur Acad Dermatol Venereol. 2014;28(Suppl 5):17-26.
32. Wilson FC, Icen M, Crowson CS, et al. Incidence and clinical predictors of psoriatic arthritis in patients with psoriasis: a population-based study. Arthritis Rheum. 2009;61:233-9.
33. Christophers E, Barker JN, Griffiths CE, et al. The risk of psoriatic arthritis remains constant following initial diagnosis of psoriasis among patients seen in European dermatology clinics. J Eur Acad Dermatol Venereol. 2010;24:548-54.
34. Zanolli MD, Wikle JS. Joint complaints in psoriasis patients. Int J Dermatol. 1992;31:488-91.
35. Anandarajah AP, Ritchlin CT. Pathogenesis of psoriatic arthritis. Curr Opin Rheumatol. 2004;16:338-43.
36. Menter A, Gottlieb A, Feldman SR, et al. Guidelines of care for the management of psoriasis and psoriatic arthritis: Section 1. Overview of psoriasis and guidelines of care for the treatment of psoriasis with biologics. J Am Acad Dermatol. 2008;58:826-50.
37. McGonagle D, Tan AL, Benjamin M. The nail as a musculoskeletal appendage—implications for an improved understanding of the link between psoriasis and arthritis. Dermatology. 2009;218:97-102.
38. Tan AL, Benjamin M, Toumi H, et al. The relationship between the extensor tendon enthesis and the nail in distal interphalangeal joint disease in psoriatic arthritis—a high-resolution MRI and histological study. Rheumatology (Oxford). 2007;46:253-6.
39. Love TJ, Gudjonsson JE, Valdimarsson H, et al. Psoriatic arthritis and onycholysis—results from the cross-sectional Reykjavik psoriatic arthritis study. J Rheumatol. 2012;39:1441-4.
40. Maejima H, Taniguchi T, Watarai A, et al. Evaluation of nail disease in psoriatic arthritis by using a modified nail psoriasis severity score index. Int J Dermatol. 2010;49:901-6.
41. Dogra A, Arora AK. Nail psoriasis: the journey so far. Indian J Dermatol. 2014;59:319-33.
42. Cantini F, Niccoli L, Nannini C, et al. Psoriatic arthritis: a systematic review. Int J Rheum Dis. 2010;13:300-17.
43. Mease PJ. Measures of psoriatic arthritis: tender and swollen joint assessment, psoriasis area and severity index (PASI), nail psoriasis severity index (NAPSI), modified nail psoriasis severity index (mNAPSI), Mander/Newcastle enthesitis index (MEI), Leeds enthesitis index (LEI), Spondyloarthritis Research Consortium of Canada (SPARCC), Maastricht Ankylosing Spondylitis Enthesis Score (MASES), Leeds Dactylitis Index (LDI), Patient Global for Psoriatic Arthritis, Dermatology Life Quality Index (DLQI), Psoriatic Arthritis Quality of Life (PsAQOL), Functional Assessment of Chronic Illness Therapy-Fatigue (FACIT-F), Psoriatic Arthritis Response Criteria (PsARC), Psoriatic Arthritis Joint Activity Index (PsAJAI), Disease Activity in Psoriatic Arthritis (DAPSA), and Composite Psoriatic Disease Activity Index (CPDAI). Arthritis Care Res (Hoboken). 2011;63(Suppl 11):S64-85.
44. Donmez S, Pamuk ON, Akker M, et al. Clinical features and types of articular involvement in patients with psoriatic arthritis. Clin Rheumatol. 2015;34:1091-6.
45. Scarpa R, Soscia E, Peluso R, et al. Nail and distal interphalangeal joint in psoriatic arthritis. J Rheumatol. 2006;33:1315-9.
46. Tan AL, Grainger AJ, Tanner SF, et al. A high-resolution magnetic resonance imaging study of distal interphalangeal joint arthropathy in psoriatic arthritis and osteoarthritis: are they the same? Arthritis Rheum. 2006;54:1328-33.
47. Coates LC, Hodgson R, Conaghan PG, et al. MRI and ultrasonography for diagnosis and monitoring of psoriatic arthritis. Best Pract Res Clin Rheumatol. 2012;26:805-22.
48. McGonagle D, Conaghan PG, Emery P. Psoriatic arthritis: a unified concept twenty years on. Arthritis Rheum. 1999;42:1080-6.
49. Dalbeth N, Pui K, Lobo M, et al. Nail disease in psoriatic arthritis: distal phalangeal bone edema detected by magnetic resonance imaging predicts development of onycholysis and hyperkeratosis. J Rheumatol. 2012;39:841-3.
50. Eulry F, Diamano J, Launay D, et al. Sausage-like toe and heel pain: value for diagnosing and evaluating the severity of spondyloarthropathies defined by Amor's criteria. A retrospective study in 161 patients. Joint Bone Spine. 2002;69:574-9.
51. Ritchlin CT, Kavanaugh A, Gladman DD, et al. Treatment recommendations for psoriatic arthritis. Ann Rheum Dis. 2009;68:1387-94.
52. Ferguson EG, Coates LC. Optimisation of rheumatology indices: dactylitis and enthesitis in psoriatic arthritis. Clin Exp Rheumatol. 2014;32:S-113-7.
53. Brockbank JE, Stein M, Schentag CT, et al. Dactylitis in psoriatic arthritis: a marker for disease severity? Ann Rheum Dis. 2005;64:188-90.
54. Gladman DD, Chandran V. Observational cohort studies: lessons learnt from the University of Toronto Psoriatic Arthritis Program. Rheumatology (Oxford). 2011;50:25-31.
55. Helliwell PS. Established psoriatic arthritis: clinical aspects. J Rheumatol Suppl. 2009;83:21-3.

56. Haddad A, Johnson SR, Somaily M, et al. Psoriatic Arthritis Mutilans: Clinical and Radiographic Criteria. A Systematic Review. J Rheumatol. 2015;42:1432-8.
57. Mc Ardle A, Flatley B, Pennington SR, et al. Early biomarkers of joint damage in rheumatoid and psoriatic arthritis. Arthritis Res Ther. 2015;17:141.
58. Jadon DR, Shaddick G, Tillett W, et al. Psoriatic Arthritis Mutilans: characteristics and natural radiographic history. J Rheumatol. 2015;42:1169-76.
59. Tan YM, Ostergaard M, Doyle A, et al. MRI bone oedema scores are higher in the arthritis mutilans form of psoriatic arthritis and correlate with high radiographic scores for joint damage. Arthritis Res Ther. 2009;11:R2.
60. McCarty DJ, O'Duffy JD, Pearson L, et al. Remitting seronegative symmetrical synovitis with pitting edema. RS3PE syndrome. JAMA. 1985;254:2763-7.
61. Olivieri I, Brandi G, Padula A, et al. Lack of association with spondyloarthritis and HLA-B27 in Italian patients with Whipple's disease. J Rheumatol. 2001;28:1294-7.
62. Gladman DD, Mease PJ, Strand V, et al. Consensus on a core set of domains for psoriatic arthritis. J Rheumatol. 2007;34:1167-70.
63. Maharaj AB, Govender J, Maharaj K, et al. Summary of Sensitivity and Specificity for Psoriatic Arthritis in a South African Cohort according to Classification Criteria. J Rheumatol. 2015;42:960-2.
64. Taylor W, Gladman D, Helliwell P, et al. Classification criteria for psoriatic arthritis: development of new criteria from a large international study. Arthritis Rheum. 2006;54:2665-73.
65. Leung YY, Tam LS, Ho KW, et al. Evaluation of the CASPAR criteria for psoriatic arthritis in the Chinese population. Rheumatology (Oxford). 2010;49:112-5.
66. Chandran V, Schentag CT, Gladman DD. Sensitivity and specificity of the CASPAR criteria for psoriatic arthritis in a family medicine clinic setting. J Rheumatol. 2008; 35:2069-70(author reply 70).
67. Ogdie A, Schwartzman S, Eder L, et al. Comprehensive treatment of psoriatic arthritis: managing comorbidities and extraarticular manifestations. J Rheumatol. 2014;41:2315-22.
68. Chiu HY, Chang WL, Huang WF, et al. Increased risk of arrhythmia in patients with psoriatic disease: a nationwide population-based matched cohort study. J Am Acad Dermatol. 2015.
69. Sharma A, Reddy MH, Sharma K, et al. Study of endothelial dysfunction in patients of psoriatic arthritis by flow mediated and nitroglycerine mediated dilatation of brachial artery. Int J Rheum Dis. 2016;19(3):300-4.
70. Sharma A, Gopalakrishnan D, Kumar R, et al. Metabolic syndrome in psoriatic arthritis patients: a cross-sectional study. Int J Rheum Dis. 2013;16:667-73.
71. Reddy SM, Anandarajah AP, Fisher MC, et al. Comparative analysis of disease activity measures, use of biologic agents, body mass index, radiographic features, and bone density in psoriatic arthritis and rheumatoid arthritis patients followed in a large U.S. disease registry. J Rheumatol. 2010;37:2566-72.
72. Ogdie A, Schwartzman S, Husni ME. Recognizing and managing comorbidities in psoriatic arthritis. Curr Opin Rheumatol. 2015;27:118-26.
73. Haroon M, Adeeb F, Devlin J, et al. A comparative study of renal dysfunction in patients with inflammatory arthropathies: strong association with cardiovascular diseases and not with anti-rheumatic therapies, inflammatory markers or duration of arthritis. Int J Rheum Dis. 2011;14:255-60.
74. McDonough E, Ayearst R, Eder L, et al. Depression and anxiety in psoriatic disease: prevalence and associated factors. J Rheumatol. 2014;41:887-96.
75. Dominguez P, Gladman DD, Helliwell P, et al. Development of screening tools to identify psoriatic arthritis. Curr Rheumatol Rep. 2010;12:295-9.
76. Azzam OA, Atta AT, Sobhi RM, et al. Fractional CO2 laser treatment vs autologous fat transfer in the treatment of acne scars: a comparative study. J Drugs Dermatol. 2013;12:e7-e13.
77. Gladman DD, Schentag CT, Tom BD, et al. Development and initial validation of a screening questionnaire for psoriatic arthritis: the Toronto Psoriatic Arthritis Screen (ToPAS). Ann Rheum Dis. 2009;68:497-501.
78. Tinazzi I, Adami S, Zanolin EM, et al. The early psoriatic arthritis screening questionnaire: a simple and fast method for the identification of arthritis in patients with psoriasis. Rheumatology (Oxford). 2012;51:2058-63.
79. Mishra S, Kancharla H, Dogra S, et al. Comparison of the four validated psoriatic arthritis screening tools in diagnosing psoriatic arthritis in patients with psoriasis (COMPAQ Study). Br J Dermatol. 2017;176(3):765-70.
80. Dhir V, Aggarwal A. Psoriatic arthritis: a critical review. Clin Rev Allergy Immunol. 2013;44:141-8.
81. Moller B, Bonel H, Rotzetter M, et al. Measuring finger joint cartilage by ultrasound as a promising alternative to conventional radiograph imaging. Arthritis Rheum. 2009; 61:435-41.
82. De Simone C, Guerriero C, Giampetruzzi AR, et al. Achilles tendinitis in psoriasis: clinical and sonographic findings. J Am Acad Dermatol. 2003;49:217-22.
83. Gutierrez M, Filippucci E, Salaffi F, et al. Differential diagnosis between rheumatoid arthritis and psoriatic arthritis: the value of ultrasound findings at metacarpophalangeal joints level. Ann Rheum Dis. 2011;70:1111-4.
84. Lin Z, Wang Y, Mei Y, et al. High-frequency ultrasound in the evaluation of psoriatic arthritis: a clinical study. Am J Med Sci. 2015;350:42-6.
85. Jadon DR, Nightingale AL, McHugh et al. Serum soluble bone turnover biomarkers in psoriatic arthritis and psoriatic spondyloarthropathy. J Rheumatol. 2015;42:21-30.

86. Menter A, Korman NJ, Elmets CA, et al. Guidelines of care for the management of psoriasis and psoriatic arthritis: section 6. American Academy of Dermatology Work Group. Guidelines of care for the treatment of psoriasis and psoriatic arthritis: case-based presentations and evidence-based conclusions. J Am Acad Dermatol. 2011;65:137-74.
87. Sharma A, Dogra S. Management of psoriatic arthritis. Indian J Dermatol Venereol Leprol. 2010;76:645-51.
88. Coates LC, Kavanaugh A, Ritchlin CT, et al. Systematic review of treatments for psoriatic arthritis: 2014 update for the GRAPPA. J Rheumatol. 2014;41:2273-6.
89. Boehncke WH, Qureshi A, Merola JF, et al. Diagnosing and treating psoriatic arthritis: an update. Br J Dermatol. 2014;170:772-86.
90. Kaltwasser JP, Nash P, Gladman D, et al. Efficacy and safety of leflunomide in the treatment of psoriatic arthritis and psoriasis: a multinational, double-blind, randomized, placebo-controlled clinical trial. Arthritis Rheum. 2004;50:1939-50.
91. Smith CH, Anstey AV, Barker JN, et al. British Association of Dermatologists' guidelines for biologic interventions for psoriasis 2009. Br J Dermatol. 2009;161:987-1019.
92. Coates LC, Helliwell PS. Psoriasis flare with corticosteroid use in Psoriatic Arthritis. Br J Dermatol. 2016;174:219-21.

16
CHAPTER

Reactive Arthritis

Riti Bhatia, Somesh Gupta

INTRODUCTION

Reactive arthritis is a form of spondyloarthropathy characterized by inflammatory arthritis that develops following an infection, although it may not be documented in most of the cases. Given the young age at onset and associated severe deformities, it may lead to a huge impact on daily life activities, hampering the productivity immensely. The cutaneous manifestations are distinctive enough to differentiate it from the other similar arthritides. The treatment, however, is a challenge for the treating physician. With the advent of biological therapeutic modalities, the approach has also shifted from disease modifying antirheumatic agents (DMARDS) to newer biological agents. However, their usefulness in the long term is yet to be seen. This chapter aims to summarize the clinical features, various investigations, and the current literature on the usefulness of existing treatment modalities in the management of reactive arthritis.

BACKGROUND

Reactive arthritis (formerly Reiter's disease) is an inflammatory arthritis affecting larger joints that usually develops after a urogenital or gastrointestinal infection. While the course and long-term prognosis has been described for reactive arthritis caused by enteric organisms, the same has not been well studied in the cases where *Chlamydia* is implicated as causative organism.

HISTORICAL ASPECTS

"Reactive arthritis" was first defined in 1969 as an arthritis which developed during or soon after an infection in the body, but in which microorganisms were not isolated from the joints.[1] The pathogens implicated in causation of reactive arthritis were not known until 1999 when, the role of *Chlamydia trachomatis, Yersinia, Salmonella, Shigella,* and *Campylobacter* was found in its causation.[2] The newer organisms implicated are *Escherichia coli, Clostridium difficile,* and *Chlamydia pneumoniae,* and rarely, intravesical bacillus-Calmette-Guerin.[2]

PATHOGENESIS

The pathogenic organisms are transferred from the genitourinary and gastrointestinal tracts to the synovial cavity either inside monocytes or during bacteremia. These reside in the synovial tissue and trigger a host-antigen reaction that eventually leads to reactive arthritis. Chlamydial heat shock protein 60, *Yersinia* adhesin, *Yersinia* outer protein and bacterial lipopolysaccharide are highly antigenic molecules that lead to apoptosis of T-cells by release of tumor necrosis factor-α (TNF-α). These also stimulate release of other pro-inflammatory cytokines, such as interleukin-6, interferon-α and nitric oxide, triggering inflammatory arthritis.

DISEASE BURDEN

Reactive arthritis is a rare disease occurring characteristically in young adult men more than women. It is reported to occur with an annual incidence of 0.6-27 per 100,000 adult population while the prevalence is around 30-40 per 100,000 adults.[2-5] The prevalence of reactive arthritis varies with the geographical location depending on the prevalence of causative organisms in that region. While *Campylobacter, Salmonella,* and *Shigella* were frequent agents in causation of reactive arthritis in adults (incidence of reactive arthritis found to be 9, 12, and 12 per 1,000 patients infected with these pathogens, respectively), *Clostridium difficile* infection was found to be causative in pediatric reactive arthritis (incidence 14 per 1,000 pediatric patients infected with this pathogen).[6]

The causative pathogens, incidence, and prevalence of reactive arthritis depend upon the geographic region. Amongst the infections caused by various pathogens, the rate of development of reactive arthritis is highest with *Chlamydia trachomatis* (4-8%).

CLINICAL PRESENTATION

Mucocutaneous Manifestations

Reactive arthritis was initially recognized as a triad of postinfectious arthritis, conjunctivitis, and urethritis.[7] However, all the features of this triad may not be seen in every patient of reactive arthritis. The recent definition of reactive arthritis is based on the following criteria:[8]
- Onset of arthritis after an interval of days-weeks (usually 1-4 weeks) after a gastrointestinal or genitourinary infection
- A typical mono- or asymmetric oligoarticular arthritis involving the lower extremities predominantly, along with associated enthesitis and dactylitis.

The preceding dysentery or urethritis, manifesting as urethral discharge, dysuria, frequency, and urgency, is usually mild and may even go unnoticed by some patients. The prognosis of reactive arthritis with symptomatic preceding urethritis or dysentery has not been shown to differ from that without symptoms of preceding infection.

While arthritis is the most common manifestation in reactive arthritis, the frequency of cutaneous and ocular involvement was found to be 15% and 20%, respectively, in a study involving 186 patients.[9]

The typical cutaneous features of reactive arthritis include a symmetrical involvement of palms and soles in the form of keratotic erythematous papules (keratoderma blennorrhagicum), circinate erosions over the glans penis and the mucosal aspect of labia majora (circinate balanitis/vulvitis) and a generalized thick keratotic papules with rupioid or ostraceous scale along with pustular lesions (Figs 1 to 8). Nail changes similar to psoriasis, including subungual hyperkeratosis, distal onycholysis and pitting, are generally seen (Fig. 9).

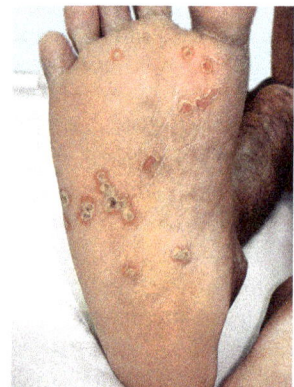

FIGURE 1: Keratoderma blenorrhegicum.

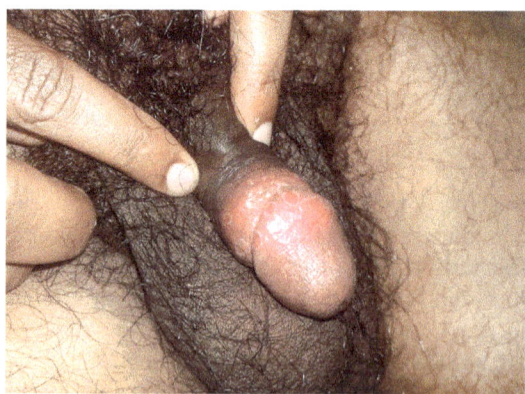

FIGURE 2: Circinate balanitis.

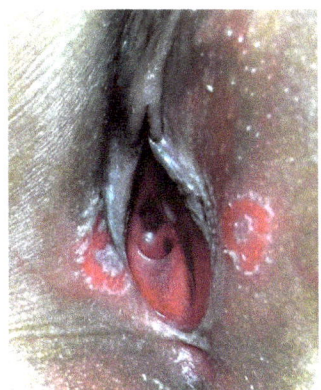

FIGURE 3: Circinate vulvitis.

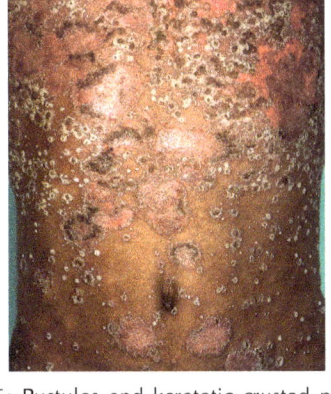

FIGURE 6: Pustules and keratotic crusted plaques on trunk.

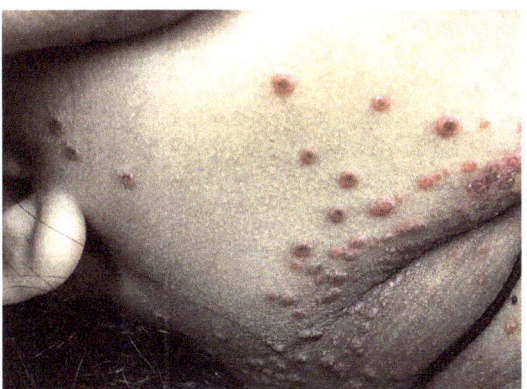

FIGURE 4: Keratotic papules on cheek.

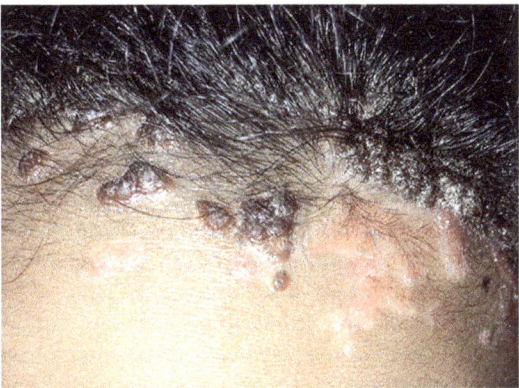

FIGURE 7: Rupioid keratotic plaques on forehead.

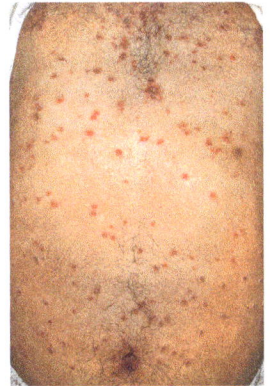

FIGURE 5: Keratotic papules on trunk.

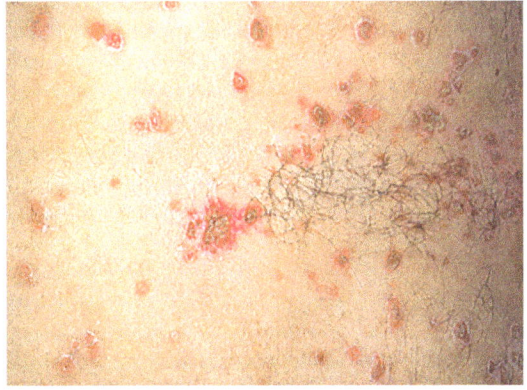

FIGURE 8: Scaly crusted papules plaques on trunk.

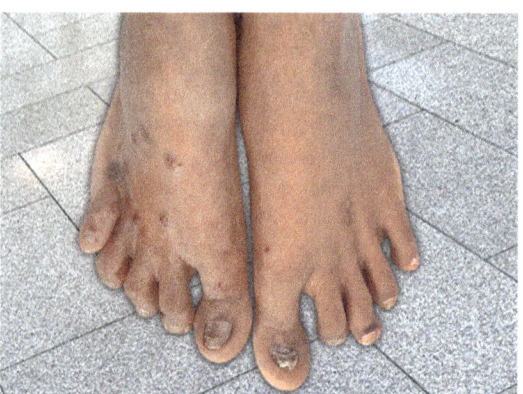

FIGURE 9: Nail changes.

Joint Manifestations

- Arthritis: Typically, an acute onset monoarthritis or asymmetric oligoarthritis, often affecting the lower extremities is seen. Approximately 50% of patients have involvement of upper extremities, with polyarthritis in the small joints in some patients. Axial arthritis, involving any part of the spine, is seen less commonly. Arthritis of more than 6 months duration is conventionally regarded as chronic reactive arthritis[10]
- Enthesitis: Enthesitis is the inflammation surrounding the enthesis, which is the site of insertion of tendons, ligaments, fascia, or joint capsule to the bone. Various studies have reported the frequency of enthesitis between 20 and 90% in the patients of reactive arthritis. Involvement of heel at the insertion of Achilles tendon and plantar fascia on the calcaneal bone, manifesting as pain and swelling of the heel, is characteristic in reactive arthritis[10]
- Dactylitis: Dactylitis, presenting as sausage digit, has been described in around 40% of patients with reactive arthritis, more so when the preceding infection is caused by *Chlamydia trachomatis*.[11]

Ocular Manifestations

Involvement of eyes is seen in the form of conjunctivitis, episcleritis, keratitis, and anterior uveitis. In one report involving 254 cases of reactive arthritis, of which 130 cases also had conjunctivitis, around one-third of cases of conjunctivitis showed positive scrapings for *Chlamydia*.[12]

Rarely, involvement of cardiac valves in the form of aortic insufficiency and pericarditis may be seen.[13]

INVESTIGATIONS

The various investigations which may show abnormalities in a patient of reactive arthritis are as follows:

- Elevation of acute inflammatory markers: There may be elevation of the acute phase reactants such as C-reactive protein (CRP) or erythrocyte sedimentation rate (ESR). However, these are not elevated in all the patients and one study found the elevation of acute phase reactants only in less than half patients[14]
- Evidence of preceding or concomitant infection: Usually, the symptoms of preceding diarrhea and urethritis subside by the time the patient develops reactive arthritis. Stool cultures for *Shigella, Salmonella, Yersinia,* and *Campylobacter* may sometimes be positive. Urethral swabs and urine samples are taken for nucleic acid amplification tests (NAATs) to detect *Chlamydia trachomatis*. Rate of pathogen identification in well-controlled studies was around 50%
- Genetic testing: Human leukocyte antigen (HLA)-B27 is found to be positive in around 30–50% of cases.[4,15] The HLA-B27 positivity is associated with a worse prognosis in some, but not all studies, with findings suggesting that patients who are HLA-B27 positive are more likely to develop a chronic spondyloarthropathy with radiographic changes[9]
- Skin biopsy: The histopathological findings in a skin biopsy done from a keratotic papule is indistinguishable from that of pustular psoriasis, showing acanthosis, parakeratosis, hypogranulosis, suprapapillary thinning, and neutrophilic abscesses in the stratum corneum (Fig. 10)
- Radiological investigations: Plain radiographs in patients of reactive arthritis show nonspecific changes of inflammatory arthritis.

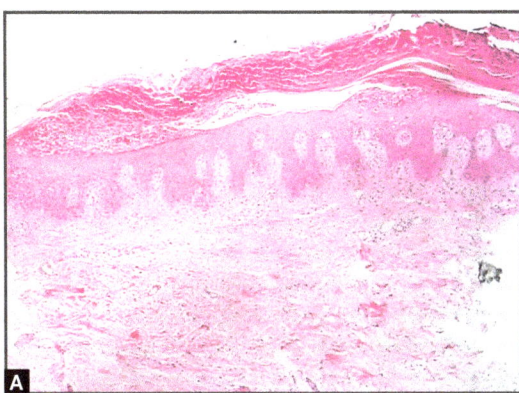 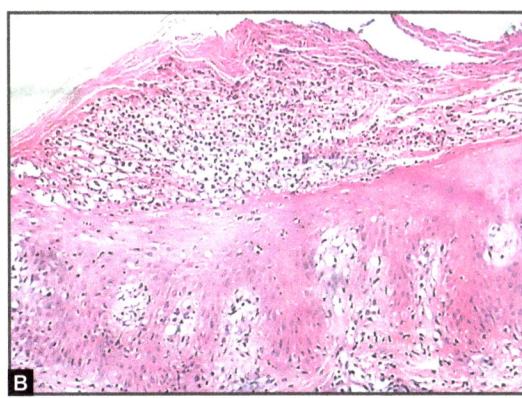

FIGURE 10: **A,** Psoriasiform hyperplasia, parakeratosis, neutrophils in stratum corneum, regular acanthosis and dilated capillaries in papillary dermis (H&E, x200); **B,** Neutrophilic abscesses in stratum corneum (H&E, x400).

Calcaneal spurs are seen in patients with heel pain but these may be seen in other inflammatory arthritides also.[16] Distinguishing reactive arthritis from psoriatic arthritis, both clinically and radiologically, may not be easy. While reactive arthritis has a predilection for joints of lower limbs, psoriatic arthritis involves joints of hands and wrists equally. Radiologically, both show a relative absence of osteoporosis and irregular periosteal bone apposition. Sacroiliitis is more commonly seen in reactive arthritis. Syndesmophytes are coarse and less symmetrical in both disorders. Other imaging modalities like magnetic resonance imaging (MRI), ultrasonography, and radionuclide bone scanning may help in early detection of inflammatory changes in the joint and enthesitis
- Joint aspiration: The findings in synovial fluid are nonspecific and are those seen in inflammatory arthritis. There is elevation of the leukocyte counts, with rise in the neutrophils.

DIFFERENTIAL DIAGNOSES

The cutaneous lesions of reactive arthritis may appear similar to psoriasis. Although heaped-up rupioid plaques are characteristically seen in reactive arthritis, these may also be a manifestation of psoriasis.

The circinate superficial scaly plaques on the glans penis may be confused with genital herpes. However, grouped vesicles with smaller superficial erosions are an indicator towards herpes. These mucocutaneous manifestations coupled with arthritis which, in some cases, is preceded by dysentery or urethritis, are fairly suggestive of reactive arthritis. On the other hand, arthritis occurring in isolation may cause diagnostic confusion, especially with other causes of mono- or oligoarthritis, like crystal-induced inflammation and bacterial synovitis. Other spondyloarthropathies, especially peripheral spondyloarthritis, may present with arthritis and enthesitis which may be difficult to distinguish from reactive arthritis.

TREATMENT

The various agents used in reactive arthritis are shown in table 1.

Approach to a patient of reactive arthritis is shown in flowchart 1.
- Nonsteroidal anti-inflammatory drugs (NSAIDs): The initial treatment of choice is NSAIDs, especially in acute reactive arthritis (defined as reactive arthritis of less than 6 months duration). A trial of at least 4 weeks may be given before switching treatment. Nonsteroidal anti-inflammatory drugs do not have any effect on the disease course
- Patients unresponsive to NSAIDs or patients with contraindications, such as renal derangement, cardiovascular or gastrointestinal disease, may be considered for steroids. In case of

involvement of few joints, intra-articular steroid injections, of triamcinolone acetonide (40 mg/mL) may bring about relief. Cases inadequately controlled by intra-articular injections or with multiple joints afflicted, may be managed by systemic steroids. Pulsed corticosteroids can help to override the intervening painful episodes and are a useful alternative to biologicals in resource poor settings. Authors have observed a significant improvement in inflammatory arthritis and cutaneous lesions of reactive arthritis with weekly dexamethasone pulses, given in dose of 100 mg and 50 mg, in adults and pediatric patients, respectively. However, these agents have not been seen to bring a change in the course of disease, necessitating the addition of a disease modifying agent

- Disease modifying antirheumatic drugs (DMARDs): Failure to respond to a dose of prednisolone of around 7.5 mg/day, continuously for 3–6 months or presence of comorbidities, such as uncontrolled diabetes, hypertension, cataract, may require switching therapy to DMARDs. Usually sulfasalazine and methotrexate are the preferred agents. Sulfasalazine is initiated at a dose of 500 mg once daily and the dose is escalated in a stepwise protocol, up to a dose of 3 g/day,

Table 1: Agents found to be useful in reactive arthritis and the levels of evidence for their usefulness

Therapeutic agent	Level of evidence
Anti-inflammatory agents	
• NSAIDs	• Grade 2B
Immunosuppressive agents	
• Steroids	
○ Intra-articular steroids	○ Grade 2C
○ Systemic steroids	○ Grade 2C
DMARDs	Grade 2B
• Biological agents	
○ TNF-α blockers	○ Grade 3

NSAIDs, nonsteroidal anti-inflammatory drugs; DMARDs, disease modifying antirheumatic drugs; TNF, tumor necrosis factor.

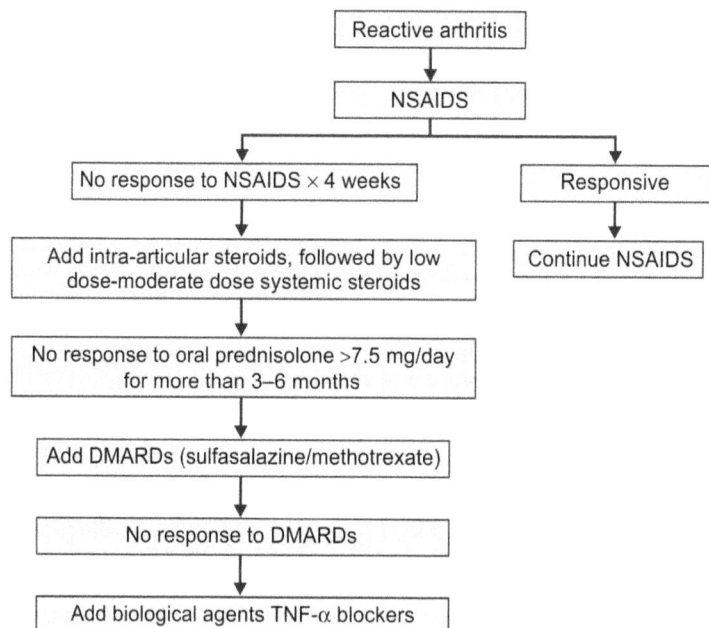

NSAIDs, nonsteroidal anti-inflammatory drugs; DMARDs, disease modifying antirheumatic drugs; TNF, tumor necrosis factor.

FLOWCHART 1: Treatment approach to a patient of reactive arthritis.

according to the response. The dosage regimen for methotrexate is similar to that in psoriatic arthritis. It is initiated at a dose of 15 mg every week and can be increased to 25 mg/week. A combination of methotrexate and sulfasalazine may be needed in some cases. Other agents found to be effective are azathioprine, cyclosporine, cyclophosphamide, leflunomide and levamisole. However, controlled trials are lacking

- Biological agents: Patients unresponsive to an adequate trial of DMARDs are best managed with biological agents. These may be initiated early in patients with contraindications to DMARDs. The efficacy of biological agents in reactive arthritis may be extrapolated from the successful use of these agents in psoriatic arthritis in a number of randomized controlled trials. The most widely used agents are TNF-α blockers. Infliximab, in a dose of 3–5 mg/kg, administered as intravenous infusion, may be the preferred TNF-α blocker. It is administered at weeks 0, 2, 6, and every 8 weeks thereafter. Etanercept is often the drug of choice in childhood reactive arthritis. An adequate trial of 3 months is usually recommended before switching to another biological agent. Failure to respond to a TNF-α blocker does not imply unresponsiveness to other TNF-α blockers. In a study, 10 patients of reactive arthritis were treated with TNF-α blockers (infliximab in 5 patients, etanercept in 4 patients, and adalimumab in 1 patient). Out of 10, 6 patients achieved remission after 7.5 months. However, there was a relapse in 3 patients, who responded to retreatment.[17]

Although there are no reports, in authors' experience, there are few patients of reactive arthritis, who are nonresponsive to most of the TNF-α blockers and also to other biological agents.

The pustular lesions and keratoderma blenorrhegicum may be treated with topical vitamin D analogs and topical steroids. For thicker papules and plaques, salicylic acid (3–6%) is used. Severe cutaneous lesions not responding to topical treatment modalities usually respond to DMARDs like methotrexate or biological agents.

Indications for Antibiotics

While patients with acute enteritis and urethritis should be given antibiotics, there is no evidence to suggest the usefulness of antibiotics in patients with no suggestion of underlying infection. In case of symptoms of chlamydial urethritis, the patients as well as their partners should receive a course of doxycycline. However, a prolonged course of doxycycline for 4 months did not help in improving the disease activity as compared to a 10-day treatment in 32 cases of *Chlamydia trachomatis*-induced reactive arthritis.[18] In a trial consisting of 186 patients of reactive arthritis, all the patients received conventional 1 g of azithromycin and then they were randomized to receive either weekly azithromycin or placebo for 3 months. The authors observed no difference between the groups in terms of arthritis, C-reactive protein, physician, and patient global assessment.[19]

Physiotherapy

An assessment of each patient is made to evaluate the degree of functional disability in daily living activities. Therapies for pain relief include hot and cold therapy, electrical stimulation, and hydrotherapy. Joint protective measures, like rest and splinting, are advocated in active joint inflammation. Based on the degree of contractures, age of the patient, and compliance, various therapeutic exercises may be advised, like range of motion (ROM) exercises, stretching, strengthening, and daily life activities.

An effort must be made to address the psychosocial aspects of patients. Details regarding any handicap in social interactions and at workplace should be sought and appropriate patient education as well as psychotherapies like self-relaxation should be advised.

PROGNOSIS

Long-term follow-up studies have shown that around 20–70% of patients have some residual joint symptoms. Approximately 15–30% of patients suffer from chronic arthritis. Radiological sacroiliitis was seen in 30% of patients with reactive arthritis in a 10-year follow-up study.[20]

CONCLUSION

Reactive arthritis is an inflammatory arthritis affecting young men more often, characteristically preceded by dysentery or urethritis, in some cases. The cutaneous manifestations are quite distinct, making the role of a dermatologist important, especially in early disease, in which joint manifestations may not be florid. Recognition of the disease early in its course helps to screen for additional extra-articular involvement, such as ocular disease and appropriate management. Considering the burden of disabilities associated with this disease, an appropriate early management in liaison with a rheumatologist, is recommended. Treatment protocol includes a step ladder approach, beginning from NSAIDs to oral and intra-articular steroids and DMARDs, with biologicals at the end. Role of rehabilitation in the form of regular physiotherapy is emphasized. Newer biological agents targeting various inflammatory mediators are being explored, providing a hope for cure in the future.

REFERENCES

1. Ahvonen P, Sievers K, Aho K. Arthritis associated with Yersinia enterocolitica infection. Acta Rheumatol Scand. 1969;15:232.
2. Townes JM. Reactive arthritis after enteric infections in the United States: the problem of definition. Clin Infect Dis. 2010;50:247.
3. Rohekar S, Pope J. Epidemiologic approaches to infection and immunity: the case of reactive arthritis. CurrOpinRheumatol 2009; 21:386.
4. Hannu T. Reactive arthritis. Best Pract Res Clin Rheumatol. 2011;25:347.
5. Leirisalo-Repo M, Sieper J. Reactive arthritis: epidemiology, clinical features, and treatment. In: Weisman MH, van der Heijde D, Reveille JD (Eds). Ankylosing spondylitis and the spondyloarthropathies. Philadelphia: Mosby/Elsevier; 2006. pp. 53.
6. Ajene AN, Fischer Walker CL, Black RE. Enteric pathogens and reactive arthritis: a systematic review of Campylobacter, salmonella and Shigella-associated reactive arthritis. J Health Popul Nutr. 2013;31:299.
7. Panush RS, Wallace DJ, Dorff RE, et al. Retraction of the suggestion to use the term "Reiter's syndrome" sixty-five years later: the legacy of Reiter, a war criminal, should not be eponymic honor but rather condemnation. Arthritis Rheum. 2007;56:693.
8. Braun J, Kingsley G, van der Heijde D, et al. On the difficulties of establishing a consensus on the definition of and diagnostic investigations for reactive arthritis. Results and discussion of a questionnaire prepared for the 4th International Workshop on Reactive Arthritis, Berlin, Germany, July 3–6, 1999. J Rheumatol. 2000;27:2185-92.
9. Kvien TK, Gaston JS, Bardin T, et al. Three month treatment of reactive arthritis with azithromycin: a EULAR double blind, placebo controlled study. Ann Rheum Dis. 2004;63:1113.
10. Leirisalo-Repo M. Reactive arthritis. Scand J Rheumatol. 2005;34:251.
11. Zeidler H, Hudson AP. New insights into Chlamydia and arthritis. Promise of a cure? Ann Rheum Dis. 2014;73:637.
12. KovalevluN, Il'in II. Ophthalmological aspects of Reiter's disease. Vestn Oftalmol. 1990;106:65.
13. Cosh JA, Gerber N, Barritt DW, et al. Proceedings: cardiac lesions in Reiter's syndrome and ankylosing spondylitis. Ann Rheum Dis. 1975;34:195.
14. Townes JM, Deodhar AA, Laine ES, et al. Reactive arthritis following culture-confirmed infections with bacterial enteric pathogens in Minnesota and Oregon: a population-based study. Ann Rheum Dis. 2008;67:1689.
15. Carter JD, Hudson AP. Reactive arthritis: clinical aspects and medical management. Rheum Dis Clin North Am. 2009; 35:21.
16. Gerster JC, Vischer TL, Bennani A, et al. The painful heel. Comparative study in rheumatoid arthritis, ankylosing spondylitis, Reiter's syndrome, and generalized osteoarthrosis. Ann Rheum Dis. 1977;36:343.
17. Meyer A, Chatelus E, Wendling D, et al. Safety and efficacy of anti-tumor necrosis factor α therapy in ten patients with recent-onset refractory reactive arthritis. Arthritis Rheum. 2011;63:1274.
18. Putschky N, Pott HG, Kuipers JG, et al. Comparing 10-day and 4-month doxycycline courses for treatment of Chlamydia trachomatis-reactive arthritis: a prospective, double-blind trial. Ann Rheum Dis 2006;65:1521-4.
19. Kvien T, Gaston J, Bardin T, et al. Three month treatment of reactive arthritis with azithromycin: a EULAR double blind, placebo controlled study. Ann Rheum Dis. 2004; 63: 1113-9.
20. Leirisalo-Repo M, Helenius P, Hannu T, et al. Long-term prognosis of reactive salmonella arthritis. Ann Rheum Dis. 1997;56:516-20.

CHAPTER 17

Rheumatoid Arthritis

Sauvik Dasgupta, Uma Kumar

INTRODUCTION

Rheumatoid arthritis (RA) is a chronic inflammatory autoimmune disease of unknown etiology, most characteristically involving small joints of hands and feet. However, RA is a systemic disease and may involve multiple organs, like skin, eyes, lungs, and heart, leading to various extra-articular manifestations.

EPIDEMIOLOGY

Rheumatoid arthritis is the most common inflammatory arthritis, with an incidence approximating 3 per 10,000 population and affecting around 0.25–1% of the world population depending on ethnicity and geographical location.[1-3] Females are thrice more commonly affected as compared to males, but the difference seems to abate with advancing age.[4,5]

PATHOGENESIS

The exact cause of RA remains unknown. The current concept in etiopathogenesis is multimodal; with environmental, immunologic, infective, and lifestyle factors, all playing a role in development of RA in genetically susceptible individuals. There appears to be a strong genetic risk factor for the predisposition of disease development. Human leukocyte antigen (HLA)-DRB1*04 cluster is the most commonly identified cluster locus with over 80% of patients expressing this locus.[6] In fact, patients expressing two HLA-DRB1*04 alleles are at an elevated risk for nodular disease and major organ involvement.[7] The disease expression is further modified by various exogenous factors such as smoking and infection, in terms of development, rate of progression and severity of RA. A wide variety of immunomodulators (cytokines and effector cells) play a role in articular and extra-articular manifestations of the disease. Activation of the innate immune response including the activation of dendritic cells by exogenous material and autologous antigens appears to be the initiating event in the pathogenesis of the disease.[7] Further, the damage is carried forward by the cells and cytokines involving adaptive immune system. The B cells contribute to RA pathogenesis via multiple mechanisms like antigen presentation, production of antibodies, autoantibodies, and cytokines.[7] The T and B cell activation results in increased production of cytokines and chemokines, which create a positive feedback loop for additional T cell, macrophage, and B cell interactions. The role of macrophages in RA cannot be overemphasized. Osteoclastogenesis, a phenomenon considered very important in inflammatory arthritis and source of cytokines, including tumor necrosis factor-α (TNF-α), Interleukin 1 (IL-1), and IL-6 are the other functions of macrophages.[7,8] Cytokines such as IL-6, IL-1, and TNF-α are the principal cytokines implicated in the pathogenesis of RA.[9] Interleukin 6, in particular, is of central importance. It not only has a paracrine effect as like other cytokines but also acts distal to the site of destruction. Interleukin 6 acts on neutrophils and contributes to inflammation and joint destruction by secreting proteolytic enzymes and reactive oxygen intermediates. Recently, IL-17 is assuming the role of the most important cytokine in the pathogenesis of RA. T helper 17 cells via production of the above mentioned cytokine plays a critical role in synovitis.[10]

CLINICAL FEATURES

The classical patient of RA presents with persistent symmetrical polyarthritis starting often with the small joints of hand or feet and later involves the larger joints, with early morning joint stiffness lasting for more than 30 minutes. The joints most frequently involved are metacarpophalangeal (MCP), proximal interphalangeal (PIP), wrists, and metatarsophalangeal (MTP) joints.[11] If left untreated, RA often leads to a progressive, debilitating, and destructive joint disease.

Synovial proliferation of tendon sheaths may give rise to "synovial proliferation cysts" on the dorsal and volar aspect of hand. Synovial proliferation may even compress the median nerve leading to carpal tunnel syndrome. The swan neck deformity describes flexion of the MCP and DIP with hyperextension of the PIP joint (Fig. 1). Conversely, boutonnière deformity results because of hyperextension at DIP joint and PIP protruding into flexion, due to avulsion of the extensor hood (Fig. 2). Weakness of the extensor carpi ulnaris muscle causes radial deviation of the wrist; with compensatory ulnar deviation of the fingers giving rise to the zigzag or Z deformity. With advancing disease, there is bony ankylosis, especially of the carpal bones. Elbow is the most common site for rheumatoid nodules (Fig. 3) and olecranon bursitis.

The midfoot and MTP joints are much more commonly involved than ankle in RA. "Cock-up" deformity of the toes may be seen consequent to downward subluxation of the metatarsal heads. It further progresses to develop a hallux valgus (bunion). Proximal intertarsal (PIT) joints protrude dorsally leading to "hammer toes". The second and third toes may deform to sit on top of the great toe and the second and third metatarsal heads become the primary weight bearers. Subtalar joint involvement is considerably common in RA and involvement of subtalar joint,

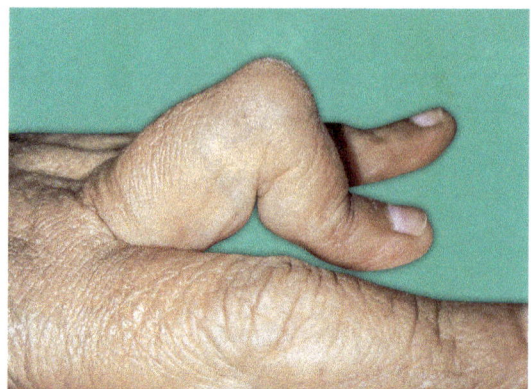

FIGURE 2: Boutonniere deformity.

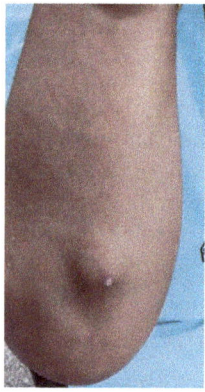

FIGURE 3: Rheumatoid nodule (White scar is skin biopsy site).

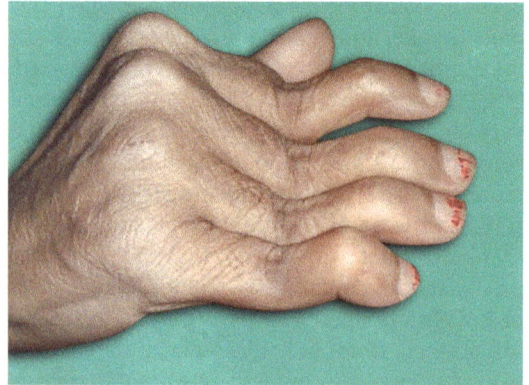

FIGURE 1: Swan neck deformity.

tibialis posterior tendon, and midfoot can lead to loss of normal arching of foot (rocker-bottom foot). Other joints like shoulder, knee, and hip also get involved during the course of illness.

Spine

Cervical spine involvement occurs late in the disease process of RA in around 25–80% of patients depending on diagnostic criteria used but neurological deficit occur only in 7–34% of patients. The C_1–C_2 vertebrae are commonly involved. Abnormalities of cervical spine in RA generally occur due to various cervical spine subluxations, of which the atlantoaxial subluxation is by far, the most common. At times, the odontoid process of axis may also migrate superiorly, through the foramen magnum; a phenomenon known as superior migration of odontoid, or cranial settling, or pseudobasilar invagination.[12] Cervical spine involvement may lead to pain in the nape of neck or occiput region, limitation of motion, instability, and the most obvious dreaded complication of progressive neurodeficit. The degree of subluxation correlates poorly with the development of neurodeficits.[13] The Ranawat classification can be used to categorize patients with rheumatoid myelopathy.[14] The importance of timely intervention in patients with neurological involvement cannot be overemphasized.

Other Joints

Cricoarytenoid joint involvement can be completely asymptomatic, or may produce symptoms of hoarseness, aspiration, or an inspiratory stridor. Temporomandibular joints are commonly involved in RA and patient may complain of pain, and masticatory difficulties. On examination, tenderness, crepitus, and subluxation of the temporomandibular joint may be appreciated.

Extra-articular Manifestations

The extra-articular manifestations usually correlate well with the duration and severity of RA. Constitutional symptoms like low grade fever, malaise, weight loss, and fatigue are the most common extra-articular manifestations; and depict a systemic inflammatory state in patients with RA.

Rheumatoid Nodule

It is seen in around 25% patients of seropositive RA. The usual site for development of rheumatoid nodule is the subcutaneous tissue, although it can develop in unusual sites, such as the sclera, vocal cords, lungs, and heart. When present in subcutaneous tissue, it is firm, nontender, located usually on the extensor surfaces or pressure points (e.g., olecranon). Pathologically, it consists of palisading fibroblasts around a central core of necrosis. Methotrexate therapy may decrease the size of nodules, or sometimes, paradoxically, increase the size, or even give rise to new nodules. Rheumatoid nodules must be differentiated from other similar subcutaneous nodules, such as gouty tophi, subcutaneous nodules of rheumatic fever, Heberden's and Bouchard's nodes, calcinosis, and xanthomatosis.

Skin

Patients can develop cutaneous vasculitis presenting as palpable purpura, gangrene (Fig. 4); pyoderma gangrenosum, palmar erythema, livedo reticularis (Fig. 5), erythema nodosum, and rarely Raynaud's phenomenon. Other extra-articular manifestations are shown in table 1.

DIAGNOSIS

Serology

The diagnosis of RA is largely clinical with serological tests like rheumatoid factor (RF) and anti-citrullinated cyclic peptide antibody (anti-CCP antibody) being only surrogate markers.

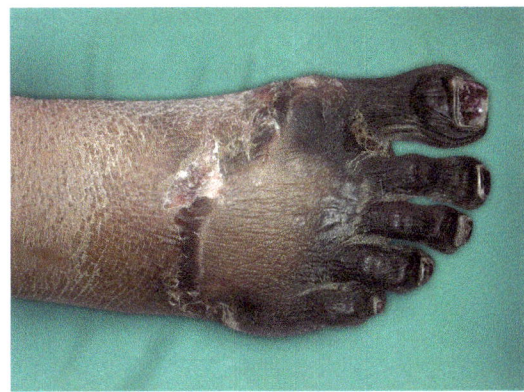

FIGURE 4: Gangrene in a patient of RA.

The sensitivity and specificity of RF varies between 50% and 90%, irrespective of the method used for testing.[15,16] Anti-CCP has almost comparable sensitivity to that of RF, although with a higher specificity of 90% or more, for the diagnosis of RA.[17] Both RF and anti-CCP are markers of poor prognosis and destructive joint disease.

Imaging

Joint imaging is an indispensable tool often used for both aiding the diagnosis, and monitoring the progression of RA. The characteristic initial radiographic finding in RA is periarticular osteopenia and soft tissue swelling around the joint. Other radiographic findings include bony subchondral erosions, joint space narrowing due to articular cartilage destruction, and subluxation (Fig. 6).

Ultrasound, by virtue of its low cost, portability, lack of radiation exposure, and sensitivity to detect early bone erosions is being increasingly used for diagnosis, monitoring disease activity, and guided intra-articular joint injection.

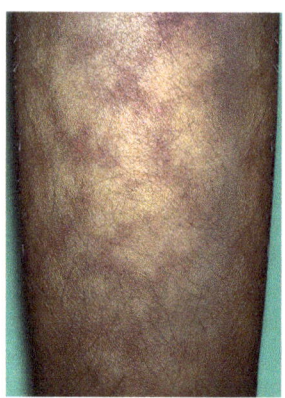

FIGURE 5: Livedo reticularis.

Table 1: Extra-articular manifestations of rheumatoid arthritis			
Organ system	Manifestation	Organ system	Manifestation
Skin	• Rheumatoid nodules • Cutaneous vasculitis: purpura, gangrene • Pyoderma gangrenosum • Palmar erythema • Livedo reticularis • Erythema nodosum • Raynaud's phenomenon	Hematologic	• Anemia • Eosinophilia • Thrombocytosis • Pure red cell aplasia • Felty's syndrome • Hematologic malignancy
Eye	• Keratoconjunctivitis sicca • Episcleritis/scleritis • Uveitis • Scleromalacia	Vascular	• Vasculitis • Visceral ischemia • Granulomatous aortitis
Lungs and pleura	• Pleurisy and pleural effusion • Interstitial lung disease • Pulmonary nodules • Small airway disease • Caplan's syndrome	Nervous system	• Central nervous system vasculitis • Cerebrovascular accident • Pachymeningitis • Mononeuritis multiplex • Peripheral neuropathy
Cardiac	• Pericarditis and pericardial effusion • Ischemic heart disease • Myocarditis and cardiomyopathy • Rheumatoid nodules • Conduction defects • Amyloidosis	Kidney	• Amyloidosis • Necrotizing glomerulonephritis
Bone	• Osteopenia/osteoporosis	–	–

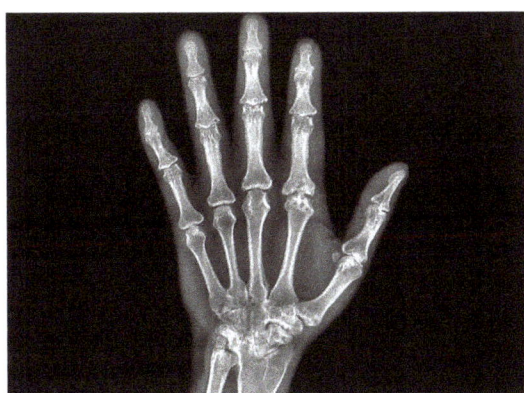

FIGURE 6: X-ray hand AP view showing periarticular osteopenia, soft tissue swelling, joint space reduction, and erosions.

Magnetic resonance imaging allows us to detect early bone edema in addition to other abnormalities detected by ultrasound, but affordability and availability are the main limiting factors for its everyday use.

The 2010 American College of Rheumatology (ACR)/European League against Rheumatism (EULAR) classification criteria that assist in making early diagnosis of RA is given in table 2.

Detailed clinical examination and relevant investigations is warranted in all patients before starting disease-modifying antirheumatic drugs (DMARDs).

MANAGEMENT

The principle of management of RA is early aggressive treatment with tight control of disease activity, where disease activity is assessed objectively by various validated disease activity indices (DAS28 ESR, DAS28 CRP, CDAI, and SDAI). This concept of "treat to target", where target is remission or at least low disease activity has revolutionized RA treatment.[18-21] Optimal treatment of RA patients comprise of pharmacological therapy, adjunctive therapy, treatment of various comorbidities, and surgical therapy, if needed. There is no gold standard drug or combination of drugs, which works for all patients, therefore, treatment must be individualized for each patient.

Table 2: The 2010 American College of Rheumatology/European League against Rheumatism classification criteria for early diagnosis of rheumatoid arthritis*

Score	
A. Joint involvement[§]	
1 large joint	0
2–10 large joints	1
1–3 small joints (with or without involvement of large joints)[#]	2
4–10 small joints (with or without involvement of large joints)	3
>10 joints (at least 1 small joint)**	5
B. Serology (at least 1 test result is needed for classification)[††]	
Negative RF and negative anti-CCP	0
Low-positive RF or low-positive anti-CCP	2
High-positive RF or high-positive anti-CCP	3
C. Acute-phase reactants (at least 1 test result is needed for classification)[‡‡]	
Normal CRP and normal ESR	0
Abnormal CRP or abnormal ESR	1
D. Duration of symptoms[§§]	
<6 weeks	0
≥6 weeks	1

RF, rheumatoid factor; CCP, citrullinated cyclic peptide; CRP, C-reactive protein; ESR, erythrocyte sedimentation rate.

*2010 ACR/EULAR Classification criteria for RA (score-based algorithm: add score of categories A–D; a score of ≥6/10 is needed for classification of a patient as having definite RA).

[§]Any swollen or tender joint on examination, or evidence of synovitis on magnetic resonance imaging or ultrasonography. distal interphalangeal, first carpometacarpal, and first metatarsophalangeal (MTP) are excluded.

[#]Metacarpophalangeal, proximal interphalangeal, 2nd–5th MTP, thumb interphalangeal, and wrist

**At least one of the involved joints must be a small joint

[††]At least one serological test and one acute phase reactant result should be available. Low positive is <3 upper limit of normal (ULN), high positive is >3 ULN. Where RF is available only as positive or negative, a positive result should be scored as low-postive for rheumatoid factor

[‡‡]As per local laboratory standard

[§§]Patient self-reported duration of symptoms of synovitis

Source: Neogi T, Aletaha D, Silman AJ, Naden RL, Felson DT, Aggarwal R, et al. The 2010 American College of Rheumatology/European League Against Rheumatism Classification Criteria for Rheumatoid Arthritis. Arthritis Rheum. 2010;62(9):2659-91.

Options for pharmacologic treatment include DMARDs, corticosteroids, nonsteroidal anti-inflammatory drugs, and immunosuppressants. The DMARDs can be classified into synthetic and biological agents. Conventional synthetic DMARDs include methotrexate (MTX), sulfasalazine, hydroxychloroquine, and leflunomide. Biologic DMARDs currently available for RA treatment are anti-TNF agents (Infliximab, Etanercept, Adalimumab, Golimumab, Certolizumab pegol); non-TNF biologics include: rituximab, an anti-CD20 B-cell antibody, abatacept, a CTLA-4 fusion molecule that blocks CD28 mediated T-cell function; and tocilizumab, an IL-6 receptor antibody. Biosimilars of Infliximab, Etanercept, Adalimumab, and Rituximab are also available in India providing cost effective alternative to innovator biologic agents. Immunosuppressants such as azathioprine, and cyclosporine too have demonstrated DMARD activity, but it is to be tried only in very desperate situations.[22-24] Both ACR and EULAR have put forth new guidelines recommending use of synthetic and biologic DMARDs, including modification, combination, and switch between various therapies. The recommendations also address other important issues like screening for latent tuberculosis infection (LTBI), immunization, treating high-risk patients, and also monitoring the clinical response and adverse effects of drug therapy.[18,19,25,26] Table 3 shows dosage, common adverse effects, and monitoring of various DMARDs used in RA.

Biologic and Biosimilar DMARDs

Biologic DMARDs have provided hope to conventional DMARDs refractory patients. Use of biologics in early RA patients have shown better short-term outcome especially in patients with poor prognostic factors.[27-29] The biggest limitation to use of biologics, especially in developing countries like India, is affordability. The advent of biosimilars into the fray has helped a great deal in partially dealing with this problem. Biosimilars are similar to, but are not identical to their originator biologics. It can be defined as a biotherapeutic product which is similar in terms of quality, safety, and efficacy to an already licensed reference biotherapeutic product.[30-32] Waning therapeutic response to biologic agents is demonstrated over period of time because of development of anti-chimeric or anti-drug antibodies in patients exposed to some of the available biologics. The use of concurrent MTX with TNF blockers helps in decreasing the immunogenicity of the later.[33,34] Reactivation of latent TB is a serious concern particularly in India. Contraindications to their use are active, recurrent, or chronic infections, the New York Heart Association (NYHA) grade III/IV heart failure, demyelinating diseases, history of nonskin malignancies in the past 5 year, pregnancy and lactation, human immunodeficiency virus (HIV), and hepatitis B and C infection.[18,26] Hence, it is recommended for all patients, who are planned for biologics to undergo screening for latent TB, hepatitis B virus, hepatitis C virus, HIV, and underlying malignancies.

Other Pharmacological Agents

Glucocorticoids in low dosage (<10 mg/day) may be used as bridging therapy for short periods of time (not more than 6 months) in combination with other DMARDs where it is found to alter disease progression and retard joint damage.[35,36]

Nonsteroidal anti-inflammatory drugs, now have limited role in RA therapy. They are primarily used for acute flares, and during initiation or modification of DMARD therapy, until DMARDs take their effect. They should be stopped as soon as their requirement ends.

Tofacitinib, a janus kinase inhibitor, is an oral synthetic small molecule that first received approval for use in RA in 2012.[37] Currently, it is recommended for patients of established RA in the dose of 5 mg BD or 11 mg OD (extended release), who are refractory to conventional DMARD monotherapy.

Other drugs that are in the pipeline and are either waiting approval, or in clinical trials are baricitinib (janus kinase inhibitor), sarilumab and sirukumab (IL-6 inhibitor), secukinumab (IL-17 inhibitor).[38-41]

Various composite measures were devised to attain a measurable, reliable, and reproducible index to determine the activity of RA (Tables 4 and 5).

Both ACR (2015) and EULAR (2013) have put forth recommendations to streamline the approach

Rheumatoid Arthritis

Table 3: Dosage, common adverse effects, and monitoring investigations of disease modifying anti-rheumatic drugs

Drug	Dosage	Side effects	Initial evaluation	Monitoring	Pregnancy and lactation
Methotrexate	• 15–30 mg/week orally or parenterally (subcutaneous/intramuscular) • Folic acid 1 mg/day to reduce toxicities	• Hepatotoxicity • Myelosuppression • Acute interstitial Pneumonitis • Pulmonary and subcutaneous nodules, • Dyspepsia/nausea • Oral ulcers • Alopecia	• Hemogram • LFT, S.Cr, HBV, HCV	• Hemogram, LFT • S.Cr every month × 3 months; then every 2–3 months	• Pregnancy category X • Contraindicated in lactation
Sulfasalazine	• 2,000–3,000 mg/day in 2–3 divided doses	• Granulocytopenia, • Hemolytic anemia • Thrombocytopenia • Nausea • Diarrhea • Rash/photosensitivity	• Hemogram, LFT • S.Cr • G6PD level	• Hemogram, LFT • S.Cr every 2–3 months	• Pregnancy category B (category D if used near term) • Relatively safe during lactation
Hydroxy-chloroquine	• 200–400 mg/day orally (5 mg/kg) in 1–2 divided doses	• Corneal deposits • Irreversible retinal damage • Rash/Skin pigmentation • Alopecia/Hair depigmentation • Neuromyotoxicity • Nausea	• Eye Examination; especially in elderly or prior ocular disease	• Complete ophthalmologic testing after 5 years of starting, and then every 1–2 years	• Pregnancy category C • Safe during lactation
Leflunomide	• 10–20 mg/day	• Diarrhea • Hepatotoxicity • Hypertension • Myelosuppression • Alopecia, weight loss • Rash	• Hemogram, LFT • S.Cr, HBV, HCV	• Hemogram, LFT • S.Cr every month × 3 months; then every 2–3 months	• Pregnancy category X • Contraindicated during lactation

Continued

Continued

Table 3: Dosage, common adverse effects, and monitoring investigations of disease modifying anti-rheumatic drugs

Drug	Dosage	Side effects	Initial evaluation	Monitoring	Pregnancy and lactation
Infliximab	• 3–5 mg/kg IV infusion at weeks 0, 2, 6, then every 8 weeks	• Risk of infections • Reactivation of latent TB • Drug-induced lupus • Neurologic deficits • Infusion reaction	• TST, IGRA, Chest X-ray, HBV, HCV, HIV	• Hemogram, LFT • S.Cr periodically	• Pregnancy category B • Unknown; best avoided during lactation
Etanercept	• 50 mg SC weekly, or • 25 mg SC biweekly	• Same as Infliximab	• Same as Infliximab	• Monitor for injection site reactions	• Pregnancy category B • Unknown; best avoided during lactation
Adalimumab:	• 40 mg SC every other week	• Same as infliximab	• Same as Infliximab	• Monitor for injection site reactions	• Pregnancy category B • Limited data indicate relative safety during lactation
Golimumab	• 50 mg SC monthly	• Same as infliximab	• Same as Infliximab	• Monitor for injection site reactions	• Pregnancy category B • Unknown; best avoided during lactation
Certolizumab	• 400 mg SC weeks 0, 2, 4 then 200 mg every other week	• Same as infliximab	• Same as Infliximab	• Monitor for injection site reactions	• Pregnancy category B • Unknown; best avoided during lactation

Abatacept	• Weight based:
	  <60 kg: 500 mg;
	  60–100 kg: 750 mg;
	  >100 kg: 1,000 mg
	  IV at week 0, 2 and 4, and then every 4 weeks
		• Increased risk bacterial, viral infections
		• Headache
		• Nausea
			• Same as Infliximab	• Monitor for infusion reactions	• Pregnancy category C
					• Unknown; best avoided during lactation

Continued

Continued

Table 3: Dosage, common adverse effects, and monitoring investigations of disease modifying anti-rheumatic drugs

Drug	Dosage	Side effects	Initial evaluation	Monitoring	Pregnancy and lactation
Rituximab	• 1,000 mg IV × 2, day 0 and 14	• Increased risk of bacterial, viral infections • Infusion reaction • Rash • Fever • Cytopenias • Hepatitis B reactivation	• Hemogram, HBV, HCV, HIV	• Hemogram at regular intervals	• Pregnancy category C • Unknown; best avoided during lactation
Tocilizumab	• 4–8 mg/kg IV monthly	• Risk of infection • Infusion reaction • LFT elevation • Dyslipidemia • Cytopenias • Heart failure	• TST, IGRA, Chest X-ray, HBV, HCV, HIV, Lipid profile	• Hemogram, LFT, lipid profile at regular intervals	• Pregnancy category C • Unknown; best avoided during lactation

SC, subcutaneous; IM, intramuscular; CBC, complete Blood Count; LFT, liver function test; S.Cr, serum creatinine; HBV, hepatitis B virus; HCV, hepatitis C virus; G6PD, glucose-6-phosphate dehydrogenase; IV, intravenous, TST, tuberculin skin test; IGRA, interferon gamma release assays.

Skin in Rheumatologic Diseases

Table 4: Various composite measures of rheumatoid arthritis disease activity

CDAI	28SJC + 28TJC + PrGA + PtGA
DAS28	
DAS28-ESR	$0.56 \times \sqrt{(28TJC)} + 0.28 \times \sqrt{(28SJC)} + 0.70 \times \ln(ESR) + 0.014 \times PtGA$
DAS28-CRP	$0.56 \times \sqrt{(28TJC)} + 0.28 \times \sqrt{(28SJC)} + 0.36 \times \ln(CRP + 1) + 0.014 \times PtGA + 0.96$
PAS	(HAQ × 3.33 + pain VAS + PtGA VAS)/3
PAS-II	(HAQ-II × 3.33 + pain VAS + PtGA VAS)/3
RAPID-3	(MDHAQ × 3.33 + pain VAS + PtGA VAS)/3
SDAI	28SJC + 28TJC + PrGA + PtGA + CRP

CDAI, Clinical Disease Activity Index; 28SJC, 28swollen joint count; 28TJC, 28 tender joint count; PrGA, provider global assessment of disease activity; PtGA, patient global assessment of disease activity; DAS28, Disease Activity Score with 28-joint counts; ESR, erythrocyte sedimentation rate; CRP, C-reactive protein; PAS, Patient Activity Scale; HAQ, Health Assessment Questionnaire; RAPID-3, Routine Assessment of Patient Index Data with 3 measures; MDHAQ, Multidimensional HAQ; SDAI, Simplified Disease Activity Index.

Table 5: Cut-off values for various disease activity measures

Disease activity measure	Scale	Remission	Low	Moderate	High
PAS/PAS II	0–10	0.00–0.25	0.26–3.70	3.71–<8.0	>8.0
RAPID-3	0–10	0–1.0	>1.0–2.0	>2.0–4.0	>4.0
CDAI	0–76	≤2.8	>2.8–10.0	>10.0–22.0	>22.0
DAS28 (ESR or CRP)	0–9.4	≤2.6	>2.6–3.2	>3.2–5.1	>5.1
SDAI	0–86	≤3.3	>3.3–11.0	>11.0–26	>26

PAS, patient activity scale; RAPID-3, routine assessment of patient index data with 3 measures; CDAI, clinical disease activity index; DAS28, disease activity score with 28-joint counts; ESR, erythrocyte sedimentation rate; CRP, C-reactive protein; SDAI, simplified disease activity index.

and strategize various treatment options for patients of RA. The following are salient features for devising a treatment strategy:[18,22,26]

- Methotrexate should be part of the first treatment strategy in patients with active RA. In cases of MTX contraindications (or early intolerance), leflunomide or sulfasalazine should be considered
- Monitoring should be frequent in active disease (every 1–3 months); if there is no response to treatment by 3 months after optimization of doses or the target has not been reached by 6 months, therapy should be adjusted
- If the treatment target is not achieved with the first DMARD strategy, in the absence of poor prognostic factors, change to another synthetic DMARD strategy should be considered; when poor prognostic factors are present, addition of a biologic DMARD should be considered. In patients responding insufficiently to MTX and/or other synthetic DMARD strategies, with or without glucocorticoids, biologic DMARDs should be commenced with MTX. Rituximab is particularly preferred in seropositive RA patients with history of lymphoma, demyelinating disorders, and high risk of TB reactivation
- If a first biologic DMARD has failed, patients should be treated with another biologic DMARD; in case of secondary anti-TNF failure, patients may receive another TNF inhibitor or a biological agent with another mode of action
- If a patient is in persistent remission after having tapered glucocorticoids, one can consider tapering biologic DMARDs, especially if this treatment is combined with a synthetic DMARD. In cases of sustained long-term remission, cautious reduction of the synthetic DMARD dose could be considered, as a shared decision between patient and physician.

REFERENCES

1. Marita C, Emma S, Damian H, Loreto C, Frederick W, Theo V, et al. The global burden of rheumatoid arthritis: estimates from the Global Burden of Disease 2010 study. Ann Rheum Dis. 2014;73(7):1316-22.
2. Charles GH, David TF, Reva CL, Sherine G, Rosemarie H, Kent K, et al. Estimates of the prevalence of arthritis and other rheumatic conditions in the United States. Arthritis Rheum. 2008;58(1):15-25.
3. Gibofsky A. Overview of Epidemiology, Pathophysiology, and Diagnosis of Rheumatoid Arthritis. Am J Manag Care. 2012;18(13 Suppl):S295-302.
4. Ahlmén M, Svensson B, Albertsson K, Forslind K, Hafström I. Influence of gender on assessments of disease activity and function in early rheumatoid arthritis in relation to radiographic joint damage. Ann Rheum Dis. 2010;69(1):230-3.
5. Areskoug-Josefsson K, Oberg U. A literature review of the sexual health of women with rheumatoid arthritis. Musculoskeletal Care. 2009;7(4):219-26.
6. Smolen JS, Aletaha D, Koeller M, Weisman MH, Emery P. New therapies for treatment of rheumatoid arthritis. Lancet. 2007;370(9602):1861-74.
7. Weyand CM, Hicok KC, Conn DL, Goronzy JJ. The influence of HLA-DRB1 genes on disease severity in rheumatoid arthritis. Ann Intern Med. 1992;117(10):801-6.
8. Smolen JS, Steiner G. Therapeutic strategies for rheumatoid arthritis. Nat Rev Drug Discov. 2003;2(6):473-88..
9. McInnes IB, Schett G. Cytokines in the pathogenesis of rheumatoid arthritis. Nat Rev Immunol. 2007;7(6):429-42.
10. Shahrara S, Huang Q, Mandelin AM 2nd, Pope RM. TH-17 cells in rheumatoid arthritis. Arthritis Res Ther. 2008;10:R93.
11. Fleming A, Crown JM, Corbett M. Incidence of joint involvement in early rheumatoid arthritis. Rheumatol Rehabil. 1976;15(2):92-6.
12. Menezes AH, VanGilder JC, Clark CR, el-Khoury G. Odontoid upward migration in rheumatoid arthritis. An analysis of 45 patients with "cranial settling". J Neurosurg. 1985;63(4):500-9.
13. Taniguchi D, Tokunaga D, Hase H, Mikami Y, Hojo T, Ikeda T, et al. Evaluation of lateral instability of the atlanto-axial joint in rheumatoid arthritis using dynamic open-mouth view radiographs. Clin Rheumatol. 2008;27(7):851-7.
14. Ranawat CS, O'Leary P, Pellicci P, et al. Cervical spine fusion in rheumatoid arthritis. J Bone Joint Surg Am. 1979;61(7):1003-10.
15. Swedler W, Wallman J, Froelich CJ, Teodorescu M. Routine measurement of IgM, IgG, and IgA rheumatoid factors: high sensitivity, specificity, and predictive value for rheumatoid arthritis. J Rheumatol. 1997;24(6):1037-44.
16. Anuradha V, Chopra A. In the era of nephlometry, latex agglutination is still good enough to detect rheumatoid factor. J Rheumatol. 2005;32:2343-4.
17. Lee DM, Schur PH. Clinical utility of the anti-CCP assay in patients with rheumatic diseases. Ann Rheum Dis. 2003;62:870-4.
18. Singh JA, Furst DE, Bharat A, Curtis JR, Kavanaugh AF, Kremer JM, et al. 2012 update of the 2008 American College of Rheumatology recommendations for the use of disease-modifying antirheumatic drugs and biologic agents in the treatment of rheumatoid arthritis. Arthritis Care Res (Hoboken). 2012;64(5):625-39.
19. Saag KG, Teng GG, Patkar NM, Anuntiyo J, Finney C, Curtis JR. American College of Rheumatology 2008 recommendations for the use of nonbiologic and biologic disease-modifying antirheumatic drugs in rheumatoid arthritis. Arthritis Rheum. 2008;59(6):762-84.
20. Tosh JC, Wailoo AJ, Scott DL, Deighton CM. Cost-effectiveness of combination nonbiologic disease-modifying antirheumatic drug strategies in patients with early rheumatoid arthritis. J Rheumatol. 2011;38(8):1593-600.
21. Aletaha D, Funovits J, Keystone EC, Smolen JS. Disease activity early in the course of treatment predicts response to therapy after one year in rheumatoid arthritis patients. Arthritis Rheum. 2007;56:3226-35.
22. Johns KR, Littlejohn GO. The safety and efficacy of cyclosporine (Neoral) in rheumatoid arthritis. J Rheumatol. 1999;26(10):2110-3.
23. Marcos JC, Maccagno A, Gutfraind E, Garsd A, Messina DO, Maldonado Cocco J, et al. Efficacy, tolerability and safety of cyclosporine for microemulsion in the treatment of active rheumatoid arthritis. Open study. Medicina (B Aires). 2000;60(4):435-40.
24. Suarez-Almazor ME, Spooner C, Belseck E. Azathioprine for treating rheumatoid arthritis. Cochrane Database Syst Rev. 2000;(4):CD001461.
25. Smolen J (on behalf of the EULAR Task Force. Session 10: update of EULAR rheumatoid arthritis management recommendations). Presented at EULAR 2013, the Annual Congress of the European League Against Rheumatism. Madrid, Spain; 2013.
26. Singh JA, Saag KG, Bridges SL Jr, Akl EA, Bannuru RR, Sullivan MC, et. al. 2015 American College of Rheumatology guideline for the treatment of rheumatoid arthritis. Arthritis Care Res (Hoboken). 2016;68(1):1-25.
27. Goekoop-Ruiterman YP, de Vries-Bouwstra JK, Allaart CF. Clinical and radiographic outcomes of four different treatment strategies in patients with early rheumatoid arthritis (the BeSt study). Arth Rheum. 2005;52:3381-90.
28. Moreland LW, O'Dell JR, Paulus HE, Curtis JR, Bathon JM, St Clair EW, et al. A randomized comparative effectiveness study of oral triple therapy versus etanercept plus methotrexate in early aggressive rheumatoid arthritis: the treatment of Early Aggressive Rheumatoid Arthritis Trial. Arthritis Rheum. 2012;64(9):2824-35.
29. Jamal S, Patra K, Keystone EC. Adalimumab response in patients with early versus established rheumatoid arthritis: DE019 randomized controlled trial subanalysis. Clin Rheumatol. 2009;28(4):413-9.
30. European Medicines Agency. Draft overarching guidelines on biosimilars: Guideline on Similar Biological Medicinal Products (Reference number: CHMP/437/04 Rev 1). European Medicines Agency. [Online] May 22, 2013.

31. World Health Organization. Expert Committee on Biological Standardization. Guidelines on Evaluation of Similar Biotherapeutic Products (SBPs). World Health Organization. [Online]. 2009.
32. U.S. Food and Drug Administration. Guidance for Industry: quality considerations in demonstration biosimilarity to a reference protein product. Washington DC: U.S. Food and Drug Administration; 2012.
33. Jani M, Barton S, Warren RB, Griffiths CE, Chinoy H. The role of DMARDs in reducing the immunogenicity of TNF inhibitors in chronic inflammatory diseases. Rheumatology (Oxford). 2014;53(2):213-22.
34. Vincent FB, Morand EF, Murphy K, Mackay F, Mariette X, Marcelli C. Antidrug Antibodies (ADAb) to Tumour Necrosis Factor (TNF)-specific Neutralising Agents in Chronic Inflammatory Diseases. Ann Rheum Dis. 2013;72(2):165-78.
35. Bijlsma JW, Hoes JN, Van Everdingen AA, Verstappen SM, Jacobs JW. Are glucocorticoids DMARDs? Ann N Y Acad Sci. 2006;1069:268-74.
36. Cutolo M, Spies CM, Buttgereit F, Paolino S, Pizzorni C. The supplementary therapeutic DMARD role of low-dose glucocorticoids in rheumatoid arthritis. Arthritis Res Ther. 2014;16(Suppl 2):S1.
37. FDA news release. November 6, 2012. (2017).
38. Smolen JS, Kremer J. Patient-Reported Outcomes from a phase 3 study of baricitinib in patients with rheumatoid arthritis (RA) and an inadequate response to tumor necrosis factor inhibitors. Ann Rheum Dis. 2015;74:785-6.
39. Genovese MC, Fleischman R, Kivitz AJ, Rell-Bakalarska M, Martincova R, Fiore S, et al. Sarilumab plus methotrexate in patients with active rheumatoid arthritis and inadequate response to methotrexate: results of a phase III study. Arthritis Rheumatol. 2015;67(6):1424-37.
40. Smolen JS, Weinblatt ME, Sheng S, Zhuang Y, Hsu B. Sirukumab, a human anti-interleukin-6 monoclonal antibody: a randomised, 2-part (proof-of-concept and dose-finding), phase II study in patients with active rheumatoid arthritis despite methotrexate therapy. Ann Rheum Dis. 2014;73(9):1616-25.
41. Genovese MC, Durez P. One-year efficacy and safety results of secukinumab in patients with rheumatoid arthritis: phase II, dose-finding, double-blind, randomized, placebo-controlled study. J Rheumatol. 2014;41(3):414-21.

18
CHAPTER

Cutaneous Association of Rheumatological Disorders

Neetu Bhari, Rahul Mahajan

INTRODUCTION

Skin is a frequently affected organ in many rheumatological diseases such as lupus erythematosus, dermatomyositis, systemic sclerosis, Sjogren syndrome, and rheumatoid arthritis. However, there are several other cutaneous diseases which although not considered as classic rheumatic diseases by themselves but are so frequently associated with them that the presence of such dermatoses warrants an investigation for an underlying rheumatologic disorder. These include panniculitides such as erythema nodosum, neutrophilic granulomatous dermatitis, and neutrophilic dermatoses such as pyoderma gangrenosum and Sweet syndrome. Although, these dermatoses are not specific to rheumatologic diseases and can be seen in association with other systemic diseases such as internal malignancy and inflammatory bowel disease, they serve as an important indicator for the correct diagnosis as well as a marker of disease activity in these disorders. Also, arthralgia is a common accompaniment of these disorders, and therefore sometimes patient presents to rheumatologists. The present chapter will focus on reviewing the etiology, clinical features, and management of these dermatoses.

ERYTHEMA NODOSUM

Erythema nodosum is a painful disorder of the subcutaneous fat. It is the most common type of panniculitis. Most commonly, it is an idiopathic condition, but it can also be a sign of underlying systemic diseases. Overall, the incidence of erythema nodosum is approximately 1–5 per 100,000 persons.[1] In adults, it is more common among women, with a male-to-female ratio of 1:6. In children, however, there is no gender preponderance. Peak incidence occurs in people between 20 and 30 years of age, although it can be seen at any age.

Etiology

Although erythema nodosum is usually idiopathic by origin, suspected possible triggers should always be ruled out. Streptococcal infections are the most common identifiable etiology, especially in children. Drug and hormonal reactions, inflammatory bowel disease, and sarcoidosis are other common causes among adults (Table 1). In a prospective study of 50 patients of erythema nodosum from Turkey, the etiology was confirmed in 27 (50.40%) patients. Primary tuberculosis was the most common cause (9) followed by poststreptococcal erythema nodosum (8), sarcoidosis (6), inflammatory bowel disease (2), Behcet's syndrome (1), and pregnancy (1).[2]

In another study of 132 patients of erythema nodosum, an etiological agent could be found in 86 patients (65.15%). Sarcoidosis was confirmed as an etiology in 37 (28%) patients, infections in 25 patients, (Epstein–Barr virus, and Cytomegalovirus in 13 patients, streptococcal infection in 8, tuberculosis in 2, and salmonellosis in 2 patients); Behcet's syndrome in 5 patients and

Skin in Rheumatologic Diseases

Table 1: Common etiological factors for erythema nodosum	
• Idiopathic (up to 55%) • Infections: Streptococcal pharyngitis (28–48%), *Yersinia spp.*, mycoplasma, chlamydia, histoplasmosis, coccidioidomycosis, mycobacteria • Sarcoidosis (11–25%) • Drugs (3–10%): Antibiotics (e.g., sulphonamides, amoxicillin), oral contraceptives • Pregnancy (2–5%) • Enteropathies (1–4%): Regional enteritis, ulcerative colitis	• Rare (less than 1%) • Infections • Viral: Herpes simplex virus, Epstein-Barr virus, hepatitis B and C viruses, human immunodeficiency virus • Bacterial: *Campylobacter spp.*, rickettsiae, *Salmonella spp.*, Psittacosis, *Bartonella spp.*, Syphilis • Parasitic: Amebiasis, giardiasis • Miscellaneous: Lymphoma, other malignancies

Sjogren's syndrome in 1; pregnancy and oral contraceptives caused erythema nodosum in 13 patients and drugs (penicillin, sulfonamides) were associated with erythema nodosum in 5 patients (3.8%).[3]

Clinical Features

Erythema nodosum is characterized by the sudden eruption of erythematous and tender nodules or plaques located mainly over the extensor aspect of lower extremities (Fig. 1). Onset of skin lesions is often preceded by a prodrome consisting of malaise, low-grade fever, cough and arthralgia with or without arthritis. This commonly occurs 1–3 weeks before the onset of erythema nodosum. Nodules range from 1 to 10 cm size in diameter and are most commonly located over the pretibial area, although the extensor surfaces of the forearm and thighs, and trunk may also be affected.

These nodules often take approximately 1–2 months to heal completely and may assume a bruise-like appearance as they fade (Fig. 2). They do not ulcerate and usually resolve without atrophy or scarring. Relapses are uncommon, but in patients with idiopathic, streptococcal or erythema nodosum associated with other upper respiratory tract infections, they are more frequent. New lesions may continue to appear for up to 6 weeks.

Clinical Variants

Clinical variants include erythema nodosum migrans, subacute nodular migratory panniculitis of Vilanova and Pinol, and chronic erythema nodosum.[4]

Erythema nodosum migrans, a disorder characterized by migrating erythematous subcutaneous nodules or plaque on the legs, was first

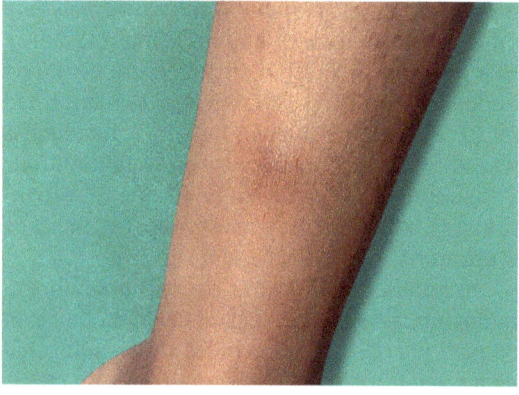

FIGURE 1: Erythematous, tender nodule over the extensor aspect of lower extremity.
Courtesy: Dr Sanjay Singh, Department of Dermatology, All India Institute of Medical Sciences, New Delhi.

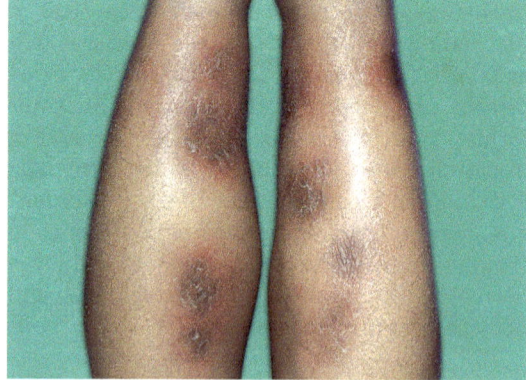

FIGURE 2: Multiple erythema nodosum lesions over both legs.

described by Bafverstedt in 1954. It was renamed as subacute nodular migratory panniculitis by Vilanova and Piñol Aguade in 1956. It is seen predominantly in women and is often unilateral in contrast to the bilateral nature of classic erythema nodosum. It initially appears as an erythematous nodule on the lateral aspects of lower legs, these nodules extend centrifugally with central clearing to form plaques with the yellow atrophic center. Lesions tend to be less tender than those of classic erythema nodosum and systemic symptoms are also less common. Chronic erythema nodosum is considered as a later stage of evolution, as inflammatory changes are less evident during this stage though some authors consider it as a different variant of erythema nodosum.[5]

Erythema induratum is also a close differential diagnosis, which presents clinically as recurrent crops of tender, violaceous nodules and plaques on the posterior lower legs. The nodules tend to ulcerate and heal with scarring and post-inflammatory hyperpigmentation. Female predominance is seen.[6]

Diagnosis

In the diagnostic workup (Box 1) after a complete history and physical examination, skin biopsy, routine hematological examination, and chest X-ray is recommended in all the patients. Chest X-ray is helpful in detecting underlying sarcoidosis or tuberculosis. Tuberculin skin test is also recommended in the diagnostic workup of erythema nodosum, although its utility in the tuberculous-endemic countries is doubtful. Some authors recommend throat culture and determination of antistreptolysin O (ASO) antibodies.[7] Histologically, erythema nodosum is characterized by septal panniculitis with no vasculitis. The septa of subcutaneous fat are thickened and infiltrated by inflammatory cells that extend to the periseptal areas of the fat lobules. The composition of the inflammatory infiltrate in the septa varies with the age of the lesion. In early lesions, edema, hemorrhage and neutrophils are responsible for the septal thickening, whereas fibrosis, periseptal granulation tissue, lymphocytes, and multinucleated giant cells are the main findings in late stage lesions of erythema nodosum (Fig. 3). A histopathologic hallmark of erythema

> **Box 1: Workup in a patient with erythema nodosum patient**
> - Detailed history (drug exposure) and complete mucocutaneous examination
> - Complete hemogram
> - Skin biopsy
> - Chest X-ray
> - Tuberculin skin test
> - Antistreptolysin O titers
> - Throat culture
> - Malignancy workup in c/o clinical suspicion
> - Stool examination

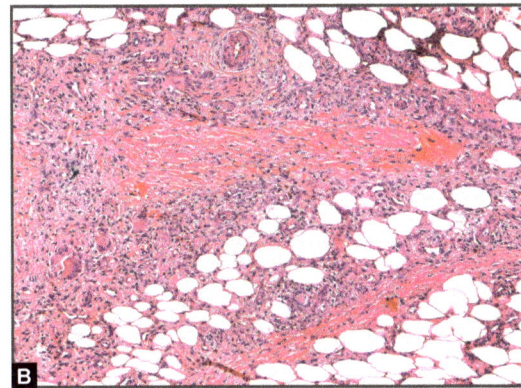

FIGURE 3: Hematoxylin and eosin stain of skin biopsy. **A,** 10x, the septa of subcutaneous fat are thickened and infiltrated by inflammatory cells that extend to the periseptal areas of the fat lobules; **B,** 40x, the composition of the inflammatory infiltrate consist of lymphocytes, histiocytes, neutrophil, eosinophil, and multinucleated giant cells associated with fibrosis.
Courtesy: Dr Ramam, Professor, Department of Dermatology, All India Institute of Medical Sciences, New Delhi.

nodosum is the presence of the Miescher's radial granulomas, which consist of small, well-defined nodular aggregations of small histiocytes arranged radially around a central cleft of variable shape. Histological examination of erythema induratum shows granulomatous septolobular panniculitis and predominant lobular involvement with primary neutrophilic vasculitis of nearby vessels.[6]

Treatment

Erythema nodosum is usually a self-limited disease. Treatment of any underlying disease and supportive therapy are the mainstay of treatment. Pain should be managed conservatively with nonsteroidal anti-inflammatory drugs (NSAIDs).[8]

Systemic steroids have been advocated as a relatively safe therapeutic option if underlying infection and malignancy have been excluded by a thorough evaluation. A general rule is 1 mg per kg body weight per day of oral prednisolone which is then slowly tapered based on the disease activity.[5]

Oral potassium iodide prepared as a supersaturated solution in a dosage of 400–900 mg per day can be given after 3–4 months of clinical improvement. In a study of 15 patients of erythema nodosum, 11 out of 15 patients showed significant improvement in their disease activity with this therapy. The effect of the drug is most marked in patients with positive C-reactive protein, joint pains and fever as the main mechanism of action is anti-inflammatory activity.[9]

Treatment may also be tailored to disease-specific regimens—steroids used in combination with hydroxychloroquine, cyclosporine, or thalidomide have been used to treat inflammatory bowel disease-associated erythema nodosum.[5] Nonsteroidal anti-inflammatory drugs should be avoided in treating erythema nodosum secondary to Crohn's disease because they may trigger a flare-up or worsen an ongoing acute bout. Colchicine has been used in patients with erythema nodosum and coexisting Behçet's syndrome, with varying results.[10] Dapsone has shown efficacy in erythema nodosum triggered by isotretinoin intake.[11] There are few reports of treatment of resistant erythema nodosum cases with biologics as etanercept and adalimumab.[12,13]

SWEET'S SYNDROME

Sweet's syndrome is classified under neutrophilic dermatosis. It usually presents with the abrupt onset of fever, peripheral neutrophilia, and tender erythematous skin lesions. It is also known as acute febrile neutrophilic dermatosis and Gomm-Button disease.

Sweet's syndrome can present in several clinical settings—classical (or idiopathic) Sweet's syndrome, malignancy-associated Sweet's syndrome, and drug-induced Sweet's syndrome.

Etiology

Sweet's syndrome is associated with a variety of underlying conditions such as infection, inflammatory disorders, pregnancy, malignancy, and drugs.

Classical Sweet's syndrome usually presents in women between the age of 30 and 50 years. It is often preceded by an upper respiratory tract infection and may be associated with inflammatory bowel disease and pregnancy. The malignancy-associated Sweet's syndrome is most commonly related to acute myelogenous leukemia, other associated solid tumors are genitourinary, breast, and gastrointestinal which are seen in around 15% of cases. Table 2 summarizes the various etiologies associated with Sweet's syndrome. Drug-induced Sweet's syndrome most commonly occurs in patients treated with the granulocyte-colony stimulating factor. Other implicated drugs

Table 2: Etiology of Sweet's syndrome

Cancer	Hematologic malignancies (acute myelogenous leukemia) and solid tumors (carcinomas of the genitourinary organs, breast, and gastrointestinal tract)
Infections	Upper respiratory tract streptococcal and gastrointestinal tract salmonella, tuberculosis, hepatitis C virus
Inflammatory bowel disease	Crohn's disease and ulcerative colitis
Medications	Granulocyte colony-stimulating factor, antibiotics, antiepileptics, retinoids
Pregnancy	–

are retinoids, minocycline, carbamazepine, and oral contraceptive.[7]

Clinical Features

Classical Sweet's Syndrome

Clinically, Sweet's syndrome presents with fever and leukocytosis. Fever is seen in more than 80% of cases. Other systemic symptoms include arthralgia, malaise, headache, and myalgia. Skin lesions are characterized by excruciatingly tender erythematous papules or nodules that may coalesce to form plaques (Fig. 4). The most common sites involved are the upper extremities, face and neck.

The lesions may be single (Fig. 5) or multiple. They show a transparent vesicle-like appearance due to the pronounced edema in the papillary dermis. With time, the lesions develop central clearing, giving annular or arcuate patterns (Fig. 6). The lesions heal without scarring. Cutaneous pathergy at sites of trauma, such as biopsy sites or venepuncture can be seen.[14]

Clinical Variants

In malignancy-associated Sweet's syndrome, lesions may appear bullous or may ulcerate. It comprises 20–25% of Sweet's syndrome cases (Fig. 7). Lesions may recur in one-third to two-thirds of patients.[15] Patients with inflammatory bowel diseases may develop a pustular variant of Sweet's syndrome.[16]

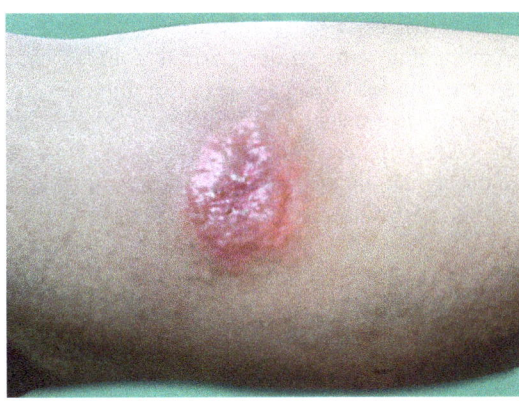

FIGURE 5: Solitary lesion of sweet syndrome over forearm.

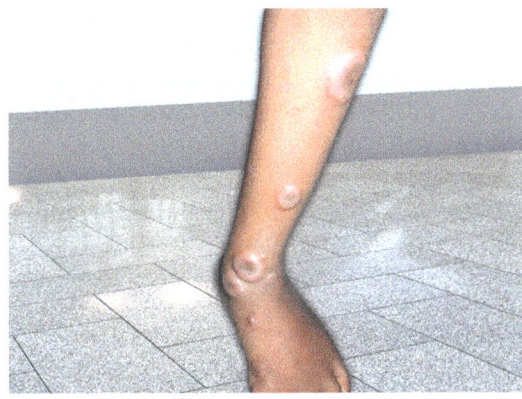

FIGURE 6: Multiple erythematous, edematous, tender plaques over lower limbs with central clearing giving an annular or arcuate pattern.

Courtesy: Dr Banwari Jangid, Department of Dermatology, All India Institute of Medical Sciences, New Delhi.

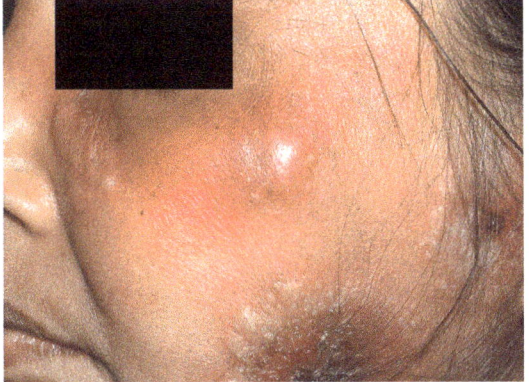

FIGURE 4: Sweet syndrome: Erythematous edematous plaques over cheek in an elderly female.

Courtesy: Dr Neena, Professor, Department of Dermatology, All India Institute of Medical Sciences, New Delhi.

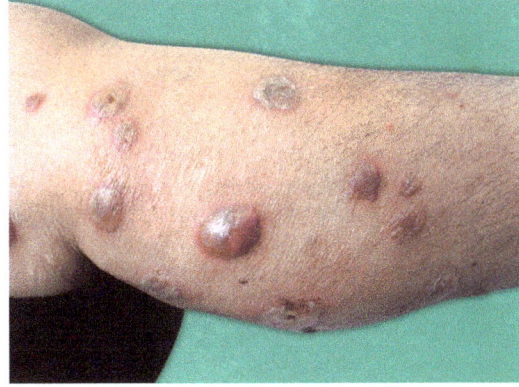

FIGURE 7: Multiple discrete, hemorrhagic fluid filled bulla over lower leg.

Courtesy: Dr Arshdeep, Postgraduate Institute of Medical Education and Research, Chandigarh.

Subcutaneous Sweet's syndrome presents as erythematous and tender dermal nodules over the extremities. Most cases are accompanied by fever, with the lower limbs being the predominant site of lesion occurrence. Histological changes in the subcutaneous tissue involve neutrophils infiltrating the lobules, the septae, or both.[17]

Extracutaneous Manifestations

Bones, central nervous system, ears, eyes, kidneys, intestines, liver, heart, lung, muscles and spleen can be the sites of extracutaneous manifestations of Sweet's syndrome. Bone and joint manifestations includes sterile arthritis, arthralgias, focal aseptic osteitis, pigmented villonodular synovitis, and osteomyelitis.[18,19] Central nervous system may be affected in the form of aseptic meningitis, acute benign encephalitis, Guillain-Barre syndrome, "neuro-Sweet disease", polyneuropathy, and psychiatric symptoms.[20]

Ocular manifestations may be the presenting feature of Sweet's syndrome. Blepharitis, conjunctivitis, episcleritis, glaucoma, iridocyclitis, iritis, peripheral ulcerative keratitis, retinal vasculitis, scleritis, and uveitis are reported associations.[21,22]

Diagnostic Criteria for Sweet's Syndrome (Table 3)

The diagnostic criteria for classical Sweet's syndrome were originally proposed by Su and Liu in 1986.[23] These criteria were modified by von den Driesch in 1994.[24]

Skin biopsy is an important adjunct in the diagnosis of Sweet's syndrome. Evaluation of underlying systemic abnormalities should be done only in the presence of associated clinical clues.

Histopathology

Sweet's syndrome is characterized by a diffuse dermal inflammatory cell infiltrate composed of mature neutrophils, in addition to papillary dermal edema. Karyorrhexis, swollen endothelial cells, and dilated small blood vessels may also be appreciated (Fig. 8).[25]

Histiocytoid Sweet Syndrome

Requana et al. in 2005, was the first to describe histiocytoid Sweet syndrome as a variant of acute febrile neutrophilic dermatosis. Although, the clinical presentation is similar to typical Sweet's

Table 3: Diagnostic criteria for Sweet's syndrome	
Classical Sweet's syndrome	**Drug-induced Sweet's syndrome**
1. Abrupt onset of painful erythematous plaques or nodules	A. Abrupt onset of painful erythematous plaques or nodules
2. Histologic evidence of a dense neutrophilic infiltrate without evidence of leukocytoclastic vasculitis	B. Histologic evidence of a dense neutrophilic infiltrates without evidence of leukocytoclastic vasculitis
3. Pyrexia >38°C	C. Pyrexia >38°C
4. Association with an underlying hematologic or visceral malignancy, inflammatory bowel disease, or pregnancy, or preceded by an upper respiratory or gastrointestinal infection or vaccination	D. Temporal relationship between drug ingestion and clinical presentation, or temporally-related recurrence after oral challenge
5. Excellent response to treatment with systemic corticosteroids or potassium iodide	E. Temporally-related resolution of lesions after drug withdrawal or treatment with systemic corticosteroids
6. Abnormal laboratory values at presentation (three of four): Erythrocyte sedimentation rate >20 mm/hour; positive C-reactive protein; >8,000 leukocytes; >70% neutrophils	

1. The presence of both major criteria (1 and 2), and two of the four minor criteria (3, 4, 5, and 6) is required in order to establish the diagnosis of classical Sweet's syndrome; the patients with malignancy-associated Sweet's syndrome are included with the patients with classical Sweet's syndrome in this list of diagnostic criteria.
2. All five criteria (A, B, C, D, and E) are required for the diagnosis of drug-induced Sweet's syndrome.

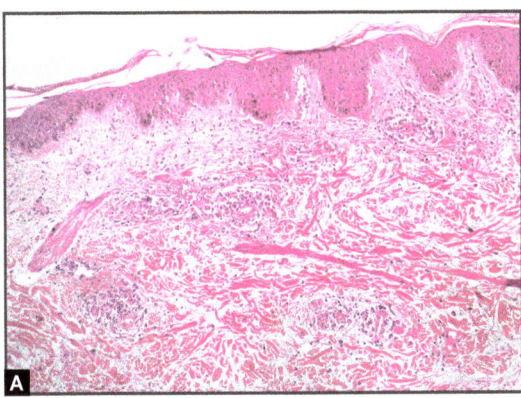 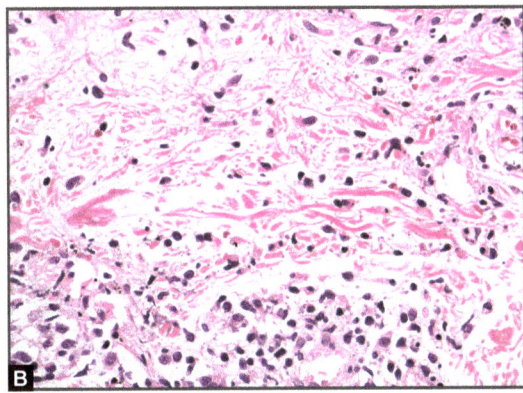

FIGURE 8: Hematoxylin and eosin stain of skin biopsy. **A,** 10x, superficial and deep dermis showing perivascular, perieccrine infiltrate; **B,** The infiltrate is composed of mainly neutrophils, lymphocytes, and histiocytes.
Courtesy: Dr Sujay Khandpur, Professor, Department of Dermatology, All India Institute of Medical Sciences, New Delhi.

syndrome, histologically there is a dense dermal infiltrate of mononuclear cells with large, slightly eccentric, elongated, kidney-shaped, basophilic nuclei that immunohistochemically stain with CD15, CD43, CD45, CD68, MAC-386, HAM56 and lysozyme. These cases are usually associated with hematologic or visceral malignancies.[26]

Treatment

Topical or Intralesional Corticosteroids

Topical or intralesional corticosteroids can be used to treat patients who have a small number of localized Sweet's syndrome lesions. Intralesional triamcinolone acetonide can be used at a dose ranging from 3 to 10 mg/mL.[27]

Systemic Corticosteroids

Systemic corticosteroids are the "gold standard" of therapy for Sweet's syndrome. Systemic corticosteroid treatment is usually started at 1 mg/kg/day dose. The dose can be tapered to 10 mg/day within 4–6 weeks. Intravenous corticosteroid therapy may be necessary in refractory cases and those with frequent recurrences.[28]

Potassium Iodide

Potassium iodide therapy results in resolution of symptoms within 1–2 days and skin lesions subside within 3–5 days. A saturated solution (1 g/mL of water) of potassium iodide is used most commonly. It is initially given at a dose of three drops three times a day. One drop equals 0.05 mL (or 50 mg if the concentration of potassium iodide is 1,000 mg/mL). Therefore, the initial dose nine drops per day equals to 450 mg of potassium iodide per day. The dose is increased by one drop three times a day, up to a maximum of 20–30 drops per day. Rhinorrhea, increased lacrimation, and hypothyroidism are potential side effects of potassium iodide.[29]

Colchicine

Several large studies have shown the efficacy of colchicine in the management of Sweet's syndrome. It is usually used in a dose of 0.5 mg orally three times each day. Maillard et al. reported 20 patients with Sweet's syndrome of whom 90% (18 individual) responded to colchicine therapy—fever resolved within 2–3 days, skin lesions improved within 2–5 days, arthralgia disappeared within 2–4 days, and leukocytosis normalized within 8–14 days. Most common adverse effect seen is gastrointestinal disturbance.[30]

Steroid Sparing Immunosuppressive Agents

Treatment with immunosuppressants such as cyclosporine (2–5 mg/kg/day), dapsone (1.5–2 mg/kg/day), azathioprine (1.5–2 mg/kg/day), cyclophosphamide (1–1.5 mg/kg/day), interferon-a, etretinate, thalidomide, and tumor necrosis factor (TNF)-α blockers have been reported to be successful in refractory cases.[31,32]

PYODERMA GANGRENOSUM

Pyoderma gangrenosum (PG) is also classified under neutrophilic dermatosis. It is characterized by extremely painful ulcers present with undermined bluish borders with surrounding erythema. It may be associated with underlying inflammatory bowel disease, connective tissue disorder, or neoplasia.

The peak incidence occurs between the ages of 20 and 50 years with women being more often affected than men. The general incidence has been estimated to be between 3 and 10 per million per year.[33] Powell et al. suggested a classification of PG into four major clinical types: (i) ulcerative, (ii) bullous, (iii) pustular, and (iv) vegetative.[34]

Etiology

About 50% of patients show an underlying disorder.[35] About 25% of patients have associated arthritis, most often seropositive rheumatoid arthritis, although the disease can occur in patients with seronegative arthritis or spondyloarthropathy. Ulcerative colitis is found in 10–15% of cases. Crohn's disease is also a commonly associated disease. On the other hand, less than 3% of patients with Crohn's disease or ulcerative colitis develop PG. Pyoderma gangrenosum is associated with paraproteinemia in up to 15% of patients, mostly of the IgA but also of the IgG and IgM types.[33] It can also occur with acute myeloblastic, myelomonocytic, chronic myeloid leukemia, and in myelodysplasia (15–25%). In a review of 18 cases, six cases (33%) had associated diseases [inflammatory bowel disease (n = 2, 11%), monoclonal gammopathy (n = 2, 11%), rheumatoid arthritis (n = 1, 6%), and diabetes mellitus (n =1, 6%)].[36] Box 2 enumerates the diseases associated with pyoderma gangrenosum.

Pyoderma gangrenosum can also occur secondary to drugs. Implicated drugs include propylthiouracil, pegfilgrastim—a granulocyte-stimulating factor, and gefitinib—an inhibitor of epidermal growth factor receptor.[35]

Clinical Features

Pyoderma gangrenosum occurs most commonly on the lower legs, preferentially involving the pretibial area (Fig. 9). Lesions have been reported on other sites of the body as well, including breast, hand, trunk, head and neck, and peristomal skin. In a review of 18 cases, anatomic locations involved were lower legs (n = 14, 78%), abdomen (n = 5, 28%), arms (n = 3, 17%), breast (n = 2, 11%),

> **Box 2: Diseases associated with pyoderma gangrenosum**
>
> - Disease of gastrointestinal tract
>   - Inflammatory bowel disease: Crohn's disease, diverticulitis, ulcerative colitis
> - Hematologic disease
>   - Myeloproliferative disease: Aplastic anemia, essential thrombocytopenia, Hodgkin's disease, leukemia, monoclonal gammopathy, myelofibrosis, myeloma, non-Hodgkin's lymphoma, polycythemia vera
> - Rheumatologic disease: Osteoarthritis, psoriatic arthritis, relapsing polychondritis, rheumatoid arthritis, seronegative arthritis, spondylitis, sterile chronic multifocal osteomyelitis, systemic lupus erythematosus, Takayasu syndrome
> - Miscellaneous rare associations: Acne conglobata, chronic active hepatitis, complement deficiency, diabetes mellitus, erythema elevatum diutinum, Fanconi's anemia, hemoglobinemia, hepatitis C, hidradenitis suppurativa, human immunodeficiency virus, Kartagener's syndrome, lung cysts, necrotizing sclerokeratitis, pyogenic arthritis, pyoderma gangrenosum, and acne syndrome, paroxysmal nocturnal hemoglobinuria, phospholipid syndrome, primary biliary cirrhosis, sarcoidosis, Vaquez disease, Wegener's granulomatosis

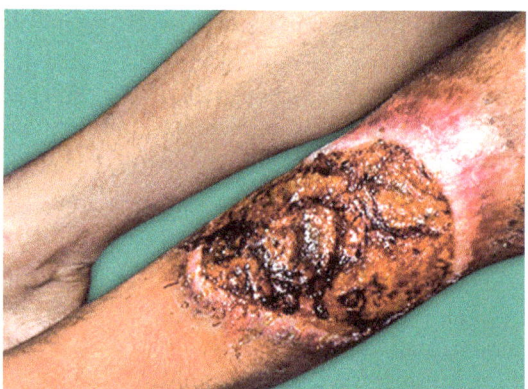

FIGURE 9: Pyoderma gangrenosum lesion over leg healing from periphery.

Courtesy: Dr Ramam, Professor, Department of Dermatology, All India Institute of Medical Sciences, New Delhi.

and buttocks (n = 1, 6%). Five patients (28%) had lesions at multiple locations (n ≥2).[36] Extracutaneous manifestations include involvement of upper airway mucosa, nodular scleritis, genital mucosal involvement causing vulvovaginal ulceration, pulmonary nodule with necrosis or splenic abscesses, and neutrophilic myositis. Multiple lesions can also be seen. In a review of 44 cases by Driesh et al., 52% of patients had one lesion, 37% had up to five and 11% had more than five lesions.[33]

Classic/Ulcerative Form

The ulcer starts as a small pustule with rapid growth followed by tissue necrosis and large ulcer. The surrounding skin becomes erythematous, edematous, and infiltrated. The ulcer borders are typically undermined and have violaceous hue (Fig. 10). The ulcer is usually malodorous due to secondary infection. Lesions are extremely painful. Patients often have constitutional symptoms such as fever, malaise, arthralgia, and myalgia. When the lesions heal the scars are often cribriform (Figs 11 and 12). Pathergy occurs in 25–50% of cases as lesions develop at the site of minor trauma.[37]

Pustular Pyoderma Gangrenosum

Pustular pyoderma is a rare variant of the disease. Lesion begins as a pustule or group of pustules that later coalesce and ulcerate. It is seen in patients with inflammatory bowel disease and tends to occur on the trunk and extensor surfaces of the limbs.[38]

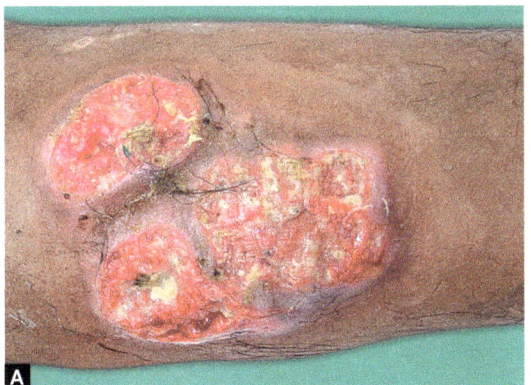
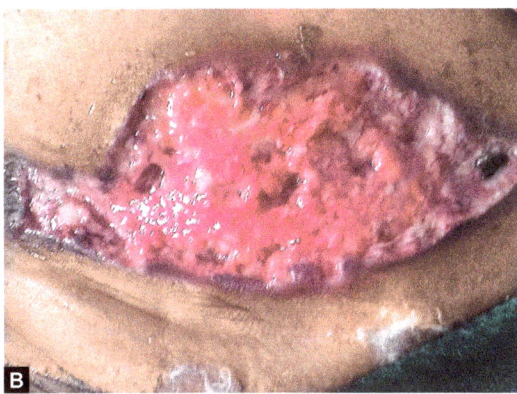

FIGURE 10: A, A well-defined large pyoderma gangrenosum (PG) ulcer over the lower leg; **B,** A PG ulcer over the abdomen, with undermined borders, hemorrhagic base, and violaceous hue.

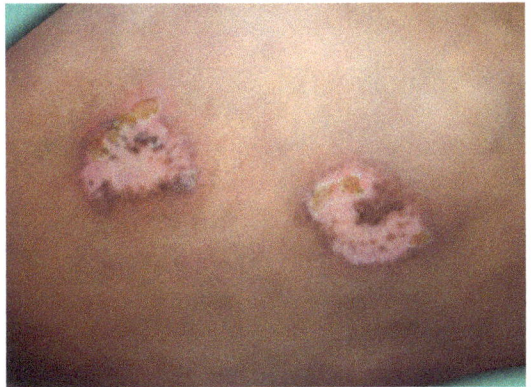
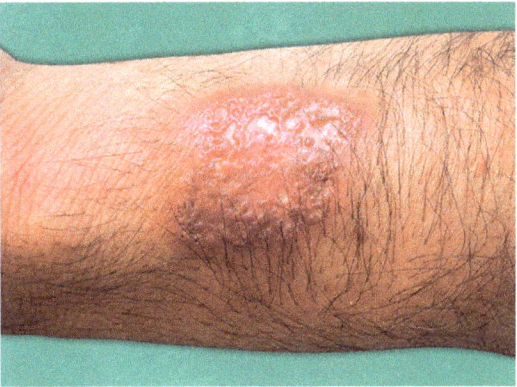

FIGURE 11: Pyoderma gangrenosum ulcer healing with scarring.

FIGURE 12: Pyoderma gangrenosum ulcer healing with cribriform scarring.

Bullous Pyoderma Gangrenosum

Bullous pyoderma gangrenosum is a superficial variant (Fig. 13). Most commonly it affects the upper limbs and face. It is associated with hematological malignancy. It presents as concentric bullous areas that spread rapidly in a concentric pattern and may break down to form superficial ulcers. Prognosis is often poor because of the underlying hematological malignancy.[39]

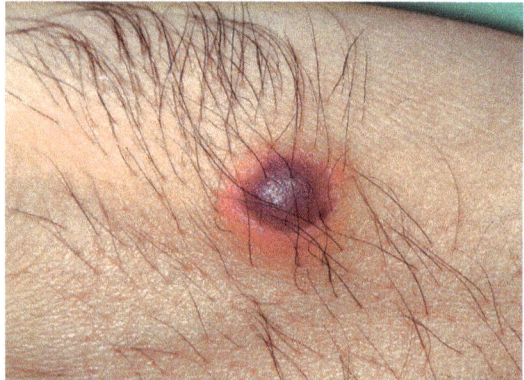

FIGURE 13: Hemorrhagic bullous pyoderma gangrenosum in an acute myeloid leukemia patient.

Vegetative Pyoderma Gangrenosum

Vegetative pyoderma gangrenosum is a superficial form of disease and is less aggressive than other variants (Fig. 14). It usually occurs as a single lesion in patients, not associated with any underlying disease and may respond to local treatment.[35] But some patients can have extensive involvement especially children (Figs 15 and 16) and may heal with disfiguring scars in them (Fig. 17).

Peristomal Pyoderma Gangrenosum

Peristomal pyoderma gangrenosum comprises about 15% of all cases of pyoderma gangrenosum. Most of these patients have inflammatory bowel

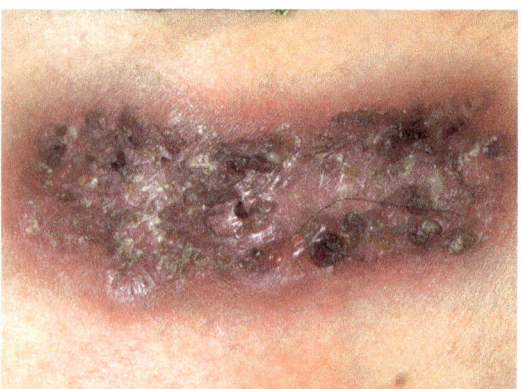

FIGURE 14: Superficial vegetative pyoderma gangrenosum.

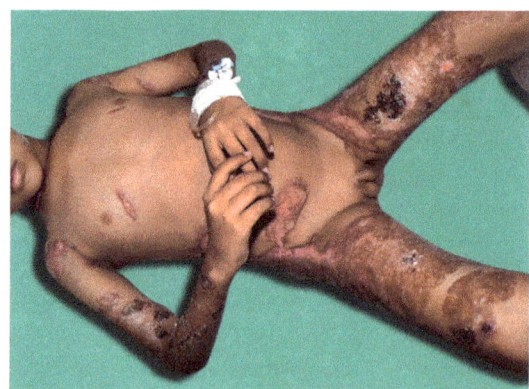

FIGURE 15: Extensive vegetative pyoderma gangrenosum in a child.

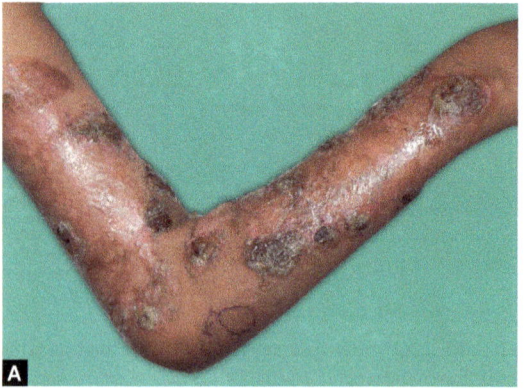
A

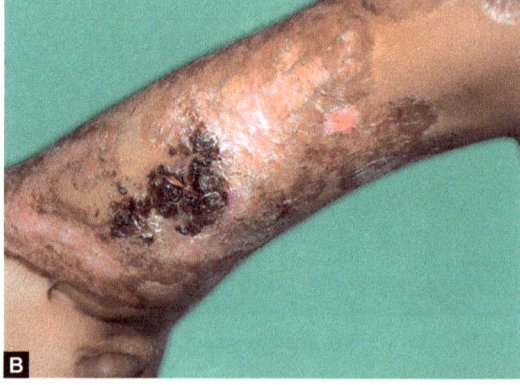
B

FIGURE 16: Vegetative pyoderma gangrenosum lesions over the limbs.

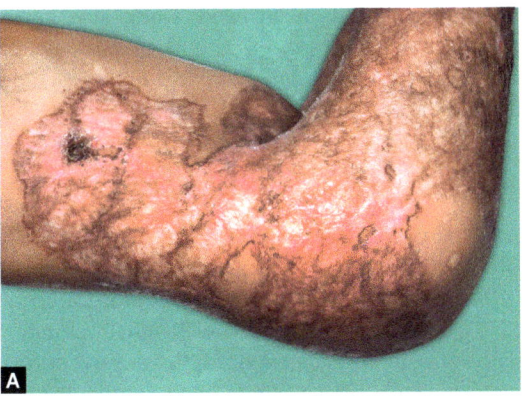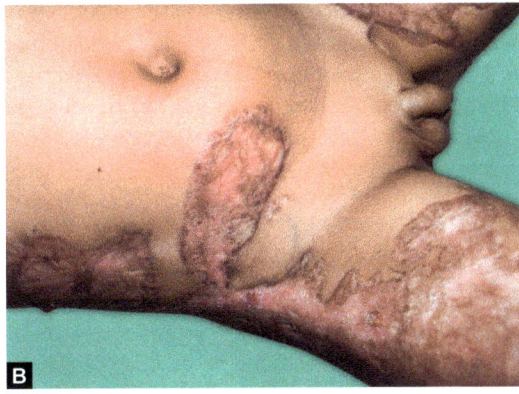

FIGURE 17: Extensive hypertrophic scars in a pyoderma gangrenosum patient.

Table 4: Diagnostic criteria for pyoderma gangrenosum	
Major criteria	**Minor criteria**
1. Rapid progression of a painful, necrotic cutaneous ulcer with an irregular, violaceous, and undermined border* 2. Other causes of cutaneous ulceration have been excluded	1. History suggestive of pathergy or clinical finding of cribriform scarring 2. Systemic diseases associated with PG 3. Histologic findings (sterile dermal neutrophilia, ± mixed inflammation, ± lymphocytic vasculitis) 4. Treatment response (rapid response to systemic steroid treatment)†

*Characteristic margin expansion of 1–2 cm/day, or a 50% increase in ulcer size within 1 month. Pain is usually out of proportion to the size of the ulceration.
†Generally responds to a dosage of 1–2 mg/kg per day, with a 50% decrease in size within 1 month.

disease, but it can also occur in patients who have had an ileostomy or colostomy for malignancy or diverticular disease. The ulcers in these patients have a similar morphology to classic pyoderma gangrenosum but bridges of normal epithelium may traverse the ulcer base.[40]

Histopathology

Histological changes are nonspecific. The early lesions show mild to moderate perivascular lymphocytic infiltrate associated with endothelial swelling. The fully developed lesions demonstrate dense neutrophil infiltration in the dermis associated with necrosis. Extravasation of erythrocytes and thrombosis can be seen occasionally. Ulceration, infarction, and abscess formation are found in the later stages of evolution. A biopsy of the advancing edge of the lesion reveals neutrophils and fibrin in superficial vessels.[41] In one large series, about 40% of patients had histologic evidence of vasculitis. Sixty-three patients with pyoderma gangrenosum were seen and studied at the Mayo Clinic from 1971 to 1980. Biopsies were taken from the erythematous border or necrotic edge of the pyoderma gangrenosum lesions and showed these characteristic features in all the cases. Immunoglobulin M, C3, and fibrin deposits in the papillary and reticular dermal vessels can be seen in direct immunofluorescence.[42]

Diagnostic Criteria for Pyoderma Gangrenosum (Table 4)

Proposed diagnostic criteria of classic, ulcerative pyoderma gangrenosum are given in table 4. Diagnosis requires both major criteria and at least two minor criteria.[43]

Treatment

Topical Therapy

Wound management is important for almost all the variants of pyoderma gangrenosum. For small lesions without secondary infection, topical high potent corticosteroids can be used. This may induce remission in the case of peristomal and vegetative pyoderma gangrenosum. Topical calcineurin inhibitors such as tacrolimus or pimecrolimus have also been used with some success.[44]

Systemic Therapy

Systemic Coritcosteroids

For patients with a more widespread disease or rapidly progressive course, systemic treatment is mandatory. Prednisolone is the drug of choice and is usually started at high doses. Prednisolone, 1–2 mg per kg per day is widely used for initial therapy. In severe cases, high-dose pulse therapy can be used to prevent progression and rapidly stop inflammation. Long-term treatment may be required in resistant cases so careful monitoring of steroid induced side effects should be done.[45]

Cyclosporine

Cyclosporine has proved to be a very helpful substitute therapy for patients in whom pyoderma gangrenosum is resistant to corticosteroid therapy or who have had serious side-effects. Doses of 2–3 mg/kg body weight per day have shown efficacy in pyoderma gangrenosum. Significant improvement occurs within weeks of oral cyclosporine and healing can be expected within 1–3 months. Renal parameters and electrolytes should be monitored carefully.[46]

Sulfa Drugs

Sulfa drugs are useful in milder cases of pyoderma gangrenosum. Sulfasalazine is used in initial daily doses of 4–6 g which are gradually reduced to maintenance levels of 0.5–1 g. Dapsone inhibits neutrophil migration and production of reactive oxygen species and exerts a variety of other anti-inflammatory effects. It can be used in a dose of 100–200 mg per day. Clofazimine has also been used in the doses of 300–400 mg per day. It exerts anti-neutrophil and anti-inflammatory activity.[47] Colchicine may be used as a single agent or in combination with prednisolone.[48]

Thalidomide: Thalidomide shows immunomodulatory activity such as suppression of TNF-α, basic fibroblast growth factor, and neutrophil chemotaxis. It has been used, along with corticosteroids in dosages ranging from 50 to 200 mg/day. Potential adverse effects include somnolence, birth defects, neuropathy, and coagulopathy.[49]

Steroid-sparing Immunosuppressive Drugs

Azathioprine (100–300 mg/day), cyclophosphamide (1.5–3.0 mg/kg/day), methotrexate (10–30 mg/week), and mycophenolate mofetil (2–3 g/day) has been used, mostly in combination with systemic corticosteroids for treating pyoderma gangrenosum. These agents have a slow onset of action and may have serious adverse effects so careful monitoring is required.

Tumor Necrosis Factor-alpha Inhibitor

Infliximab is reported to be effective in pyoderma gangrenosum associated with inflammatory bowel disease at a dosage of 5 mg/kg body weight. It is given by infusion at weeks 0, 2 and 6, and every 8 weeks thereafter. In Crohn's disease, it has been used in combination with low-dose methotrexate. Since infusion reactions can occur in 3–17% of patients with Crohn's disease that are antibody associated, the concurrent administration of steroids and the use of immunosuppressant such as methotrexate or azathioprine has been recommended.[50,51]

Etanercept has also shown its efficacy in pyoderma gangrenosum lesions. It is given by subcutaneous injections of 50 mg twice weekly. Because there is a risk of reactivation of tuberculosis during anti-tumor necrosis factor alpha therapy, patients have to be screened for tuberculosis before and during treatment.[52]

Alefacept is a recombinant protein that blocks the LFA-3/CD2 interaction, resulting in inhibition of T-lymphocyte function. In an open-label pilot study, it has shown to reduce pyoderma gangrenosum severity levels.[53]

Since pyoderma gangrenosum is a neutrophilic disease, removal of activated neutrophils should improve the symptoms. Leukocytapheresis, where white blood cells are removed extracorporeally, and granulocyte adsorptive apheresis, a more selective procedure, have been used in isolated cases with success. These methods have been used in cases unresponsive to systemic standard therapy with success.[54]

PALISADED AND NEUTROPHILIC GRANULOMATOUS DERMATITIS

Palisaded and neutrophilic granulomatous dermatitis (PNGD) is a rare inflammatory dermatosis. Synonyms are Churg-Strauss granuloma, interstitial granulomatous dermatitis with arthritis, linear subcutaneous bands, rheumatoid papules, linear granuloma annulare, rheumatoid granuloma, superficial ulcerating rheumatoid necrobiosis, necrobiotic granuloma, palisading granuloma, and cutaneous extravascular necrotizing granuloma.[55]

Etiology

Box 3 enumerates the disease associations of PNGD. This disorder is associated with immune-mediated diseases such as rheumatoid arthritis, systemic lupus erythematosus (SLE), systemic vasculitis, Behçet's disease, as well as with lymphoproliferative conditions, bacterial endocarditis, diabetes mellitus and celiac disease, sarcoidosis, and drugs such as allopurinol.[55]

Clinical Features

Clinically, PNGD presents with asymptomatic, occasionally tender, skin-colored to erythematous and violaceous papules, nodules, plaques, and annular plaques (Fig. 18) with or without central ulceration and crusting on the extensor parts of extremities, medial thighs, trunk, and hands (Fig. 19), sometimes linearly arranged.[56]

Palisaded and neutrophilic granulomatous dermatitis is a heterogeneous entity, and some authors claim that interstitial granulomatous disease (IGD) represents a separate entity. Interstitial granulomatous disease is clinically characterized by erythematous plaques or linear cords over lateral chest and axilla and histologically shows interstitial and palisaded granulomatous patterns around tiny foci of degenerated collagen with neutrophils. Interstitial granulomatous disease never shows leukocytoclastic vasculitis. Meanwhile, PNGD is clinically typified by umbilicated papules or nodules over the elbows

Box 3: Disease associations of palisaded and neutrophilic granulomatous dermatitis

- Connective tissue disease: Rheumatoid arthritis, systemic lupus erythematosus, vasculitis, Wegener's granulomatosis
- Systemic vasculitis: Periarteritis nodosa, Takayasu's aortitis
- Malignancy: Lymphoma (Hodgkin's and non-Hodgkin's), Prostate adenocarcinoma, metastatic
- Systemic disease: Sjogren's syndrome, sarcoidosis, Behcet's disease, Still's disease, multiple sclerosis, celiac disease and type 1 diabetes mellitus, limited systemic sclerosis, chronic active hepatitis, Raynaud's phenomenon, chronic ulcerative colitis
- Others: Hemolytic uremic syndrome, thrombotic thrombocytopenic purpura, streptococcal infection, bloody diarrhea, seronegative erosive arthritis, acquired immunodeficiency syndrome, subacute bacterial endocarditis, pleuropericarditis, autoimmune thyroiditis, polyarthritis

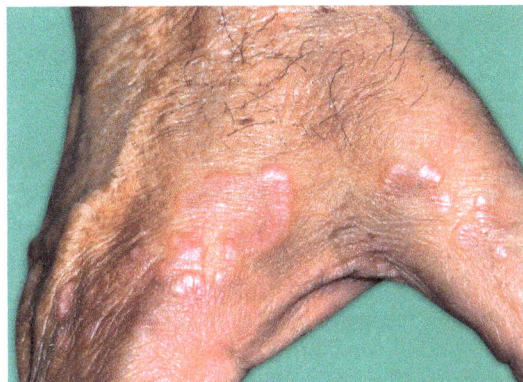

FIGURE 18: Palisaded neutrophilic granulomatous dermatitis annular plaque over the dorsum of hand.

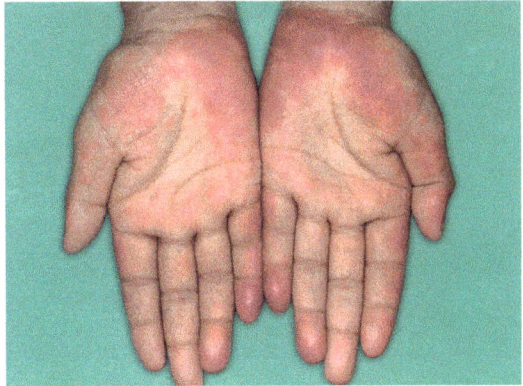

FIGURE 19: Erythematous infiltrated plaques of palisaded neutrophilic granulomatous dermatitis on the palms.

and digits and is histologically associated with palisaded necrotizing granuloma with neutrophils. Palisaded and neutrophilic granulomatous dermatitis sometimes shows leukocytoclastic vasculitis. However, overlapping clinical and histological features exist between PNGD and IGD. The patients with PNGD can have erythematous plaques on the flank as well as nodules on the digits or elbows, and the nodular lesions of PNGD on the digits or elbows can show the identical histological features as IGD.[57]

Histopathology

Histopathology of PNGD shows a spectrum of findings dependent on the duration of lesions—early lesions display leukocytoclastic vasculitis, dense neutrophilic infiltrate, and degenerated collagen; fully developed lesions appear as palisaded granulomas with neutrophils (Fig. 20). Resolving lesions show palisaded granulomas with dermal fibrosis and scant neutrophilic debris.[58]

Treatment

Lesions are self-limiting, but the condition may persist for several months to a few years. Treatment is focused on the underlying disorder. Improvement has been reported with topical corticosteroids, low-dose prednisolone and dapsone. Variable responses have been reported to cyclosporine, methotrexate, cyclophosphamide, colchicine, hydroxychloroquine, NSAIDs, and infliximab.[56]

KIKUCHI-FUJIMOTO DISEASE

Kikuchi-Fujimoto disease (KFD) is a benign, self-limited, and inflammatory disorder. It was first reported in Japan and is more prevalent among women in the third decade of life. This condition is also known as "subacute cervical necrotizing lymphadenitis" and it is characterized by persistent cervical lymphadenopathy. It is usually followed by persistent fever. Other rare presentations include leukopenia, atypical lymphocytes on peripheral smear, liver dysfunction, bone marrow involvement, fatigue, hepatosplenomegaly, and skin rash.[59] Skin rash is known to occur in around 40% of the cases and the most common skin manifestations are erythematous macules, papules, plaques, nodules, and ulcers, localized on the face, on the upper and lower extremities and on the trunk.[60]

The etiology of KFD is unknown, although viral agents as Epstein-Barr (EB) virus, parvovirus B19, and human herpesvirus-8 are implicated in pathogenesis by many authors.[61,62] A definite diagnosis of KFD is made via histological analysis which shows necrotizing granulomatous lymphadenitis.[63]

This disease usually resolves within 1–3 months and recurrence is noted in 3% of the cases. In a retrospective review, overall mortality due to KFD was estimated to be 2.1%.[61]

It seems that individuals with patients with Kikuchi disease are more susceptible to develop SLE. In a retrospective review, 55 cases of KFD

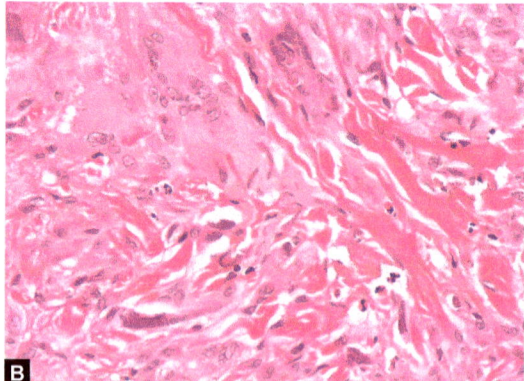

FIGURE 20: Hematoxylin and eosin stain of skin biopsy. **A,** 10X, presence of degenerated collagen surrounded with dense infiltrate in superficial, mid, and deep dermis; **B,** The infiltrate is composed of palisading granuloma and neutrophils.
Courtesy: Dr Ramam, Professor, Department of Dermatology, All India Institute of Medical Sciences, New Delhi.

occurring in the context of definite connective tissue disease were reviewed, 50 of which were associated with SLE. Of the 55 cases, 22 (40%) had simultaneous onset with, 19 (35%) predated the onset of, and 14 (25%) developed after the associated connective tissue disease.[64] Kikuchi-Fujimoto disease occurring in the context of connective tissue disease does not usually take the benign self-limiting course.

CONCLUSION

This chapter describes some rare cutaneous associations of rheumatologic diseases. Recognizing these entities is of utmost importance as it may indicate underlying associated systemic diseases as inflammatory bowel disease or an occult malignancy. Skin biopsy is usually helpful in the diagnosis. Anti-inflammatory and immunosuppressive drugs are used in the management based on the disease severity, though, most of the diseases exhibit a chronic remitting-relapsing course.

REFERENCES

1. Schwartz RA, Nervi SJ. Erythema Nodosum: a sign of systemic disease. Am Fam Physician. 2007;75:695-700.
2. Mert A, Ozaras R, Tabak F, et al. Erythema nodosum: an experience of 10 years. Scand J Infect Dis. 2004;36:424-7.
3. Psychos DN, Voulgari PV, Skopouli FN, et al. Erythema nodosum: the underlying conditions. Clin Rheumatol. 2000;19:212-6.
4. Horio T, Imamura S, Danno K, et al. Potassium iodide in the treatment of erythema nodosum and nodular vasculitis. Arch Dermatol. 1981;117:29-31.
5. Requena L, Requena C. Erythema nodosum. Dermatol Online J. 2002;8:4.
6. Gilchrist H, Patterson JW. Erythema nodosum and erythema induratum (nodular vasculitis): diagnosis and management. Dermatol Ther. 2010;23:320-7.
7. González-Gay MA, García-Porrúa C, Pujol RM, et al. Erythema nodosum: a clinical approach. Clin Exp Rheumatol. 2001;19:365-8.
8. Mokhtari F, Abtahi-Naeini B, Pourazizi M. Erythema nodosum migrans successfully treated with indomethacin: A rare entity. Adv Biomed Res. 2014;3:264.
9. Horio T, Imamura S, Danno K, et al. Potassium iodide in the treatment of erythema nodosum and nodular vasculitis. Arch Dermatol. 1981;117:29-31.
10. De Coninck P, Baclet JL, Di Bernado C, et al. Treatment of erythema nodosum with colchicine. Presse Med. 1984;13:680.
11. Tan BB, Lear JT, Smith AG. Acne fulminans and erythema nodosum during isotretinoin therapy responding to dapsone. Clin Exp Dermatol. 1997;22:26-7.
12. Boyd AS. Etanercept treatment of erythema nodosum. Skin Med. 2007;6:197-9.
13. Quin A, Kane S, Ulitsky O. A case of fistulizing Crohn's disease and erythema nodosum managed with adalimumab. Nat Clin Pract Gastroenterol Hepatol. 2008;5:278-81.
14. Cohen PR. Sweet's syndrome—a comprehensive review of an acute febrile neutrophilic dermatosis. Orphanet J Rare Dis. 2007;2:34.
15. Bourke JF, Keohane S, Long CC, et al. Sweet's syndrome and malignancy in the UK. Br J Dermatol. 1997;137:609-13.
16. Sarkany RP, Burrows NP, Grant JW, et al. The pustular eruption of ulcerative colitis: a variant of Sweet's syndrome. Br J Dermatol. 1998;138:365-6.
17. Cohen PR. Subcutaneous Sweet's syndrome: a variant of acute febrile neutrophilic dermatosis that is included in the histologic differential diagnosis of neutrophilic panniculitis. J Am Acad Dermatol. 2005;52:927-8.
18. Trentham DE, Masi AT, Bale GF. Arthritis with an inflammatory dermatosis resembling Sweet's syndrome: report of a unique case and review of the literature on arthritis associated with inflammatory dermatoses. Am J Med. 1976;61:424-32.
19. Gosheger G, Hillmann A, Ozaki T, et al. Sweet's syndrome associated with pigmented villonodular synovitis. Acta Orthop Belg 2002, 68:68-71.
20. Balass S, Duparc A, Zaid S, et al. Aseptic meningitis during Sweet syndrome. Ann Dermatol Venereol. 2005,132:1003-6.
21. Cohen PR. Sweet's syndrome presenting as conjunctivitis. Arch Ophthalmol. 1993;111:587-8.
22. Chen TC, Goldstein DA, Tessler HH, et al. Scleritis associated with acute febrile neutrophilic dermatosis (Sweet's syndrome). Br J Ophthalmol. 1998;82:328-9.
23. Su WP, Liu HN. Diagnostic criteria for Sweet's syndrome. Cutis. 1986;37:167-74.
24. von den Driesch P. Sweet's syndrome (acute febrile neutrophilic dermatosis). J Am Acad Dermatol. 1994;31:535-6.
25. Going JJ, Going SM, Myskow MW, et al. Sweet's syndrome: histological and immunohistochemical study of 15 cases. J Clin Pathol. 1987;40:175-9.
26. Requena L, Kutzner H, Palmedo G, et al. Histiocytoid Sweet syndrome: a dermal infiltration of immature neutrophilic granulocytes. Arch Dermatol. 2005;141:834-42.
27. Cohen PR, Kurzrock R. Treatment of Sweet's syndrome. Am J Med. 1990;89:396.
28. Case JD, Smith SZ, Callen JP. The use of pulse methylprednisolone and chlorambucil in the treatment of Sweet's syndrome. Cutis. 1989;44:125-9.
29. Sterling JB, Heymann WR. Potassium iodide in dermatology: a 19th century drug for the 21st century—uses, pharmacology, adverse effects, and contraindications. J Am Acad Dermatol. 2000;43:691-7.

30. Maillard H, Leclech C, Peria P, et al. Colchicine for Sweet's syndrome. A study of 20 cases. Br J Dermatol. 1999;140:565-6.
31. Yamuauchi PS, Turner L, Lowe NJ, et al. Treatment of recurrent Sweet's syndrome with coexisting rheumatoid arthritis with the tumor necrosis factor antagonist etanercept. J Am Acad Dermatol. 2006;54:S122-6.
32. Browning CE, Dixon JE, Malone JC, et al. Thalidomide in the treatment of recalcitrant Sweet's syndrome associated with myelodysplasia. J Am Acad Dermatol. 2005;53:S135-8.
33. von den Driesch P. Pyoderma gangrenosum: a report of 44 cases with follow-up. Br J Dermatol. 1997;137:1000-5.
34. Powell FC, Su WP, Perry HO. Pyoderma gangrenosum: classification and management. J Am Acad Dermatol. 1996; 34:395-409.
35. Bhat RM. Pyoderma gangrenosum. An update. Indian Dermatol Online J. 2012;3:7-13.
36. Hasselmann DO, Bens G, Tilgen W, et al. Pyoderma gangrenosum: clinical presentation and outcome in 18 cases and review of the literature. J Dtsch Dermatol Ges. 2007;5:560-4.
37. Bhat RM, Nandakishore B, Sequeira FF, et al. Pyoderma gangrenosum: an Indian perspective. Clin Exp Dermatol. 2011;36:242-7.
38. Shankar S, Sterling JC, Rytina E. Pustular pyoderma gangrenosum. Clin Exp Dermatol. 2003;28:600-3.
39. Caughman W, Stern R, Haynes H. Neutrophilic dermatosis of myeloproliferative disorders. Atypical forms of pyoderma gangrenosum and Sweet's syndrome associated with myeloproliferative disorders. J Am Acad Dermatol. 1983; 9:751-8.
40. Hughes AP, Jackson JM, Callen JP. Clinical features and treatment of peristomal pyoderma gangrenosum. JAMA. 2000;284:1546-8.
41. Callen JP. Pyoderma gangrenosum. Lancet. 1998;351:581-5.
42. Su WP, Schroeter AL, Perry HO, et al. Histopathologic and immunopathologic study of pyoderma gangrenosum. J Cutan Pathol. 1986;13:323-30.
43. Su WP, Davis MD, Weenig RH, et al. Pyoderma gangrenosum: clinicopathologic correlation and proposed diagnostic criteria. Int J Dermatol. 2004;43:790-800.
44. Bhat RM. Management of pyoderma gangrenosum—an update. Indian J Dermatol Venereol Leprol. 2004;70:329-35.
45. Johnson RB, Lazarus GS. Pulse therapy: therapeutic efficacy in the treatment of pyoderma gangrenosum. Arch Dermatol. 1982;118:76-84.
46. Matis WL, Ellis CN, Griffiths CEM, et al. Treatment of pyoderma gangrenosum with cyclosporin. Arch Dermatol. 1992; 28:1060-4.
47. Arbiser JL, Moschella SL. Clofazimine: a review of its medical uses and mechanisms of action. J Am Acad Dermatol. 1995;32:241-7.
48. Kontochristopoulos GJ, Stavropoulos PG, Gregoriou S, et al. Treatment of pyoderma gangrenosum with low-dose colchicine. Dermatology. 2004;209:233-6
49. Peuckmann V, Fisch M, Bruera E. Potential novel uses of thalidomide: focus on palliative care. Drugs. 2000;60:273-92.
50. Schmidt C, Wittig BM, Moser C, et al. Cyclophosphamide pulse therapy followed by azathioprine or methotrexate induces long-term remission in patients with steroid-refractory Crohn's disease. Aliment Pharmacol Ther. 2006; 24:343-50.
51. Daniels NH, Callen JP. Mycophenolate mofetil is an effective treatment for peristomal pyoderma gangrenosum. Arch Dermatol. 2004;140:1427-9.
52. Roy DB, Conte ET, Cohen DJ. The treatment of pyoderma gangrenosum using etanercept. J Am Acad Dermatol. 2006; 54:S128-34.
53. Foss CE, Clark AR, Inabinet R, et al. An open-label pilot study of alefacept for the treatment of pyoderma gangrenosum. J Eur Acad Dermatol Venereol. 2008;22:943-9.
54. Fujimoto E, Fujimoto N, Kuroda K, et al. Leukocytapheresis treatment for pyoderma gangrenosum. Br J Dermatol. 2004; 151:1090-2.
55. Paštar Z, Radoš J, Pavić I, et al. Palisaded neutrophilic and granulomatous dermatitis in association with subcutaneous nodular and systemic sarcoidosis. Acta Dermato venerol Croat. 2013;21:245-9.
56. Al-Daraji W, Coulson I, Howat A. Palisaded neutrophilic and granulomatous dermatitis. Clin Experiment Dermatol. 2005; 30:578-9.
57. Coutinho I, Pereira N, Gouveia M, et al. Interstitial Granulomatous Dermatitis: A Clinicopathological Study. Am J Dermatopathol. 2015;37:614-9.
58. Chu P, Connolly K, LeBoit PE. The histopathologic spectrum of palisaded neutrophilic and granulomatous dermatitis in patients with collagen vascular disease. Arch Dermatol. 1994;130:1278.
59. Hutchinson CB, Wang E. Kikuchi-Fujimoto disease. Arch Pathol Lab Med. 2010;134:289-93.
60. Resende C, Araújo C, Duarte Mda L, et al. Kikuchi's disease of the xanthomatous type with cutaneous manifestations. An Bras Dermatol. 2015;90:245-7.
61. Lee HY, Huang YC, Lin TY, et al. Primary Epstein-Barr virus infection associated with Kikuchi's disease and hemophagocytic lymphohistiocytosis: a case report and review of the literature. J Microbiol Immunol Infect. 2010;43:253-7.
62. Atarashi K, Yoshimura N, Nodera H, et al. Recurrent histiocytic necrotizing lymphadenitis (Kikuchi's disease) in a human T lymphotropic virus type I carrier. Intern Med. 1996; 35:821-5.
63. Papla B, Urbańczyk K, Gałazka K. Histiocytic necrotizing lymphadenitis without granulocytic infiltration (the so called Kikuchi-Fujimoto disease). Pol J Pathol. 2008;59:55-61.
64. Sharma V, Rankin R. Fatal Kikuchi-like lymphadenitis associated with connective tissue disease: a report of two cases and review of the literature. Springer plus. 2015;4:167.

CHAPTER 19

Approach to a Patient with Livedo Reticularis

Prasan D Rath, Silas S Nelson, Ajaz K Khan

INTRODUCTION

Livedo reticularis (LR) refers to the purple or red-violaceous reticular mottled lace-like appearance of the skin mostly involving the lower limbs (Fig. 1) and sometimes the upper limbs resulting from a narrowing or occlusion of the small and medium arteries or arterioles at the dermis-subcutis border.

It derives its name from the latin words *liviere* meaning bluish and *reticular* meaning net-like in appearance.

HISTORICAL

In 1955, Feldaker et al.[1] described what is now termed livedoid vasculopathy as livedo reticularis with summer ulcerations. In 1967, Bard and Winkelmann[2] used segmental hyalinizing vasculitis and livedo vasculitis to describe livedoid vasculopathy. In 1998, Papi et al.[3] described that platelet and lymphocyte activation was present in livedoid vasculopathy, whereas the levels of inflammatory mediators were in the normal range. They noted increased expression of platelet P-selectin.

ETIOLOGY

It is caused by an interruption of blood flow in the dermal arteries/arterioles, either due to spasm, inflammation, or vascular obstruction and is associated with diseases of varying etiology and severity.

Livedoid vasculopathy lesions can occur at any age, but livedoid vasculopathy is most commonly a disease of adulthood. Women are affected more often than men. Livedoid vasculopathy, although painful, is not associated with any loss of life or limb.

HISTOLOGY

Biopsy of lesions shows segmental hyalinizing vascular involvement of thickened dermal blood vessels, endothelial proliferation, and focal thrombosis without nuclear dust. There is no true vasculitis. Direct immunofluorescence study reveals immunoglobulin and complement components in the superficial, mid-dermal,

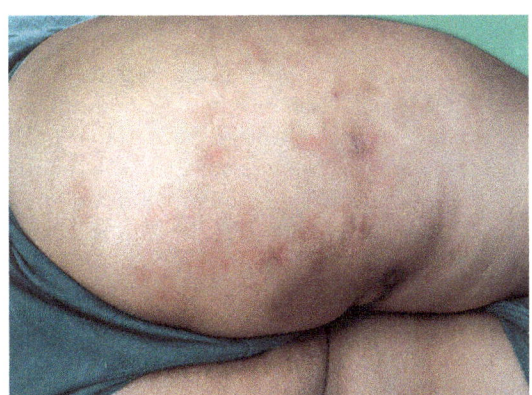

FIGURE 1: Livedo reticularis over the right buttock in a female patient with partial thrombosis of right internal iliac artery in the anterior division.

and deep dermal vessels. Pathogenesis involves hyalinization and thrombosis rather than leukocytoclastic vasculitis.

Ackerman et al.[4] described the histopathologic findings of livedoid vasculopathy.

Histopathologic findings in the early stage include the following:
- Sparse perivascular infiltrate of lymphocytes
- Frequently there is fibrin within the walls and fibrin thrombi within the lumen of venules in the upper part of the dermis
- Sometimes there is involvement of the lower half of the dermis.

Histopathologic findings at the full stage of disease include the following (Fig. 2):
- Moderately dense, superficial, and deep perivascular infiltrate of lymphocytes
- Sparse neutrophils in the upper dermis
- Fibrin in the walls of venules, in particular in the upper dermis
- Thrombi occluding the lumen of venules in the upper dermis
- Fibrin in the wall and thrombi in the lumen of the same venules in one or more venules
- Large numbers of extravasated red blood cells in the upper part of the dermis
- Edema of the papillary dermis
- Spongiosis and ballooning sometimes resulting in intraepidermal vesiculation
- Epidermal necrosis.

Histopathologic findings in the late stage include the following:
- Sparse infiltrate of lymphocytes mostly in the upper part of the dermis
- Sclerosis in the upper part of the dermis
- Numerous telangiectasias in the upper part of the dermis
- Epidermis thinned markedly and largely lacking rete ridges.

Under the electron microscopy in the early purpuric stage, fibrinoid material can be seen in the upper dermis in the capillary walls and the lumina along with trapped erythrocytes and platelets within the fibrin. Other changes at this stage are endothelial proliferation and thickened walls. Deeper dermal and subcutaneous vessels are not involved at this stage. Later there is dilatation of capillaries (with a diameter up to 100 μm), with a thin endothelium, together with obliterated capillaries. Vessels are present in a dense, fibrotic connective tissue. Fibrin deposition with occlusion of the lumina of superficial blood vessels can be present. Endothelial cells are replaced by heavy fibrin depositions in older lesions.

Atrophie blanche appears in the late scarring phase of the vasculopathy. The epidermis is thinned and the fibrinoid material replaces the dermal vessels. There is scarce or no cellular infiltrate. The upper dermis is more involved than the deeper dermis, and in other cases, the deeper layers show more of the changes mentioned above.

PATHOPHYSIOLOGY

A reduction of blood flow in the arterioles can cause livedo reticularis. A complete interruption of this flow due to blockage of the lumen can cause hemorrhagic infarcts which present as reticular purpuric lesions (retiform purpura) that can become ecchymotic (Fig. 3) with extensive areas of necrosis and secondary ulceration.

Necrotic lesions and ulcers caused by arterial or arteriolar occlusion tend to have reticular, stellate margins. Severe inflammatory reactions of the vascular wall and perivascular dermis cause painful subcutaneous nodules, located either in the same area as the reticular lesions or along the path of the vessel.

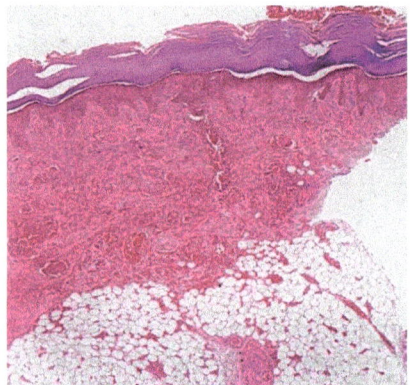

FIGURE 2: Histopathology of livedoid vasculopathy- Fibrin deposition and thrombi formation seen in upper and mid dermal vessels.

Courtesy- Dr Sujay Khandpur, Dermatology, AIIMS, Delhi.

Approach to a Patient with Livedo Reticularis

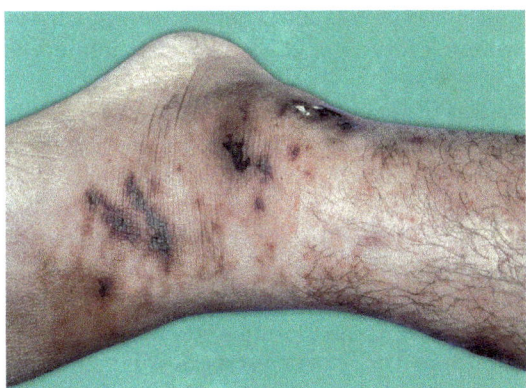

FIGURE 3: Reticular purpuric, ecchymotic and necrotic lesions.

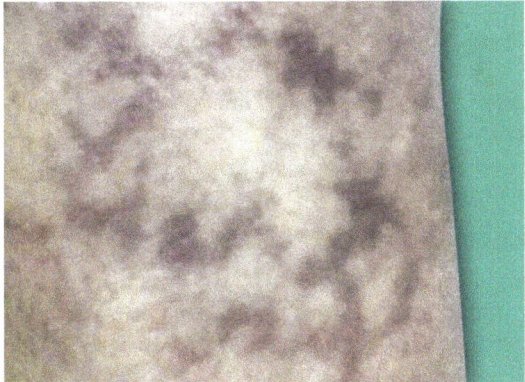

FIGURE 4: Livedo reticularis with complete rings of erythema.

Table 1: Causes of livedo reticularis	
Arteriolar spasm	Response to cold, drug induced (ergotamine, cocaine)
Vessel inflammation noninfectious (vasculitis)	• Systemic polyarteritis nodosa • Cutaneous polyarteritis nodosa • Wegener granulomatosis • Churg-Strauss syndrome • Microscopic polyangiitis • Drug-induced vasculitis (thiouracil) • Vasculitis associated with SLE or RA
Vessel inflammation infectious	• Lucio's phenomenon
Vascular obstruction-thrombosis (without inflammation)	• Antiphospholipid syndrome • Sneddon syndrome • Livedoid vasculopathy • SLE, RA • Coumarin-induced necrosis • Disseminated intravascular coagulation • Dysproteinemia (type I cryoglobulinemia) • Procoagulant genetic factors (factor V) • Sickle cell anemia • Drugs
Embolization	• Atrial myxoma • Cholesterol emboli
Vessel wall disorders	• Calciphylaxis • Hyperoxaluria

RA, rheumatoid arthritis; SLE, systemic lupus erythematosus.

In livedo reticularis there is a purplish-blue erythema, reticulated (small and complete meshes) (Fig. 4) in contrast to livedo racemosa (large broken circular segments), which is considered by some as more organic than functional. This is related to a secondary slowdown of the blood flow in the dermic venules. These venules form adjacent circles communicating with each other, parallel to the skin surface. The slowdown of blood flow may be due to a local vasoconstriction (vasomotor livedo) or to an arteriolar occlusion. Arteriolar occlusion may be related to blood abnormalities (thrombosis, high viscosity, and embolus) or to increased parietal thickness (vasculitis, calcic deposition, and intimal hyperplasia). It is not always possible to clinically distinguish a vasomotor livedo from those associated with diseases.

Livedo reticularis has many possible causes (Table 1).

APPROACH TO A PATIENT WITH LIVEDO RETICULARIS

A detailed history can provide useful information and should include questioning about drugs, associated diseases (such as renal failure, arteriosclerosis, systemic autoimmune diseases, and monoclonal gammopathy), recent surgery (catheterization, angioplasty), and history of spontaneous abortion. It is also essential to determine the course of the disease (chronic, acute, or fulminant), and associated symptoms like fever, dyspnea, and arthralgia.

Fever may be due to an infectious process, or due to an inflammatory process such as systemic lupus erythematosus or systemic vasculitis.

Laboratory investigations which are useful are complete blood count, coagulation studies, kidney function tests, urinary sediment, proteinuria, antinuclear antibodies, complement levels, antineutrophil cytoplasmic antibodies (ANCAs), cryoglobulin and cryofibrinogen levels, antiphospholipid antibodies, and hepatitis B and C serology. Other helpful investigations are coagulation factors protein C and S levels, factor V Leiden mutations, prothrombin G20210A gene mutations, homocysteine levels, and the C677T mutation of the methylenetetrahydrofolate reductase gene.[5,6]

In a patient with livedo reticularis with purpura, necrosis, or subcutaneous nodules, a full thickness skin biopsy reaching hypodermis, should be taken from the erythematous-violaceous or purpuric areas, the margin of a necrotic lesion, or a nodule. A punch biopsy may be sufficient if the biopsy site is chosen correctly. Pathologic analysis will show whether the lesion is inflammatory or noninflammatory and can provide a clue to the etiology.

If there is inflammation, it is important to identify the size of the affected vessels and see if it is in superficial or deep plexus. Also the types of cells of the inflammatory infiltrate (polymorphonuclear neutrophils, mononuclear cells, or giant cells) are seen. If the deep plexus is involved with polymorphonuclear neutrophils infiltrate the diagnosis favors polyarteritis nodosa. Small superficial plexus vessels involvement explains the presence of palpable purpura in Wegener granulomatosis, Churg-Strauss syndrome, and microscopic polyangiitis. In small vessel vasculitis both superficial and deep plexus are involved.

In polyarteritis nodosa, microscopic polyangiitis, and lupus-related polyangiitis, the infiltrate is of polymorphonuclear neutrophils. However, in Wegener granulomatosis and Churg-Strauss syndrome, it has granulomatous features, with macrophages and lymphocytes. In Churg-Strauss syndrome, there are also numerous eosinophils.

If it is noninflammatory, the biopsy findings will help to identify the cause of vessel obstruction (e.g., clot, cholesterol crystals, calcium, endothelial proliferation, and hyalinization). In noninflammatory lesions with clot the differential diagnosis can be antiphospholipid syndrome, Sneddon syndrome, disseminated intravascular coagulation, coumarin-induced necrosis, hemoglobin S, and drugs. A noninflammatory lesion with calcium in vessel walls is found in calciphylaxis. Birefringent crystals are seen in hyperoxaluria, eosinophilic material in type 1 cryoglobulinemia, cholesterol crystals in cholesterol embolization, positive alcian blue staining with myxoma, and hyalinization in livedoid vasculopathy.

Isolated livedo reticularis can be caused by arteriolar spasm which is due to vasoconstriction as a response to cold or certain drugs.

Inflammation of the Blood Vessels

Noninfectious (Vasculitis)

Vasculitides (Figs 5 and 6) like polyarteritis nodosa (systemic and cutaneous), Wegener granulomatosis, Churg-Strauss syndrome, microscopic polyangiitis, vasculitis of systemic lupus erythematosus, and rheumatoid arthritis, and certain types of vasculitis induced by drugs such as thiouracil can involve the arterioles of the skin.

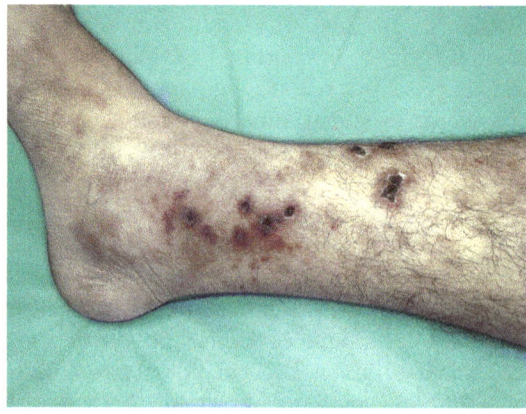

FIGURE 5: Superficial purpuric and necrotic lesion due to vasculitis. Note reticular erythema in the background.

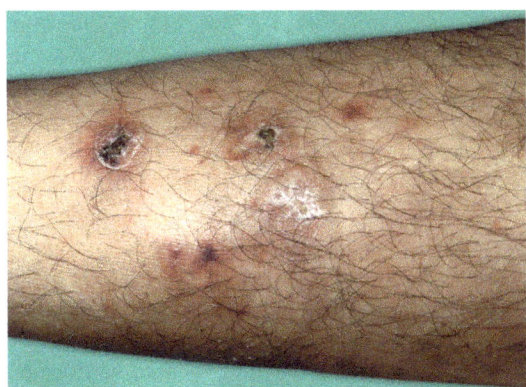

FIGURE 6: Superficial necrotic ulceration healing with atrophie blanche like scars in a vasculitis patient.

They can present with dermatological manifestations like livedo reticularis, inflammatory subcutaneous nodules, palpable purpura, necrosis, and secondary ulceration. A full thickness skin biopsy will help determine the type of blood vessels affected and the nature of the inflammatory infiltrate.[7]

A good clinical history, examination for systemic involvement, looking at lab investigations for evidence of systemic inflammation like leukocytosis, thrombocytosis, urine microscopy for nephritic sediments, chest X rays, and CT scans to pick up cavitations, nodules, and alveolar hemorrhages, etc., electrophysiological studies to pick up mononeuritis multiplex and ANCA determinations help pick up type of small vessel vasculitis and making early diagnosis.

Inflammation (Vasculitis) due to an Infection

Infectious diseases can cause inflammation of blood vessels by hematogenous dissemination of bacteria. Inflammation of vessel due to direct or contiguous infection, type II or immune complex reaction, cell-mediated hypersensitivity, or inflammation due to immune dysregulation triggered by bacterial toxin or superantigen, can compromise vascular integrity resulting in end organ damage.

It is a septic process characterized by the appearance of erythematous, purpuric, or pustular papules. Infectious processes generally affect the vessels of the superficial plexus, causing thrombosis and a polymorphonuclear infiltrate. Clinical manifestations can be like that of primary vasculitis like nonspecific constitutional symptoms, pyrexia, skin lesions and major organ infarction.

The microbial pathogens implicated are viral, bacterial, mycobacteria, fungus, parasites, rickettsiae and mycoplasma.

Vascular Obstruction in the Absence of Inflammation

Noninflammatory vascular disorders can mimic vasculitis but it is important to differentiate between them as their treatment is different. The vascular endothelium appears to play a central role in the pathogenesis though vascular obstruction has many different causes. Livedo reticularis without inflammation is associated with signs of hemorrhagic infarction (retiform purpura), necrosis, and the subsequent formation of ulcers with reticular or stellate margins. Occlusion of vessel lumen can occur due to thrombosis or embolization or vessel wall disorder.

Thrombosis

Thromboembolic events in the arterioles of the skin usually follow hypercoagulable states and can give rise to livedo reticularis and extensive skin necrosis.

Antiphospholipid syndrome is an autoimmune thrombophilic state characterized by the presence of antiphospholipid antibodies, thrombosis affecting the arteries or veins (thrombophlebitis, pulmonary thromboembolism, and cerebrovascular accidents), and recurrent spontaneous abortion. It may be a primary disorder or secondary often associated with systemic lupus erythematosus and other autoimmune diseases. Patients may present with various cutaneous manifestations some of which can be mistaken for vasculitis like purpura, necrosis, superficial thrombophlebitis, chronic ulcers on the legs, atrophie blanche, perniosis, subungual hemorrhage, and digital infarcts.[8] Sneddon syndrome is characterized by generalized livedo reticularis with thromboembolic events.

Livedoid vasculopathy is characterized by livedo reticularis and painful purpuric, necrotic lesions with stellate margins on both legs simultaneously, mainly in the malleolar region (Figs 7 and 8) and on the soles of the feet. Lesions heal leaving atrophic scars with telangiectasias and pigmented borders (atrophie blanche) (Fig. 9). Other clinical features include Raynaud's phenomenon, acrocyanosis, signs of peripheral venous insufficiency, and collagen vascular diseases like systemic lupus erythematosus and scleroderma.

Livedoid vasculopathy can be found in association with carcinomas, lymphoma, and myeloma. Histopathology findings include thrombosis and hyalinization of dermal vessels with no evidence of vasculitis.

Many patients with livedoid vasculopathy have coagulation disorders, mainly due to procoagulant factors and diseases like antiphospholipid antibodies, cryofibrinogen, decreased antithrombin III activity, heterozygous factor V mutations,[9] protein C deficiency,[10] increased platelet aggregation, cryoglobulinemia[11] and increased levels of plasminogen activator inhibitor-1.[12]

In type I cryoglobulinemia, there is an accumulation of monoclonal immunoglobulin G or M. This dysproteinemia is associated with B-cell lymphoproliferative disorders such as myeloma, B-cell lymphoma, and macroglobulinemia. These immunoglobulins tend to precipitate in the cold.

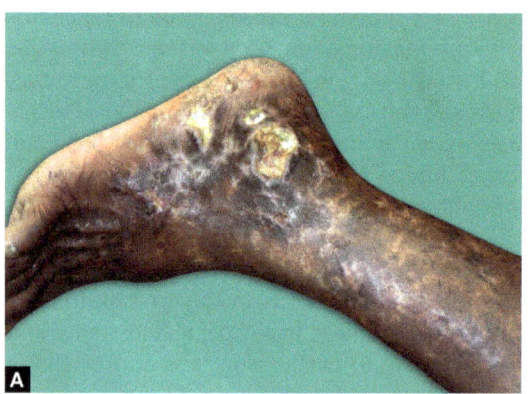 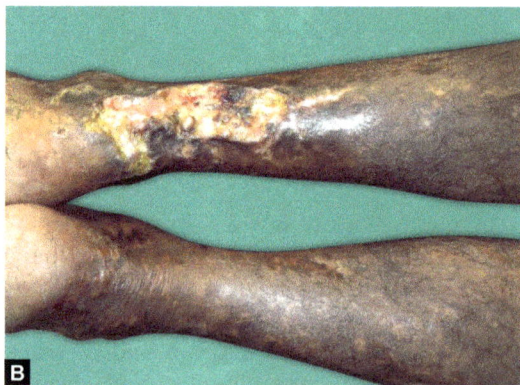

FIGURE 7: Livedoid vasculopathy patient with active ulcerative lesions over the right lateral malleoli and achilles tendon.

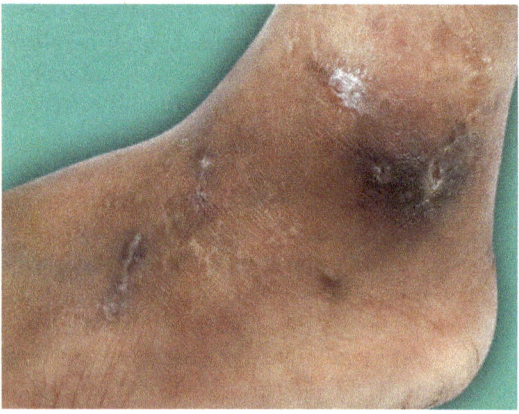 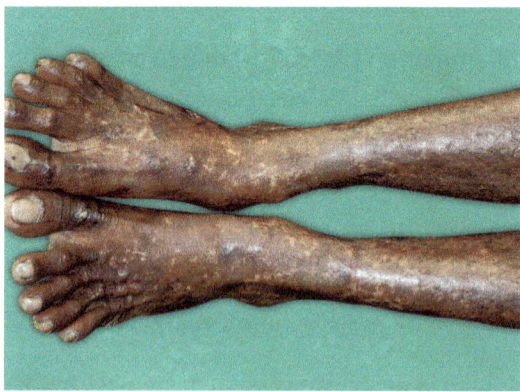

FIGURE 8: Livedoid vasculopathy patient with healing ulcer over left lateral malleoli.

FIGURE 9: Livedoid vasculopathy patient with extensive multiple reticulate healed scars on dorsum of feet and lower leg.

Intravascular precipitation of immunoglobulins causes arterial occlusion; the precipitates are visualized as amorphous, eosinophilic material within the vascular lumen, with no evidence of inflammation. The main organs affected in this type of cryoglobulinemia are the skin, kidneys, liver, and nervous system. Skin lesions can be one of the first signs of the disease, manifesting as acrocyanosis, distal necrosis of the legs, and Raynaud's phenomenon.

Livedo reticularis can occur with disseminated intravascular coagulation. Skin involvement is generalized, with well-demarcated, stellate, hemorrhagic, and necrotic plaques.

Disseminated intravascular coagulation is caused by the sudden intravascular activation of coagulation mechanisms resulting in depletion of platelets and various coagulation factors such as fibrinogen, prothrombin, factor V, factor VIII, and protein C. Purpura fulminans is an acute condition characterized by the appearance of extensive areas of hemorrhagic necrosis during or immediately after an infectious process (meningococcus, group A *Streptococcus*, *Staphylococcus*, pneumococcus) or other serious clinical conditions such as multiple trauma, obstetric conditions, and toxic syndromes.

Complication associated with the use of coumarins is the appearance of extensive areas of stellate ecchymoses and necrotic skin lesions with well delimited borders occurring symmetrically on the chest, buttocks, thighs, and arms (Fig. 10). A biopsy performed at the edge of lesions will show thrombosis of the dermal vessels but no inflammation. The condition is rare and occurs in subjects with congenital or acquired protein C deficiencies.

Sickle cell anemia is caused by homozygosity for hemoglobin S. The clinical features are caused by the occlusion of microvessels by sickle-shaped red blood cells. It affects young individuals and can affect all organs. The disease causes persistent chronic ulcers in the malleolar region that do not heal.

The coadministration of diphenhydramine and the sedative pyrithyldione can cause livedo reticularis, nodules, and necrotic lesions. The manifestations are secondary to massive

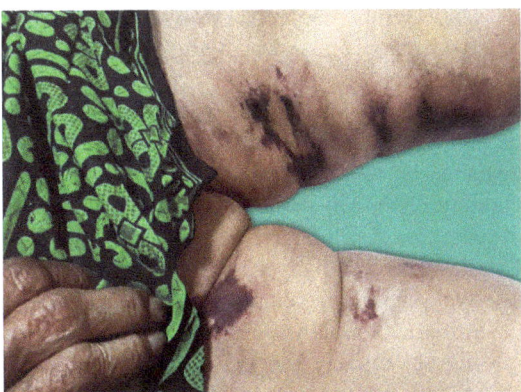

FIGURE 10: Coumrin-induced cutaneous and subcutaneous fat necrosis over medial aspect of both thigh. Note extensive area of necrosis with reticulate erythema at the margins of necrotic area.

thrombosis of the dermal vessels and without evidence of vasculitis.

Patients with myeloproliferative diseases receiving long-term treatment with hydroxyurea can present with painful necrotic lesions and secondary ulcers with atrophic, fibrous borders in the malleolar region of the legs or on the feet.

Generalized livedo reticularis, without vasculitis or thrombosis, can also occur in systemic lupus erythematosus and rheumatoid arthritis. In these, the condition may be secondary to a slowing of the blood flow (due to increased viscosity or thrombophilic states), to an intense vasoconstrictor reaction induced by cold, or to a combination of both mechanisms.

Embolism

Emboli can cause livedo reticularis and necrosis. Emboli originate from atrial myxomas or atheromatous plaques and can obstruct peripheral arteries or arterioles.

Myxomas are benign tumors usually found in the left atrium and originate in endothelial cell.

Tumor fragments can disseminate, causing distal emboli and results in characteristic symptoms such as livedo reticularis, necrosis, distal cyanosis, and splinter hemorrhages. A skin lesion biopsy will show obstruction of the arteriolar lumen by an amorphous, basophilic myxoid material.

Cholesterol emboli are caused by the rupture of atheromatous plaques in the aorta or other great arteries, spontaneously or after procedures like catheterization, angioplasties, angiography, or following initiation of treatment with anticoagulants or thrombolytic agents. Patients with cholesterol emboli often have leukocytosis with eosinophilia, thrombocytopenia, elevated levels of C reactive protein, high erythrocyte sedimentation rates, and signs of secondary acute inflammation.

Embolization can occur in the blood vessels of different organs. The first sign of cholesterol embolization are the skin lesions secondary to the presence of emboli in skin arteries and arterioles. The lesions manifest as livedo reticularis (which becomes accentuated when the patient is standing), a bluish discoloration of the feet, a faint reticular pattern on the soles of the feet, retiform purpura, necrosis, ulcers, nodules, and cyanosis.[13]

Cholesterol embolization can be confirmed by skin biopsy which shows occlusion of the arteries and arterioles of the deep plexus. The lumen of the vessels contains needle shaped biconcave spaces, occupied by the crystals inside the embolism. Histopathology shows an inflammatory infiltrate consisting of neutrophils, eosinophils, and lymphocytes in the early stages and of giant cells in the late stages.

Vessel Wall Disorders

In patients with advanced renal failure and secondary hyperparathyroidism, disorders of calcium and phosphorus metabolism can cause metastatic calcifications in the arteries, soft tissues, joints, and organs. Calciphylaxis is a very serious and often fatal condition.

The onset of lesion is usually located in the fatty areas of the lower limbs. The lesion may also occur on the trunk, abdomen, thighs, and buttocks although calciphylaxis on these areas tend to be more serious than the development of lesions in the lower limbs.

Calciphylaxis causes calcification of the media of arteries and can cause sudden appearance of livedo reticularis, hemorrhagic infarcts, necrosis, ulcers, and violaceous plaques on the limbs. Plaques are well delimited and extremely painful and sometimes have an orange-peel skin appearance.[14] There is a high risk of calciphylaxis when the calcium-phosphorus product is high. Diagnosis is made by the identification of calcium in the walls of the superficial and deep dermal vessels.[15]

Calciphylaxis is characterized based on the involvement of calcification and its characteristics such as:
- Systemic medial calcification of the arteries more commonly in the tunica media
- Small vessel mural calcification either with or without the presence of endovascular fibrosis, vascular thrombosis, and extravascular calcification that can result to tissue ischemia and skin ischemia or skin necrosis.

The cause of calciphylaxis is not clear but it has been suggested that it requires the combination of an increased calcium-phosphorus product and vessel wall disorders secondary to renal failure. Hyperparathyroidism is an excessive parathyroid hormone in the blood as a consequence of hyperactivity in the parathyroid glands. Excessive levels of parathyroid hormone are potentially harmful to the bones and this condition is being associated to the onset of calciphylaxis.

Some patients have been found to have a protein C deficiency, which might act as a predisposing factor or as a marker for other disorders responsible for triggering the disease.

Primary hyperoxaluria is an autosomal recessive hereditary disease caused by a deficiency of either of the following liver enzymes: (i) alanine-glyoxylate aminotransferase (type I hyperoxaluria or glycolic aciduria) or (ii) D-glyceric dehydrogenase (type II hyperoxaluria or L-glyceric aciduria). These deficiencies increase the levels of calcium oxalate in the body, causing crystal precipitation in the joints, kidneys, heart, eyes, and skin.[16] The disease can affect children, adolescents, and adults. Patients can have renal failure or kidney stones. Vascular complications manifest on the skin as livedo reticularis, retiform purpura, necrosis, ulcers, and acrocyanosis. Skin biopsy will reveal aggregates of yellowish-gray crystals in the dermis, subcutaneous tissue, and walls of blood vessels. Dilated vessels, thrombosis, and foci of necrotic fatty tissue may also be seen.

TREATMENT FOR LIVEDO RETICULARIS

As there is a high risk of serious consequences with inappropriate treatment, each patient should be carefully investigated, monitored, and treated.[17]

The treatment is mainly directed at the underlying cause. Systemic vasculitis is treated with corticosteroids and immunosuppressants. Serious organ dysfunction requires the use of corticosteroids and cyclophosphamide pulse therapy for induction and the combination of low doses of corticosteroids with methotrexate or azathioprine for maintenance treatment.

There is no effective treatment for generalized livedo reticularis in antiphospholipid syndrome or Sneddon syndrome. Lifestyle modifications like quitting up of smoking are important. Treatments like the use of aspirin, pentoxifylline, dipyridamole and hyperbaric oxygen have been used in various case scenarios. Hydroxychloroquine is also a very effective and safe drug for treatment of livedo reticularis specially in patients with antiphospholipid syndrome.[18,19] Skin lesions due to thrombosis can often be treated with low doses of aspirin or antiplatelet therapy, although some experts advocate the use of anticoagulants for refractory or severe lesions.[20] Alprostadil (prostaglandin E1) and intravenous immunoglobulin have been used in difficult to treat patients. Sometimes these drugs are combined with immunosuppressants for better results.[21]

Danazol or stanozolol can be prescribed to patients with cryofibrinogenemia and coumarins or low molecular weight heparin may be indicated for hypercoagulable states.

Patients with methylenetetrahydrofolate reductase mutation can be treated with folic acid while those with plasminogen-1 activator inhibitor abnormalities can be administered an intravenous infusion of tissue plasminogen activator.

There are no clearly effective treatments for embolic diseases like calciphylaxis, or hyperoxaluria, all of which can lead to obstruction of the renal arteries and subsequent renal failure, which requires specific treatment. Systemic corticosteroids should be recommended for treatment of cholesterol emboli as they halt the secondary inflammatory cascade that can have fatal consequences.

CONCLUSION

Livido reticularis is a vasculopathy leading to a purplish reticular lace like mottled appearance of the skin of extremities which happens because of sluggishness of blood flow in the subdermal arteries/arterioles due to varied etiologies some of which can lead to serious consequences if not detected early. Hence it is important to recognize this sign and through a careful history, examination, and investigation identify and treat the underlying cause.

REFERENCES

1. Feldaker M, Hines EA Jr, Kierland RR. Livedo reticularis with summer ulcerations. AMA Arch Derm. 1955;72(1):31-42.
2. Bard JW, Winkelmann RK. Livedo vasculitis. Segmental hyalinizing vasculitis of the dermis. Arch Dermatol. 1967;96(5):489-99.
3. Papi M, Didona B, De Pità O, et al. Livedo vasculopathy vs small vessel cutaneous vasculitis: cytokine and platelet P-selectin studies. Arch Dermatol. 1998;134(4):447-52.
4. Ackerman AB, Chongchitnant N, Sanchez J. Histologic Diagnosis of Inflammatory Skin Diseases: An Algorithmic Method Based on Pattern Analysis, 2nd edition. Baltimore, Md: Williams and Wilkins; 1997.
5. Callen JP. Livedoid Vasculopathy: What it is and how the patient should be evaluated and treated. Arch Dermatol. 2006;142:1481-2.
6. Hairston BR, Davis M, Pittelkow MR, et al. Livedoid vasculopathy: further evidence for procoagulant pathogenesis. Arch Dermatol. 2006;142:1413-8.
7. Carlson JA, Chen KR. Cutaneous vasculitis update: neutrophilic muscular vessel and eosinophilic, granulomatous, and lymphocytic vasculitis syndromes. Am J Dermatopathol. 2007;29:32-43.
8. Grob JJ, Bonerandi JJ. Cutaneous manifestations associated with the presence of the lupus anticoagulant. A report of two cases and a review of the literature. J Am Acad Dermatol.1986;15:211-9.
9. Calamia KT, Balabanova M, Perniciario C, et al. Livedo (livedoid) vasculitis and the factor V Leiden mutation: additional evidence for abnormal coagulation. J Am Acad Dermatol. 2002;46:133-7.
10. Boyvat A, Kundakci N, Babikir MO, et al. Livedoid vasculopathy associated with heterozygous protein C deficiency. Br J Dermatol. 2000;143:840-2.
11. Tran MD, Becherel PA, Cordel N, et al. Idiopathic white atrophy. Ann Dermatol Venereol. 2001;128:1003-7.

12. Deng A, Gocke CD, Hess J, et al. Livedoid vasculopathy associated with plasminogen activator inhibitor-1 promoter homozygosity (4G/4G) treated successfully with tissue plasminogen activator. Arch Dermatol. 2006;142:1466-9.
13. Jucgla A, Moreso F, Muniesa C, et al. Cholesterol embolism: still an unrecognized entity with a high mortality rate. J Am Acad Dermatol. 2006;55:786-93.
14. Nahm WK, Badiavas E, Touma DJ, et al. Calciphylaxis with peau d'orange induration and absence of classical features of purpura, livedo reticularis and ulcers. J Dermatol. 2002;29:209-13.
15. Kyttaris VC, Timbil S, Kalliabakos D, et al. Calciphylaxis: a pseudo-vasculitis syndrome. Semin Arthritis Rheum. 2007;36:264-7.
16. Bogle MA, Teller CF, Tschen JA, et al. Primary hyperoxaluria in a 27-year-old woman. J Am Acad Dermatol. 2003;49:725-8.
17. Ribi C, Mauget D, Egger JF, et al. Pseudovasculitis and corticosteroid therapy. Clin Rheumatol. 2005;24:539-43.
18. Amato L, Chiarini C, Berti S, et al. Idiopathic atrophie blanche. Skinmed. 2006;5:151-4.
19. Sepp N. Other vascular disorders. In: Bolognia JL, Jorizzo J, Rapini RP. Dermatology. London: Mosby; 2003. pp. 1651-9.
20. Lee SS, Ang P, Tan SH. Clinical profile and treatment outcome of livedoid vasculitis: a case series. Ann Acad Med Singapore. 2003;32:835-9.
21. Schanz S, Ulmer A, Fierlbeck G. Intravenous immunoglobulin in livedo vasculitis: a new treatment option? J Am Acad Dermatol. 2003;49:555-6.

20 CHAPTER

Dermatological Manifestations of Large and Medium Vessel Vasculitides: Rheumatologists' Perspective

Arvind Ganapathi, Sramana Mukhopadyay, Renu George, Debashish Danda

CASE VIGNETTE

A 23-year-old gentleman presented with recurrent painful nonhealing ulcers on both lower limbs for 2 years along with pregangrenous changes in the great toe of right foot. He did not have any other characteristic features suggestive of systemic vasculitis. Biopsy taken earlier revealed features of necrotizing vasculitis involving dermal medium vessels. He had received two doses of 1 g rituximab biosimilar 15 days apart, along with oral deflazacort at 1 mg/kg/day of prednisolone equivalent dose. It was tapered off rapidly and mycophenolate mofetil was started as maintenance immunosuppressant. The ulcers had responded to this line of management. Eleven months following rituximab biosimilar therapy, similar ulcers recurred on both lower limbs including a large necrotic ulcer over right lateral malleolus and a few on both the feet. On examination, he had multiple superficial ulcerations on both the feet with surrounding livedoid skin changes as well as a tender, large circular ulcer on the right lateral malleolus measuring 6 × 6 cm with sloping margins and necrotic base (Fig. 1A). Skin biopsy revealed infiltration of lymphocytes in the walls of arteries and arterioles of subcutaneous tissue with fibrinoid necrosis in the vessel wall. Since there was no other systemic features of vasculitis, a diagnosis of cutaneous polyarteritis nodosa was made and he was given two more doses of rituximab biosimilar 15 days apart with 1 mg/kg/day of steroids with a fast taper as before. Mycophenolate mofetil was continued at optimum dose after checking 6-hour area under the curve levels in blood. Ulcers again healed with this therapeutic strategy (Fig. 1B). Plan is to check CD19+ B cells, to look for efficacy of the biosimilar as well as any possible early B cell repopulation to consider optimum timing for repeat doses of rituximab in future.

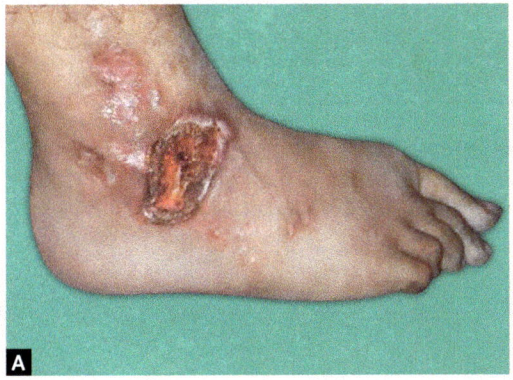 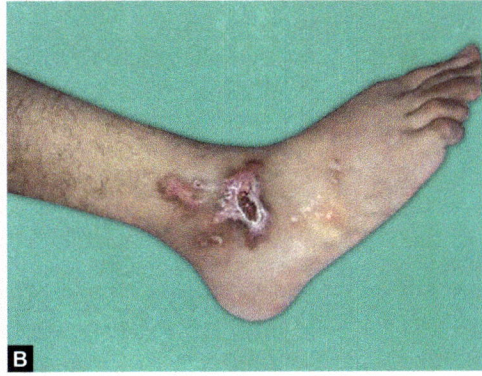

FIGURE 1: A, Ulcerative nodular cutaneous polyarteritis nodosa lesions; **B,** Lesions healed with two doses of rituximab biosimilar at 15 days interval (1 g each) along with a short course of 1 mg/kg/day of steroids with rapid tapering and maintenance with mycophenolate mofetil.

Skin in Rheumatologic Diseases

INTRODUCTION

Vasculitides are a heterogeneous group of disorders characterized by inflammation of blood vessels of varying sizes. Vascular inflammation causes obstruction of the vascular lumen, leading to ischemia and infarction of the tissue supplied by the vessels. Since blood vessels of any caliber in any organ system may be involved, the resultant clinical manifestations may be protean. Skin manifestations related to these group of disorders often herald the onset of systemic inflammation and provide vital clues for an accurate diagnosis, more so in small vessel vasculitides followed by medium and large vessel vasculitic disorders in that order.

Based on the type of the vessels involved, these disorders are commonly classified as large, medium and small vessel vasculitides. Aorta and its main branches at origin are called large vessels; vessels beyond the origin from aorta till they lose muscle coat on their walls are called medium vessels and further distally, the branches devoid of any muscle coat are small vessels. A vessel diameter below 50 μm, 50–150 μm, and more than 150 μm are also used by some experts as cutoff to define small, medium, and large vessels, respectively. However, absolute size of the vessel does not always determine if the vessel belongs to large, medium, or small category. For example, vasa nervorum on a sural nerve is a medium vessel as it has muscle coat on its wall, in spite of its tiny diameter.

In addition, a vasculitic disorder and its consequences may be categorized either as primary or it may be a secondary manifestation of other diseases.

CLASSIFICATION

Classification of vasculitides has been revised over the years. Despite attempts to devise a classification system that is inclusive of clinical features, vessel site, histopathological features, laboratory findings, and possible etiologic factors, such an ideal classification has not yet been established. Recently proposed working classification for vasculitides adopted at the International Chapel Hill Consensus Conference (CHCC) 2012 is currently considered as the gold standard in this regard (Table 1).[1]

The earlier ill-defined entity of polyangiitis overlap syndrome, with predominant large and medium vessel involvement in the same patient has been currently redefined as an unclassifiable, broad spectrum subset and mentioned in figure 2.

Table 1: Classification adopted at the 2012 International Chapel Hill Consensus Conference on the Nomenclature of vasculitides[1]			
Large vessel vasculitis	• Takayasu arteritis • Giant cell arteritis		
Medium vessel vasculitis	• Classic polyarteritis nodosa • Kawasaki disease		
Small vessel vasculitis (SVV)	• Antineutrophil cytoplasmic antibody (ANCA)-associated vasculitis		• Immune complex SVV
	1. Microscopic polyangiitis 2. Granulomatosis with polyangiitis (earlier known as Wegener's granulomatosis) 3. Eosinophilic granulomatosis with polyangiitis (earlier known as Churg-Strauss syndrome)		1. Antiglomerular basement membrane disease 2. Cryoglobulinemic vasculitis 3. IgA vasculitis or IgAV (earlier known as Henoch-Schönlein purpura)
Variable vessel vasculitis	• Behçet's disease • Cogan's syndrome		
Single-organ vasculitis	• Cutaneous leukocytoclastic angiitis • Cutaneous arteritis • Primary central nervous system vasculitis • Isolated aortitis • Others		

Continued

Continued

Table 1: Classification adopted at the 2012 International Chapel Hill Consensus Conference on the Nomenclature of vasculitides[1]	
Vasculitis associated with systemic disease	• Lupus vasculitis • Rheumatoid vasculitis • Sarcoid vasculitis • Others
Vasculitis associated with probable etiology	• Hepatitis C virus-associated cryoglobulinemic vasculitis • Hepatitis B virus-associated vasculitis • Syphilis-associated aortitis • Drug-associated immune complex vasculitis • Drug-associated ANCA-associated vasculitis • Cancer-associated vasculitis • Others

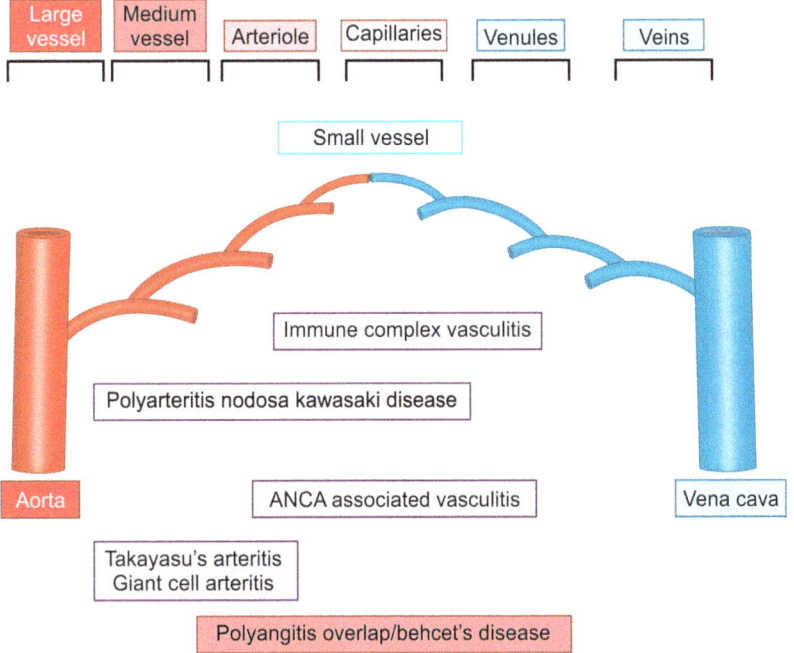

ANCA, antineutrophil cytoplasmic antibody.

FIGURE 2: Classification of vasculitic disorders by blood vessel size.

This chapter focuses on elucidation of dermatological manifestations that are associated with large and medium vessel vasculitides classified under CHCC 2012 classification. Isolated primary cutaneous vasculitis and other skin manifestations of small vessel vasculitides are discussed elsewhere in this book.

GIANT CELL ARTERITIS

Giant cell arteritis (GCA) is a systemic disease characterized by a granulomatous pan-arteritis involving predominantly the large arteries along with medium-sized arterial involvement in contiguity. Giant cell arteritis typically affects women above the age of 50 years and is more common in the northern hemisphere, predominantly amongst the descendants of the Norwegian ancestry. It is remarkably rare in Asian Indian population.

Clinical Features

New onset severe headache, jaw claudication, constitutional features like fever, malaise including polymyalgia rheumatica with painful, stiff shoulders and/or hip girdles are notable presenting symptoms. Classically, a swollen, tender, pulseless, and thick temporal artery is a suggestive sign of GCA.

Cutaneous involvement in giant cell arteritis is uncommon.[2,3] Dermatological manifestations include either tender nodules in the distribution of the superficial temporal arteries or alopecia, urticaria, livedoid changes, and hyperpigmentation of the skin mostly involving the scalp. In the lower extremities, purpura, necrotic ulcers, and gangrene as ischemic sequelae have been reported.[4] Occasionally, lingual artery involvement may present as a red, sore, atrophied, or gangrenous tongue.

Diagnosis

While temporal artery biopsy may reveal diagnostic features of the condition, color duplex sonography can be used as a surrogate to biopsy in identifying and monitoring patients on treatment in GCA.[5] Along with clinical suggestions mentioned above, a markedly elevated erythrocyte sedimentation rate (ESR) in absence of other explanations acts as an important clue for the disease.

Treatment

Skin manifestations usually respond to the standard of care in GCA that is high dose glucocorticoids. Prednisolone 1 mg/kg body weight per day (or other steroids in equivalent doses) is continued for 2-4 weeks or till the reversal of signs and symptoms whichever is later. After an initial taper to 20 mg/day in 2 months, further taper is usually very slow over a period of 9-12 months to avoid a relapse.

The evidence on use of methotrexate in GCA has shown conflicting results[6] and tumor necrosis factor (TNF) α inhibitors also have shown lack of efficacy in GCA.[7,8]

TAKAYASU'S ARTERITIS

Takayasu's arteritis (TA) is a large vessel vasculitis which causes granulomatous inflammation of aorta and its major branches at their points of origin. This rare disease is more commonly seen in Japan, India, Southeast Asia, and Mexico.[9] The exact cause is unknown. Experts believe that TA and GCA represent a spectrum within the same disease.

Clinical Features

Takayasu's arteritis is predominantly a disease of young women in their second or third decades of life. Its initial manifestations are unsuspectingly nonspecific including constitutional features, which are commonly missed out as possible clues for TA. Later in the pulseless stage of the disease, however, patients present with bruits, loss of arterial pulses, asymmetry of blood pressure recordings between upper limbs, and symptoms of ischemia in the involved vessel territories.

Cutaneous manifestations in patients with TA vary greatly from country to country. The frequency of skin lesions in TA is estimated to be between 2.8% and 28% of cases. In Europe and North America, acute inflammatory nodules or erythema nodosum like lesions are the most commonly observed skin lesions.[10-12]

Skin in the ischemic limbs is usually dry, atropic, devoid of hair due to circulatory disturbance. While pyoderma gangrenosum (PG) (Figs 3A and 4) and papulonecrotic lesions are described in the occlusive stage of the disease,[13] acute and subacute erythema nodosum like cutaneous nodules (Fig. 3B) are reported early in the course of TA. Regardless of the disease stage, the occurrence of cutaneous lesions is strongly related to persistent disease activity as well as tapering of glucocorticoid treatment. However, no report exists in literature showing correlation beween location of skin lesions and angiographically involved large vessel territory.[11,14]

In a series of 60 TA patients by Rocha et al. 19 patients (31.6%) had various cutaneous manifestations (Table 2).[15]

Dermatological Manifestations of Large and Medium Vessel Vasculitides...

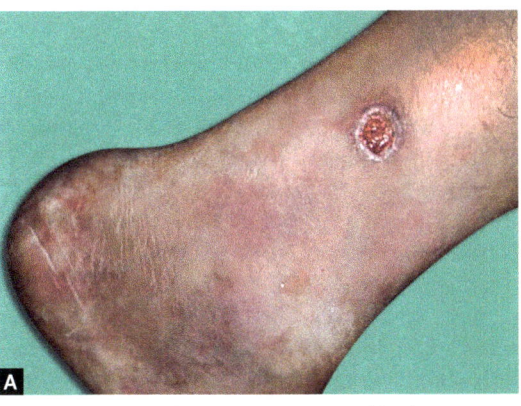
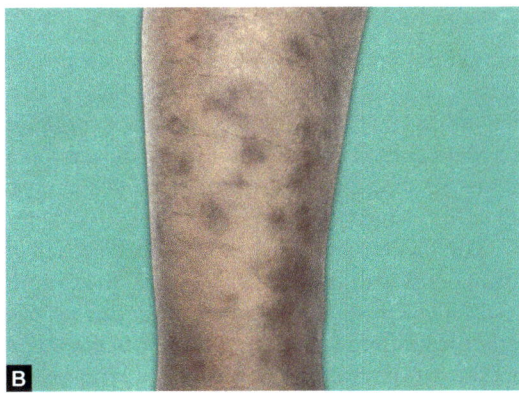

FIGURE 3: A, Pyoderma gangrenosum like lesion in a patient with Takayasu's arteritis (TA); **B,** Multiple erythema nodosum lesions in a TA patient.

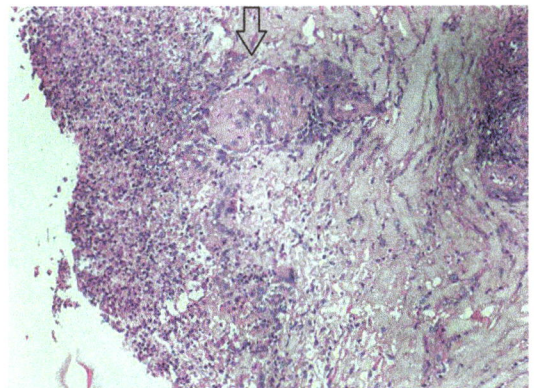

FIGURE 4: Photomicrograph of the lesion in figure 3A showing superficial granulomatous type of pyoderma gangrenosum with epidermal ulceration and superficial dermal dense neutrophilic infiltrate, histiocytic aggregates, and occasional multinucleate giant cells (H&E, 100x).

Table 2: Dermatologic manifestations of Takayasu's arteritis (Rocha et al.[15])

Cutaneous manifestation	Number of patients (n)
Erythema nodosum-like lesions	3
Raynaud's syndrome	3
Psoriasis	2
Eczema	2
Lupus erythematosus	1
Lichen planopilaris	1
Pityriasis versicolor	2
Viral warts	2
Seborrheic dermatitis	3

Pathology

Skin lesions of TA may variably show features of necrotizing vasculitis with fibrinoid changes, granulomatous vasculitis with giant cells, and panniculitis.[16]

Treatment

The skin manifestations of the disease usually respond to management of systemic disease, i.e., systemic corticosteroids at initial 0.5–1 mg/kg body weight/day. Cyclosporine may be effective in managing TA with pyoderma gangrenosum.[17,18] In authors' experience, intravenous immunoglobulin (IVIG) infusions followed by mycophenolate for maintenance seems to be a very effective, steroid sparing, and safe treatment strategy for PG in special situations; it is, however, an expensive option.

POLYARTERITIS NODOSA

Polyarteritis nodosa (PAN) is a rare, severe necrotizing vasculitis of medium-sized arteries with or without involvement of small sized arteries; arterioles, capillaries or venules are usually spared in its classic form. Vasculitic process in PAN affects multiple organ systems. Although immune complex mediated pathogenesis is one of the oldest theories behind classic PAN, immune deposits have been variably reported in literature including reports of few or no deposit.[19] While most cases of PAN are idiopathic, one-third of the cases are associated with hepatitis B infection.

Clinical Features

Polyarteritis nodosa presents with nonspecific constitutional as well as ischemic symptoms in one or more organ systems. In a Swedish series, common manifestations at disease onset were constitutional (65–80%), nervous system (55%), skin (44%), abdominal (33%) and renal symptoms (11%).[20]

Skin involvement can be found in about half of the patients with systemic PAN. Palpable purpura associated with erythema on the lower extremities is the most common presentation.[21] Subcutaneous nodule or group of nodules of varying sizes ranging from 0.5 to 2 cm, predominantly on the lower limbs in close proximity to vessels are also reported in classic PAN. Nodules may become pulsatile due to fibrosis resulting in weakness of the vessel wall and occasionally, they may also get secondarily ulcerated.[22] Livedo reticularis may occur, with or without ulceration; gangrene and ulceration of the digits or penis have also been described in PAN.

Histopathology

The histopathological picture of PAN is that of leukocytoclastic vasculitis. The initial inflammatory infiltrate is neutrophil rich, which subsequently becomes lymphocyte/histiocyte rich. Fibrinoid necrosis of the medium-sized vessel wall is often the rule. The vasculitis may cause development of microaneurysms which may rupture or lead to luminal thrombosis, obliteration, and tissue necrosis.[23]

Other Investigations

No specific laboratory test is available to diagnose PAN; presence of anemia, elevated ESR/CRP (C-reactive protein), elevated serum creatinine, abnormal liver enzymes, seropositivity for hepatitis B virus (HBV) in a likely clinical scenario, however, may support a diagnosis of PAN. Till date, American College of Rheumatology classification remains to be the most useful clinical guide to suspect PAN. Magnetic resonance angiography or computed tomographic angiography are less sensitive than conventional or digital subtraction angiography in detecting multiple small aneurysms, vessel ectasia, and focal occlusive lesions in the renal and mesenteric arteries.

Treatment

Cutaneous manifestations of classic PAN are usually responsive to immunosuppressive agents used to control systemic disease. Hepatitis B related PAN usually responds well to antiviral therapy, plasma exchange, and/or glucocorticoids. In a cohort of 115 patients included in a study conducted between 1972 and 2002, such a treatment regimen achieved remission in 81% of patients with a subsequent relapse rate of only 10%.[24] Principles of management of non-HBV PAN should be dictated by severity of the disease as defined by the five-factor prognostic score; this policy implies that aggressive immunosuppression with corticosteroids and cyclophosphamide is a must in patients with five-factor score of 2 or more.[25]

The relapse rate over a period of 6 years is reported to be 22% (28% in non-HBV-related PAN vs 11% in HBV PAN). According to published literature, the overall mortality rate is 25% (20% in non-HBV PAN vs 34% in HBV-PAN). Five-year relapse-free survival for HBV-related PAN is 67% versus 59% in non-HBV PAN. Amongst the patients with skin manifestations, non-HBV PAN usually has worse prognosis.[26]

CUTANEOUS POLYARTERITIS NODOSA

Cutaneous polyarteritis nodosa (C-PAN) is a variant of PAN restricted to the skin. Controversy exists on whether it represents an early or more limited form of PAN.[27] Diagnosis of C-PAN usually needs exclusion of visceral involvement. In spite of persistent and relapsing nature of the lesions in C-PAN, a relatively better prognosis is expected due to lack of visceral involvement. Occasional extracutaneous involvement is usually limited to adjacent muscles, nerves or joints manifesting as myalgia, peripheral neuropathy and arthralgias respectively, sometimes with accompanying fever.[28]

Clinical Features

Nodular lesions, pink to purple-red in color, are most commonly located on the distal lower extremities near the malleoli and may extend proximally to the thighs, buttocks, arms, or

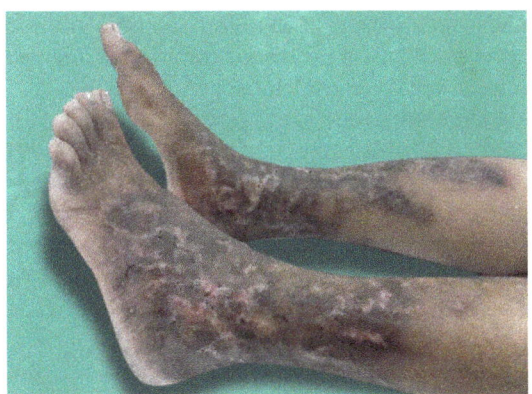

FIGURE 5: Livedoid vasculopathy characterized by the triad of "livedo racemosa", "crusted ulcerations," and "atrophie blanche" as well as postinflammatory hyperpigmentation in a patient of cutaneous polyarteritis nodosa with recurring lesions in the disease course. She received two courses of intravenous immunoglobulin and currently on maintenance with mycophenolate mofetil.

hands. Tenderness may be an associated feature. Nodules may ulcerate and occasional crops of lesions can be appreciated on a background of livedo reticularis.[28] "Atrophie blanche" may be the manifestation in such a setting (Fig. 5). Gangrene of digits has been known to occur in the setting of C-PAN, most commonly in children.[29]

Histopathology

Early in the course of C-PAN, lesions show leukocytoclastic vasculitis as in the systemic form, affecting the walls of medium-sized arteries and arterioles in the septae of the subcutaneous fat. The involved vessels typically demonstrate a target-like appearance due to a ring of fibrinoid necrosis. Similar to systemic PAN, there is predominant infiltration of lymphocytes and histiocytes later in the disease process.[22]

Direct immunofluorescence studies may show positivity for IgM and C3, either alone or in combination and sometimes, it may be detectable only in superficial and uninvolved dermis.

Treatment

No randomized controlled trial has been conducted in this condition. Corticosteroids, at a dosage of 0.8–1 mg/kg/day can usually control C-PAN lesions.[30] Low-dose weekly methotrexate (7.5–20 mg/week) has been used in patients who are not responsive to corticosteroids.[31] In view of frequent recurrences, second-line immunosuppressants like cyclophosphamide, azathioprine, and mycophenolate are often needed in many patients as well as in specific situations.[32] Other treatment options according to recently documented anecdotal reports include warfarin,[33] rituximab,[34,35] and infliximab.[36] There are reports of benefit in ulcer healing with antibiotics including penicillins, particularly in the juvenile onset post streptococcal C-PAN setting.[37]

KAWASAKI DISEASE

Kawasaki disease (KD) is a multisystem and mostly self-limiting vasculitic disorder of children associated with mucocutaneous lymphadenopathy syndrome. Medium and small arteries are predominantly affected in KD.

Mucocutaneous signs make up four out of the five clinical criteria needed for the diagnosis of Kawasaki disease. Therefore, dermatologists have an important role to play in early diagnosis of this disease, as delay in diagnosis is fraught with potential morbidity and mortality.

Clinical Features

An erythematosus rash, usually appearing during the acute phase, is part of KD diagnostic criteria. It is transient, may last 1 week or more and may be missed. It has been described as nonspecific, nonpruritic, nonvesicular, nonbullous, and noncrusting, but may be purpuric.[38,39] At times it has also been described as scarlatiniform or morbilliform exanthemata as well as urticarial and erythema multiforme-like targetoid lesions.[40] During the acute phase, conjunctival injection (Fig. 6) is reported to be the second most common feature after fever; there is usually erythema or non-pitting edema of the extremities at this stage. These findings can be subtle and confined to the fingertips. Characteristic acral desquamation (Fig. 7) is often a late sign[41] and waiting for this feature to make a diagnosis may lead to major complications as discussed in the subsequent paragraphs.

High spiking fever is known to occur despite antibiotics, but usually it resolves after 1-2 weeks, even in the absence of treatment. If untreated, 20-25% patients develop coronary artery aneurysms[42] along with occasional rupture, myocarditis, conduction defects, pericarditis, valvulitis, and sudden death. Long-term sequelae include coronary artery stenosis and thrombosis leading to myocardial ischemia or infarction.[38]

Different types of psoriasis like plaques including pustular and guttate varieties have been described to coexist in acute as well as convalescent phases of Kawasaki disease. A bacterial superantigen or proinflammatory cytokines might trigger the appearance of psoriasiform lesions in Kawasaki syndrome if the patient also has genetic predisposition to psoriasis.[43]

The characteristic desquamation of the fingers and toes that helps confirm the diagnosis, typically occurs in the second week of the illness, during the convalescent phase. It is typically not present within the first 10 days of illness, when it is necessary to initiate treatment. A series of 58 patients showed that 39 patients (67%) had a perineal eruption.[44] This is described as confluent erythematous macules or plaques that spare the groin folds. Desquamation of these eruptions occurs earlier than those in fingers and toes.

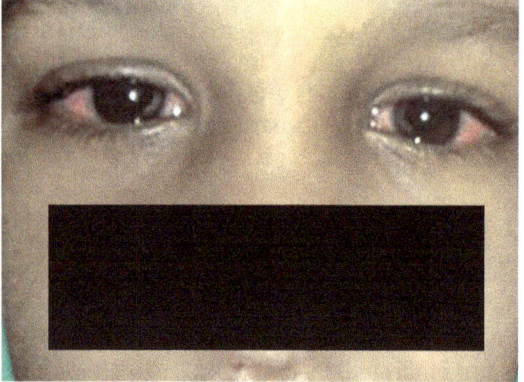

FIGURE 6: Conjunctival injection in both eyes of a patient with Kawasaki disease.

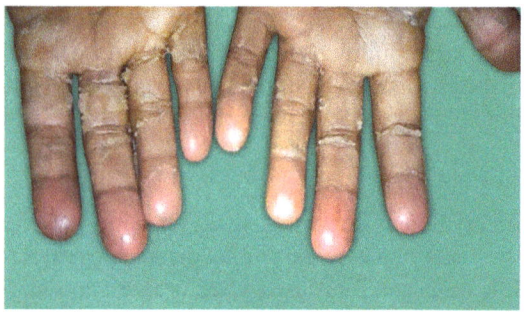

FIGURE 7: Acral desquamation in a patient with Kawasaki disease.

Diagnosis

There is no single specific laboratory test that can be used to diagnose Kawasaki disease. Rather, clinical diagnostic criteria are applied for this purpose. A flowchart is designed by the authors to facilitate an optimum diagnostic approach (Flowchart 1).[45]

An incomplete or atypical variant of Kawasaki disease is described with fever for at least 5 days along with fewer than four clinical criteria.[46]

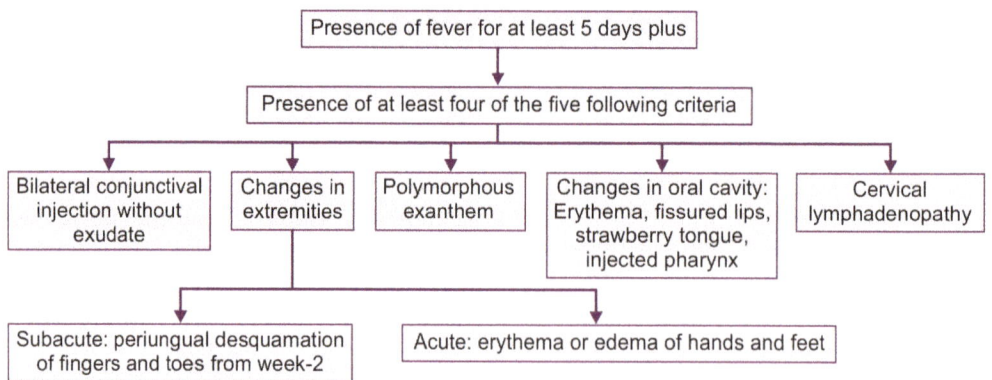

FLOWCHART 1: Algorithm for utilizing the diagnostic criteria of Kawasaki disease[45]

Histopathology

Histopathological features of the skin lesions have not been well described, as biopsies are infrequently performed due to transient nature of the rash. Typically the findings are as nonspecific as the clinical nature of the rash. Papillary dermal edema with a perivascular infiltrate of lymphocytes and mononuclear cells have been most commonly described.[47] Degenerative endothelial necrosis and subendothelial edema have also been described.[48] Psoriatic epidermal hyperplasia and intraepidermal subcorneal abscesses are noted in the psoriasiform and pustular eruptions, respectively.

Treatment

Skin manifestations are transient and per se do not warrant treatment. They disappear with institution of therapy for the systemic vasculitis, however some skin lesions have been reported to be resistant to conventional line of management. Treatment with IVIG (2 g/kg body weight given over 10-12 hours) and high-dose aspirin (80-100 mg/kg body weight/24 hours in divided doses) have been well established as effective therapy for Kawasaki disease. Treatment given early in the course of the disease (within the first 10 days of the onset of fever) not only results in a faster resolution of fever, but decreases the risk of coronary artery involvement.[49]

ANTINEUTROPHIL CYTOPLASMIC ANTIBODY-ASSOCIATED VASCULITIS (ALSO REFER TO CHAPTER 21)

Antineutrophil cytoplasmic antibody (ANCA)-associated vasculitides (AAVs) are a group of primary systemic vasculitides involving small and medium-sized vessels associated with autoantibodies that target cytoplasmic antigens in neutrophils (ANCAs).[50] The skin is a common target organ in AAV. Skin lesions may present as the initial manifestation or may coexist with other systemic vasculitic features. Skin lesions occur in 60% of patients with eosinophilic granulomatosis with polyangiitis (EGPA),[51-53] 40% of patients with microscopic polyangiitis (MPA),[52,54] and 20% of patients with granulomatosis with polyangiitis (GPA).[55] Skin manifestations in AAV are of two types: (i) vasculitic and (ii) nonvasculitic.[56] Figure 8 enumerates cutaneous lesions of AAV under these two categories. Clinical photographs of various such lesions in AAV are depicted in figure 9.

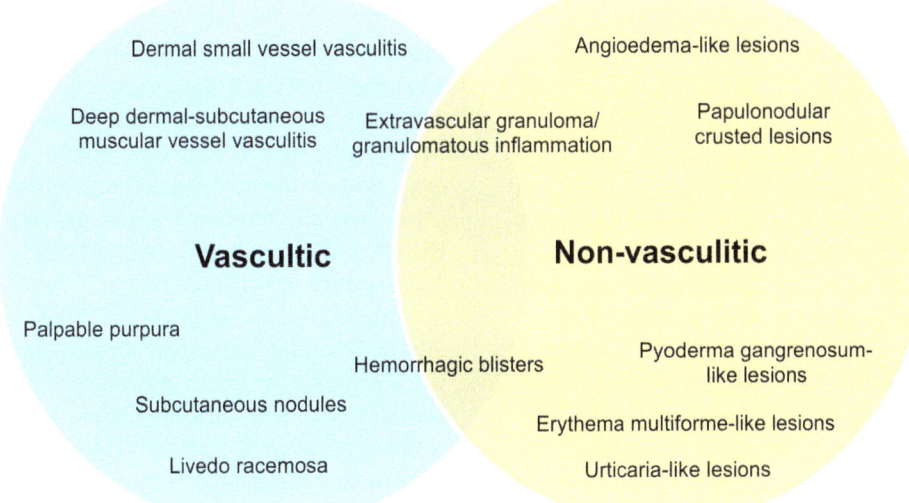

FIGURE 8: Picture depicting various skin lesions in antineutrophil cytoplasmic antibody-associated vasculitis.

Skin in Rheumatologic Diseases

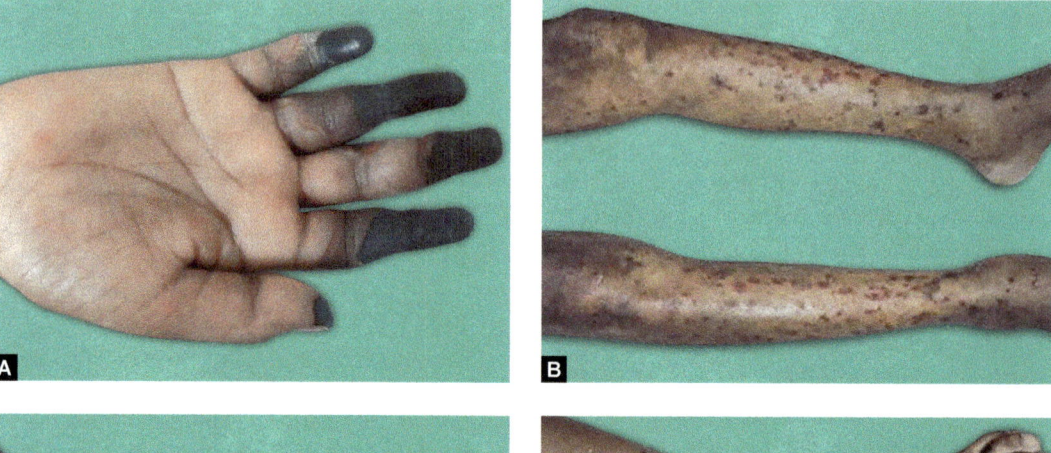

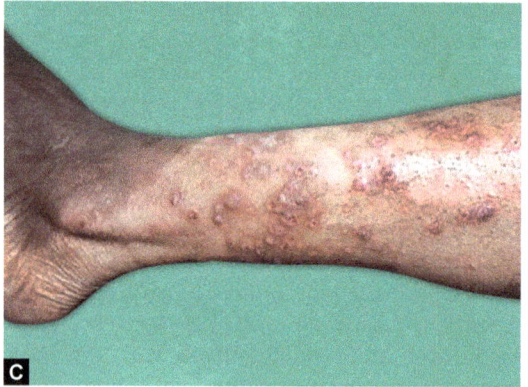

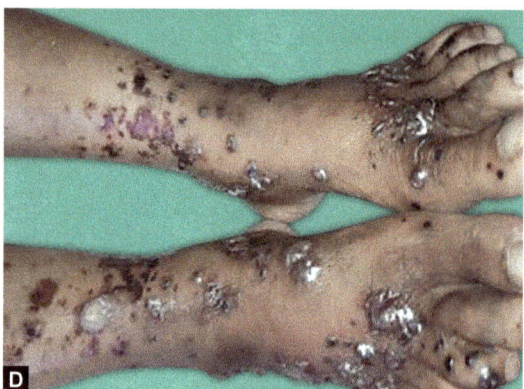

FIGURE 9: A, Gangrene of digits in patient of eosinophilic granulomatosis with polyangiitis; **B,** Cutaneous vasculitis with left foot drop (partially visible) in a patient of microscopic polyangiitis; **C,** Healing crusted papulonodular lesions in a patient of granulomatosis with polyangiitis; and **D,** Bullous lesions in a patient of antineutrophil cytoplasmic antibody-associated vasculitis.

Clinical Features

Cutaneous vasculitis in MPA, GPA, or EGPA generally affect dermal venules and arterioles (less commonly) presenting clinically as palpable purpura in the legs (51-55) as well as other dependent parts. Vasculitis of cutaneous medium vessels in AAV is relatively uncommon and may present clinically as livedo racemosa, nodular erythema, or subcutaneous nodules.[51,57]

Histopathology

Leukocytoclastic vasculitis, characterized by a predominant infiltrate of neutrophils mixed nuclear dust, is the most common histopathologic feature of both MPA and GPA; it is also an occasional feature of EGPA. Leukocytoclastic vasculitis of GPA is surrounded by a granuloma or granulomatous inflammation. In EGPA, two distinct types of vasculitis are present—either neutrophilic vasculitis or eosinophilic vasculitis, depending on the predominant inflammatory cells in a mixed infiltrate of neutrophils and eosinophils. Histological evolution of vasculitic skin lesions in AAV are depicted in figure 10.

Subcutaneous arteritis in MPA has the identical clinico-histopathologic features of C-PAN. However, the coexistence of overlying dermal venulitis in the same biopsy, seen in MPA is not present in C-PAN.[52,58] Figures 11 and 12 show histopathological features of eosinophilic panniculitis in EGPA and leukocytoclastic vasculitis in GPA, respectively.

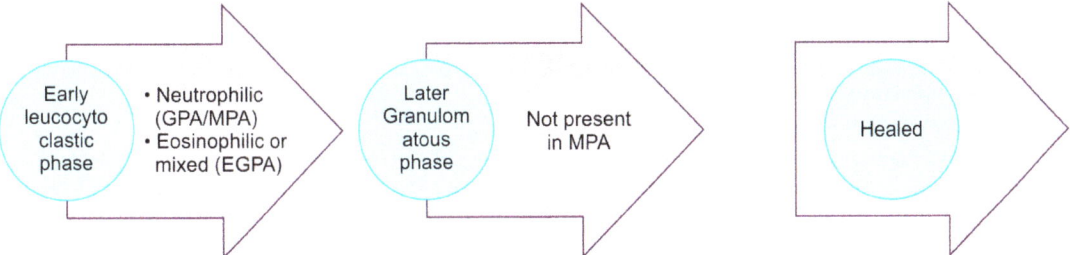

MPA, microscopic polyangiitis; GPA, granulomatosis with polyangiitis; EGPA, eosinophilic granulomatosis with polyangiitis.

FIGURE 10: Picture depicting morphologic evolution of histopathological features in cutaneous arteritis of antineutrophil cytoplasmic antibody)-associated vasculitis.

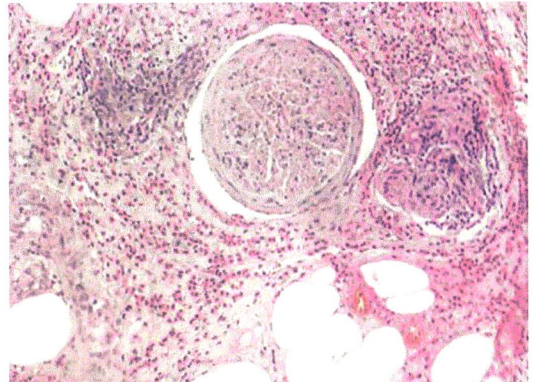

FIGURE 11: Histopathological examination showing eosinophilic panniculitis and focal granulomatous inflammation and entrapped nerve bundles displaying perineural fibrosis (H&E 10x), in a patient who presented with erythema nodosum like lesions on the extremities. This patient was subsequently diagnosed as eosinophilic granulomatosis with polyangiitis when she developed foot drop and gangrene of digits.

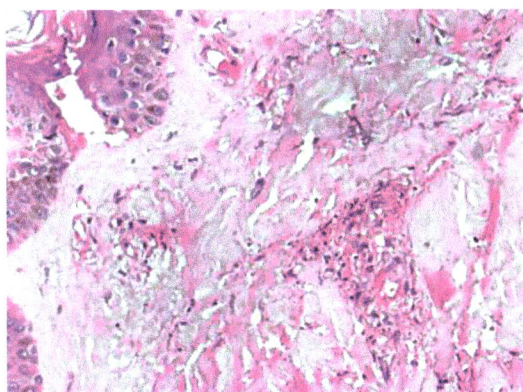

FIGURE 12: Transmural inflammation with prominent fibrinoid necrosis of superficial dermal small vessels in leukocytoclastic vasculitis (H&E, 200x), in a patient of antineutrophil cytoplasmic antibody-associated vasculitis (GPA) who presented with targetoid skin lesions on the extremities.

Nonvasculitic Skin Lesions in Associated Vasculitis

Nonvasculitic lesions show a montage of clinical features without any evidence of fibrinoid necrosis, a clear marker of vasculitis. Common cutaneous manifestations include bullae or vesicles, urticaria-like lesions, erythematous papules or plaques, erythema-multiforme-like lesions, and angioedema-like lesions in EGPA, PG-like lesions in GPA, and papules or nodules with an ulcerated or crusted center in GPA as well as in EGPA. Box 1 lists these lesions with clinico-histological correlations as available in literature.

Treatment

Treatment depends on whether skin manifestations are a part of organ threatening or non-organ threatening systemic disease. Flowchart 2 describes a practical treatment approach in AAV.

Cutaneous manifestations in medium vasculitides may predict a poorer outcome. In a retrospective study on outcome of cutaneous ischemia and gangrene in systemic necrotizing vasculitides that include PAN, GPA, EGPA, and MPA, patients with cutaneous ischemia had a higher relapse (56.9%) and mortality rates (27.7%) as compared to those without cutaneous ischemia (38.4 and 15.9% respectively) ($p < 0.04$).[61]

Box 1: Characteristics of various nonvasculitic skin lesions in antineutrophil cytoplasmic antibody-associated vasculitis[59,60]

Type of nonvasculitic lesions
- Dermal perivascular infiltrate of neutrophils or eosinophils
- Basophilic palisading granuloma: It occurs most often in eosinophilic granulomatosis with polyangiitis (EGPA) and granulomatosis with polyangiitis (GPA). Papules or nodules with central crusted or ulcerated lesions on frictional areas, such as elbows, knees, finger joints, or buttocks are commonly seen as its manifestations. Histopathology of these lesions reveal palisaded histiocytic granuloma with a central zone of basophilic degenerated collagen fibers mixed with nuclear dust and neutrophils
- Eosinophilic palisading granuloma (red granuloma, Churg-Strauss granuloma): It is associated with extravascular lesions of internal organs in EGPA
- Dermal granulomatous inflammation with or without granuloma formation
- Pyoderma gangrenosum-like lesions: Characteristic feature of GPA and may appear on the face. Palisaded granuloma surrounding a large central zone of a geographic necrosis, with marked neutrophilic abscess formation and hemorrhage are histopathologic hallmarks

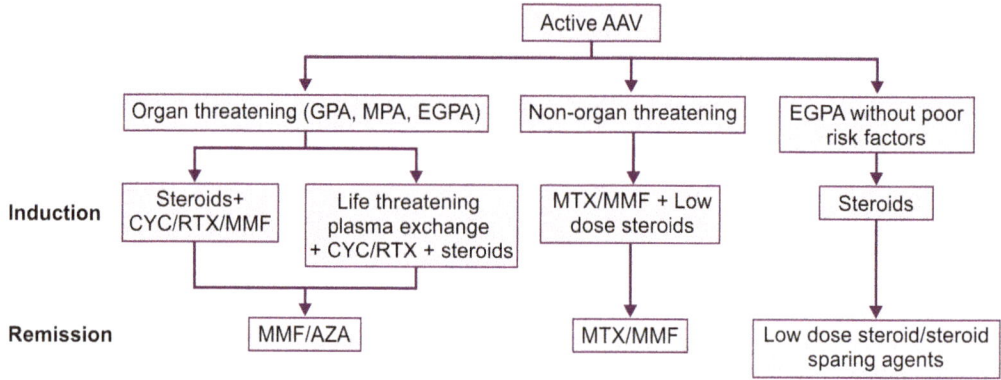

CYC, cyclophosphamide; RTX, rituximab; MMF, mycophenolate; MTX, methotrexate; AZA, azathioprine; AAV, associated vasculitis; MPA, microscopic polyangiitis; GPA, granulomatosis with polyangiitis; EGPA, eosinophilic granulomatosis with polyangiitis.

FLOWCHART 2: The flowchart of regimens used in antineutrophil cytoplasmic antibody-associated vasculitis based on organ involvement.

CONCLUSION

The dermatological manifestations of large and medium vessel vasculitides are protean; these features often herald the onset of a vasculitic disorder and provide vital clues for an accurate diagnosis.

Giant cell arteritis (GCA): Skin manifestations in GCA are rare and include tender nodules in the distribution of the superficial temporal arteries or alopecia, livedoid changes, and hyperpigmentation of the skin mostly involving the scalp.

Takayasu's arteritis: Between 2.8 and 28% of TA cases may have skin lesions. Erythema nodosum like nodules occur early in the course of TA; PG and papulonecrotic lesions occur in late occlusive stage of the disease. Occurrence of cutaneous lesions is strongly related to persistent disease activity. There is no correlation between location of skin lesions and involved large vessel territory.

Polyarteritis nodosa: Skin involvement is seen in 50% pateints with systemic PAN. Palpable purpura is the most common presentation; other lesions described include subcutaneous nodules in close proximity to involved vessels, ulceration on a background of livedo reticularis and gangrene of the digits. Cutaneous PAN is a variant of PAN restricted to the skin and its diagnosis requires exclusion of visceral involvement. Skin lesions in C-PAN, in spite of sparing internal visceral organs, tend to have persistent, refractory, and relapsing course unless immunosuppressants are added.

Kawasaki disease: Mucocutaneous signs like polymorphous exanthem, conjunctival congestion, acral desquamation, and changes in oral cavity make up four out of the five clinical criteria needed for the diagnosis of Kawasaki disease. Perineal skin lesions may appear earlier than acral exfoliations. Early recognition and treatment is crucial to prevent serious morbidities and mortality.

Antineutrophil cytoplasmic antibody-associated vasculitis: Skin lesion occurs in 60, 40, and 20% of patients with EGPA, MPA, and GPA respectively. Skin manifestations in AAV are of 2 types: (i) Vasculitic features like palpable purpura, subcutaneous nodule, and livedo racemosa and (ii) Nonvasculitic presentations like bullae or vesicles, urticaria-like lesions, erythematous papules or plaques, erythema-multiforme-like lesions, angioedema-like lesions, PG-like lesions, and papulonodular lesions with crusted ulceration.

Treatment: The skin manifestations in LVV and medium vessel vasculitis usually respond to steroids used for management of systemic features of vasculitis. Some vasculitic skin lesions per se, are steroid nonresponsive and need addition of other steroid sparing second-line immunosuppresives like cyclosporine, mycophenolate mofetil, methotrexate, azathioprine and on occasion, TNF-α inhibitors and B cell depleting agents.

ACKNOWLEDGMENT

We thank Dr Sathish Kumar (Professor, Paediatric Rheumatology Unit, CMC, Vellore), Dr Aswin M Nair, Dr Santosh Kumar Mandal, Dr Nikhil Gupta, and Dr Suvrat Arya (Senior Postgraduate Registrars, Department of Clinical Immunology and Rheumatology, CMC, Vellore) for providing clinical images and Dr Mandeep Singh Bindra (Department of Pathology, CMC, Vellore) for providing the histopathology pictures.

REFERENCES

1. Jennette JC, Falk RJ, Bacon PA, et al. 2012 revised International Chapel Hill Consensus Conference Nomenclature of Vasculitides. Arthritis Rheum. 2013;65:1-11.
2. Hitch JM. Dermatologic manifestations of giant-cell (temporal, cranial) arteritis. Arch Dermatol. 1970;101:409-15.
3. Baum EW, Sams WM, Payne RR. Giant cell arteritis: a systemic disease with rare cutaneous manifestations. J Am Acad Dermatol. 1982;6:1081-8.
4. Kinmont PD, Mccallum DI. The aetiology, pathology and course of giant-cell arteritis. The possible role of light sensitivity. Br J Dermatol. 1965;77:193-202.
5. Karahaliou M, Vaiopoulos G, Papaspyrou S, et al. Colour duplex sonography of temporal arteries before decision for biopsy: a prospective study in 55 patients with suspected giant cell arteritis. Arthritis Res Ther. 2006;8:R116.
6. Hoffman GS, Cid MC, Hellmann DB, et al. A multicenter, randomized, double-blind, placebo-controlled trial of adjuvant methotrexate treatment for giant cell arteritis. Arthritis Rheum. 2002;46:1309-18.
7. Hoffman GS, Cid MC, Rendt-Zagar KE, et al. Infliximab for maintenance of glucocorticosteroid-induced remission of giant cell arteritis: a randomized trial. Ann Intern Med. 2007;146:621-30.
8. Martínez-Taboada VM, Rodríguez-Valverde V, Carreño L, et al. A double-blind placebo controlled trial of etanercept in patients with giant cell arteritis and corticosteroid side effects. Ann Rheum Dis. 2008;67:625-30.
9. Kerr GS, Hallahan CW, Giordano J, et al. Takayasu arteritis. Ann Intern Med. 1994;120:919-29.
10. Pascual-López M, Hernández-Núñez A, Aragüés-Montañés M, et al. Takayasu's disease with cutaneous involvement. Dermatol Basel Switz. 2004;208:10-5.
11. Francès C, Boisnic S, Blétry O, et al. Cutaneous manifestations of Takayasu arteritis. A retrospective study of 80 cases. Dermatologica. 1990;181:266-72.
12. Skaria AM, Ruffieux P, Piletta P, et al. Takayasu arteritis and cutaneous necrotizing vasculitis. Dermatol Basel Switz. 2000;200:139-43.
13. Arend WP, Michel BA, Bloch DA, et al. The American College of Rheumatology 1990 criteria for the classification of Takayasu arteritis. Arthritis Rheum. 1990;33:1129-34.
14. Hidano A, Watanabe K. [Pyoderma gangraenosum and cardio-vasculopathies, particularly Takayasu arteritis. Review of the Japanese literature (author's transl)]. Ann Dermatol Vénéréologie. 1981;108:13-21.
15. Rocha LK, Romitti R, Shinjo S, et al. Cutaneous manifestations and comorbidities in 60 cases of Takayasu arteritis. J Rheumatol. 2013;40:734-8.
16. Perniciaro CV, Winkelmann RK, Hunder GG. Cutaneous manifestations of Takayasu's arteritis. A clinicopathologic correlation. J Am Acad Dermatol. 1987;17:998-1005.

17. Ujiie H, Sawamura D, Yokota K, et al. Pyoderma gangrenosum associated with Takayasu's arteritis. Clin Exp Dermatol. 2004;29:357-9.
18. Fearfield LA, Ross JR, Farrell AM, et al. Pyoderma gangrenosum associated with Takayasu's arteritis responding to cyclosporin. Br J Dermatol. 1999;141:339-43.
19. Jennette JC, Falk RJ, Andrassy K, et al. Nomenclature of systemic vasculitides. Proposal of an international consensus conference. Arthritis Rheum. 1994;37:187-92.
20. Mohammad AJ, Jacobsson LTH, Mahr AD, et al. Prevalence of Wegener's granulomatosis, microscopic polyangiitis, polyarteritis nodosa and Churg-Strauss syndrome within a defined population in southern Sweden. Rheumatol Oxf Engl. 2007;46:1329-37.
21. Decleva I, Marzano AV, Barbareschi M, et al. Cutaneous manifestations in systemic vasculitis. Clin Rev Allergy Immunol. 1997;15:5-20.
22. Jorizzo JL. Clinical dermatol. In: Demis DJ (Ed). Philadelphia: Lippincott; 1991.
23. Shaumberg-Lever G LW. Histopathology of the skin, 7th edition. Philadelphia: Lippincott; 1900.
24. Guillevin L, Mahr A, Callard P, et al. Hepatitis B virus-associated polyarteritis nodosa: clinical characteristics, outcome, and impact of treatment in 115 patients. Medicine (Baltimore). 2005;84:313-22.
25. Gayraud M, Guillevin L, le Toumelin P, et al. Long-term followup of polyarteritis nodosa, microscopic polyangiitis, and Churg-Strauss syndrome: analysis of four prospective trials including 278 patients. Arthritis Rheum. 2001;44:666-75.
26. Pagnoux C, Seror R, Henegar C, et al. Clinical features and outcomes in 348 patients with polyarteritis nodosa: a systematic retrospective study of patients diagnosed between 1963 and 2005 and entered into the French Vasculitis Study Group Database. Arthritis Rheum. 2010;62:616-26.
27. Minkowitz G, Smoller BR, McNutt NS. Benign cutaneous polyarteritis nodosa. Relationship to systemic polyarteritis nodosa and to hepatitis B infection. Arch Dermatol. 1991;127(10):1520-3.
28. Marzano AV, Vanotti M, Alessi E. Widespread livedoid vasculopathy. Acta Derm Venereol. 2003;83:457-60.
29. Kumar L, Thapa BR, Sarkar B, et al. Benign cutaneous polyarteritis nodosa in children below 10 years of age—a clinical experience. Ann Rheum Dis. 1995;54:134-6.
30. Siberry GK, Cohen BA, Johnson B. Cutaneous polyarteritis nodosa. Reports of two cases in children and review of the literature. Arch Dermatol. 1994;130:884-9.
31. Jorizzo JL, White WL, Wise CM, et al. Low-dose weekly methotrexate for unusual neutrophilic vascular reactions: cutaneous polyarteritis nodosa and Behçet's disease. J Am Acad Dermatol. 1991;24:973-8.
32. AN Malaviya, B Sharma, S Kapoor, et al. Twenty-three patients with cutaneous polyarteritis nodosa (C-PAN)—do rheumatologists see a more severe form of the disease? IJR. 2006;1:99-106.
33. Kawakami T, Soma Y. Use of warfarin therapy at a target international normalized ratio of 3.0 for cutaneous polyarteritis nodosa. J Am Acad Dermatol. 2010;63:602-6.
34. Sonomoto K, Miyamura T, Watanabe H, et al. [A case of polyarteritis nodosa successfully treated by rituximab]. Nihon Rinshō Meneki Gakkai Kaishi. 2008;31:119-23.
35. Bansal NK, Houghton KM. Cutaneous polyarteritis nodosa in childhood: a case report and review of the literature. Arthritis. 2010;2010:687547.
36. Vega Gutierrez J, Rodriguez Prieto MA, Garcia Ruiz JM. Successful treatment of childhood cutaneous polyarteritis nodosa with infliximab. J Eur Acad Dermatol Venereol JEADV. 2007;21:570-1.
37. Till SH, Amos RS. Long-term follow-up of juvenile-onset cutaneous polyarteritis nodosa associated with streptococcal infection. Br J Rheumatol. 1997;36:909-11.
38. Newburger JW, Takahashi M, Gerber MA, et al. Diagnosis, treatment, and long-term management of Kawasaki disease: a statement for health professionals from the Committee on Rheumatic Fever, Endocarditis and Kawasaki Disease, Council on Cardiovascular Disease in the Young, American Heart Association. Circulation. 2004;110:2747-71.
39. Burns JC, Glodé MP. Kawasaki syndrome. Lancet. 2004; 364:533-44.
40. Frieden IJ, Resnick SD. Childhood exanthems. Old and new. Pediatr Clin North Am. 1991;38:859-87.
41. Hicks RV, Melish ME. Kawasaki syndrome. Pediatr Clin North Am. 1986;33:1151-75.
42. Suzuki A, Kamiya T, Kuwahara N, et al. Coronary arterial lesions of Kawasaki disease: cardiac catheterization findings of 1100 cases. Pediatr Cardiol. 1986;7:3-9.
43. Eberhard BA, Sundel RP, Newburger JW, et al. Psoriatic eruption in Kawasaki disease. J Pediatr. 2000;137:578-80.
44. Friter BS, Lucky AW. The perineal eruption of Kawasaki syndrome. Arch Dermatol. 1988;124:1805-10.
45. Ayusawa M, Sonobe T, Uemura S, et al. Revision of diagnostic guidelines for Kawasaki disease (the 5th revised edition). Pediatr Int Off J Jpn Pediatr Soc. 2005;47:232-4.
46. Rosenfeld EA, Corydon KE, Shulman ST. Kawasaki disease in infants less than one year of age. J Pediatr. 1995;126:524-9.
47. Weston WL, Huff JC. The mucocutaneous lymph node syndrome: a critical re-examination. Clin Exp Dermatol. 1981;6:167-78.
48. Hirose S, Hamashima Y. Morphological observations on the vasculitis in the mucocutaneous lymph node syndrome. A skin biopsy study of 27 patients. Eur J Pediatr. 1978;129:17-27.
49. Tse SML, Silverman ED, McCrindle BW, et al. Early treatment with intravenous immunoglobulin in patients with Kawasaki disease. J Pediatr. 2002;140:450-5.
50. Falk RJ, Jennette JC. ANCA disease: where is this field heading? J Am Soc Nephrol JASN. 2010;21:745-52.
51. Chen KR, Carlson JA. Clinical approach to cutaneous vasculitis. Am J Clin Dermatol. 2008;9:71-92.

52. Jennette JC, Falk RJ. Small-vessel vasculitis. N Engl J Med. 1997;337:1512-23.
53. Guillevin L, Cohen P, Gayraud M, et al. Churg-Strauss syndrome. Clinical study and long-term follow-up of 96 patients. Medicine (Baltimore). 1999;78:26-37.
54. Guillevin L, Durand-Gasselin B, Cevallos R, et al. Microscopic polyangiitis: clinical and laboratory findings in eighty-five patients. Arthritis Rheum. 1999;42:421-30.
55. Duna GF, Galperin C, Hoffman GS. Wegener's granulomatosis. Rheum Dis Clin North Am. 1995;21:949-86.
56. Chen KR. Skin involvement in ANCA-associated vasculitis. Clin Exp Nephrol. 2013;17:676-82.
57. Chen KR, Sakamoto M, Ikemoto K, et al. Granulomatous arteritis in cutaneous lesions of Churg-Strauss syndrome. J Cutan Pathol. 2007;34:330-7.
58. Ishibashi M, Kudo S, Yamamoto K, et al. Churg-Strauss syndrome with coexistence of eosinophilic vasculitis, granulomatous phlebitis and granulomatous dermatitis in bullous pemphigoid-like blisters. J Cutan Pathol. 2011;38:290-4.
59. Daoud MS, Gibson LE, DeRemee RA, et al. Cutaneous Wegener's granulomatosis: clinical, histopathologic, and immunopathologic features of thirty patients. J Am Acad Dermatol. 1994;31:605-12.
60. Reed WB, Jensen AK, Konwaler BE, et al. The cutaneous manifestations in Wegener's granulomatosis. Acta Derm Venereol. 1963;43:250-64.
61. Lega JC, Seror R, Fassier T, et al. Characteristics, prognosis, and outcomes of cutaneous ischemia and gangrene in systemic necrotizing vasculitides: a retrospective multicenter study. Semin Arthritis Rheum. 2014;43:681-8.

CHAPTER 21

Antinuclear Cytoplasmic Antibody-associated Small Vessel Vasculitis

Aman Sharma, Shankar Naidu, Kusum Sharma

INTRODUCTION

Systemic vasculitides are a complex heterogeneous medical disorders often presenting with skin as one of the commonly involved organs. The classification is mostly based upon the size and type of vessel involved. There are seven main subgroups according to the revised Chapel Hill consensus conference (CHCC) nomenclature system namely large vessel vasculitis, medium vessel vasculitis, small vessel vasculitis, variable vessel vasculitis, single organ vasculitis, vasculitis associated with systemic diseases, and vasculitis associated with probable etiology. Some of these groups have been further divided into subgroups and contain various different types of vasculitides. The small vessel vasculitis group is subdivided into two subgroups—(i) antineutrophil cytoplasm antibodies (ANCA)-associated vasculitis (AAV), and (ii) immune complex vasculitis. The present chapter will have details of AAV. The types of AAV are granulomatosis with polyangiitis (GPA), microscopic polyangiitis (MPA), and eosinophilic granulomatosis with polyangiitis (EGPA).

Box 1: Key Clinical features of granulomatosis with polyangiitis

- Prevalence—variable in different regions of world, no gender predilection
- Genetic factors, infections, drugs, environmental exposure to toxic compounds—all play role in pathogenesis
- HPE—triad of granuloma, vasculitis, and necrosis.
- Severity variable—localized granulomatous inflammation to widespread angiitis
- Constitutional symptoms accompany more generalized and extensive disease
- Nasal, laryngeal, tracheal mucosa, and paranasal sinuses are commonly affected—inflammation, erosion, ulceration, later scaring
- Lung—commonly affected, mainly as nodules solid or cavitary, single or multiple. Sometimes as lung hemorrhage, atelectasis, and consolidation. Pleura and lymph node rarely affected
- Kidney—involved in one-fifth of the patients as crescentic glomerulonephritis, can result in renal failure
- Skin involved in almost half of patients; nodules, palpable purpura, ulcers, hemorrhagic bullae, and pyoderma gangrenosum-like lesions
- Other organ affected—eyes, peripheral and central nervous system

GRANULOMATOSIS WITH POLYANGIITIS

Previously known as Wegener's granulomatosis (WG), GPA is a multisystem disease with a wide spectrum of clinical manifestations (Box 1). Classical histopathology triad consists of granulomatous inflammation, tissue necrosis, and vasculitis. Granulomatosis with polyangiitis was first described by Heinz Klinger in 1931.[1] However, it was Wegener, who after demonstration of histopathological changes on autopsy of three patients proposed that it was a distinct entity.[2]

CLASSIFICATION AND NOMENCLATURE

The American College of Rheumatology (ACR) set down the classification criteria for seven types of vasculitis including GPA (WG) in 1990.[3] A diagnosis of GPA (WG) could be made if at least two of these four criteria were present.
1. Nasal or oral inflammation: Development of painful or painless oral ulcers or purulent or bloody nasal discharge
2. Abnormal chest radiograph: Chest radiograph showing the presence of nodules, fixed infiltrates, or cavities
3. Urinary sediment: Microhematuria (>5 red blood cells per high power field) or red cell casts in urine sediment
4. Granulomatous inflammation on biopsy: Histologic changes showing granulomatous inflammation within the wall of an artery or in the perivascular or extravascular area (artery or arteriole).

These criteria had a sensitivity of 88.2% and a specificity of 92.0%. The CHCC nomenclature system provided the definition of GPA in 1994. According to this nomenclature system, GPA was characterized by granulomatous inflammation of the respiratory tract, along with necrotizing vasculitis of small and medium sized vessels (capillaries, venules, arterioles, and arteries).[4]

The GPA has an association with ANCA and in the revised CHCC nomenclature system proposed in 2012, it has been put in a subgroup of ANCA associated vasculitis along with MPA and EGPA.[5]

EPIDEMIOLOGY

The estimates of prevalence of GPA have varied depending upon the study designs. A population based study, from England, reported an annual incidence of 8.5 per million.[6] The incidence of GPA seems to have increased after introduction of ANCA testing. However, studies done subsequently showed a stable incidence with no significant change during the 22 year observation period of the Norwich Vasculitis Cohort.[7]

CLINICAL FEATURES

Clinically, the disease shows very diverse manifestations ranging from a localized granulomatous respiratory inflammation to widespread systemic necrotizing granulomatous angiitis. The characteristic clinical phenotype is in the form of multisystem involvement with upper airway inflammation, lung nodules, and glomerulonephritis. This must be considered amongst the differential diagnosis of renopulmonary syndrome.

Fever, arthralgia, weight loss, and other constitutional symptoms are common in the generalized phase of the disease. The transition from limited to generalized disease is usually associated with constitutional symptoms, elevated laboratory markers of inflammation, and evidence of major organ involvement.

Articular involvement is usually in the form of arthralgia but true arthritis with active synovitis may also occur. The pattern of joint involvement may vary from oligoarticular, predominantly large joint involvement to symmetrical additive inflammatory small joint polyarthritis.

Upper Airways and Nose

The involvement of nose and paranasal sinuses is very common, seen in up to 60% patients.[8] The symptoms can be in the form of nasal congestion, nasal obstruction, rhinorrhea, pain over the dorsum of nose, anosmia, recurrent epistaxis, and epiphora.[9] Chronic sinusitis is common and may present with headache, postnasal drip, chronic cough, and sinus tenderness.[10] Examination may reveal ulceration of nasal mucosa, nasal crusting, and septal perforation (Fig. 1). Nasal endoscopy

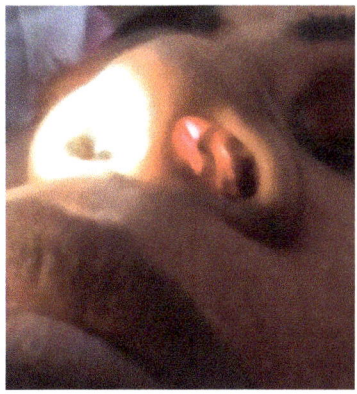

FIGURE 1: Granulomatosis with polyangiitis patient having nasal septal perforation.

may show purulent discharge in the middle meatus, crusting over the septum and turbinates, friable nasal mucosa, and rarely, nasal polyps.[11] Granulomatous inflammation may eventually result in "saddle nose deformity" (Fig. 2) and nasal airway stenosis. Involvement of larynx and trachea is also common.[12] Airway involvement is more common in the younger patients under 30 years of age and in females.[13] There may be ulceration, granuloma formation, pseudo membranes, and cobble stone appearance of the mucosa of larynx and trachea. The symptoms are in the form of recurrent cough, change in voice, respiratory difficulty, and hemoptysis. Subglottic stenosis is a rare complication and manifests as hoarseness of voice and stridor and can require emergency tracheostomy.[14] It is more commonly seen in association with generalized GPA. Biopsy from the subglottic area may occasionally confirm the diagnosis of GPA.[15]

Oral Manifestations

Oral cavity involvement at presentation occurs in less than or equal to 6% of patients. "Strawberry" gingivitis, reddish to pinkish hyperplastic gingivitis with numerous petechiae, associated with pain and bleeding gums, is a classical manifestation. Mucosal ulcers over the tongue, buccal mucosa (Fig. 3), gums or palate, cobblestone-like lesion over the palate, nonhealing extraction socket, and oroantral fistula may be the other manifestations. Submandibular or parotid gland sialadenitis may be a presenting feature and simulate Sjögren syndrome.[16,17]

Pulmonary Involvement

Pulmonary manifestations frequently dominate the clinical presentation. Lung involvement may vary from asymptomatic lung nodules to catastrophic pulmonary hemorrhage. Nodules may be single or multiple (Fig. 4), solid or cavitary, fixed or migratory and can mimic lung abscess or even lung cancer (Fig. 5). Reticular or reticulonodular opacities, atelectasis, and consolidation are less common. Pulmonary hemorrhage, due to capillaritis, may present with hemoptysis and pulmonary infiltrates (Fig. 6).

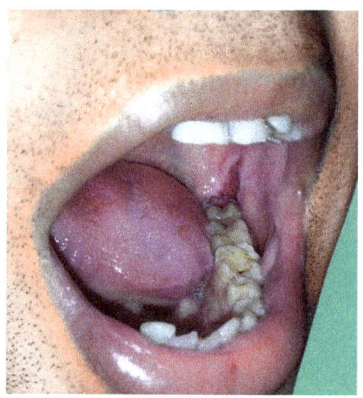

FIGURE 3: Mucosal ulcer over the buccal cavity in granulomatosis with polyangiitis patient.

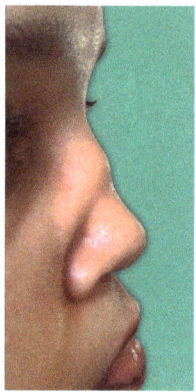

FIGURE 2: Collapsed nasal bridge in a granulomatosis with polyangiitis patient.

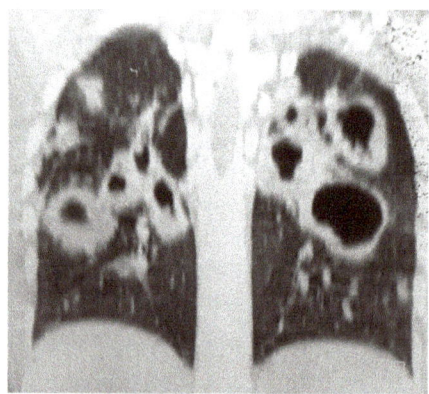

FIGURE 4: Multiple cavitating nodules seen in bilateral lung fields in granulomatosis with polyangiitis patient.

Antinuclear Cytoplasmic Antibody-associated Small Vessel Vasculitis

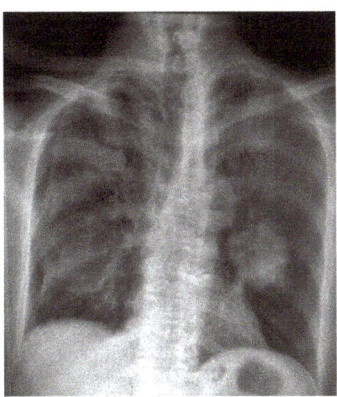

FIGURE 5: Chest X-ray mimicking bronchogenic carcinoma in a patient with granulomatosis with polyangiitis.

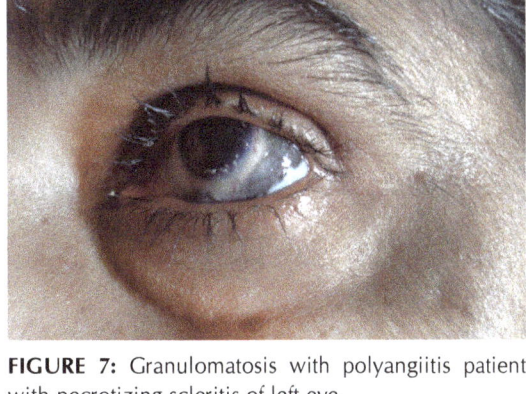

FIGURE 7: Granulomatosis with polyangiitis patient with necrotizing scleritis of left eye.

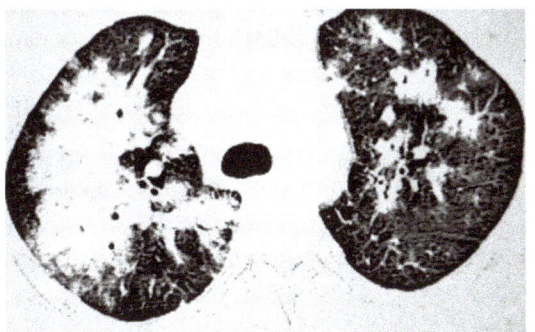

FIGURE 6: Computed tomography scan showing diffuse alveolar hemorrhage in bilateral lung parenchyma (right > left).

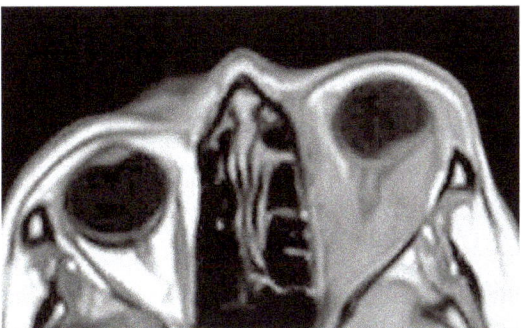

FIGURE 8: Pseudotumor of the orbit in a granulomatosis with polyangiitis patient.

Renal Manifestations

Kidney involvement is another major clinical manifestation. The most sinister presentation is in the form of rapidly progressive renal failure characterized by oliguria, microscopic hematuria, red blood cell casts, and rapidly rising serum creatinine.

Eyes

The eyes may be involved in several ways. Necrotizing scleritis (Fig. 7), peripheral ulcerative keratitis, and orbital pseudotumor (Fig. 8) are among the most prominent manifestations. Scleritis may begin with pain and redness and eventually cause "scleromalacia perforans" and loss of vision. Peripheral ulcerative keratitis can also result in vision loss due to "corneal melt" resulting in perforation. The orbital pseudotumor like presentation can cause proptosis, pain, and vision loss. This is usually refractory to therapy. The description, of GPA from India, is in the form of small case series and case reports.[18-21]

Skin

Skin lesions appear in an around half of the GPA patients and the morphology of lesions is varied. Most commonly patients present with nodules, palpable purpura, ulcers, hemorrhagic bullae, and pyoderma gangrenosum-like lesions (Fig. 9), or digital infarcts. Usually, skin involvement parallels the systemic disease activity and skin biopsy findings help in establishing the diagnosis.

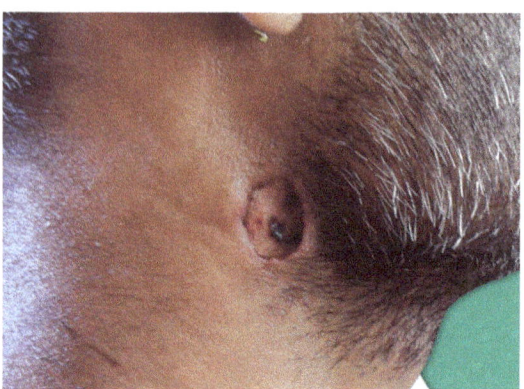

FIGURE 9: Pyoderma gangrenosum-like lesion in a granulomatosis with polyangiitis patient.

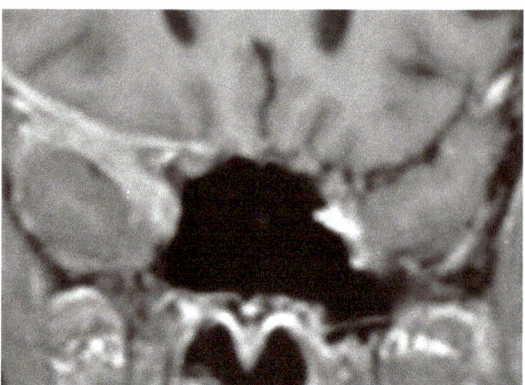

FIGURE 10: Pachymeningitis of central nervous system in a granulomatosis with polyangiitis patient.

Other Manifestations

Neurological manifestations include peripheral nervous system (PNS) or central nervous system (CNS) involvement. The PNS involvement is more common and usually manifests as mononeuritis multiplex or distal sensorimotor neuropathy. The CNS involvement is rare, usually in the form of cranial neuropathies, pachymeningitis (Fig. 10), or mass lesions. Rarer manifestations include diabetes insipidus due to pituitary involvement, bowel manifestations resembling ischemic bowel and inflammatory bowel disease, prostatic vasculitis, and "mass" lesions in the muscles and breasts.[22]

DIAGNOSIS

In the absence of validated diagnostic criteria, the diagnosis of GPA is clinical. The key to the diagnosis is high index of suspicion in the appropriate clinical settings, especially when there is multisystem involvement. This is supported by ANCA along with histopathological evidence of GPA. Disseminated infection like infective endocarditis is a close clinical mimic and must be reasonably excluded.

Laboratory Tests

Acute phase reactants such as erythrocyte sedimentation rate and C-reactive protein are generally elevated. There may be leukocytosis and thrombocytosis. Rheumatoid factor may be positive in up to 50% patients. Urinalysis and renal function tests show abnormalities in case of renal involvement. Mild increase in transaminases may also be observed. The international consensus statement on reporting of ANCA recommends both indirect immunofluorescence (IIF) and enzyme-linked immunosorbent assay (ELISA) assay as 5% of IIF negative results are ELISA positive.[23] The main target antigens of ANCA are located in the neutrophils and monocytes cytoplasm.[24] Two main target antigens are proteinase 3 (PR3) and myeloperoxidase (MPO).[25,26]

Imaging

Computed tomography (CT) of nose and paranasal sinuses may show bone destruction with generalized mucosal thickening. Bone destruction typically commences in the midline affecting the nasal septum and turbinates initially, spreading laterally, symmetrically to involve the maxillary antrum and other sinuses with sclerotic changes of the walls.[27] The end result is single large cavity with loss of nasal septum, turbinates, and walls of the maxillary antrum.[28]

Magnetic resonance imaging (MRI) shows high signal intensity of T1 weighted sequence and evidence of fat signal from the sclerotic walls of the sinus.[29] Though conventional X-rays would show nodules and infiltrates in widespread disease, CT scan of the chest has a better sensitivity than plain chest X-ray in demonstrating changes in patients with milder involvement. High resolution CT of chest can show changes like small nodules, linear opacities, and ground glass opacities.

MEASUREMENT OF DISEASE ACTIVITY

This helps in planning therapy, and preventing undue immunosuppression as some symptoms may be due to accrual damage, rather than disease activity. Birmingham vasculitis activity score (BVAS) is a validated measure of disease activity. The BVAS version 3 is presently being used. There is a shorter GPA specific BVAS score. The validated measure of disease damage is vasculitis damage index. A recent study on relevance of monitoring PR3-ANCA titers in predicting relapse in GPA patients showed that no strict clinical-immunological correspondence was observed for 25% of the patients. It was concluded that GPA management cannot be based on ANCA levels alone.

TREATMENT

With the currently available treatment, this once invariably fatal condition has changed into a relapsing remitting, chronic disease. The present therapeutic concerns include the prevention of relapse, and minimizing damage due to disease activity and drugs.

Current treatment recommendations are based upon the disease severity. The European Vasculitis Study Group (EUVAS) recommends five grades of disease severity of AAV. These are: (i) localized—upper or lower airway disease without other systemic involvement or constitutional symptoms, (ii) early systemic disease—or systemic disease without organ or life-threatening disease, (iii) generalized—renal or other organ threatening disease, serum creatinine level less than or equal to 5.6 mg/dL, (iv) severe-renal or other organ failure, serum creatinine more than or equal to 5.6 mg/dL, (v) refractory-progressive disease unresponsive to glucocorticoids (GCs) and cyclophosphamide (CYC).[30]

Remission induction: In generalized or severe disease, the drug of choice for remission induction remains CYC. The dose is modified in the presence of renal failure and in old age. Mesna should be used to decrease bladder toxicity of CYC, especially if oral CYC is used. In patients who have contraindication for CYC, such as cytopenia, intolerance, malignancy or fertility protection, rituximab (RTX) may be used as an alternative agent for remission induction.

Rituximab is a chimeric anti-CD20 monoclonal antibody shown to be effective to induce remission in GPA. The two back to back randomized controlled trials "the rituximab for ANCA associated vasculitis (RAVE)" and "rituximab versus CYC in ANCA associated renal vasculitis" were published in 2010.[31,32] Both these trails showed that in non-life threatening disease, RTX was not inferior to CYC for induction of remission. Long-term follow-up of RAVE study showed that those patients who achieved remission with a single course of RTX remained in remission for long.[33] In patients with mild localized disease, a combination of methotrexate 15–25 mg/week and prednisolone may be tried.

Remission maintenance: Once remission is achieved, its maintenance can be achieved with drugs like azathioprine, mycophenolate mofetil, or methotrexate. Rituximab has also been used in remission maintenance at 4-6 monthly intervals.[34,35] Maintain remission of ANCA-associated vasculitides study has shown that after the initial induction with CYC, RTX (initial 1 g followed by 500 mg every 6 months) is better than azathioprine in remission maintenance.[36] The RTX can be planned provided IgG levels are more than or equal to 7 g/L, otherwise there may be increased risk of infections.

Plasma Exchange

The MEPEX trial showed that plasma exchange improved the chances of renal recovery in patients with serum creatinine more than or equal to 5.8 mg/dL. There was, however, no survival benefit. Its role in patients with lower serum creatinine and diffuse alveolar hemorrhage is uncertain.[37]

A recent meta-analysis did not show any survival benefit or decrease in progression to end stage renal disease.[38]

MORBIDITY

Despite significant advances in management, significant morbidity, and mortality associated with AAV in patients, compared to matched background population, persists.[39] Increased morbidity is due to both the disease per se, and the treatment received. There are increased chances of deep venous thrombosis.[40] Despite control of disease activity, these patients have poor quality of life, with fatigue being a major contributor.[41] There are increased chances of infection such as *Pneumocystis jirovecii*, *Herpes zoster varicella*. The RTX has been associated with increased risk of progressive multifocal leukoencephalopathy. The predictors for development of infection are age, severity of renal dysfunction, leukopenia, and intensity and duration of immunosuppression.[42,43]

MICROSCOPIC POLYANGIITIS

Microscopic polyangiitis (MPA) was traditionally considered to be part of polyarteritis nodosa. The terms polyarteritis nodosa, microscopic polyarteritis, and microscopic polyangiitis were often used interchangeably (Box 2).[44] At the 1994 Chapel Hill Consensus Conference, microscopic polyangiitis was formally recognized as a distinct entity and the nomenclature was accepted universally.[4] Microscopic polyangiitis is characterized by the presence of antibodies directed against antigenic targets in the neutrophil cytoplasm—the ANCA. Microscopic polyangiitis is defined as a necrotizing vasculitis, with few or no immune deposits, predominantly affecting small vessels. Necrotizing arteritis involving small and medium arteries may be present. Necrotizing glomerulonephritis is very common. Pulmonary capillaritis often occurs. Granulomatous inflammation is absent.[5]

EPIDEMIOLOGY

Microscopic polyangiitis has an annual incidence of 2.5–10/million.[45] Microscopic polyangiitis may have a latitudinal variation in incidence in the northern hemisphere, with increasing incidence in the more southern latitudes.[46]

DIAGNOSIS

There are no diagnostic criteria for establishing the diagnosis of MPA. The diagnosis is based on grounds of clinical evidence of small vessel vasculitis (purpura, mononeuritis multiplex, alveolar hemorrhage, nephritic proteinuria, and hematuria, etc.). Once small vessel vasculitis is suspected, it is recommended that the classification of the vasculitis is performed as set out by Watts et al.[47]

CLINICAL FEATURES

Constitutional symptoms are common at diagnosis. Fever more than 38°C, weight loss more than 2 kg, arthralgia, myalgia are reported in the majority of patients. About 80% of patients with MPA present with renal involvement. Rapidly progressive glomerulonephritis can be a presenting feature. Most patients will have early hematuria and proteinuria with few other clinical manifestations which may flare explosively. The presence of glomerulosclerosis on kidney biopsy at diagnosis is suggestive of the presence of smoldering disease prior to clinical presentation. Patients may present with oliguria/anuria and need dialysis at diagnosis. Proteinuria in the nephrotic range is not usual but is seen in about 15% of patients.[48]

Pulmonary involvement can be catastrophic, in the form of alveolar hemorrhage.[49] It is seen in about 10% of patients,[50] and has a poor prognosis. Most patients with pulmonary hemorrhage

> **Box 2: Key clinical features of Microscopic polyangiitis**
>
> - It is a pauci-immune necrotizing vasculitis, predominantly affecting small vessels in the absence of granuloma
> - Prevalence variable in different regions, but it is the most common of the three AAV and its incidence is increasing
> - Majority have constitutional symptoms at the time of presentation
> - Renal involvement in 80%—mild renal insufficiency to full blown renal failure, necrotizingionon of the glomerulonephritis
> - Lung—infiltrates, alveolar hemorrhage, lung fibrosis
> - Skin—purpura, ulcers, necrotizing nodules, livedo reticularis, digital ischemia, and gangrene
> - Other organ—nervous system, gut, eye, and heart may be involved
>
> AVV, anti-neutrophil cytoplasm antibodies (ANCA) associated vasculitis.

have coexistent glomerulonephritis. Pulmonary fibrosis is seen in about a third of patients with MPA,[50] and may be a function of the MPO-ANCA serotype.[51] Computed tomography scan imaging show ground glass changes, consolidation, and thickening of bronchovascular bundles.[51]

Neurological involvement is usually in the form of mononeuritis multiplex, which is observed in the majority of patients at diagnosis. Axonal sensorimotor neuropathy and cranial nerve involvement have also been documented.[48]

Cutaneous involvement is seen in almost half of the patients and includes cutaneous changes such as maculopapular purpura over the limbs, ulcers (Fig. 11), vesicles, necrotizing nodules (Fig. 12), splinter hemorrhages, livedo reticularis, digital ischemia, and gangrene; mucosal involvement such as mouth or genital ulcers. Leukocytoclastic vasculitis is common. The nodules are due to arteriolar and small vessel involvement in deep dermis and subcutis.

Ocular involvement in the form of retinal vasculitis, scleritis, episcleritis, blepharitis, conjunctivitis, keratitis, uveitis; rarely heart involvement in the form of pericarditis, myocardial infarction, congestive cardiac failure; gastrointestinal involvement in the form of mesenteric ischemia, gastrointestinal bleeding, and perforation.

INVESTIGATIONS

Anemia and thrombocytosis are common. Renal abnormality of some form is nearly universal. The mean serum creatinine in the largest cohort of patients with MPA was 2.54 (SD 2.96) mg/dL at diagnosis.[48] The creatine kinase may be elevated in a small number of patients with muscle involvement.

Urine analysis abnormalities include hematuria, varying degrees of proteinuria, and red-cell casts.

Antineutrophil cytoplasm antibodies are present in most patients at diagnosis. Indirect immunofluorescence uptake in a perinuclear (P) pattern or a diffuse cytoplasmic (C) pattern may be seen. Enzyme-linked immunosorbent assay is usually positive for MPO or PR3. Perinuclear/MPO ANCA or a C/PR3 ANCA is over 98% specific for a diagnosis of AAV.[52] Antibodies directed against lysosomal associated membrane protein-2 have been shown to be pathogenic and maybe of value in serial monitoring, but is currently of academic interest and requires further work.[53]

Chest imaging in the form of plain radiographs and CT scan is of value in documenting silent chest disease.

Renal biopsy is highly sensitive for the diagnosis and when possible should be preferentially sampled. Sural nerve, muscle, and skin can be biopsied as well. The characteristic changes of MPA include focal segmental glomerulonephritis in the kidney with presence of crescents in nearly all patients. There is little or no immune complex deposition. Granulomas are not a feature of MPA.

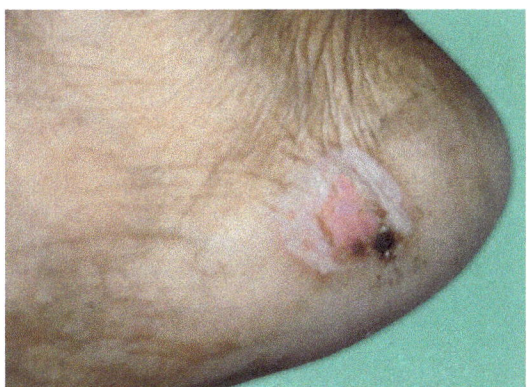

FIGURE 11: Ulcerative skin lesion in a patient with microscopic polyangiitis.

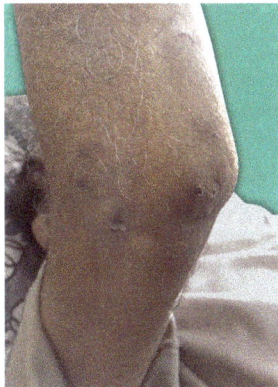

FIGURE 12: Nodular skin lesions over the elbow in a patient with microscopic polyangiitis.

DIAGNOSTIC APPROACH

Microscopic polyangiitis should be suspected in patients with involvement of more than one organ-system which includes the kidneys. Patients are typically unwell, and may have been investigated for chronic symptoms like the case above who was being investigated for anemia.

In the absence of a diagnostic test, every effort should be made to obtain tissue biopsy prior to initiating treatment. In patients with an inconclusive/negative biopsy and negativity for P/MPO or C/PR3 ANCA, alternative differentials include systemic lupus erythematosus, infective endocarditis, cancer, antiglomerular basement membrane disease, and the other AAV. Management is on the similar lines as GPA

EOSINOPHILIC GRANULOMATOSIS WITH POLYANGIITIS (CHURG-STRAUSS SYNDROME)

Eosinophilic granulomatosis with polyangiitis, formerly also named Churg-Strauss syndrome, is a small-sized vessel systemic necrotizing vasculitis (Box 3).[4,5,54,55] It is the rarest of the three main ANCA-associated vasculitides and whether it should remain part of this vasculitis subgroup is increasingly discussed.[56-58] Epidemiologically, most characteristic manifestations of EGPA, such as asthma and eosinophilia, and the main pathogenic mechanisms of EGPA differ from those of MPA and GPA. In addition, ANCAs, mainly antimyeloperoxidase (anti-MPO) ANCAs, are detected in the sera of only 30–40% of EGPA patients, whose clinical features differ from those of ANCA-negative patients.[59-61]

EPIDEMIOLOGY

Eosinophilic granulomatosis with polyangiitis is one of the rarest primary systemic necrotizing vasculitides. Eosinophilic granulomatosis with polyangiitis prevalence ranges from 7 to 22 per million inhabitants. A few studies have reported a slightly higher prevalence in northern versus southern Europe and urban versus rural regions, but in general, the geographical distribution shows no pattern.[45,48] A few epidemiological studies of ANCA-associated vasculitis suggested that EGPA is rare in Asia, but some large series have recently been reported from Japan and Korea.[45,58,62,63]

In asthma patients, the average annual incidence is not surprisingly higher, because asthma can be considered a predisposing condition for EGPA or a first phase of the disease; the EGPA incidence has been estimated at about 34 per million patients with asthma and up to 60–64.4 per million in those requiring a leukotriene-receptor antagonist or other nonleukotriene-modifying asthma drugs.[64-67] A recent study suggested an association of the human leukocyte antigen DRB4 (HLA-DRB4) and severe asthma, sinusitis, nasal polyposis, and eosinophils, which may help in the early identification of some patients at risk of EGPA.[68] The presence of blood eosinophilia in a patient with difficult-to-control

---

Box 3: Key clinical features of eosinophilic granulomatosis with polyangiitis

- Eosinophilic granulomatosis with polyangiitis is a systemic necrotizing vasculitis of small-sized vessels characterized by blood eosinophilia and late onset difficult to control asthma
- Prevalence—least incidence among three AAV, rare in Asia, mean age at diagnosis around 50 years, and no sex preponderance
- Exact cause unknown
- Constitutional symptoms frequently present at diagnosis
- Lung infiltrates in 35–75%, sometimes pleural effusion and hilar and/or mediastinal lymphadenopathy, while alveolar hemorrhage and nodules are rare
- Skin (30–75% cases)-most commonly as palpable purpura or urticarial macula-papular rash
- Peripheral nervous system—mononeuritis multiplex, polyneuropathy is rare
- Cardiac (10–50%)—cardiomyopathy, ischemic changes due to coronary artery, and small myocardial vessel vasculitis
- Kidney—mainly focal segmental and pauci-immune glomerulonephritis
- Other organ—CNS, eye, GIT, venous thromboembolic event

AVV, anti-neutrophil cytoplasm antibodies (ANCA) associated vasculitis; CNS, central nervous system; GIT, gastrointestinal tract.

and late-onset asthma or allergic sinusitis should certainly alert physicians but is not sufficient to establish a diagnosis of EGPA. Late-onset asthma is almost always present in EGPA patients and preceded the first vasculitis manifestations by a mean of 6.7–8.9 years in the French studies and a median of 4 years in the study by Keogh et al.[59,69,70]

Mean age at diagnosis of EGPA patients is about 50 years. Diagnosis of EGPA in children is rare, but a few case series have been reported, as well as in older adults.[63,71]

The exact cause(s) of EGPA remains unknown. Inhaled allergens, desensitization, or drugs (e.g., macrolides, carbamazepine, and quinine) have been implicated as potential triggers and/or precipitating cofactors for EGPA onset or flares as have been several medications to treat asthma such as leukotriene-receptor antagonists or omalizumab.[67,72,73] A direct triggering role of these latter antiasthma drugs cannot be excluded, but more likely in reported cases, they provided the opportunity for substantial tapering or withdrawal of GCs in patients with asthma, thereby unmasking an underlying "forme fruste" of EGPA, which had been controlled by GCs. For a long time, vaccinations have been considered potential triggers of EGPA or EGPA flare. Recent studies of vaccinations in vasculitis patients have been more reassuring.[74,75]

Asthma often clusters in families, whereas familial cases of EGPA are exceptional.

DIAGNOSIS

In a patient presenting with classical symptoms, the diagnosis of EGPA can be relatively simple. However, in many patients, especially ANCA-negative patients and/or those without histological evidence of (granulomatous and eosinophilic) vasculitis, several alternative diagnoses must be considered and ruled out. The most difficult diagnoses to exclude are primary hypereosinophilic syndrome, mainly with its lymphocytic subsets, and lymphomas, mostly T-cell types.

CLINICAL FEATURES

The diagnostic criteria for Churg-Strauss syndrome devised by Lanham in the mid-1980s are too broad and not specific.[76,77] However, they remain of interest because they underscored, probably for the first time clearly, the three prototypical successive phases of the disease. The prodromal phase begins with asthma and allergic manifestations; the second stage is characterized by blood eosinophilia more than 10% (1,500/mm^3) and tissue eosinophilia affecting visceral organs such as the lung; and the last stage involves the development of vasculitis features (involving two or more extrapulmonary organs) such as those affecting the skin (purpura) and peripheral nerves. The three phases do not systematically occur successively, because they can overlap in time. In the absence of overt clinical vasculitis manifestations (third phase), the diagnosis of EGPA remains uncertain and should likely not be concluded. We lack other diagnostic criteria at this time, although international efforts to develop criteria are under way.[78] The 1990 American College of Rheumatology classification criteria of Churg-Strauss vasculitis are for classification purposes.[54] The 2012 revised Chapel Hill nomenclature of EGPA provided an updated definition of the disease.[5] Importantly, none of these criteria should be used to support a diagnostic impression because they are not diagnostic criteria and are specific to only patients with already established and proven vasculitis.

Constitutional symptoms such as arthralgias, myalgias, weight loss, and/or fever are frequent at diagnosis. Ear, nose, and throat (ENT) manifestations, such as rhinitis or sinus polyposis, and/or asthma are present in almost all EGPA patients. Lung infiltrates, which would be predominantly eosinophilic if a bronchoalveolar lavage fluid examination is performed, is present in 35–75% of patients, depending on the series, and eosinophilic pleural effusion is present in 7–30%. Hilar and/or mediastinal lymphadenopathy are possible, although their presence should raise concerns about a possible underlying lymphoproliferative disorder. Alveolar hemorrhage and nodules are rare in EGPA. Interstitial lung fibrosis is a rare complication of anti-MPO ANCA-associated vasculitis, including MPA and EGPA.[79]

Skin and peripheral nerve involvement are the next most common manifestations, the former occurring in 30–75% of patients, mainly palpable purpura or maculopapules, often with a urticarial appearance and, sometimes, migratory pattern (Figs 13 and 14). Cutaneous nodules, livedo reticularis, ulcerations, erythema multiforme, scalp erythematous, macular lesions (Fig. 15), nail-fold infarctions, vesicles or bullae, toe or finger ischemia, deep pannicular vasculitis, and facial edema have been reported.

Mononeuritis multiplex, with asymmetric motor and/or sensory signs, is the most frequent and characteristic feature of peripheral nerve involvement. The peroneal and tibial branches of the sciatic, ulnar, and median nerves are the most commonly affected nerves. Polyneuropathy, symmetrical or not, is rarer.

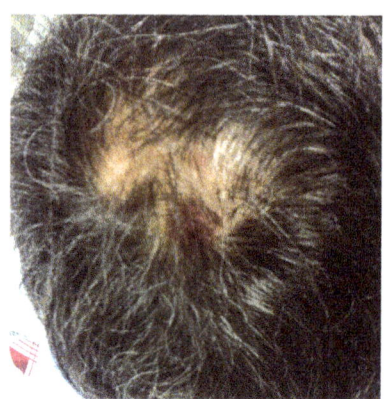

FIGURE 15: Erythematous-macular skin lesions of the scalp, superficially eroded, in a patient with eosinophilic granulomatosis with polyangiitis.

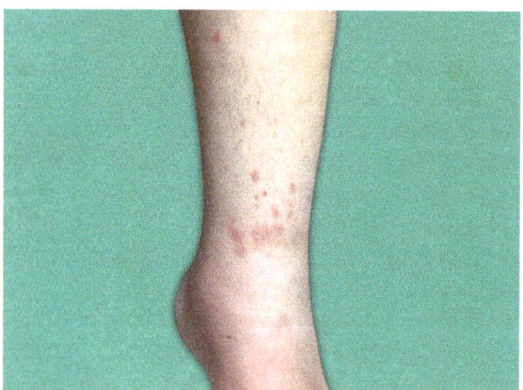

FIGURE 13: Purpuric papules and reddish macular skin lesions on the leg, above the ankle, in a patient with eosinophilic granulomatosis with polyangiitis.

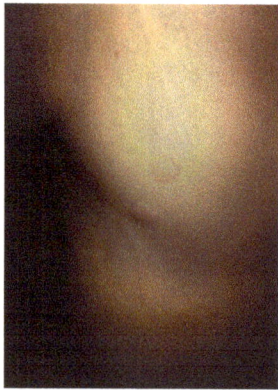

FIGURE 14: Maculopapular pseudourticarial lesion in the scapular area in a patient with eosinophilic granulomatosis with polyangiitis.

Cardiac manifestations occur in 10–50% of patients, depending on the series, with definitions and/or cardiac investigations described.[77,80,81] The mechanisms of EGPA cardiac manifestations may combine eosinophilic and/or granulomatous infiltration of the myocardium, eosinophil-derived protein toxicity in heart tissues, possibly leading to fibrosis, and/or coronary artery and small myocardial vessel vasculitis, causing ischemic lesions. Cardiomyopathy has been associated with increased mortality in earlier series of EGPA and justifies an aggressive therapeutic management. Eosinophilic pericardial effusion is frequent, in up to 20% of patients, as are conduction disorders and supraventricular arrhythmias. Intraventricular thrombi, dysautonomic manifestations, or cardiac valve involvement are rare.[82]

Other possible manifestations include cranial nerve palsy, central nervous system involvement (intracranial and/or subarachnoid hemorrhage, cerebral infarction, pachymeningitis), which usually occurs later during the course of the disease, and gastrointestinal manifestations (abdominal pain, vomiting or diarrhea, eosinophilic granulomatous colitis or esogastritis, and of more concern, bleeding, mesenteric artery branches vasculitis, with the risk of bowel infarction and perforation).

Kidney involvement (mainly focal segmental and pauci-immune glomerulonephritis) and urological manifestations (urethral or ureteral stenosis, prostatitis) are not as frequent as in

GPA. Ophthalmologic manifestations (uveitis, episcleritis, or retinal vasculitis) and venous thromboembolic events, including pulmonary embolism, mainly during the active phase of the vasculitis, are other possible manifestations.[83,84]

Outcomes for patients seem similar regardless of ANCA status at diagnosis but with a limited follow up of 3–5 years; some studies with a longer follow-up suggested a possible higher relapse rate of the vasculitis manifestations (differentiated from "simple" asthma exacerbations) but lower mortality in ANCA-positive than negative patients.[60,69,85]

INVESTIGATIONS

Blood eosinophilia is almost constant during active disease, usually more than 1,000/mm^3, and can exceed 50,000/mm^3. Serum IgE level is elevated in most patients, as a simple surrogate marker of eosinophilia (its measurement does not seem to add much to the diagnosis or monitoring disease). Anti-neutrophil cytoplasmic antibodies can be detected in up to 40% of EGPA patients, usually generating a perinuclear immunofluorescent-labeling pattern, most frequently anti-MPO, on ELISA.[57,69,70]

RADIOLOGY

Imaging of the sinus may reveal nondestructive sinusitis and/or sinus polyposis (Fig. 16). Chest radiographs can show pulmonary infiltrates, most often transient, labile and patchy, with an alveolar pattern (Figs 17 and 18). A diffuse interstitial infiltrative pattern or massive bilateral nodular infiltrates may be seen, as well as pleural effusion. Cardiac imaging should probably be systematic at diagnosis with ultrasound and/or MRI (Fig. 19).

HISTOPATHOLOGY

When possible, the diagnosis of EGPA should be substantiated by biopsy of an involved tissue. The three main histological lesions of EGPA include—(i) vessel wall infiltrates (mainly with eosinophils) with fibrinoid necrosis (vasculitis), (ii) extravascular eosinophilic infiltrates, and (iii) extravascular necrotizing granulomas (mainly with eosinophils). However, these three types of histological lesions are found together in only a few cases.[86]

Skin biopsies are easy to obtain when patients have cutaneous lesions. Lung and/or muscle and peripheral nerve biopsies are more invasive. The yield of ENT biopsies is low; the histology of polyps is often nonspecific (eosinophilic infiltrates, as in more common allergic polyposis).

DIAGNOSTIC APPROACH

Diagnosis relies on the combination of suggestive clinical manifestations, as described earlier, and

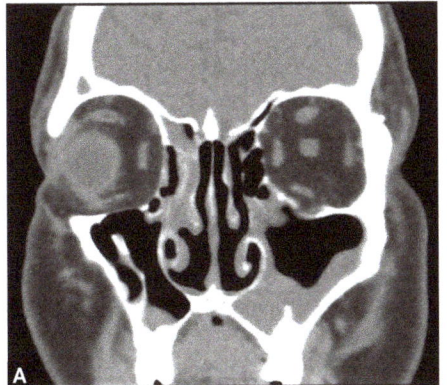
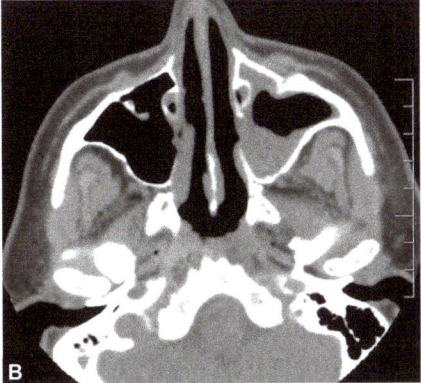

FIGURE 16: Sinus computed tomography of a patient with eosinophilic granulomatosis with polyangiitis, coronal and horizontal views) showing bilateral, non-erosive sinusitis (clearly predominating on the left maxillary sinus, with some fluid consolidation in right ethmoido-sphenoidal sinus).

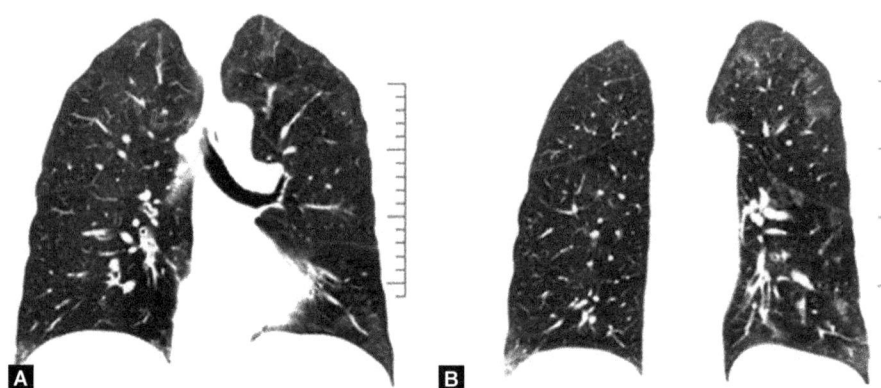

FIGURE 17: Chest computed tomography of a patient with eosinophilic granulomatosis with polyangiitis (frontal views) showing multiple patchy ground-glass opacities, mainly in the left apex and basis.

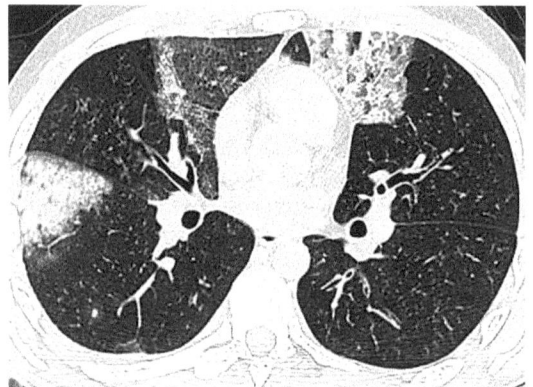

FIGURE 18: Chest computed tomography of a patient with eosinophilic granulomatosis with polyangiitis (horizontal view) showing multiple patchy opacities and consolidation are seen in bilateral lung fields.

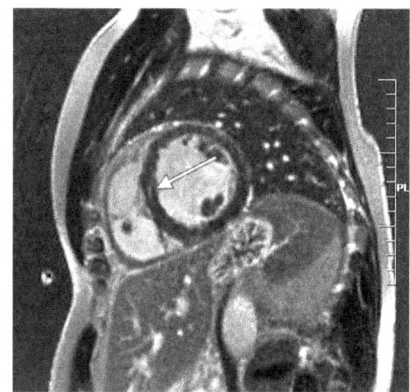

FIGURE 19: Cardiac magnetic resonance imaging of a patient with eosinophilic granulomatosis with polyangiitis and cardiac involvement (parasagittal view, late postgadolinium phase-sensitive inversion recovery sequence). The left-ventricular volume is in the upper limit of normal. A small, linear, late gadolinium enhancement (arrow) in the basal and mid-septum involves the mesocardium. Dynamic sequences reveal mild reduction in left ventricle systolic function with mild hypokinesis of the septum consistent with mild dilated cardiomyopathy.

biological parameters, including eosinophilia and, in up to 40% of patients, positive ANCA test results. Ideally, diagnosis is supported by biopsy findings when feasible. Sometimes, diagnosis of EGPA can be confirmed and that of chronic eosinophilic pneumonia or primary eosinophilic syndrome ruled out only after several months or years of follow-up. Circulating lymphocyte immunophenotyping, T-cell clonal and cytogenetic studies, and molecular analyses to detect Fip1-like 1 (FIP1L1)-platelet-derived growth factor receptor-α (PDGFRA) gene fusion should be performed for patients with suspected EGPA but who are ANCA-negative and/or without histologically proven vasculitis to detect lymphoid or myeloid neoplasms associated with eosinophilia. However, these screening tests are not entirely sensitive and the presence of a circulating but simply reactive T-cell clone is possible during active phases of obvious EGPA.[57,87] More specific tests and screening for other PDGFRA, PDGFRB, or FGFR1 fusion gene should be discussed with hematologists.

Once the diagnosis of EGPA is established, disease severity should be thoroughly evaluated. Importantly, investigations to search for cardiac (echocardiography and ECG systematically and, perhaps, MRI and Holter-ECG) and renal (serum creatinine and urine analysis and microscopy) are mandatory. Treatment for patients with life-threatening and/or major organ involvement must not be delayed.

MANAGEMENT

Treatment should be adapted to the type and severity of disease and should combine immunosuppressants as needed and local anti-asthma therapies (inhaled GCs and/or bronchodilators). Several patients in apparent clinical remission may show persistently mild, isolated, and fluctuating eosinophilia.

Patients without severe manifestations can initially receive GCs alone.[88,89] Whether adding a GC-sparing agent such as azathioprine, methotrexate, mycophenolate mofetil or leflunomide for patients with GC-dependent asthma, is effective is not known, although this is common in practice; if they are effective, which is more effective is not clearly demonstrated.[90,91]

Patients with severe manifestations must receive a combination of GCs [starting with a prednisone-equivalent dose of 1 mg/kg/day, preceded by methylprednisolone intravenous (IV) pulses 0.5–1 g/day for 1–3 consecutive days in most severe cases, then gradually tapered to 20 mg/day at about month 3, then 5 mg/day at month 5 if possible] and a potent immunosuppressant, primarily CYC, for induction (CYC, 15 mg/kg IV every 2 weeks for 1 month, then every 3 weeks or 2 mg/kg/day when given orally, adjusted for age and renal function).[92] Similar to treatment for MPA and GPA, CYC should be switched after a maximum of 3–6 months to a less toxic immunosuppressant, such as azathioprine (orally, 2 mg/kg/day) or methotrexate (orally or subcutaneously, 0.3 mg/kg/week with a maximum dose of 25 mg/week), once remission has been achieved. The optimal duration of this entire staged strategy is unknown but should be at least 18–24 months. Intravenous Ig (2 g/kg/month) may be an alternative to immunosuppressants in pregnant women and have been beneficial in few patients with refractory EGPA.[93] Plasma exchange should be considered in patients with severe glomerulonephritis and/or alveolar hemorrhage.[94-97]

Interferon-alpha (3 MU thrice weekly, up to 21 MU/week) can reverse Th2-mediated immune responses and has been used in a few patients with refractory EGPA. However, the treatment has potential cardiac toxicity and responses were generally only transient.[98,99] Omalizumab, a murine monoclonal antibody directed against human IgE, can be used to treat allergic asthma and showed some benefits for asthma control in few EGPA patients. However, development of full-blown EGPA in patients with "common" asthma after receiving omalizumab has been reported, likely due to the GC-sparing effect of the biologic agent that allowed EGPA with a "forme fruste" of EGPA to become overt, similar to what was previously reported with antileukotriene-receptor antagonists.[100-104] Rituximab was used in a few CSS patients, mainly, but not only, ANCA-positive positive, with some interesting results.[105] Conversely, the drug was found ineffective and caused severe bronchospasms in two ANCA-negative patients.[106] One randomized controlled study of mepolizumab, a humanized monoclonal anti-IL-5 antibody, is including patients with refractory, relapsing, or GC-dependent EGPA manifestations after promising results were observed in small open studies of such patients.[107-109]

REFERENCES

1. Klinger H. Grenzforman der Periarteriitis nodosa. Frankfurter Zeitschrift fürPathologie. 1931;42:455.
2. Wegener F. Über generalisierte, septische gefäßerkrankungen. Verh Dtsch Ges Pathol. 1936;29:202-10.
3. Leavitt RY, Fauci AS, Bloch DA, et al. The American College of Rheumatology 1990 criteria for the classification of Wegener's granulomatosis. Arthritis Rheum. 1990;33:1101-7.
4. Jennette JC, Falk RJ, Andrassy K, et al. Nomenclature of systemic vasculitides. Proposal of an international consensus conference. Arthritis Rheum. 1994;37:187-92.
5. Jennette JC, Falk RJ, Bacon PA, et al. 2012 revised International Chapel Hill Consensus Conference Nomenclature of Vasculitides. Arthritis Rheum. 2013;65:1-11.

6. Watts RA, Carruthers DM, Scott DG. Epidemiology of systemic vasculitis: changing incidence or definition? Semin Arthritis Rheum. 1995;25:28-34.
7. Watts RA, Mooney J, Skinner J, et al. The contrasting epidemiology of granulomatosis with polyangiitis (Wegener's) and microscopic polyangiitis. Rheumatology (Oxford). 2012;51:926-31.
8. Rasmussen N. Management of the ear, nose, and throat manifestations of Wegener granulomatosis: an otorhinolaryngologist's perspective. Curr Opin Rheumatol. 2001;13:3-11.
9. McDonald TJ, DeRemee RA. Wegener's granulomatosis. Laryngoscope. 1983;93:220-31.
10. Prokopakis E, Nikolaou V, Vardouniotis A, et al. Nasal manifestations of systemic diseases. B-ENT. 2013;9:171-84.
11. McDonald TJ, DeRemee RA, Kern EB, et al. Nasal manifestations of Wegener's granulomatosis. Laryngoscope. 1974;84:2101-12.
12. Lebovics RS, Hoffman GS, Leavitt RY, et al. The management of subglottic stenosis in patients with Wegener's granulomatosis. Laryngoscope. 1992;102:1341-5.
13. Alaani A, Hogg RP, Drake Lee AB. Wegener's granulomatosis and subglottic stenosis: management of the airway. J Laryngol Otol. 2004;118:786-90.
14. Langford CA, Sneller MC, Hallahan CW, et al. Clinical features and therapeutic management of subglottic stenosis in patients with Wegener's granulomatosis. Arthritis Rheum. 1996;39:1754-60.
15. Devaney KO, Travis WD, Hoffman G, et al. Interpretation of head and neck biopsies in Wegener's granulomatosis. A pathologic study of 126 biopsies in 70 patients. Am J Surg Pathol. 1990;14:555-64.
16. Ah-See KW, McLaren K, Maran AG. Wegener's granulomatosis presenting as major salivary gland enlargement. J Laryngol Otol. 1996;110:691-3.
17. Specks U, Colby TV, Olsen KD, et al. Salivary gland involvement in Wegener's granulomatosis. Arch Otolaryngol Head Neck Surg. 1991;117:218-23.
18. Bambery P, Sakhuja V, Bhusnurmath SR, et al. Wegener's granulomatosis: clinical experience with eighteen patients. J Assoc Physicians India. 1992;40:597-600.
19. Bambery P, Sakhuja V, Gupta A, et al. Wegener's granulomatosis in north India. An analysis of eleven patients. Rheumatol Int. 1987;7:243-7.
20. Malaviya AN, Kumar A, Singh YN, et al. Wegener's granulomatosis in India: not so rare. Br J Rheumatol. 1990; 29:499-500.
21. Kumar A, Pandhi A, Menon A, et al. Wegener's granulomatosis in India: clinical features, treatment and outcome of twenty-five patients. Indian J Chest Dis Allied Sci. 2001;43:197-204.
22. Sharma A, Gopalakrishan D, Nada R, et al. Uncommon presentations of primary systemic necrotizing vasculitides: the Great Masquerades. Int J Rheum Dis. 2014;17: 562-72.
23. Savige J, Gillis D, Benson E, et al. International Consensus Statement on Testing and Reporting of Antineutrophil Cytoplasmic Antibodies (ANCA). Am J ClinPathol. 1999; 111:507-13.
24. Bartunkova J, Tesar V, Sediva A. Diagnostic and pathogenetic role of antineutrophil cytoplasmic autoantibodies. Clin Immunol. 2003;106:73-82.
25. Falk RJ, Jennette JC. Anti-neutrophil cytoplasmic autoantibodies with specificity for myeloperoxidase in patients with systemic vasculitis and idiopathic necrotizing and crescentic glomerulonephritis. N Engl J Med. 1988;318:1651-7.
26. Jenne DE, Tschopp J, Ludemann J, et al. Wegener's autoantigen decoded. Nature. 1990;346:520.
27. Lloyd G, Lund VJ, Beale T, et al. Rhinologic changes in Wegener's granulomatosis. J Laryngol Otol. 2002;116: 565-9.
28. Simmons JT, Leavitt R, Kornblut AD, et al. CT of the paranasal sinuses and orbits in patients with Wegener's granulomatosis. Ear Nose Throat J. 1987;66:134-40.
29. Provenzale JM, Allen NB. Wegener granulomatosis: CT and MR findings. Am J Neuroradiol. 1996;17:785-92.
30. Mukhtyar C, Guillevin L, Cid MC, et al. EULAR recommendations for the management of primary small and medium vessel vasculitis. Ann Rheum Dis. 2009;68:310-7.
31. Stone JH, Merkel PA, Spiera R, et al. Rituximab versus cyclophosphamide for ANCA-associated vasculitis. N Engl J Med. 2010;363:221-32.
32. Jones RB, Tervaert JW, Hauser T, et al. Rituximab versus cyclophosphamide in ANCA-associated renal vasculitis. N Engl J Med. 2010;363:211-20.
33. Specks U, Merkel PA, Seo P, et al. Efficacy of remission-induction regimens for ANCA-associated vasculitis. N Engl J Med. 2013;369:417-27.
34. Rhee EP, Laliberte KA, Niles JL. Rituximab as maintenance therapy for anti-neutrophil cytoplasmic antibody-associated vasculitis. Clin J Am SocNephrol. 2010;5:1394-400.
35. Smith RM, Jones RB, Guerry MJ, et al. Rituximab for remission maintenance in relapsing antineutrophil cytoplasmic antibody-associated vasculitis. Arthritis Rheum. 2012; 64:3760-9.
36. Terrier B, Pagnoux C, Karras A, et al. Rituximab versus azathioprine for maintenance in antineutrophil cytoplasmic antibodies (ANCA)-associated vasculitis (MAINRITSAN): follow-up at 34 months. La PresseMedicale. 2013;42: 778-9.
37. Jayne DR, Gaskin G, Rasmussen N, et al. Randomized trial of plasma exchange or high-dosage methylprednisolone as adjunctive therapy for severe renal vasculitis. J Am SocNephrol. 2007;18:2180-8.
38. Walsh M, Catapano F, Szpirt W, et al. Plasma exchange for renal vasculitis and idiopathic rapidly progressive glomerulonephritis: a meta-analysis. Am J Kidney Dis. 2011;57:566-74.

39. Flossmann O, Berden A, de Groot K, et al. Long-term patient survival in ANCA-associated vasculitis. Ann Rheum Dis. 2011;70:488-94.
40. Merkel PA, Lo GH, Holbrook JT, et al. Brief communication: high incidence of venous thrombotic events among patients with Wegener granulomatosis: the Wegener's Clinical Occurrence of Thrombosis (WeCLOT) Study. Ann Intern Med. 2005;142:620-6.
41. Basu N, Jones GT, Fluck N, et al. Fatigue: a principal contributor to impaired quality of life in ANCA-associated vasculitis. Rheumatology (Oxford). 2010;49:1383-90.
42. Harper L, Savage CO. ANCA-associated renal vasculitis at the end of the twentieth century--a disease of older patients. Rheumatology (Oxford). 2005;44:495-501.
43. Charlier C, Henegar C, Launay O, et al. Risk factors for major infections in Wegener granulomatosis: analysis of 113 patients. Ann Rheum Dis. 2009;68:658-63.
44. Niles JL. Value of tests for antineutrophil cytoplasmic autoantibodies in the diagnosis and treatment of vasculitis. Curr Opin Rheumatol. 1993;5:18-24.
45. Mohammad AJ, Jacobsson LT, Westman KW, et al. Incidence and survival rates in Wegener's granulomatosis, microscopic polyangiitis, Churg-Strauss syndrome and polyarteritis nodosa. Rheumatology (Oxford). 2009;48:1560-5.
46. Gibson A, Stamp LK, Chapman PT, et al. The epidemiology of Wegener's granulomatosis and microscopic polyangiitis in a Southern Hemisphere region. Rheumatology (Oxford). 2006;45:624-8.
47. Watts R, Lane S, Hanslik T, et al. Development and validation of a consensus methodology for the classification of the ANCA-associated vasculitides and polyarteritis nodosa for epidemiological studies. Ann Rheum Dis. 2007;66:222-7.
48. Guillevin L, Durand-Gasselin B, Cevallos R, et al. Microscopic polyangiitis: clinical and laboratory findings in eighty-five patients. Arthritis Rheum. 1999;42:421-30.
49. Lauque D, Cadranel J, Lazor R, et al. Microscopic polyangiitis with alveolar hemorrhage. A study of 29 cases and review of the literature. Grouped'Etudeset de Recherchesur les Maladies "Orphelines" Pulmonaires (GERM"O"P). Medicine (Baltimore). 2000;79:222-33.
50. Tzelepis GE, Kokosi M, Tzioufas A, et al. Prevalence and outcome of pulmonary fibrosis in microscopic polyangiitis. EurRespir J. 2010;36:116-21.
51. Ando Y, Okada F, Matsumoto S, et al. Thoracic manifestation of myeloperoxidase-antineutrophil cytoplasmic antibody (MPO-ANCA)-related disease. CT findings in 51 patients. J Comput Assist Tomogr. 2004;28:710-6.
52. Choi HK, Liu S, Merkel PA, et al. Diagnostic performance of antineutrophil cytoplasmic antibody tests for idiopathic vasculitides: metaanalysis with a focus on antimyeloperoxidase antibodies. J Rheumatol. 2001;28:1584-90.
53. Kain R, Exner M, Brandes R, et al. Molecular mimicry in pauci-immune focal necrotizing glomerulonephritis. Nat Med. 2008;14:1088-96.
54. Masi AT, Hunder GG, Lie JT, et al. The American College of Rheumatology 1990 criteria for the classification of Churg-Strauss syndrome (allergic granulomatosis and angiitis). Arthritis Rheum. 1990;33:1094-100.
55. Churg J, Strauss L. Allergic granulomatosis, allergic angiitis, and periarteritis nodosa. Am J Pathol. 1951;27:277-301.
56. Kallenberg CG. Churg-Strauss syndrome: just one disease entity? Arthritis Rheum. 2005;52:2589-93.
57. Pagnoux C, Guillevin L. Churg-Strauss syndrome: evidence for disease subtypes? Curr Opin Rheumatol. 2010;22:21-8.
58. Mahr A, Moosig F, Neumann T, et al. Eosinophilic granulomatosis with polyangiitis (Churg-Strauss): evolutions in classification, etiopathogenesis, assessment and management. Curr Opin Rheumatol. 2014;26:16-23.
59. Comarmond C, Pagnoux C, Khellaf M, et al. Eosinophilic granulomatosis with polyangiitis (Churg-Strauss): clinical characteristics and long-term followup of the 383 patients enrolled in the French Vasculitis Study Group cohort. Arthritis Rheum. 2013;65:270-81.
60. Sinico RA, Di Toma L, Maggiore U, et al. Prevalence and clinical significance of antineutrophil cytoplasmic antibodies in Churg-Strauss syndrome. Arthritis Rheum. 2005;52:2926-35.
61. Baldini C, Della Rossa A, Grossi S, et al. Churg-Strauss syndrome: outcome and long-term follow-up of 38 patients from a single Italian centre. Reumatismo. 2009;61:118-24.
62. Kim MY, Sohn KH, Song WJ, et al. Clinical features and prognostic factors of Churg-Strauss syndrome. Korean J Intern Med. 2014;29:85-95.
63. Uchiyama M, Mitsuhashi Y, Yamazaki M, et al. Elderly cases of Churg-Strauss syndrome: case report and review of Japanese cases. J Dermatol. 2012;39:76-9.
64. Harrold LR, Andrade SE, Eisner M, et al. Identification of patients with Churg-Strauss syndrome (CSS) using automated data. Pharmacoepidemiol Drug Saf. 2004; 13:661-7.
65. Harrold LR, Andrade SE, Go AS, et al. Incidence of Churg-Strauss syndrome in asthma drug users: a population-based perspective. J Rheumatol. 2005;32:1076-80.
66. Harrold LR, Patterson MK, Andrade SE, et al. Asthma drug use and the development of Churg-Strauss syndrome (CSS). Pharmacoepidemiol Drug Saf. 2007;16:620-6.
67. Wechsler ME, Pauwels R, Drazen JM. Leukotriene modifiers and Churg-Strauss syndrome: adverse effect or response to corticosteroid withdrawal? Drug Saf. 1999;21:241-51.
68. Bottero P, Motta F, Bonini M, et al. Can HLA-DRB4 Help to Identify Asthmatic Patients at Risk of Churg-Strauss Syndrome? ISRN Rheumatol. 2014;2014:843804.
69. Keogh KA, Specks U. Churg-Strauss syndrome: clinical presentation, antineutrophil cytoplasmic antibodies, and leukotriene receptor antagonists. Am J Med. 2003;115:284-90.

70. Keogh KA, Specks U. Churg-Strauss syndrome: update on clinical, laboratory and therapeutic aspects. SarcoidosisVasc Diffuse Lung Dis. 2006;23:3-12.
71. Zwerina J, Eger G, Englbrecht M, et al. Churg-Strauss syndrome in childhood: a systematic literature review and clinical comparison with adult patients. Semin Arthritis Rheum. 2009;39:108-15.
72. Wechsler ME, Finn D, Gunawardena D, et al. Churg-Strauss syndrome in patients receiving montelukast as treatment for asthma. Chest. 2000;117:708-13.
73. Wechsler ME, Wong DA, Miller MK, et al. Churg-strauss syndrome in patients treated with omalizumab. Chest. 2009; 136:507-18.
74. Kostianovsky A, Charles P, Alves JF, et al. Immunogenicity and safety of seasonal and 2009 pandemic A/H1N1 influenza vaccines for patients with autoimmune diseases: a prospective, monocentre trial on 199 patients. ClinExpRheumatol. 2012;30:S83-9.
75. Duggal T, Segal P, Shah M, et al. Antineutrophil cytoplasmic antibody vasculitis associated with influenza vaccination. Am J Nephrol. 2013;38:174-8.
76. Lanham JG, Cooke S, Davies J, et al. Endomyocardial complications of the Churg-Strauss syndrome. Postgrad Med J. 1985;61:341-4.
77. Lanham JG, Elkon KB, Pusey CD, et al. Systemic vasculitis with asthma and eosinophilia: a clinical approach to the Churg-Strauss syndrome. Medicine (Baltimore). 1984; 63:65-81.
78. Luqmani RA, Suppiah R, Grayson PC, et al. Nomenclature and classification of vasculitis - update on the ACR/EULAR diagnosis and classification of vasculitis study (DCVAS). Clin Exp Immunol. 2011;164Suppl 1:11-3.
79. Hervier B, Pagnoux C, Agard C, et al. Pulmonary fibrosis associated with ANCA-positive vasculitides. Retrospective study of 12 cases and review of the literature. Ann Rheum Dis. 2009;68:404-7.
80. Marmursztejn J, Guillevin L, Trebossen R, et al. Churg-Strauss syndrome cardiac involvement evaluated by cardiac magnetic resonance imaging and positron-emission tomography: a prospective study on 20 patients. Rheumatology (Oxford). 2013;52:642-50.
81. Mavrogeni S, Tsirogianni AK, Gialafos EJ, et al. Detection of myocardial inflammation by contrast-enhanced MRI in a patient with Churg-Strauss syndrome. Int J Cardiol. 2009;131:e54-5.
82. Pagnoux C, Guillevin L. Cardiac involvement in small and medium-sized vessel vasculitides. Lupus. 2005;14:718-22.
83. Allenbach Y, Seror R, Pagnoux C, et al. High frequency of venous thromboembolic events in Churg-Strauss syndrome, Wegener's granulomatosis and microscopic polyangiitis but not polyarteritis nodosa: a systematic retrospective study on 1130 patients. Ann Rheum Dis. 2009;68:564-7.
84. Ames PR, Roes L, Lupoli S, et al. Thrombosis in Churg-Strauss syndrome. Beyond vasculitis? Br J Rheumatol. 1996; 35:1181-3.
85. Sable-Fourtassou R, Cohen P, Mahr A, et al. Antineutrophil cytoplasmic antibodies and the Churg-Strauss syndrome. Ann Intern Med. 2005;143:632-8.
86. Noth I, Strek ME, Leff AR. Churg-Strauss syndrome. Lancet. 2003;361:587-94.
87. Gotlib J. World Health Organization-defined eosinophilic disorders: 2014 update on diagnosis, risk stratification, and management. Am J Hematol. 2014;89:325-37.
88. Samson M, Puechal X, Devilliers H, et al. Long-term outcomes of 118 patients with eosinophilic granulomatosis with polyangiitis (Churg-Strauss syndrome) enrolled in two prospective trials. J Autoimmun. 2013;43:60-9.
89. Ribi C, Cohen P, Pagnoux C, et al. Treatment of Churg-Strauss syndrome without poor-prognosis factors: a multicenter, prospective, randomized, open-label study of seventy-two patients. Arthritis Rheum. 2008;58:586-94.
90. Metzler C, Hellmich B, Gause A, et al. Churg Strauss syndrome--successful induction of remission with methotrexate and unexpected high cardiac and pulmonary relapse ratio during maintenance treatment. Clin Exp Rheumatol. 2004;22:S52-61.
91. Iatrou C, Zerbala S, Revela I, et al. Mycophenolatemofetil as maintenance therapy in patients with vasculitis and renal involvement. Clin Nephrol. 2009;72:31-7.
92. Cohen P, Pagnoux C, Mahr A, et al. Churg-Strauss syndrome with poor-prognosis factors: A prospective multicenter trial comparing glucocorticoids and six or twelve cyclophosphamide pulses in forty-eight patients. Arthritis Rheum. 2007;57:686-93.
93. Danieli MG, Cappelli M, Malcangi G, et al. Long term effectiveness of intravenous immunoglobulin in Churg-Strauss syndrome. Ann Rheum Dis. 2004;63:1649-54.
94. Cordier JF, Cottin V. Alveolar hemorrhage in vasculitis: primary and secondary. SeminRespirCrit Care Med. 2011;32:310-21.
95. Guillevin L, Pagnoux C. Indications of plasma exchanges for systemic vasculitides. Ther Apher Dial. 2003;7:155-60.
96. Guillevin L, Lhote F, Cohen P, et al. Corticosteroids plus pulse cyclophosphamide and plasma exchanges versus corticosteroids plus pulse cyclophosphamide alone in the treatment of polyarteritis nodosa and Churg-Strauss syndrome patients with factors predicting poor prognosis. A prospective, randomized trial in sixty-two patients. Arthritis Rheum. 1995;38:1638-45.
97. Guillevin L, Lhote F. Treatment of polyarteritis nodosa and Churg-Strauss syndrome: indications of plasma exchanges. Transfus Sci. 1994;15:371-88.
98. Metzler C, Lamprecht P, Hellmich B, et al. Leucoencephalopathy after treatment of Churg-Strauss syndrome with interferon {alpha}. Ann Rheum Dis. 2005;64:1242-3.
99. Metzler C, Schnabel A, Gross WL, et al. A phase II study of interferon-alpha for the treatment of refractory Churg-Strauss syndrome. Clin Exp Rheumatol. 2008;26:S35-40.

100. Giavina-Bianchi P, Agondi R, Kalil J. One year administration of anti-IgE to a patient with Churg-Strauss syndrome. Int Arch Allergy Immunol. 2008;146:176.
101. Giavina-Bianchi P, Giavina-Bianchi M, Agondi R, et al. Omalizumab and Churg-Strauss syndrome. J Allergy ClinImmunol. 2008;122:217; author reply -8.
102. Giavina-Bianchi P, Giavina-Bianchi M, Agondi RC, et al. Anti-IgE in Churg-Strauss syndrome. Thorax. 2009;64:272-3.
103. Pabst S, Tiyerili V, Grohe C. Apparent response to anti-IgE therapy in two patients with refractory "formefruste" of Churg-Strauss syndrome. Thorax. 2008;63:747-8.
104. Hanania NA, Wenzel S, Rosen K, et al. Exploring the effects of omalizumab in allergic asthma: an analysis of biomarkers in the EXTRA study. Am J RespirCrit Care Med. 2013;187:804-11.
105. Jones RB, Ferraro AJ, Chaudhry AN, et al. A multicenter survey of rituximab therapy for refractory antineutrophil cytoplasmic antibody-associated vasculitis. Arthritis Rheum. 2009;60: 2156-68.
106. Bouldouyre MA, Cohen P, Guillevin L. Severe bronchospasm associated with rituximab for refractory Churg-Strauss syndrome. Ann Rheum Dis. 2009;68:606.
107. Kim S, Marigowda G, Oren E, et al. Mepolizumab as a steroid-sparing treatment option in patients with Churg-Strauss syndrome. J Allergy ClinImmunol. 2010;125:1336-43.
108. Herrmann K, Gross WL, Moosig F. Extended follow-up after stopping mepolizumab in relapsing/refractory Churg-Strauss syndrome. Clin Exp Rheumatol. 2012;30:S62-5.
109. Moosig F, Gross WL, Herrmann K, et al. Targeting interleukin-5 in refractory and relapsing Churg-Strauss syndrome. Ann Intern Med. 2011;155:341-3.

22
CHAPTER

Small Vessel Vasculitis of the Skin

Neetu Bhari, Tanvi Dev, Gomathy Sethuraman

INTRODUCTION

Vasculitis is defined as inflammatory cell infiltration and destruction of the blood vessels. According to the International Chapel Hill Consensus conference 2012, vasculitis can be classified into large, medium, small, and variable vessel and single organ vasculitis. Large vessel vasculitis affects primarily the larger arteries like aorta and temporal arteries. Medium vessels are small muscular arteries that are present either in the subcutaneous tissue or at the junction between dermis and subcutaneous tissue. Hence, inflammation of medium vessels manifests as large subcutaneous nodules with deep punched out ulcers along with livedoid changes. It is often associated with systemic arteritis such as renal and mesenteric arteritis. Small vessel vasculitis affects the arterioles and postcapillary venules present in the papillary dermis, which manifests as palpable purpura. Often, there is an overlap between the medium and small vessel vasculitis.

Small vessel vasculitis is further classified into antineutrophil cytoplasmic antibody (ANCA) associated vasculitis and immune complex vasculitis. Wegener's granulomatosis, microscopic polyangiitis, and eosinophilic granulomatosis with polyangiitis are the major forms in the former while Henoch-Schönlein purpura, cryoglobulinemic vasculitis, antiglomerular basement membrane disease, and hypocomplementemic vasculitis are included in the latter group. Cutaneous leukocytoclastic vasculitis or hypersensitivity angiitis in included under single organ vasculitis. In this chapter, we mainly focus on cutaneous leukocytoclastic vasculitis, Henoch-Schönlein purpura, and drug-induced vasculitis.

SMALL VESSEL VASCULITIS OF THE SKIN (CUTANEOUS LEUKOCYTOCLASTIC VASCULITIS)

Small vessel vasculitis of the skin has also been referred as "cutaneous leukocytoclastic vasculitis," or simply "leukocytoclastic vasculitis," "hypersensitivity vasculitis," "cutaneous leukocytoclastic angiitis," and "cutaneous small vessel vasculitis." The term skin-limited small vessel vasculitis is favored in the revised 2012 Chapel Hill Consensus Criteria.[1]

Small vessel vasculitis of the skin is most often acute and self-limited, and its prognosis is favorable, particularly when internal involvement is absent, however, internal organ involvement must be ruled out in every case as it affects the prognosis and management.

Epidemiology

Small vessel vasculitis of the skin affects both the sexes equally and patients of all ages. In a population-based retrospective study for biopsy proven leukocytoclastic vasculitis, an incidence rate of 4.5 per 100,000 person-years was observed.[2] The medical records of 57 adult patients (>18 years) with biopsy-proven cutaneous leukocytoclastic vasculitis were reviewed and

21 (36.8%) were classified as having primary cutaneous small vessel vasculitis.[3] Cutaneous small-vessel vasculitis was diagnosed in 38 (45%) patients, while 25 (30%) showed immunoglobulin A (IgA) vasculitis.

Pathophysiology

Small vessel vasculitis of the skin is mediated by immune complex deposition in affected vessels. Circulating antigens due to medications, infections, connective tissue disease, or neoplasia are bound by antibodies, forming immune complexes that become lodged and trapped within small vessels in the superficial dermis, most frequently in dependent areas, the joints, the gastrointestinal tract, or the glomeruli. These complexes, in turn, activate complement and induce an inflammatory response that leads to vessel destruction and extravasation of red blood cells.[4] In the case of palpable purpura in the skin, this small vessel involvement accounts for the small size of the lesions; the complement cascade and subsequent inflammation account for the palpability and symptomatology of the lesions; and the red blood cell extravasation results in nonblanching purpura.

Etiology

About half of the cases are idiopathic. The remainders are most often either drug-induced or postinfectious. Antibiotics, β-lactams in particular, are common culprits. Among infectious causes, upper respiratory infections (such as β-hemolytic streptococcus group A) and hepatitis C are commonly implicated; however, numerous infectious triggers have been described.[5] Small vessel vasculitis may be a presenting sign of underlying connective tissue diseases such as systemic lupus erythematosus, Sjögren, syndrome, rheumatoid arthritis, or dermatomyositis.[6] This group of vasculitis is more commonly associated with significant internal organ involvement. A small percentage of patients (<5%) may have an underlying hematologic or solid organ malignancy.[7]

Clinical Features

It classically presents with crops of purpuric, round, 1–3 mm papules (palpable purpura) that

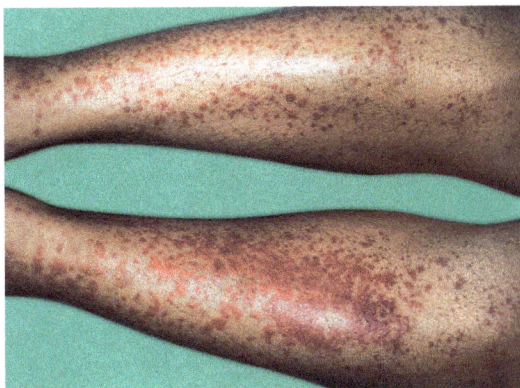

FIGURE 1: Small vessel vasculitis of skin; showing multiple erythematous discrete and confluent palpable purpura over the lower extremities.

appear on dependent areas (Fig. 1). The number of lesions may vary from dozens to hundreds. These lesions resolve over 2–3 weeks, leaving behind postinflammatory hyperpigmentation.[4]

Besides typical palpable purpura, vesicles, pustules, small hemorrhagic bullae, and even ulcers can be seen. The presence of subcutaneous nodules, livedo reticularis, retiform purpura, larger hemorrhagic bullae, and more significant ulceration and necrosis is indicative of underlying medium vessel vasculitis.[8]

The patients may complain of burning, itching, or pain sensation. They may experience aching and uncomfortable swelling of the affected limbs, or they may be completely asymptomatic. In most cases of small vessel vasculitis of the skin, significant systemic manifestations are unlikely, though, a detail history regarding fever, weight loss, and other constitutional symptoms; arthralgias or arthritis; myalgias; abdominal pain, melena, or hematochezia; cough, hemoptysis, or dyspnea; hematuria or frothy urine; sinusitis or rhinitis; and paresthesias, weakness, or foot drop should be taken.

Laboratory Investigations

After a thorough history and physical examination, a systematic and targeted laboratory workup should be done. The workup should aim to elucidate the underlying cause and extent of organ involvement and should be guided by clinical signs and symptoms. In a basic work-up, complete blood count, metabolic panel, and urinalysis (with microscopy) should be performed. Fecal occult blood testing should be done in all patients, more so if the patient has abdominal symptoms or gastrointestinal bleeding. Other organ-specific targeted workup should be done based on clinical symptoms and physical examination.

If there is no obvious history of infection or drug prior to the onset of vasculitis, a detailed workup should be done to look for underlying cause. Infectious serologies including hepatitis B and C, human immunodeficiency virus and antistreptolysin-O; autoimmune workup, including antinuclear antibody and rheumatoid factor, serum protein electrophoresis with immunofixation to look for evidence of a paraprotein; serum C3 and C4 complement levels, ANCAs, and cryoglobulin levels can be performed as directed by history and physical examination.

Histologic Findings

A skin biopsy from the active lesion should be performed to confirm the diagnosis. Ideally, a representative lesion should be sampled and since the findings depends on the age of the lesion and a biopsy performed too early or too late may be nondiagnostic, a lesion roughly 24–48 hours old should be selected for the histologic evaluation. If "deeper" lesions, such as subcutaneous nodules or retiform purpura, are present, an appropriately deep punch or wedge biopsy should be performed to rule out the presence of a medium or small-to-medium vessel vasculitis.

The prototypical findings of leukocyte common antigen include a neutrophilic infiltrate of superficial and mid-dermal small blood vessels (Fig. 2), nuclear dust (leukocytoclasis), fibrinoid necrosis, and disruption of vessel walls and extravasation of red blood cells into the surrounding tissue.[9] A mixed inflammatory infiltrate may also be present, particularly in older lesions. Cutaneous small-vessel vasculitis associated with solid-organ malignancies tends to have deeper dermal involvement and a different cellular milieu from cases not associated with solid-organ malignancies.[10] The presence of tissue eosinophilia suggests the vasculitis may be

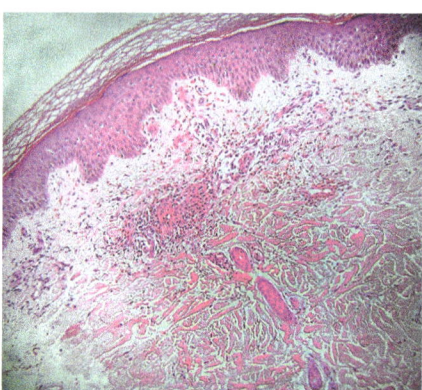

FIGURE 2: Small vessel vasculitis of skin; perivascular infiltrate of neutrophils along with extravasation of red blood cells.

drug-induced.[11] The presence of granulomatous vasculitis is suggestive of granulomatosis with polyangiitis or eosinophilic granulomatosis with polyangiitis.

A second biopsy should be performed for direct immunofluorescence studies. Biopsies for direct immunofluorescence should be taken from lesional skin (within 8–24 hour of onset), should be chosen as the subsequent inflammatory cascade, destroys the immune complexes resulting in falsely negative test in older lesions. Detection of immune complex deposition may be seen in small vessel vasculitis.

Management

Once systemic involvement has been excluded, the treatment of cutaneous small vessel vasculitis should be focused on symptom management. Identifiable triggers should be eliminated or treated. Prolonged standing should be avoided. Rest and elevation and use of compression stockings can be helpful to decrease stasis-related immune complex deposition and accelerate healing of ulcers on the lower legs. More than half of patients require no systemic treatment.

Systemic therapies are indicated for severe, intractable, or recurrent disease. For patients with chronic small vessel vasculitis of the skin, often anti-inflammatory medications work without the need for systemic glucocorticoids.

Initially, long-term treatment options include colchicine (0.6 mg 2-3 times/day). This medication has been reported useful for skin and joint symptoms in open label studies, inducing prompt resolution of cutaneous vasculitis. Dosing may be limited by gastrointestinal side effects.[12]

The use of dapsone (50-200 mg/day) is supported by anecdotal case reports and small case series. It may be combined with colchicine when response to monotherapy with either medication is incomplete.[13]

Other options include hydroxychloroquine (200-400 mg/day), pentoxifylline (400-1,200 mg/day), and nonsteroidal anti-inflammatory agents such as indomethacin, which may provide symptomatic relief.[14]

Systemic corticosteroids in doses of 0.5-1 mg/kg/day of prednisone are recommended for those with severe, necrotic vasculitis lesions, or serious systemic involvement such as renal or gastrointestinal involvement.[15]

If the vasculitis is chronic or refractory, immunosuppressive medications such as azathioprine (50-200 mg/day), methotrexate (15-25 mg/week), and mycophenolate mofetil (2-3 g/day) can be considered.[16,17] The tumor necrosis factor (TNF) inhibitors, especially infliximab, has shown to be effective in small vessel vasculitis of the skin.[18] Rituximab has also been used in some refractory cases.[19]

Prognosis

Most episodes of small vessel vasculitis of the skin are self-limited, resolve over 3-4 weeks with residual hyperpigmentation. Prognosis depends on the severity of organ involvement as well as any underlying associated medical disorder. A certain number of patients, perhaps 8-10%, develop chronic or recurrent vasculitis.

HENOCH-SCHÖNLEIN PURPURA

A specific subset of small vessel vasculitis is immunoglobulin IgA vasculitis (Henoch-Schönlein purpura), which is an IgA-mediated syndrome characterized by cutaneous, gastrointestinal, joint, and/or kidney involvement. Cutaneous manifestations include palpable purpuras and nephritis is the most severe clinical involvement with a risk of progression to end stage renal disease.

The European League Against Rheumatism/Paediatric Rheumatology International Trials Organisation/Pediatric Rheumatology European Society (EULAR/PRINTO/PRES) criteria for Henoch-Schönlein purpura include having purpura and at least one of the four following phenomenon: (i) abdominal pain, (ii) histopathologically leukocytoclastic vasculitis or proliferative glomerulonephritis with IgA deposits, (iii) arthritis or arthralgia, and (iv) renal involvement.[20] American College of Rheumatology Criteria requires two of the following four features: (i) palpable purpura, nonthrombocytopenic, (ii) age less than or equal to 20 years at disease onset, (iii) bowel angina, and (iv) histology showing granulocytes in the wall of arteriole and venule.[21]

Epidemiology

Henoch-Schönlein purpura primarily affects children of age 10-14 years. Its annual incidence is 6.1-26.7 cases per 100,000 per year in children compared to 1.3 cases per 100,000 per year.[22] We studied 61 patients of cutaneous vasculitis and observed that hypersensitivity vasculitis [23 (37.7%)] and Henoch-Schönlein purpura [16 (26.2%)] were the two most common forms.[23] In a retrospective study from Zagreb, 180 children with vasculitis were reviewed.[24] Most of the children (155 or 86%) were diagnosed with Henoch-Schönlein purpura, isolated cutaneous leukocytoclastic vasculitis was seen only in 5 (2.8%) children. Adult onset Henoch-Schönlein purpura is increasingly recognized.[25]

Etiology

Viral upper respiratory tract infection (URTI) or *Streptococcal pharyngitis* frequently precedes the onset of IgA vasculitis by 1-2 weeks. In a retrospective review of 86 children with Henoch-Schönlein purpura, a history of preceding URTI and drugs were reported to occur in 41% and 30% children, respectively.[26] Paraneoplastic associations have been seen in adults.[27] As with small vessel cutaneous vasculitis as a whole, a significant fraction of cases have no identifiable cause.

Pathogenesis

Antigen antibodies complexes (IgA) are formed as result of bacterial and viral infection, drug or vaccination. These immune complexes are deposited in the small blood vessels of skin, gastrointestinal tract, renal tissue, and joints, resulting in activation of neutrophils and subsequent inflammation.[28] C3 and properdin were found in the glomerular deposits of 75–100% of patients with Henoch-Schönlein purpura and activated complement C3 has been found to be associated with subsequent deterioration of renal function.[29] In addition, glomerular deposits of components of the lectin pathway, mannose-binding lectin (MBL) and MBL-associated serine protease (MASP) as well as C3b/C3c, C5b-9 and C4-binding protein (C4bp), were detected in eight of 10 patients with HSP, and it was suggested that complement activation through the lectin pathway was also involved in the onset of Henoch-Schönlein purpura nephritis.[30] According to the studies, several proinflammatory cytokines, including TNF-α, interleukin (IL)-1b, IL-2, IL-6, IL-8, transforming growth factor-β and vascular endothelial growth factor have been reported to be involved in the pathogenesis of Henoch-Schönlein purpura. Recently, genetic predisposition has been shown in the children with Henoch-Schönlein purpura. Human leukocyte antigen-DRB1 polymorphisms were associated with an increased risk of Henoch-Schönlein purpura in Turkish children.[31]

Clinical Features

In IgA vasculitis, the most common cutaneous feature is palpable purpura. Lower extremities are the most commonly affected sites in children while adults have shown more common involvement of upper extremities (Fig. 3).[31] Systemic features include the presence of gastrointestinal symptoms, such as abdominal pain and gastrointestinal bleeding in 40–65%, arthralgia or arthritis with periarticular swelling in 50–63%, and renal involvement with microscopic or gross hematuria in 50–70%. These studies have shown more frequent and severe systemic involvement in adult cases of Henoch-Schönlein purpura than in childhood HSP. Uppal et al. compared 20 adults with 82 children of Henoch-Schönlein purpura and found that adults have more frequent nephropathy (90% vs. 52.4%) than children.[25] Similar observation was also noted by Kang et al. who retrospectively reviewed 112 children and 48 adults of Henoch-Schönlein purpura and found significant higher renal involvement in adults compared to children (79.2% versus 30.4%).[32] Both these studies noted a higher joint involvement in children compared to adult. Central nervous system (CNS) manifestations can occur rarely in Henoch-Schönlein purpura, and possible neurologic features include headache, altered mentality, seizures, visual disturbance, verbal disability, peripheral neuropathy, facial palsy, encephalopathy, intracranial hemorrhage, and Guillain-Barre´ syndrome.[33] Pulmonary

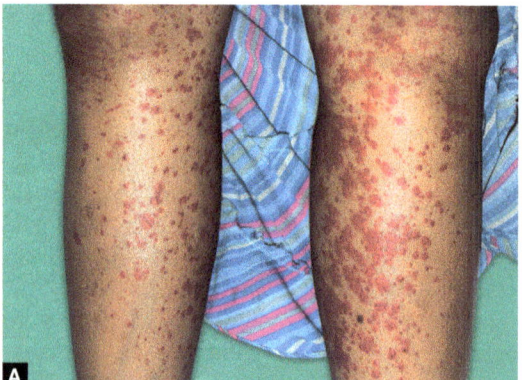 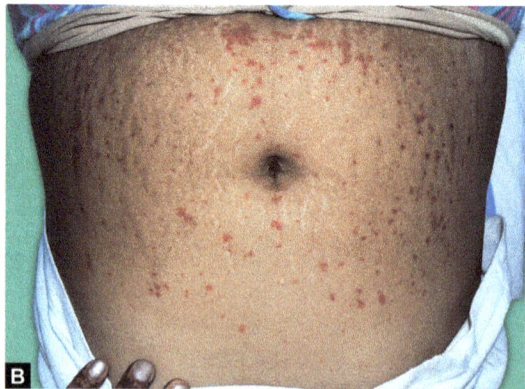

FIGURE 3: Henoch–Schönlein purpura. **A,** Showing multiple erythematous discrete and confluent palpable purpura over the lower extremities; **B,** Similar lesions over the anterior abdominal wall.

hemorrhage is a rare and life-threatening complication.[34] Recently, there are numerous reports of scrotal involvement in Henoch-Schönlein purpura with a reported incidences varying from 2 to 38%.[35]

Investigations

Skin biopsy shows identical features as of small vessel vasculitis of skin (Fig. 4), though the deposition of IgA on direct immunofluorescence is highly diagnostic. Other findings include anemia, thrombocytosis, hematuria, proteinuria and positive occult blood in stool. In cases of persistent hematuria and proteinuria, renal biopsy may show mesangioproliferative IgA nephropathy.

Treatment

Henoch-Schönlein purpura is a self-limiting disease in most of the cases. Intensive treatment is only required in the presence of systemic involvement. Nonsteroidal anti-inflammatory drugs can be used in mild cases. Oral corticosteroids provide quick symptomatic relief, ameliorate joint and abdominal pain and seem to accelerate the resolution of renal symptoms, but they do not seem to prevent renal complications and hence their prophylactic use is not recommended.[36] Ronkainen et al. treated 171 patients of Henoch-Schönlein purpura with prednisone 1 mg/kg/day for 2 weeks followed by weaning in next 2 weeks. There was significant improvement in abdominal and joint complaint and improvement of renal symptoms in 61% of patients compared to 34% of placebo, though it did not prevent development of new renal symptoms.[37] High dose of intravenous pulse steroids are recommended in nephrotic range of proteinuria and mesenteric vasculitis.[38] A combination of immunosuppressive drugs as azathioprine, cyclosporine, cyclophosphamide and corticosteroid had been used successfully in severe cases of renal involvement.[39,40] Methotrexate was used as a steroid sparing agent in a chronic case of Henoch-Schönlein purpura.[41] Biologics as rituximab has been used recently in the management of adult patients of IgA vasculitis with biopsy proven nephritis.[42] Plasmapheresis or high dose intravenous immunoglobulin therapy is recommended in progressively worsening renal functions, hemorrhage in lung or brain, and a refractory severe disease.[43]

Prognosis

The usual duration of IgA vasculitis is between several weeks to a few months (average of 4 weeks). Up to one-third of patients have persistent or recurrent disease for as long as 6 months. The prognosis of IgA vasculitis is generally favorable but depends mostly on the severity of renal disease. Stewart et al. followed-up 270 patients of Henoch-Schönlein purpura over 13 years and found that overall prognosis was good with less than 1% of morbidity and 1% of renal involvement.[44] Progressive glomerular disease and renal failure may occur in 1–3%, so patients with hematuria or proteinuria should be carefully followed for late deterioration of renal function. Predicting the progression of renal disease is difficult. Bunchmann et al. reviewed 16 patients of anaphylactoid purpura with renal failure and compared them with children of Henoch-Schönlein purpura with reversible renal involvement and concluded that a creatinine clearance of more than 125 mL/min/1.73 cm^2 predicted recovery while a clearance of less than 70 mL/min/1.73 cm^2 predicted progression to end-stage renal failure.[45] In addition, older age, hypertension, presence of abdominal symptoms, arthralgia, hematuria, proteinuria, and nephrotic syndrome at the time of diagnosis predicts

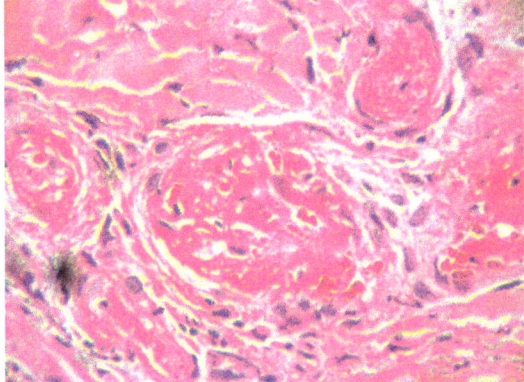

FIGURE 4: Henoch-Schönlein purpura. Photomicrograph showing fibrinoid necrosis of the blood vessel in the dermis.

increased risk of progression to end stage renal failure.[39] Renal insufficiency and long-term sequelae are more common in adults.

DRUG-INDUCED VASCULITIS

Drug-induced vasculitis is defined as any case of inflammatory vasculitis in which a specific drug including toxins is established as a causal agent of the disease when other forms of vasculitis are excluded. It is important to diagnose drug-induced vasculitis as the clinical course, and treatment is different from the idiopathic variety.[46]

Types of Drug-induced Leukocytoclastic Vasculitis

Drug-induced leukocytoclastic vasculitis can be classified into drug associated immune complex vasculitis and drug associated ANCA related vasculitis.[46,47]

Drug Associated Immune Complex Vasculitis

Drug associated immune complex vasculitis can present as cutaneous leukocytoclastic vasculitis or hypersensitivity vasculitis in the skin and clinically it presents as palpable purpura that may be associated with nonspecific constitutional symptoms such as fever, arthralgia and myalgia. There may be lymphadenopathy. The usual latent period between the drug intake and the onset of purpura is about a week. Withdrawal of the causative drugs leads to complete recovery of the illness. Usually, there is no systemic involvement.[46,47]

Drug Associated Antineutrophil Cytoplasmic Antibody Related Vasculitis

Some of the drug-induced vasculitis can manifest as systemic vasculitic syndrome with involvement of kidneys, lungs, liver, and CNS, features related to an idiopathic ANCA related vasculitis such as Wegener's granulomatosis. The most frequently implicated drugs are hydralazine, antithyroid drugs (propylthiouracil, methimazole, carbimazole), minocycline. The other uncommon causative drugs include allopurinol, penicillamine, procainamide, phenytoin, antituberculous drugs (rifampicin, isoniazid), indomethacin, and TNF-α blocking biologicals.[48-50]

In contrast to the idiopathic ANCA related vasculitis, patients with drug associated ANCA related vasculitis produce ANCA to more than one neutrophil antigen, the most common being granule proteins myeloperoxidase (MPO), human leukocyte elastase (HLE), cathepsin G, and lactoferrin. It is possible that the activated neutrophils in the presence of hydrogen peroxidase released MPO convert these drugs into cytotoxic products that become immunogenic for T cells. They in turn activate the B cells to produce ANCA. In addition the drugs and their metabolites accumulate within the neutrophils and modify the configuration of MPO with subsequent intermolecular determinants spreading the autoimmune response to other autoantigens and turning several of the neutrophil proteins immunogenic. Some of the drugs can also cause neutrophil apoptosis with translocation of ANCA antigens to the cell surface leading to production of ANCA.[46]

The initial clinical manifestations include nonspecific symptoms such as fever, malaise, arthralgia, loss of appetite, and weight loss. If the causal drugs are not withdrawn, systemic involvement is more likely to develop. Kidney is the most common organ involved that may manifest as hematuria, proteinuria, etc. Some patients may develop pulmonary intra-alveolar hemorrhage, which presents as cough, hemoptysis, and breathlessness. Other rarer manifestations include pyoderma gangrenosum, serositis and CNS vasculitis.[47,48]

The diagnosis of drug-induced ANCA associated vasculitis is based on the temporal correlation between the drug intake and appearance of vasculitis. The presence of multispecific ANCA is highly diagnostic. These neutrophil specific antibodies will show perinuclear pattern on immunofluorescence (p-ANCA) and can be directed to MPO, HLE, cathepsin G, lactoferrin, and azurocidin. Sometimes drug-induced ANCA associated vasculitis shares clinical and serological features of drug-induced lupus (DIL), which also manifests as fever, arthritis, myalgias and serositis. However, renal and systemic features are much more common and severe in the later. Autoantibodies to neutrophil autoantigens can also be found in DIL. Antinuclear, antihistone, and antiphospholipid antibodies can be found in both the conditions. The causative medications are also same for both. Hence, it is difficult at times to distinguish between these two drug-induced syndromes.[46-48]

Management

The laboratory workup for drug-induced vasculitis include the baseline hemogram, routine biochemistry, acute phase reactants, urine and stool examination, skin biopsy, and chest screening. Serological and immunological assays including ANCA assays using indirect immunofluorescence and antigen specific enzyme-linked immunosorbent assay need to be done. For milder cases without systemic features, immediate withdrawal of the suspected drug is the only intervention required. Patients with more severe disease should be treated with systemic corticosteroids and/or immunosuppressive drugs such as cyclophosphamide. For massive pulmonary hemorrhage, plasmapheresis may be required. Since drug-induced vasculitis usually has a milder course compared to idiopathic vasculitis, long-term maintenance may not be necesaary.[46-48]

REFERENCES

1. Jennette JC. Overview of the 2012 revised International Chapel Hill Consensus Conference nomenclature of vasculitides. Clin Exp Nephrol. 2013;17(5):603-6.
2. Arora A, Wetter DA, Gonzalez-Santiago TM, et al. Incidence of leukocytoclastic vasculitis, 1996 to 2010: A population-based study in Olmsted County, Minnesota. Mayo Clin Proc. 2014;89:1515-24.
3. Al-Mutairi N. Spectrum of cutaneous vasculitis in adult patients from the Farwaniya region of Kuwait. Med Princ Pract. 2008;17(1):43-8.
4. Chimenti MS, Ballanti E, Triggianese P, et al. Vasculitides and the complement system: A comprehensive Review. Clin Rev Allergy Immunol. 2015;49(3):333-46.
5. Greco F, Sorge A, Salvo V, et al. Cutaneous vasculitis associated with Mycoplasma pneumoniae infection: case report and literature review. Clin Pediatr (Phila). 2007;46:451.
6. Barile-Fabris L, Hernandez-Cabrera MF, Barragan-Garfias JA. Vasculitis in systemic lupus erythematosus. Curr Rheumatol Rep. 2014;16(9):440.
7. Loricera J, Calvo-Rio V, Ortiz-Sanjuan F, et al. The spectrum of paraneoplastic cutaneous vasculitis in a defined population: incidence and clinical features. Medicine (Baltimore). 2013; 92(6):331-43.
8. Xu LY, Esparza EM, Anadkat MJ, et al. Cutaneous manifestations of vasculitis. Semin Arthritis Rheum 2009; 38(5):34-60.
9. Johnson EF, Wetter DA, Lehman JS, et al. Leukocytoclastic vasculitis in children: clinical characteristics, subtypes, causes and direct immunofluorescence findings of 56 biopsy-confirmed cases. J Eur Acad Dermatol Venereol. 2017;31(3):544-9.
10. Podjasek JO, Wetter DA, Wieland CN, et al. Histopathologic Findings in Cutaneous small-Vessel Vasculitis Associated With Solid-Organ Malignancy. Br J Dermatol 2 014;171(6):1397-401.
11. Bahrami S, Malone JC, Webb KG, et al. Tissue eosinophilia as an indicator of drug-induced cutaneous small-vessel vasculitis. Arch Dermatol 2006;142:155-61.
12. Sais G, Vidaller A, Jucgla A. Colchicine in the treatment of cutaneous leukocytoclastic vasculitis. Results of a prospective, randomized controlled trial. Arch Dermatol 1995;131:1399.
13. Fredenberg MF, Malkinson FD. Sulfone therapy in the treatment of leukocytoclastic vasculitis. Report of three cases. J Am Acad Dermatol 1987;16(4):772-8.
14. Lopez LR, Davis KC, Kohler PF, et al. The hypocomplementemic urticarial vasculitis syndrome: therapeutic response to hydroxychloroquine. J Allergy Clin Immunol 1984;73:600-3.
15. Villa-Forte A. European League Against Rheumatism. European Vasculitis Study Group. European League Against Rheumatism/European Vasculitis Study Group recommendations for the management of vasculitis. Curr Opin Rheumatol. 2010;22(1):49-53.
16. Jorizzo JL, White WL, Wise CM, et al. Low dose weekly methotrexate for unusual neutrophilic vascular reactions: cutaneous polyarteritis nodosa and Behcet's disease. J Am Acad Dermatol. 1991;24:973-8.
17. Haeberle MT, Adams WB, Callen JP. Treatment of severe cutaneous small-vessel vasculitis with mycophenolate mofetil. Arch Dermatol. 2012;148(8):887-8.
18. Mang R, Ruzicka T, Stege H. Therapy for severe necrotizing vasculitis with infliximab. J Am Acad Dermatol. 2004;51:321.
19. Chung L, Funke AA, Chakravarty EF, et al. Successful use of rituximab for cutaneous vasculitis. Arch Dermatol. 2006;142(11):1407-10.
20. Ozen S, Pistorio A, Iusan SM, et al. EULAR/PRINTO/PRES criteria for Henoch–Schönlein purpura, childhood polyarteritis nodosa, childhood Wegener granulomatosis and childhood Takayasu arteritis: Ankara 2008. Part II: Final classification criteria. Ann Rheum Dis. 2010;69:798-806.
21. Mills JA, Michel BA, Bloch DA, et al. The American College of Rheumatology 1990 criteria for the classification of Henoch–Schönlein purpura. Arthritis Rheum. 1990;33:1114-21.
22. Aalberse J, Dolman K, Ramnath G, et al. Henoch–Schönlein purpura in children: an epidemiological study among Dutch

paediatricians on incidence and diagnostic criteria. Ann Rheum Dis. 2007;66(12):1648-50.
23. Khetan P, Sethuraman G, Khaitan BK, et al. An aetiological and clinicopathological study on cutaneous vasculitis. Indian J Med Res. 2012;135:107-13.
24. Jelusić M, Kostić L, Frković M, et al. Vasculitides in childhood: a retrospective study in a period from 2002 to 2012 at the department of paediatrics, university hospital centre Zagreb. Reumatizam. 2015;62(2):6-10.
25. Uppal SS, Hussain MA, Al-Raqum HA et al. Henoch-Schönlein's purpura in adults versus children/adolescents: a comparative study. Clin Exp Rheumatol. 2006;24(2 Suppl 41): S26-30.
26. Gonzalez-Gay MA, Calviño MC, Vazquez-Lopez ME, et al. Implications of upper respiratory tract infections and drugs in the clinical spectrum of Henoch-Schönlein purpura in children. Clin Exp Rheumatol. 2004;22(6):781-4.
27. Fox MC, Carter S, Khouri IF, Giralt SA, et al. Adult Henoch-Schönlein purpura in a patient with myelodysplastic syndrome and a history of follicular lymphoma. Cutis. 2008;81(2):131-7.
28. Sohagia AB, Gunturu SG, Tong TR, et al. Henoch-schonlein purpura-a case report and review of the literature. Gastroenterol Res Pract. 2010;2010:597648.
29. Zwirner J, Burg M, Schulze M, et al. Activated complement C3: a potentially novel predictor of progressive IgA nephropathy. Kidney Int. 1997;51(4):1257-64.
30. Hisano S, Matsushita M, Fujita T, et al. Activation of the lectin complement pathway in Henoch-Schönlein purpura nephritis. Am J Kidney Dis. 2005;45(2):295-302.
31. Soylemezoglu O, Peru H, Gonen S, et al. HLA-DRB1 alleles and Henoch-Schonlein purpura: susceptibility and severity of disease. J. Rheumatol. 2008;35(6):1165-8.
32. Kang Y, Park JS, Ha YJ, et al. Differences in clinical manifestations and outcomes between adult and child patients with Henoch-Schönlein purpura. J Korean Med Sci. 2014;29(2):198-203.
33. Iannetti L, Zito R, Bruschi S, et al. Recent understanding on diagnosis and management of central nervous system vasculitis in children. Clin Dev Immunol. 2012;2012:698327.
34. Rajagopala S, Shobha V, Devaraj U, et al. Pulmonary haemorrhage in Henoch Schonlein purpura: case report and systematic review of the English literature. Semin. Arthritis Rheum. 2013;42(4):391-400.
35. Aaron S, Al-Watban L, Manca D. Scrotal involvement in an adult with Henoch-Schonlein purpura. Clin Rheumatol. 2013;32(Suppl. 1):S93-5.
36. Chartapisak W, Opastirakul S, Hodson EM, et al. Interventions for preventing and treating kidney disease in Henoch-Schonlein purpura (HSP). Cochrane Database Syst Rev. 2009;(3):CD005128.
37. Ronkainen J, Koskimies O, Ala-Houhala M, et al. Early prednisone therapy in Henoch-Schönlein purpura: a randomized, double-blind, placebo-controlled trial. J Pediatr. 2006;149(2):241-7.
38. Segura Torres P, Borrego Utiel FJ, Pérez Del Barrio P, et al. Complete remission of nephrotic syndrome with methylprednisolone pulses in an adult with Schönlein-Henoch purpura. Nefrologia. 2007;27(1):96-8.
39. Shin JI, Park JM, Shin YH, et al. Can azathioprine and steroids alter the progression of severe Henoch-Schönlein nephritis in children? Pediatr Nephrol. 2005;20:1087-92.
40. Oner A, Tinaztepe K, Erdogan O. The effect of triple therapy on rapidly progressive type of Henoch-Schönlein nephritis. Pediatr Nephrol. 1995;9(1):6-10.
41. Rettig P, Cron RQ. Methotrexate used as a steroid-sparing agent in non-renal chronic Henoch-Schönlein purpura. Clin Exp Rheumatol. 2003;21(6):767-9.
42. Fenoglio R, Naretto C, Basolo B, et al. Rituximab therapy for IgA-vasculitis with nephritis: a case series and review of the literature. Immunol Res. 2017;65(1):186-92.
43. Chaudhary K, Shin JY, Saab G, et al. Successful treatment of Henoch-Schonlein purpura nephritis with plasma exchange in an adult male. NDT Plus. 2008;1(5):303-6.
44. Stewart M, Savage JM, Bell B, et al. Long term renal prognosis of Henoch-Schönlein purpura in an unselected childhood population. Eur J Pediatr. 1988;147(2):113-5.
45. Bunchman TE, Mauer SM, Sibley RK, et al. Anaphylactoid purpura: characteristics of 16 patients who progressed to renal failure. Pediatr Nephrol. 1988;2(4):393-7.
46. Wiik A. Drug induced vasculitis. Curr Opin Rheumatol. 2008;20:35-9.
47. Radic M, Kaliterna DM, Radic J. Drug induced vasculitis: a clinical and pathological review. Neth J Med. 2012;70: 12-7.
48. Merkel PA. Drugs associated with vasculitis. Curr Opin Rheumatol. 1998;10:45-50.
49. Pendergraft WF, Niles JL. Trojan horses: drug culprits associated with antineutrophil cytoplasmic autoantibody (ANCA) vasculitis. Curr Opin Rheumatol. 2014;25:42-9.
50. Keaaberry J, Frazier J, Isbel NM, et al. Hydralazine induced antineutrophil cytoplasmic antibody positive renal vasculitis presenting with a vasculitic syndrome, acute nephritis and a puzzling skin rash: a case report. J Med Case Rep. 2013;7:1-5.

23 CHAPTER

Behçet's Disease

Iffat Hassan, Yasmeen Jabeen Bhat, Debashish Danda

INTRODUCTION

The first description of the Behçet's disease (BD) is attributed to the Turkish dermatologist Hulusi Behçet in 1937, although, Hippocrates first described the symptomatology of the disease.[1,2] The Greek ophthalmologist Benediktos Adamantiades, in 1930, reported a patient with inflammatory arthritis, oral and genital ulcers, phlebitis, and iritis.[3] Many names have been given in the past for this condition, including triple symptom complex, syndrome de Behçet, Adamantiades-Behçet's syndrome, Behçet's multiple symptom complex, Behçet's syndrome, Adamantiades-Behçet's disease, mucocutaneous-ocular syndrome, mouth and genital ulcers with inflamed cartilage syndrome, and pseudo-Behçet's syndrome, but BD is the most commonly used terminology.[4-7]

EPIDEMIOLOGY

Behçet's disease is prevalent worldwide, with the higher incidence in the Mediterranean, the Middle East, and the Far East, Turkey having the highest prevalence (Table 1).[8] The disease is more frequent in men, except in Japan and Korea where women are more commonly affected.[9-12] Males with poor prognosis, such as those with ocular, gastrointestinal, neurologic, and vascular involvement, have younger age of onset than in females.[13] The association of BD with the "Silk Route", the ancient trading route, and the distribution of human leukocyte antigens (HLA)-B5 and its subtype HLA-B51 provides important clues to its origin. Behçet's disease is more prevalent between the latitudes 30°N and 45°N in Eurasian populations.[10-12]

Behçet's disease typically occurs in the third or fourth decade of life, and has been rarely seen in children or patients aged above 50 years. The clinical courses of childhood onset BD and late onset BD are relatively benign.[9,14-17] Familial cases have been reported.[18] The outcome of BD in pregnancy is varied with exacerbation in 67% and improvement in 33%. In about 78% of cases who experience worsening of the disease during pregnancy, clinical exacerbation occurred mostly during the first trimester.[12,13]

Table 1: Countries with high prevalence of Behçet's disease

Country	Prevalence per 10^5
Turkey (Istanbul)	420
Israel (Druze)	146.4
Northern China	110
Iran	80
Korea	30.2
Japan (Hokkaido)	22
Saudi Arabia	20
Iraq	17
Morocco	>15
Egypt	7.6

ETIOPATHOGENESIS

The exact etiopathogenesis of BD is unclear, however, the disease may be triggered by environmental factors such as infectious agents or pollution, in patients who are genetically susceptible (Fig. 1).[19-21] Exposure to an infectious agent, including herpes simplex virus, *Streptococcus* species, *Staphylococcus* species, and *Escherichia coli*, the commensals in the oral cavity, may trigger a cross-reactive immune response.

Sixty percent of patients with BD test positive for HLA-B51, showing a strong association with it within the major histocompatibility complex region of chromosome 6.[22-24] The common variants of interleukin 10 (IL-10), IL-23 receptor, and *IL-12β2* genes are strongly associated with BD.[24] The proinflammatory cytokine IL-23 stimulates T-helper 17 (Th17) proliferation, increases the production of inflammatory cytokines and increases the expression of IL-23 p19 messenger RNA in erythema nodosum-like skin lesions in patients with BD.[22,25] The anti-inflammatory cytokine IL-10 inhibits the action of proinflammatory cytokines, and the upregulation of the $CD4^+$ and $CD25^+$ regulatory T cells, thereby improving the symptoms of BD.[26]

Immunoglobulin M (IgM) type anti-endothelial cell antibodies (AECA) target the antigen α-enolase in the endothelial cells of blood vessels in patients with BD causing the clinical presentation of vasculitis and thrombosis. The AECA bind to the endothelial cells, resulting in cell activation, secretions of chemoattractants and cytokines as well as secretion or inhibition of prostacyclin, complement-dependent cytotoxicity, and antibody-dependent cellular toxicity.[27] Heat shock proteins (HSPs) may be contributory as human HSP-60 and HSP-65 share greater than 50% homology with mycobacterial HSP, eliciting enhanced T cell response with exposure to both bacterial and human homogenates in BD patients.[28]

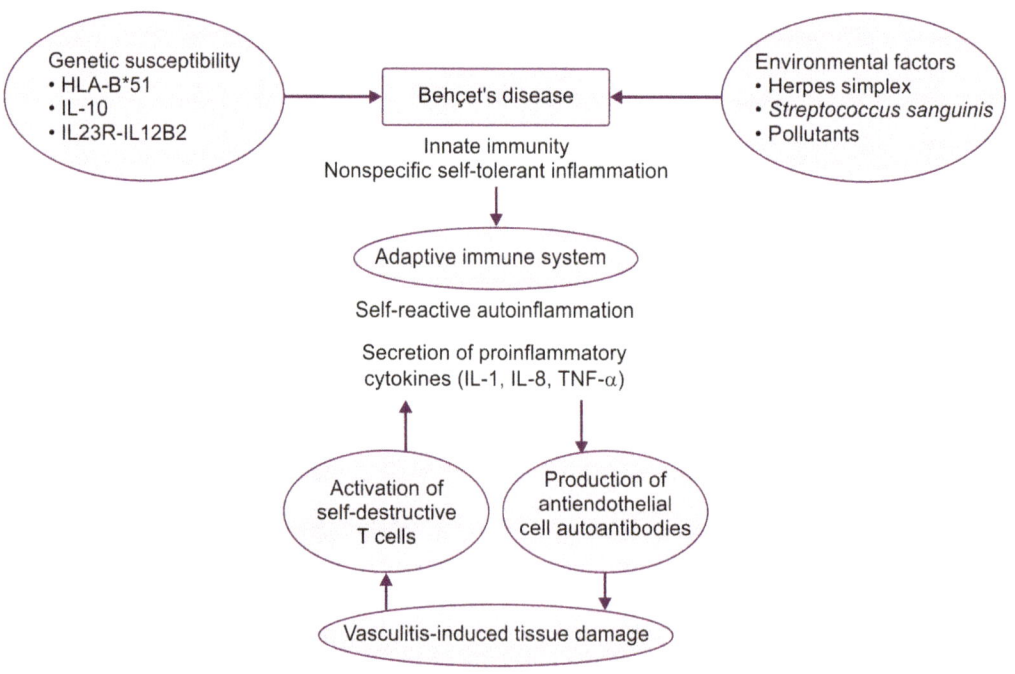

HLA, Human leukocyte antigen; CD86, Cluster of Differentiation 86; PD-L1, Programmed death-ligand 1 IL, interleukin; TNF-α, tumor necrosis factor α; CTLA-4, cytotoxic T-lymphocyte-associated protein 4.

FIGURE 1: Diagram representing etiopathogenesis of Behçet's disease.

CLINICAL FEATURES

Skin and Mucous Membrane Manifestations

Painful oral lesions (aphthous or herpetiform) are one of the criteria for diagnosis and may be the first manifestation (70% of cases). Oral lesions are commonly found in keratinized areas of the oropharynx, often excluding the nonkeratinized surfaces of the dorsal tongue, gums, and hard palate (Fig. 2). The lesions are usually not distinguishable from those due to other causes but often have a high recurrence rate [often more than five times per year, despite only three times per year as specified in International Study Group (ISG) criteria] and appear as multiple lesions or crops (often more than six simultaneous lesions at a given time). They can be very painful, can last up to 3-5 weeks, and can vary in size. Large ulcers (>10 mm in diameter) heal with scarring, as do their genital counterparts.

Skin lesions often occur in the genital region of both sexes. In males, scrotal involvement is most characteristic; however, lesions can also develop on the penile shaft (Fig. 3). In females, the labial area is most commonly involved, with lesions occasionally developing in the vagina and on the perineum (Fig. 4). Genital ulcerations typically last longer than oral ulcers, heal with scarring, and are more painful in men. Development of ulcerations in women may correlate with menstruation.

Extragenital ulcerations affect only 3% of patients, heal with scarring, and are very specific for BD (Fig. 5). They can be found in the axillae, neck, breast, interdigital skin of the feet, and groin.

Nodules that resemble erythema nodosum are more common in the lower extremities of females

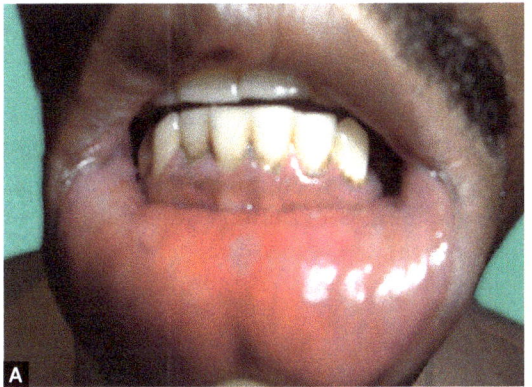
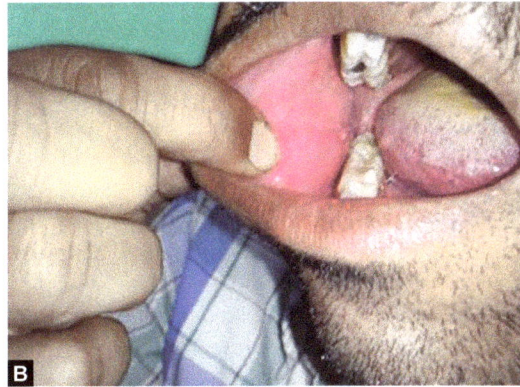

FIGURE 2: Oral aphthous ulcer in Behçet's disease patient.

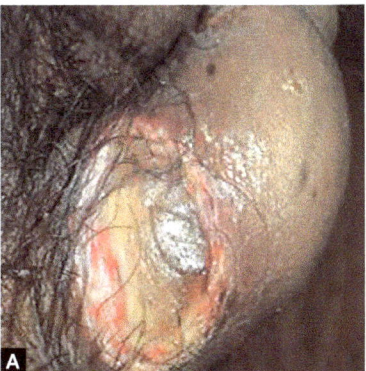
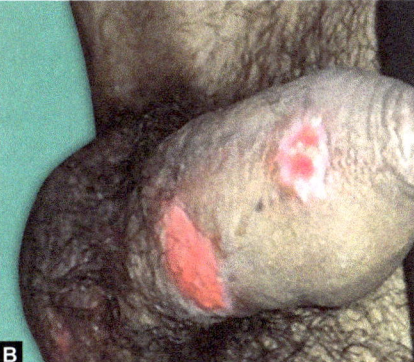
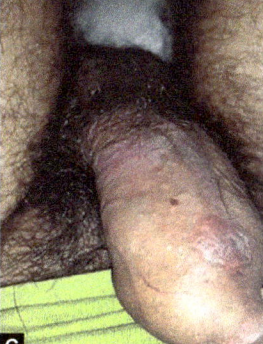

FIGURE 3: Showing recalcitrant genital aphthous ulcer in a patient with Behçet's disease before treatment and showing gradual healing after two doses of 3mg/kg infliximab infusion.

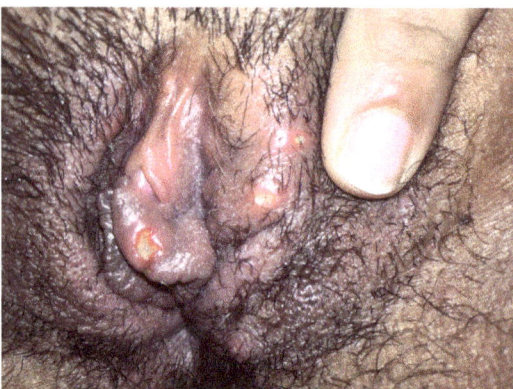

FIGURE 4: Aphthous ulcer over labia.

(Fig. 6). They are tender, erythematous, and usually resolve after 2–3 weeks but often recur. Erythema nodosum may be an indicator of mild BD.

Papulopustular lesions (folliculitis or pseudo-folliculitis) are more common in men and are usually found on the trunk and extremities but can occur over other body parts also (Fig. 7). They are more prevalent in Turkish and Europeans.

Prevalence of positive pathergy test in patients with BD was found to vary between 50 and 80% in Turkey, 44% in Japan and between 12 and 52% in Europe. Pathergy test positivity is also more common in patients with ophthalmologic and neurologic manifestations.

The extracutaneous systemic manifestations of BD are summarized in table 2.

DIAGNOSIS OF BEHÇET'S DISEASE

In 1990, the ISG for Behçet's disease clarified criteria for the diagnosis of BD.[29] The ISG group compared the clinical findings of 914 patients with a history of aphthous ulcers with those of controls. The Revised International Classification Criteria for BD is given in box 1.[30]

DIFFERENTIAL DIAGNOSIS OF BEHÇET'S DISEASE

- Sarcoidosis
- Drug reactions
- Amyloidosis
- Antiphospholipid syndrome
- Sweet's syndrome
- Inflammatory bowel disease
- Paraneoplastic syndrome
- Polyarteritis nodosa
- Systemic lupus erythematosus
- Wegener's granulomatosis.

INVESTIGATIONS

Histopathology

A review of the pathological features of vasculitides described three main types of reaction in BD,[31] namely:

1. Vascular, including:
   a. A lymphocytic or granulomatous vasculitis with or without thrombosis, necrosis, and fibrinoid deposition
   b. A paucicellular thrombogenic vasculopathy
   c. A neutrophilic vascular reaction that may affect capillaries as well as arteries or veins of any size, and that includes a leukocytoclastic vasculitis and a Sweet's syndrome-like reaction
2. Extravascular with or without vasculopathy, including a mononuclear cell or neutrophil-predominant inflammation of the dermis and/or panniculus, or a histiocytic panniculitis
3. A suppurative or mixed suppurative/granulomatous folliculitis comprising of acneiform lesions.

Laboratory findings are nonspecific and reflect the inflammatory state. The C-reactive protein (CRP) levels, erythrocyte sedimentation rate (ESR), leukocyte count, complement components, and acute-phase reactants may all be elevated during an acute attack. Serum ESR, CRP, and *S100A12*, related to neutrophil hyperactivity, have been used to assess disease activity and clinical responses to treatment in BD.[32,33] Levels of IgA, IgG, α-2 globulin, IgM, and immune complexes may be elevated. Other investigations to find antiphospholipid antibodies like lupus anticoagulant, anticardiolipin antibodies, and dilute Russell viper venom test, should be done to rule out alternate causes of thrombosis. Serum calprotectin levels have been found elevated in patients with BD, but it does not correlate with scores on the Behçet Disease Current Activity

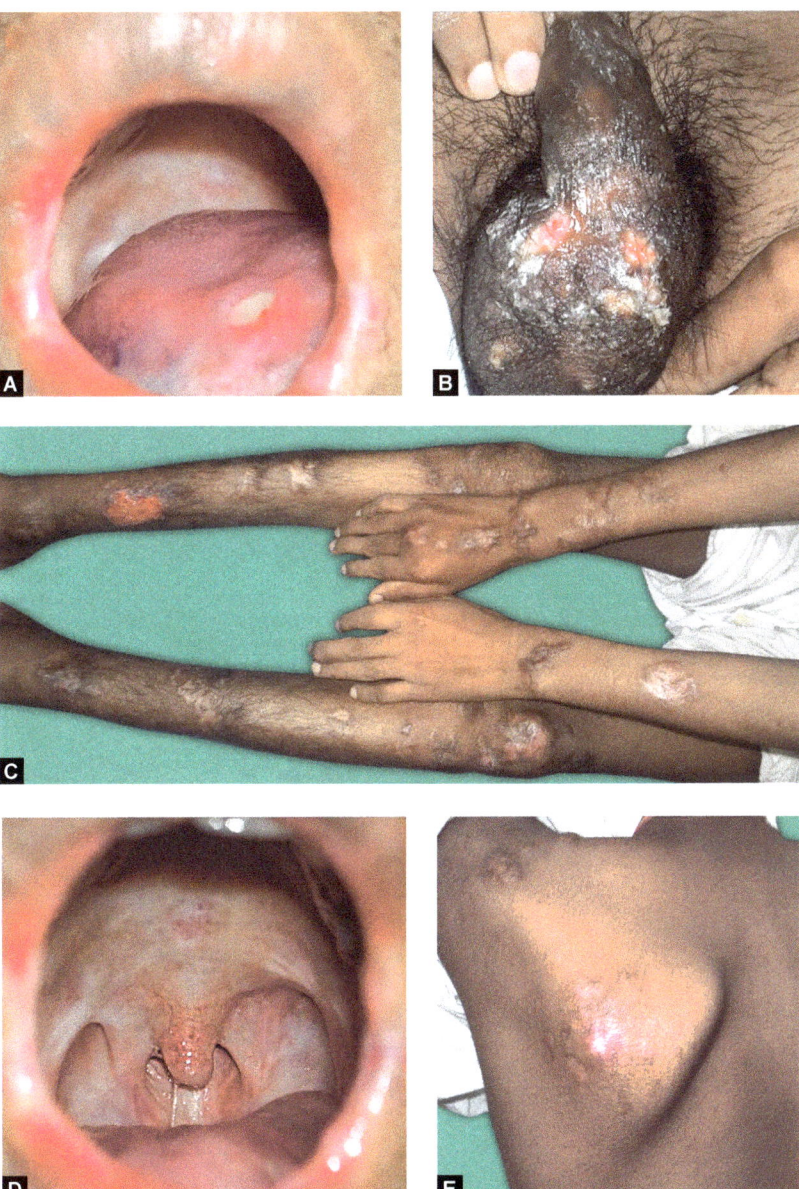

FIGURE 5: Behçet's disease patient had major aphthe appearing in oral cavity, pharynx, esophagus, and scrotum. Lesions healed with significant scarring leading to restricted mouth opening, pharyngeal scarring, and difficulty in swallowing. He also had pustular lesions and pyoderma gangrenosum like erosions appearing over the limbs, scapula, and buttocks which are also healed with significant scarring.

Courtesy: Dr B K Khaitan, Professor, Department of Dermatology and Venereology, AIIMS, New Delhi.

Form.[34] Perinuclear antineutrophil cytoplasmic antibody (p-ANCA) may be positive in these patients but has no role in prognosis or treatment.

Synovial fluid usually is cloudy with variable viscosity, the white blood cell counts are 300–36,000/µL, polymorphonuclear leukocytes and

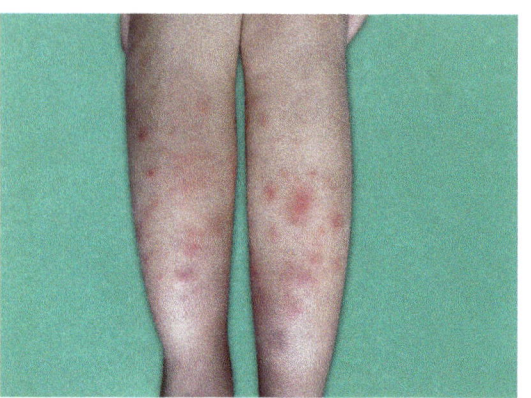

FIGURE 6: Erythema nodosum in Behçet's disease patient.

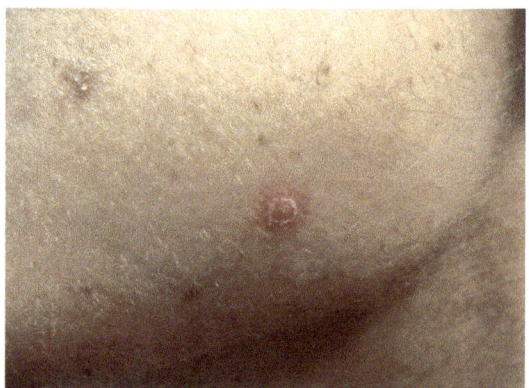

FIGURE 7: Recurrent pustular lesion appeared over face and trunk and healed without scarring.

Table 2: Extracutaneous manifestations of Behçet's disease	
Ocular (Fig. 8)	**Neurologic**
• Occurs in 90% of patients; favors men, in whom it is more severe • Symptoms include blurred vision, periorbital pain, photophobia, sclera injection, and excessive lacrimation • Can be painful and may lead to blindness • Retinal vasculitis (more frequently associated with blindness) • Posterior uveitis (most characteristic ocular finding) • Anterior uveitis, hypopyon • Secondary glaucoma, cataracts • Conjunctivitis, scleritis, keratitis, vitreous hemorrhage, optic neuritis • Leaky retinal vessels revealed by fluorescein angiography, leading to atrophy and fibrosis in some cases	• Usually appears later during the evolution of the disease • Associated with a poor prognosis • Acute meningoencephalitis which may resolve spontaneously • Cranial nerve palsies • Brainstem lesions that can induce swallowing difficulties, laughter, and crying • Pyramidal or extrapyramidal signs • Memory tends to be affected in most cases, particularly affecting recall and learning • Seizures and bulbar signs with ophthalmoplegia are less common • Peripheral nerve involvement is rare
Musculoskeletal	**Vascular**
• Approximately 50% of patients develop arthritis • In majority (~80% of patients), duration of attacks is less than 2 months • Monoarthritic or polyarthritic and nonerosive • Most commonly knees, wrists, and ankles • Symptoms relapse and remit, and rarely become chronic	• Aneurysmal or occlusive arterial disease • Venous involvement (usually in the form of superficial thrombophlebitis) is more common than arterial • Presents in a linear fashion with overlying erythema and tenderness • In males, formation of these linear areas of vasculopathy leads to string-like thickening in affected areas • Deep venous thrombosis develops in some cases manifesting as local tenderness or as disparity in limb girth

Continued

Continued

Table 2: Extracutaneous manifestations of Behçet's disease	
Gastrointestinal	**Cardiopulmonary**
• Abdominal pain and/or hemorrhage may be difficult to distinguish from inflammatory bowel disease. • Ulcerations develop within the small bowel (in particular the ileocecal region) as well as the transverse and ascending colon and esophagus; perforation can occur	• Coronary arteritis, valvular disease, pericarditis, myocarditis • Recurrent ventricular arrhythmias • Pulmonary artery aneurismal involvement is associated with right-sided cardiac thromboses • Can manifest as hemoptysis, cough, chest pain, or dyspnea
Genitourinary	**Renal**
• Genitourinary involvement can include epididymitis, neurogenic bladder, and sterile urethritis	• Occurs in 1–29% of patients • Nephritic-range proteinuria • Crescentic and proliferative glomerulonephritis, as well as immunoglobulin A nephritis • Associated amyloidosis may develop

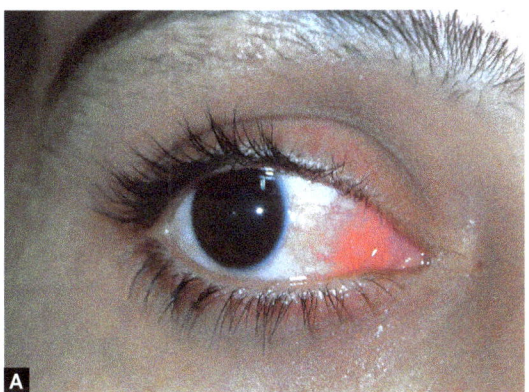 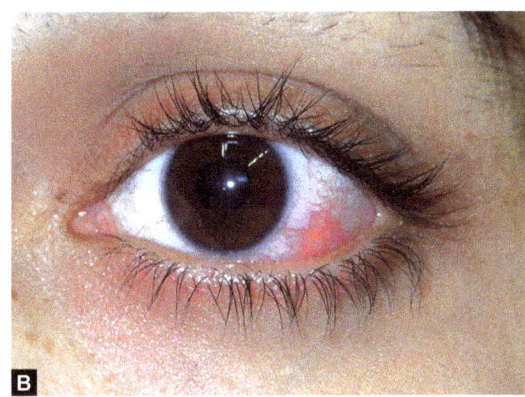

FIGURE 8: Nodular episcleritis in right eye and sectoral episcleritis in left eye in Behçet's disease patient.

Box 1: International Study Group criterion for diagnosis of Behçet's disease

Major plus more than or equal to two minor criteria
- Major Criteria
  - Recurrent oral ulceration: Aphthous oral ulceration (idiopathic) observed by patient or physician, recurring at least three times in a 12-month period
- Minor Criteria
  - Recurrent genital ulceration: Aphthous genital ulceration or scarring, observed by physician or patient
  - Eye lesions: Anterior or posterior uveitis; cells in the vitreous by slit-lamp examination, or retinal vasculitis observed by ophthalmologist
  - Cutaneous lesions: Erythema nodosum-like lesions observed by physician or patient; papulopustular lesions or pseudofolliculitis; or acneiform nodules observed by physician in a postadolescent patient not on any corticosteroids
  - Positive pathergy test: Formation of a sterile erythematous papule 2 mm in diameter or larger that appears 48 hours following a skin prick with a sharp sterile needle

protein are elevated but the glucose levels are near normal. Synovial fluid analysis helps to rule out the presence of aseptic joint, crystal-induced arthropathy, or other alternative identifiable cause.

Radiographs may show soft-tissue swelling, effusions or sacroiliitis, although magnetic resonance imaging (MRI) may delineate changes much earlier. Cerebral vasculopathy and ischemia can be identified using brain MRI or magnetic resonance angiography.

MONITORING ACTIVITY OF MUCOCUTANEOUS DISEASE

Mumcu et al., have devised a patient reported composite index of oral ulcers, genital ulcers, and erythema nodosum to detect mucocutaneous activity in BD. With the use of questionnaire, mucocutaneous index (MI) score was found to be sensitive to changes of symptoms. Scores of inactive patients were zero and almost all of the active patients had oral ulcers. Persistence of activity or worsening of mucocutaneous lesions was associated with poor scores of MI, as compared to patients with resolved or significantly decreased lesions.[35]

TREATMENT

The management of BD may involve a combined approach by dermatologist, rheumatologist, urologist, neurologist, ophthalmologist, gastroenterologist, surgeon, nephrologist, and rarely pulmonologist or cardiologist. The treatment of BD is symptomatic and empirical and depends on the individual patient, severity of disease and major organ involvement. Diet has no role in management. The European League against Rheumatism (EULAR) recommendations related to the eye, skin/mucosa, and arthritic diseases are mainly evidence based, but recommendations on vascular, neurological, and gastrointestinal involvement are based largely on expert opinion and uncontrolled evidence from open trials and observational studies. The therapeutic ladder for BD is summarized in fig. 9. Corticosteroids are commonly used to treat clinical manifestations of BD as a monotherapy or in combination with immunosuppressants. Although they have beneficial effects against acute inflammation, no definite evidence has indicated that they are effective for controlling progression of the disease, and the adverse effects of long-term use must always be considered.

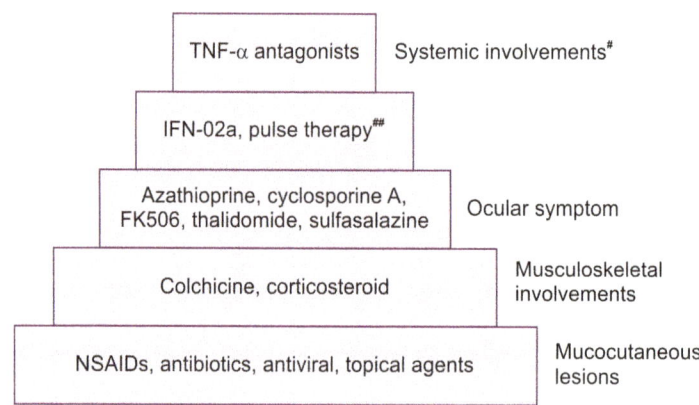

#CNS, GI, CVS symptoms
Corticosteroid, cyclophosphamide

TNF-α, tumor necrosis factor a; IFN, interferon; CNS, central nervous system; CVS, cardiovascular system; GI, gastrointestinal; NSAIDs, non-steroidal anti-inflammatory drugs.

FIGURE 9: Therapeutic approach to Behçet's disease.

For mild isolated oral and genital ulcerations, topical steroids, or sucralfate solution are the first-line treatments. For severe mucocutaneous lesions, systemic corticosteroids, azathioprine, pentoxifylline, dapsone, interferon-α, colchicine, and thalidomide are helpful. Colchicine has also been used to prevent mucocutaneous relapse.[36,37] Cutaneous disease with erythema nodosum may be treated with colchicine or dapsone.

For mild ocular disease, azathioprine is the initial agent while for severe disease (significant drop in visual acuity, retinal vasculitis, or macular involvement), either cyclosporine A or infliximab may be used in combination with azathioprine and corticosteroids.[38-40] Interferon-α, alone or in combination with corticosteroids, is the second choice in eye disease.[41]

Musculoskeletal manifestations generally respond to oral corticosteroids and nonsteroidal anti-inflammatory drugs, and occasionally colchicine. Severe exacerbation in joints may require intra-articular corticosteroids. Interferon-α, azathioprine, and tumor necrosis factor α (TNF-α) blockers may be tried in difficult cases with resistant, prolonged, and disabling attacks.

Major vessel disease with thrombotic events is treated with systemic anticoagulants in addition to corticosteroids, azathioprine, cyclophosphamide, or cyclosporine A. Pulmonary arterial aneurysms are treated with cyclophosphamide and corticosteroids. Gastrointestinal manifestations are managed with 5-amino salicylic acid derivatives, including sulfasalazine or mesalamine; systemic corticosteroids, and azathioprine.

TUMOR NECROSIS FACTOR-α INHIBITORS IN BEHÇET'S DISEASE

Infliximab has been shown to be effective in reducing the various mucocutaneous manifestations of the disease in various case reports.[42-44] Etanercept is the only TNF-α inhibitor evaluated in a randomized controlled trial of 4-weeks duration, in which 20 patients received etanercept 25 mg twice a week and 20 others received placebo injections. Without suppressing the pathergy reaction, etanercept decreased the frequency of oral ulcers, papulopustular lesions, and arthritis with a moderate effect on the size and frequency of genital ulcers and nodular lesions.

Tumor necrosis factor α inhibitors have also shown varying degrees of success in treating cases of severe gastrointestinal, ocular, and central nervous system manifestations of BD and have the added benefit of improving mucocutaneous manifestations and polyarthritis.[40,45] Infliximab was reported to successfully treat a case of BD in pregnancy.[46] Case reports have described successful treatment of refractory BD with alemtuzumab[47] and golimumab.[48]

Surgical Care

Few complications of BD require surgical care. Gastrointestinal manifestations requiring surgical intervention include intestinal stenosis, lesions unresponsive to medical therapy, fistula formation, perforation, and severe bleeding. Pulmonary aneurysms, ventricular aneurysms, coronary thrombosis, and areas that incur ischemic damage due to vasculitis or thrombosis may require resection. Neurosurgery may be required to correct central nervous system aneurysms and clots. Ophthalmological complications like glaucoma, cataracts, and retinal detachment also require surgical intervention.

REFERENCES

1. Behçet H. Über rezidivierende, aphthöse, durch ein Virus verursachte Geschwüre am Auge, und an den Genitalien. Dermatol Wochenschr. 1937;105:1152-7.
2. Feigenbaum A. Description of Behçet's syndrome in the Hippocratic third book of endemic diseases. Br J Ophthalmol. 1956;40(6):355-7.
3. Adamantiades B. A case of recurrent hypopyon iritis. Med Soc Athens. 1930;586-93.
4. Lee S, Bang D, Lee ES, , et al. Behçet's Disease: A Guide to its Clinical Understanding, 1st edition. Berlin, Heidelberg, New York: Springer Verlag; 2001.
5. Lee S. Behçet's disease or Behçet's syndrome-considerations for the unified diagnosis related terminology. In: Bang D, Lee ES, Lee S (Eds). Behçet's Disease: Proceedings of the Ninth International Conference on Behçet's Disease, held in Seoul, Korea, May 27-29, 2000. Seoul: Design Mecca; 2000. pp. 40-2.
6. Barnes CG. History and diagnosis. In: Yazici Y, Yazici H (Eds). Behçet's Syndrome, 1st edition. New York: Springer; 2010. pp. 7-33.

7. Cho SB, Cho S, Bang D. New insights in the clinical understanding of Behçet's disease. Yonsei Med J. 2012; 53(1):35-42.
8. Levine JA, O'Duffy JD. Pseudo-Behçet's syndrome-a description of twenty-three cases. In: Godeau P, Wechsler B (Eds). Behçet's Disease: Proceedings of the Sixth International Conference on Behçet's Disease, held in Paris, France, June 30 to July 1, 1993. Amsterdam: Elsevier Science Publishers; 1993. pp. 295-8.
9. Yurdakul S, Yazici Y. Epidemiology of Behçet's syndrome and regional differences in disease expression. In: Yazici Y, Yazici H (Eds). Behçet's Syndrome, 1st edition. New York: Springer; 2010. pp. 35-52.
10. Verity DH, Marr JE, Ohno S, et al. Behçet's disease, the Silk Road and HLA-B51: historical and geographical perspectives. Tissue Antigens. 1999; 54(3):213-20.
11. Davatchi F, Shahram F, Chams-Davatchi C, et al. Behcet's disease: from East to West. Clin Rheumatol. 2010;29(8):823-33.
12. Bang D, Lee ES, Lee S. Behçet's disease. In: Eun HC, Kim SC, Lee WS (Eds). Asian Skin and Skin Diseases: Special Book of the 22nd World Congress of Dermatology, held from May 24 to 29, 2011 in Seoul, Korea. Seoul: MEDrang Inc.; 2011. pp. 313-25.
13. Bang DS, Oh SH, Lee KH, et al. Influence of sex on patients with Behçet's disease in Korea. J Korean Med Sci. 2003;18(2):231-5.
14. Tugal-Tutkun I. Behçet disease in the developing world. Int Ophthalmol Clin. 2010;50(2):87-98.
15. Yesudian PD, Edirisinghe DN, O'Mahony C. Behçet's disease. Int J STD AIDS. 2007;18(4):221-7.
16. Kim DK, Chang SN, Bang D, Lee , et al. Clinical analysis of 40 cases of childhood-onset Behçet's disease. Pediatr Dermatol. 1994;11(2):95-101.
17. Sungur G, Hazirolan D, Hekimoglu E, , et al. Late-onset Behçet's disease: demographic, clinical, and ocular features. Graefes Arch Clin Exp Ophthalmol. 2010; 248(9):1325-30.
18. Fietta P. Behçet's disease: familial clustering and immunogenetics. Clin Exp Rheumatol. 2005;23(4 Suppl 38):S96-105.
19. Sakane T, Takeno M, Suzuki N, , et al. Behçet's disease. N Engl J Med. 1999;341(17):1284-91.
20. Ohno S, Ohguchi M, Hirose S, , et al. Close association of HLA-Bw51 with Behçet's disease. Arch Ophthalmol. 1982;100(9):1455-8.
21. Kaneko F, Oyama N, Yanagihori H, , et al. The role of streptococcal hypersensitivity in the pathogenesis of Behçet's Disease. Eur J Dermatol. 2008; 18(5):489-98.
22. Wallace GR, Niemczyk E. Genetics in ocular inflammation--basic principles. Ocul Immunol Inflamm. 2011;19(1):10-8.
23. Mizuki N, Meguro A, Ota M, et al. Genome-wide association studies identify IL23R-IL12RB2 and IL10 as Behçet's disease susceptibility loci. Nat Genet. 2010;42(8):703-6.
24. Remmers EF, Cosan F, Kirino Y, et al. Genome-wide association study identifies variants in the MHC class I, IL10, and IL23R-IL12RB2 regions associated with Behçet's disease. Nat Genet. 2010; 42(8):698-702.
25. Lew W, Chang JY, Jung JY, et al. Increased expression of interleukin-23 p19 mRNA in erythema nodosum-like lesions of Behçet's disease. Br J Dermatol 2008;158(3):505-11.
26. Shim J, Lee ES, Park S, , et al. CD4(+) CD25(+) regulatory T cells ameliorate Behçet's disease-like symptoms in a mouse model. Cytotherapy. 2011;13(7):835-47.
27. Lee KH, Chung HS, Kim HS, et al. Human alpha-enolase from endothelial cells as a target antigen of anti-endothelial cell antibody in Behçet's disease. Arthritis Rheum. 2003;48(7):2025-35.
28. Kaneko S, Suzuki N, Yamashita N, et al. Characterization of T cells specific for an epitope of human 60-kD heat shock protein (hsp) in patients with Behçet's disease (BD) in Japan. Clin Exp Immunol. 1997;108(2):204-12.
29. International Study Group for Behçet's Disease. Criteria for diagnosis of Behçet's disease. International Study Group for Behçet's Disease. Lancet. 1990;335(8697):1078-80.
30. Davatchi F, Calamia KT, Schirmer M, et al. International Team for the Revision of the International Criteria for Behçet's Disease, "Evaluation and Revision of the International Study Group Criteria for Behçet's Disease". Boston, Mass, USA: Proceedings of the American College of Rheumatology Meeting; 2007.
31. Sakane T, Suzuki N, Takeno M. Innate and Acquired Immunity in Behçet's Disease, 8th International Congress on Behçet's Disease. Reggio Emilia, Italy, 7-9 October 1998. Program and Abstracts: 56.
32. Coskun B, Saral Y, Gödekmerdan A, et al. Activation markers in Behçet's disease. Skinmed. 2005; 4(5):282-6.
33. Han EC, Cho SB, Ahn KJ, et al. Expression of Proinflammatory Protein S100A12 (EN-RAGE) in Behçet's Disease and Its Association with Disease Activity: A Pilot Study. Ann Dermatol. 2011;23(3):313-20.
34. Oktayoglu P, Mete N, Caglayan M, et al. Elevated serum levels of calprotectin (MRP8/MRP14) in patients with Behçet's disease and its association with disease activity and quality of life. Scand J Clin Lab Invest. 2015;75(2):106-12.
35. Mumcu G, Inanc N, Taze A, , et al. A new Mucocutaneous Activity Index for Behçet's disease. Clin Exp Rheumatol. 2014;32(4 Suppl 84):S80-6.
36. Aktulga E, Altac M, Muftüoglu A, et al. A double blind study of colchicine in Behçet's disease. Haematologica. 1980;65(3):399-402.
37. Calis M, Ates F, Yazici C, Kose K, Kirnap M, Demir M, et al. Adenosine deaminase enzyme levels, their relation with disease activity, and the effect of colchicine on adenosine deaminase levels in patients with Behçet's disease. Rheumatol Int. 2005;25(6):452-6.
38. Markomichelakis N, Delicha E, Masselos S, , et al. Intravitreal infliximab for sight-threatening relapsing uveitis in Behçet disease: a pilot study in 15 patients. Am J Ophthalmol. 2012;154(3):534-41.
39. Keino H, Okada AA, Watanabe T, et al. Decreased ocular inflammatory attacks and background retinal and

disc vascular leakage in patients with Behcet's disease on infliximab therapy. Br J Ophthalmol. 2011;95(9): 1245-50.
40. Hatemi G, Silman A, Bang D, et al. EULAR recommendations for the management of Behçet disease. Ann Rheum Dis. 2008;67(12):1656-62.
41. Deuter CM, Zierhut M, Mohle A, et al. Long-term remission after cessation of interferon-a treatment in patients with severe uveitis due to Behçet's disease. Arthritis Rheum. 2010;62(9):2796-805.
42. Robertson LP, Hickling P. Treatment of recalcitrant orogenital ulceration of Behçet's syndrome with infliximab. Rheumatology (Oxford). 2001;40(4):473-4.
43. Connolly M, Armstrong JS, Buckley DA. Infliximab treatment for severe orogenital ulceration in Behçet's disease. Br J Dermatol. 2005;153(5):1073-5.
44. Almoznino G, Ben-Chetrit E. Infliximab for the treatment of resistant oral ulcers in Behçet's disease: a case report and review of the literature. Clin Exp Rheumatol. 2007;25(4 Suppl 45):S99-102.
45. Estrach C, Mpofu S, Moots RJ. Behçet's syndrome: response to infliximab after failure of etanercept. Rheumatology (Oxford). 2002;41(10):1213-4.
46. Takayama K, Ishikawa S, Enoki T, et al. Successful treatment with infliximab for Behçet disease during pregnancy. Ocul Immunol Inflamm. 2013;21(4):321-3.
47. Perez-Pampin E, Campos-Franco J, Blanco J, et al. Remission induction in a case of refractory Behçet disease with alemtuzumab. J Clin Rheumatol. 2013;19(2):101-3.
48. Mesquida M, Victoria Hernández M, Llorenç V, et al. Behçet disease-associated uveitis successfully treated with golimumab. Ocul Immunol Inflamm. 2013;21(2):160-2.

24 CHAPTER

Miscellaneous Rheumatological Disorders with Skin Manifestations

Savita Yadav, Vishal Gupta

INTRODUCTION

The number of rheumatological disorders is very vast. In this book, the authors have tried to cover the disorders with significant cutaneous manifestations. In this chapter, some miscellaneous group of rheumatological disorders which have some skin involvement and have not been covered elsewhere in the book are presented (Box 1).

AUTOINFLAMMATORY SYNDROMES

Autoinflammatory syndromes (Box 2) are a group of rare disorders of innate immunity characterized by repeated episodes of seemingly unprovoked inflammation. They differ from autoimmune disease as there is lack of high titer autoantibodies and also antigen specific T cells.

The predominant effector cells are the monocytes and the neutrophils rather than the lymphocytes.

Clinically, these may manifest as recurrent fevers, skin lesions, joint pains, and other systemic features during childhood. Many of these disorders have an increased risk of amyloidosis due to chronic inflammation. Laboratory investigations show evidence of chronic inflammation—anemia of chronic disease, neutrophilic leukocytosis, raised C-reactive protein (CRP), and erythrocyte sedimentation rate (ESR). Recently, genetic basis has been identified for many of these diseases and inflammasomes have been brought into focus in their pathogenesis, thus paving the way for newer

---

Box 1: Miscellaneous rheumatological disorders

- Autoinflammatory syndromes: Periodic fever syndromes, PAPA syndrome, SAPHO syndrome, Blau syndrome, Still's disease*
- Gout
- Palisaded and neutrophilic granulomatous dermatitis
- Interstitial granulomatous dermatitis with arthritis
- Relapsing polychondritis
- Multicentric reticulohistiocytosis
- Juvenile hyaline fibromatosis and infantile systemic hyalinosis
- Stiff skin syndrome

*PAPA, pyogenic arthritis, pyoderma gangrenosum, and acne; SAPHO, synovitis, acne, pustulosis, hyperostosis, and osteitis.

Box 2: Autoinflammatory syndromes

- Childhood or adolescence onset
- Positive family history of similar illness
- Recurrent febrile episodes at regular or irregular intervals
- Atypical urticarial rash or other distinctive skin lesions
- Systemic features, e.g., serositis, arthralgias, organomegaly, ocular, or neurologic involvement
- A similar course in all episodes or flares
- Increased risk of amyloidosis due to chronic systemic inflammation
- Anemia of chronic disease, neutrophilic leukocytosis, raised ESR, and CRP (elevated acute phase reactants) on laboratory evaluation
- Better response to IL-1 or TNF-α antagonist than conventional immunosuppressants

ESR, erythrocyte sedimentation rate; CRP, C-reactive protein; IL-1, interleukin 1; TNF-α, tumor necrosis factor alpha.

targeted therapies. Interleukin 1 (IL-1) and tumor necrosis factor alpha (TNF-α) blockers have been found to be more effective than the conventional immunosuppressives in their treatment.[1-3] Some of the autoinflammatory syndromes with prominent skin and joint involvement are briefly described here.

Periodic Fever Syndromes

Some of the autoinflammatory syndromes show a periodicity in the pattern of fever, and are called periodic fever syndromes. Familial Mediterranean fever (FMF) is the prototype periodic fever syndrome (with recurrent febrile episodes lasting 1–3 days) as the key symptom. Other examples of this group are TNF-receptor associated periodic syndrome (TRAPS, fever duration 1–3 weeks), cryopyrin-associated periodic syndrome (CAPS; fever duration can be less than 1 day in familial cold autoinflammatory syndrome, 1–3 days in Muckle-Wells syndrome and daily in neonatal-onset multisystem inflammatory disease or chronic infantile neurologic, cutaneous, and arthritis), and hyperimmunoglobulin D syndrome (HIDS, fever duration 3–7 days).[3]

Erythematous edematous skin lesions (urticarial eruption) are one of the most common and earliest findings in many autoinflammatory syndromes. Urticarial rash is the characteristic cutaneous manifestation of CAPS, while it may also be seen in TRAPS, HIDS, and other autoinflammatory diseases. Though the urticarial rash of autoinflammatory syndrome may be nearly indistinguishable from those seen in urticaria patients, certain features may provide a clue for the suspecting clinician[4] (Table 1).

Other cutaneous manifestations which can provide a clue to the diagnosis include erysipelas-like eruption (in FMF),[5] distal migratory rash on extremities (in TRAPS),[6] and morbilliform eruption (in HIDS). Nonspecific skin lesions may also be present, like purpura, annular erythema, subcutaneous inflammatory nodules, oral, and genital ulcers. Like fever and cutaneous manifestations, systemic features are also episodic, and can include myalgias, serositis, arthritis, acute abdomen, testicular pain and lymphadenopathy.[1-3]

Pyogenic Arthritis, Pyoderma Gangrenosum and Acne Syndrome

Pyogenic arthritis, pyoderma gangrenosum, and acne syndrome (PAPA syndrome) shows autosomal dominant inheritance. Genetic defect lies in *PSTPIP1* (proline-serine-threonine phosphatase interacting protein 1), also known as *CD2BP1*, which causes increased binding of the pyrin protein to the pyrin domain of *NLRP*, leading to inflammasome activation.[7]

Clinical Features

It is the triad of pyoderma gangrenosum, acne vulgaris, and pyogenic arthritis. Pyoderma

Table 1: Distinguishing features between the urticarial rash of urticaria and autoinflammatory syndromes	
Urticarial rash in urticaria patients	**Urticarial rash in autoinflammatory syndromes**
Monomorphic urticarial lesions	Polymorphic lesions erythematous patches, purpuric lesions, and nodules in addition to the classic urticarial papules
Wheal-and-flare appearance of lesions	No flare surrounding the wheals
Angioedema may be associated	No associated angioedema
Severely itchy lesions	Largely asymptomatic, minimally itchy, or have a burning sensation
Lasts for few minutes to hours	Lasts for hours up to 24 hours
Asymmetrical distribution of lesions	Symmetrical distribution of lesions
Can affect any body site	Usually on the trunk and extremities, with relative sparing of face
Usually respond to antihistaminics	Poor response to antihistaminics
Skin biopsy shows dermal edema and perivascular eosinophilic infiltrates	Skin biopsy shows neutrophilic (or sometimes nonspecific) infiltrate, without significant dermal edema

gangrenosum and arthritis (painful, recurrent, and sterile monoarticular arthritis with prominent neutrophilic infiltrate commonly affecting the knees, elbows, and ankles) typically present in early childhood, whereas severe nodulocystic acne often begins during puberty.[8] Other dermatologic manifestations described are hidradenitis suppurativa, rosacea, and psoriasis.

Treatment

The most consistent response has been seen with the use of TNF-α antagonists like infliximab and etanercept. Response to anakinra is variable, but seems to be more effective in the management of joint manifestations rather than cutaneous disease. Topical and systemic retinoids have been effective in combination with biological agents for the management of cystic acne. Control of inflammation can sometimes be achieved with prednisone.[9]

Synovitis, Acne, Pustulosis, Hyperostosis and Osteitis Syndrome

Synovitis, acne, pustulosis, hyperostosis and osteitis syndrome (SAPHO syndrome) is characterized by pustular skin lesions and osteoarticular manifestations. The usual age of onset is in childhood. The genetic basis of SAPHO is still unknown.

Clinical Features

Palmoplantar pustulosis is the most common cutaneous finding, affecting up to 60% of patients, followed by acne conglobata, acne fulminans (in approximately 25% patients), and hidradenitis suppurativa.[10,11] Rarely, pyoderma gangrenosum and Sweet's syndrome may occur. Osteoarticular manifestations are the hallmark of SAPHO syndrome, and occur regardless of the presence of dermatologic manifestations.[12] Osteitis (sterile inflammation of cortical bone) manifests as bone pain and commonly affects the anterior chest wall, followed by the spine, particularly the thoracic spine. Sacroileitis may also occur, and mandibular lesions can be seen in up to 10% of adults. Hyperostosis manifests as enlargement of the bony ends, most commonly affecting the sternoclavicular joint. Synovitis distant from sites of bony involvement is seen in up to 30% of adults but is rarely noted in children.

Treatment

Nonsteroidal anti-inflammatory drugs (NSAIDs) and intra-articular corticosteroids have been useful in the management of joint inflammation. Systemic corticosteroids in combination with disease-modifying antirheumatic drugs (DMARDs) such as methotrexate and azathioprine have been used with some benefit for the management of bony and cutaneous disease. Anti-TNF-α agents, including etanercept, adalimumab, and infliximab, have shown promise in the management of bone disease in SAPHO syndrome, with generally rapid improvement in bone pain as early as after the first treatment.[9]

Blau Syndrome

Blau syndrome is an autosomal dominant granulomatous disorder characterized by the triad of cutaneous lesions, symmetric polyarthritis, and ocular manifestations (Fig. 1). Blau syndrome and early-onset sarcoidosis are thought to be the same condition, with the differentiating factor being that Blau is the familial manifestation and early-onset sarcoidosis is the sporadic manifestation of the disease. Mutations in *NOD2/CARD15* gene are implicated.[13]

Clinical Features

Most patients present before 4–5 years of age, usually with arthritis and skin manifestations, and later with ocular manifestations, usually between 7 and 12 years of age. Skin lesions appear as nonpruritic, generalized, and pinpoint erythematous papules that can become confluent. There is symmetric polyarthritis of the hands and feet with boggy joint swelling, erythema, warmth, and tenderness. Flexion contractures of the fingers and toes, known as camptodactyly, and decreased motion of large joints may develop in later stages. Ocular manifestations include uveitis, iritis, vitritis, and closed-angle glaucoma.[14,15]

Diagnosis

Skin biopsy reveals noncaseating granulomas. The definitive diagnosis of Blau is made with evidence of mutation in the *NOD2* gene.[14,15]

Miscellaneous Rheumatological Disorders with Skin Manifestations

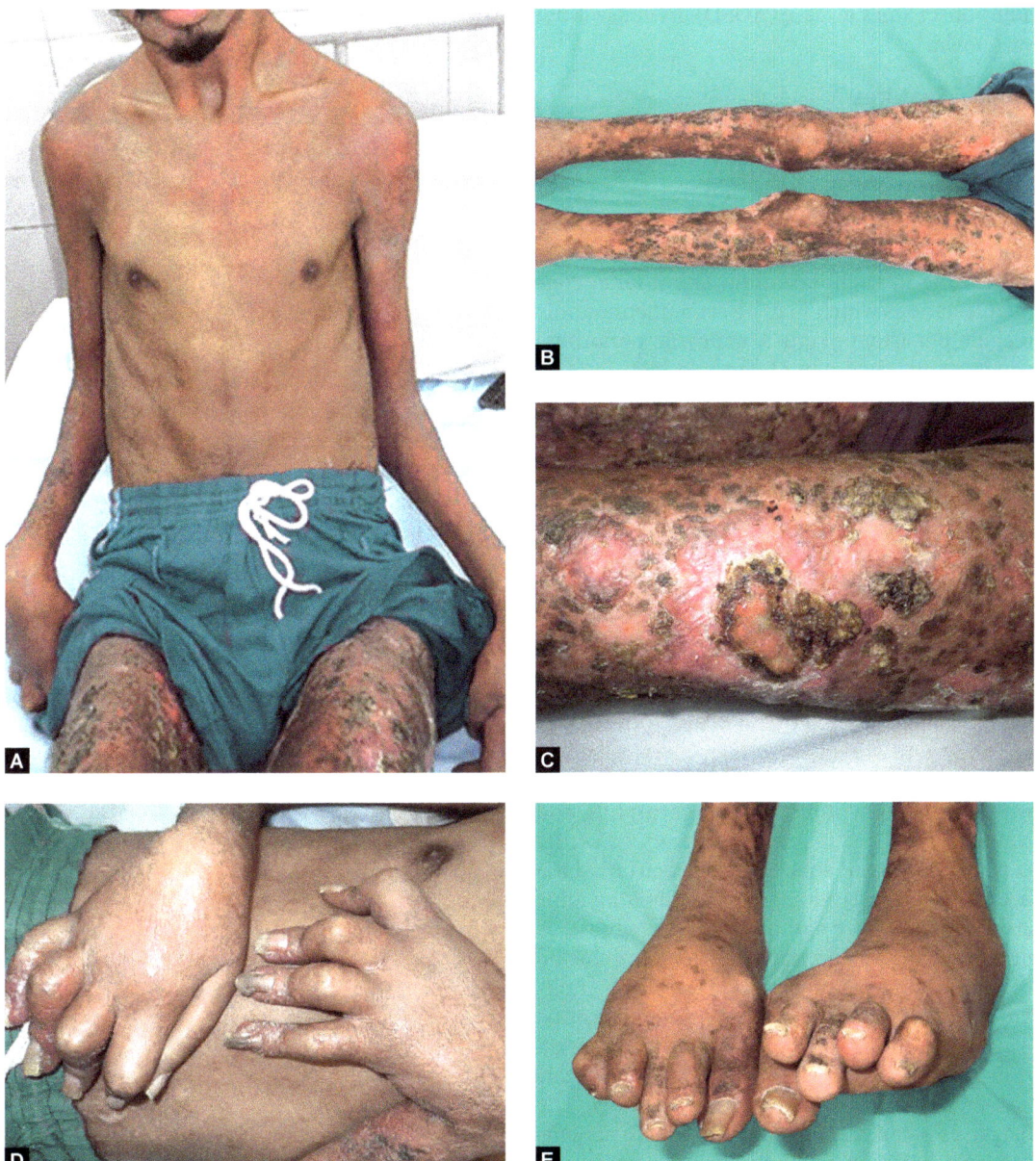

FIGURE 1: Young male with granulomatous dermatitis of the skin, arthritis since infancy and uveitis fit clinically into spectrum of Blau syndrome (genetic analysis could not be done).

Treatment

Response to targeted anti-IL-1 therapy is inconsistent. Infliximab and thalidomide have been used with moderate success, whereas treatment with prednisone may be necessary to control ocular inflammation. Surgical intervention is an option for advanced glaucoma.

Still's Disease

Still's disease, also known as systemic-onset juvenile idiopathic arthritis, is now considered to be an autoinflammatory syndrome and is characterized by daily spiky fever, polyarthritis, evanescent skin rash, and other systemic manifestations. Its adult counterpart is known as adult-onset Still's disease (AOSD). Its cause is not yet known.

Clinical Features

Skin lesions are classically described as evanescent nonpruritic erythematous macules and papules affecting the trunk and proximal extremities, commonly the waist and axillae, and often coincide with febrile episodes. The lesions can be linear, due to koebnerization. Other cutaneous manifestations which may be seen uncommonly include persistent plaques, urticaria, periorbital edema and rheumatoid nodule-like lesions. Spiky fever (≥39°C, quotidian) is seen in almost all the patients, usually manifesting in the afternoon or early evening. The arthritis is symmetric polyarthritis affecting the knees, ankles, hips, and small joints of hands. Systemic manifestations include myalgias, weight loss, serositis (pleuritis, pericarditis, etc.), generalized lymphadenopathy, and hepatosplenomegaly.[16-18]

Diagnosis

Complete blood count shows leukocytosis, anemia, elevated ESR, and CRP. Antinuclear antibody and rheumatoid factor are negative. Skin biopsy shows superficial dermal edema with perivascular infiltrate of neutrophils and lymphocytes.[19] A systemic inflammatory disorder is often considered a part of the spectrum of the better-known systemic-onset juvenile idiopathic arthritis, with later age onset. The diagnosis is primarily clinical and necessitates the exclusion of a wide range of mimicking disorders. Adult-onset Still's disease is a heterogeneous entity, usually presenting with high fever, arthralgia, skin rash, lymphadenopathy and hepatosplenomegaly accompanied by systemic manifestations. The diagnosis is clinical and empirical, where patients are required to meet inclusion and exclusion criteria with negative immunoserological results. There are no clear-cut diagnostic radiological or laboratory signs. Complications of AOSD include transient pulmonary hypertension, macrophage activation syndrome, diffuse alveolar hemorrhage, thrombotic thrombocytopenic purpura, and amyloidosis. Common laboratory abnormalities include neutrophilic leukocytosis, abnormal liver function tests, and elevated acute-phase reactants (ESR, CRP and ferritin).

Treatment

Nonsteroidal anti-inflammatory drug may be used for mild attacks, however, majority patients require systemic corticosteroids and DMARDs (methotrexate, cyclosporine, and azathioprine) to control systemic disease activity. Tumor necrosis factor-α blockers and anakinra are also associated with good results.[19]

GOUT

Gout, a common crystal-induced arthropathy, is a metabolic disorder characterized by deposition of monosodium urate crystals in the soft tissue, caused by the precipitation of urate crystals from supersaturated body fluids (Box 3).

Clinical Features

The arthritis of gout is usually monoarticular. The most common joint to be affected is the first metatarsophalangeal joint (podagra), which becomes red, swollen, and painful. Other joints are less commonly involved, and include knee, ankle, elbows, wrists, and hands (Fig. 2). Urate crystals deposited in the skin and soft tissue, known as "tophi," are usually seen in patients with chronic gout (usually appear on an average of 10 years after the development of gout). However, there are reports of tophus as the first presenting sign of gout.[20] Clinically, tophi manifest as skin-colored to yellowish firm dermal papules or subcutaneous nodules with a smooth or lobulated surface. Sometimes, they may ulcerate with discharge of chalky material. The common sites are skin around joints, ear helix, olecranon, bursa and tragus. Intradermal urate deposits presenting as multiple tiny papules on an erythematous base have been called "miliarial" gout.[21]

Box 3: Gout

- Monoarticular arthritis, usually of the first metatarsophalangeal joints
- Urate crystal deposits in skin known as "tophus," common in periarticular skin, ear helix, olecranon bursa, and tragus
- Synovial aspirates show sodium urate crystals; needle-shaped clefts surrounded by palisaded granulomas characterize the histology of tophus

Miscellaneous Rheumatological Disorders with Skin Manifestations

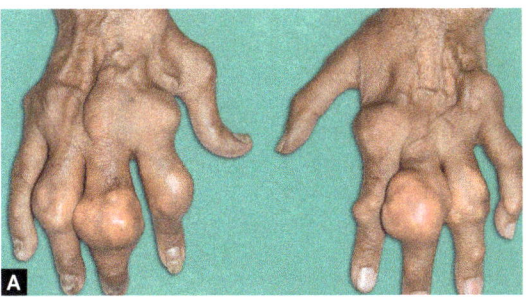
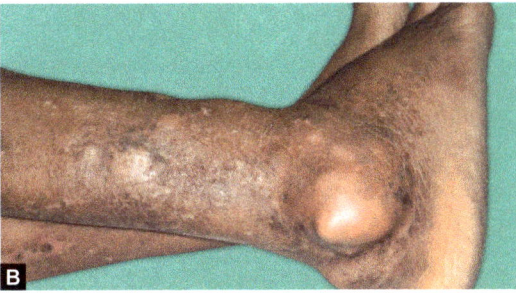

FIGURE 2: Gouty tophi present over small joints of hand and ankle.

Diagnosis

The diagnosis relies on the typical clinical features, supported by demonstration of monosodium urate crystals in the synovial aspirate. Histological examination of the tophus shows deposition of amorphous material containing needle-shaped clefts, surrounded by a palisade of histiocytes, lymphocytes, and multinucleated giant cells. Serum uric acid level may be within the normal range.[22]

Treatment

Nonsteroidal anti-inflammatory drug, colchicine, and sometimes systemic corticosteroids are needed to treat the acute attacks. Xanthine oxidase inhibitors like allopurinol and febuxostat are used in the long-term therapy of gout. Tophi may also reduce in size with treatment.[23,24]

PALISADED AND NEUTROPHILIC GRANULOMATOUS DERMATITIS

Palisaded and neutrophilic granulomatous dermatitis (PNGD) is an uncommon dermatosis which may be seen in patients with autoimmune connective tissue diseases (Box 4). It is referred with other names as well—rheumatoid papules and Churg-Strauss granuloma. The most commonly described associations are rheumatoid arthritis, systemic lupus erythematosus, and Wegener's granulomatosis.

Clinical Features

The skin lesions appear as largely asymptomatic skin-colored to erythematous papules; symmetrically distributed on the extensors of extremities, typically the periarticular locations (Fig. 3). Elbows and fingers are the common sites. The skin lesions may have central umbilication or crust, sometimes there may be ulceration.[25,26] The appearance of the skin lesions may coincide with worsening of the underlying systemic disease.[25]

> **Box 4: Palisaded and neutrophilic granulomatous dermatitis**
> - Usually seen in the setting of a connective tissue disease like rheumatoid arthritis, systemic lupus erythematosus, and Wegener's granulomatosis
> - Periarticular skin-colored to erythematous papules on the extensors of extremities
> - Histology shows palisading of histiocytes around altered collagen, along with neutrophils and fibrinoid deposition on the vessel walls

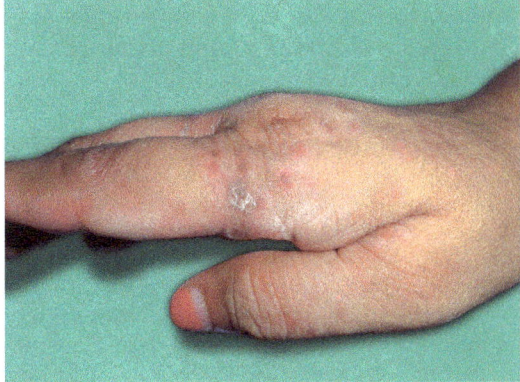

FIGURE 3: Palisaded and neutrophilic granulomatous dermatitis lesions over the extremities.

Diagnosis

Skin biopsy from a fully developed lesion shows a palisade (the term "palisade" refers to a pattern of arrangement of histiocytes where the histiocytes lie surrounding a central focus, with their long axis parallel to each other) of histiocytes around central degenerated basophilic (altered) collagen. There are neutrophils and leukocytoclasia within the infiltrate. Fibrinoid deposition on the vessel walls is usually seen, while frank changes of leukocytoclastic vasculitis may be seen during the early stage of the lesion.[26] Once the diagnosis of PNGD has been established, a search for an underlying connective tissue disease should be made.

Treatment

It usually has a self-limited course and does not require specific therapy. Improvement in skin lesions has been reported with topical and intralesional corticosteroids, dapsone, and hydroxychloroquine sulfate.

INTERSTITIAL GRANULOMATOUS DERMATITIS WITH ARTHRITIS (ACKERMAN'S SYNDROME)

The term "interstitial granulomatous dermatitis (IGD) with arthritis" was first coined by Ackerman in 1993[27] and is considered by many to belong to the same spectrum as PNGD; noninfectious granulomatous dermatitis occurring in the setting of a connective tissue disease (Box 5). The common associations of IGD include rheumatoid arthritis, systemic lupus erythematosus, and autoimmune thyroiditis.[28-30]

> **Box 5: Interstitial granulomatous dermatitis with arthritis**
> - Erythematous-violaceous papules, nodules, annular plaques; linear subcutaneous cord-like structure extending from the axilla to flank
> - Considered by many to be in the same spectrum as palisaded and neutrophilic granulomatous dermatitis, due to similar histopathology and clinical setting

Clinical Features

The skin lesions are characterized by erythematous-to-violaceous papules, nodules, or annular plaques present symmetrically over the trunk, buttocks, and thighs. A linear subcutaneous cord extending from the axilla to the flank, the so-called "rope sign," is the hallmark cutaneous finding.[27]

Diagnosis

The histology of the skin lesions is characterized by interstitial as well as palisading granulomas, which is often "bottom-heavy." "Rosette" of palisading granulomas around fragmented collagen is quite characteristic of IGD. Like in PNGD, neutrophils may be present; however, features of vasculitis are usually not seen.[31]

Treatment

In the absence of a standard treatment, various therapeutic modalities have been tried with variable success, including NSAIDs, topical corticosteroids, systemic corticosteroids, and TNF-α blockers.

RELAPSING POLYCHONDRITIS

Relapsing polychondritis (Box 6) is a rare autoimmune disease affecting a variety of cartilaginous structures. The most characteristic manifestation is the episodic inflammation of the ear and nose cartilage, however, it may lead to progressive multiorgan damage. It may be associated with another autoimmune disorder or a myelodysplastic syndrome. The peak age of onset is in the fifth decade of life, though both extremes of age may be affected.[32] Females may be more commonly affected than males.[33]

> **Box 6: Relapsing polychondritis**
> - Multisystem autoimmune disease characterized by episodic inflammation of ear and nose cartilage
> - Joints, larynx, bronchi, eyes, and other internal organs can be affected as a part of systemic involvement
> - Can be associated with other autoimmune diseases or myelodysplastic syndromes

Clinical Features

The most common clinical feature is the inflammation of the pinna (only the cartilaginous portion of the external ear is involved and the ear lobe, which lacks cartilage, is spared) manifesting as redness, swelling, and pain (Fig. 4) affecting the pinna (in about 90% cases). The repeated episodes of inflammation may lead to destruction of cartilage, and the ear may lose its shape and may appear soft, flabby, or like a cauliflower (Fig. 5).[32,34] Episodes of external ear inflammation may be accompanied by hearing impairment and symptoms of vestibular dysfunction. The second most common symptom is arthralgia (seen in about 80%), which may or may not be accompanied by arthritis. The arthritis is usually nonerosive and episodic. Though any joint can be involved, usually the metacarpophalangeal, interphalangeal, and knee joints are affected.[34,35] Inflammation of the nasal cartilage presents as pain, rhinorrhea, stuffiness, or epistaxis. Repeated attacks may give rise to the characteristic "saddle-nose deformity" (Fig. 6). Respiratory tract involvement can extend from the larynx to bronchi and is potentially fatal. It can manifest as cough, dyspnea, wheezing, stridor, or tenderness over the thyroid cartilage or trachea. Complications can include upper airway collapse, strictures, and secondary pulmonary infections. Eye manifestations include scleritis, episcleritis, conjunctivitis, and corneal ulcers. A variety of nonspecific cutaneous lesions are known to occur

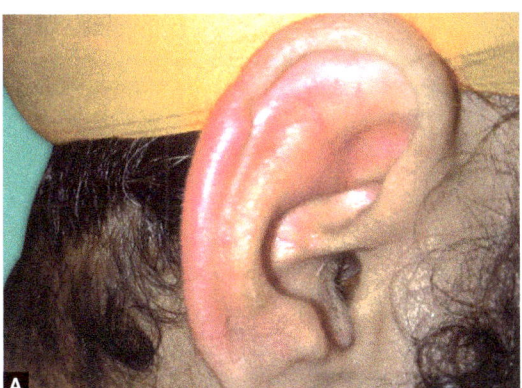 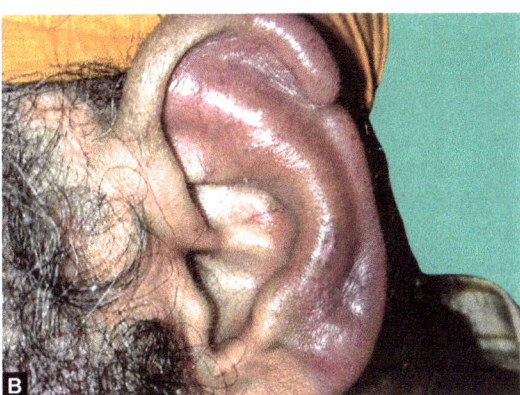

FIGURE 4: Redness, swelling of ear pinna in a relapsing polychondritis patient.

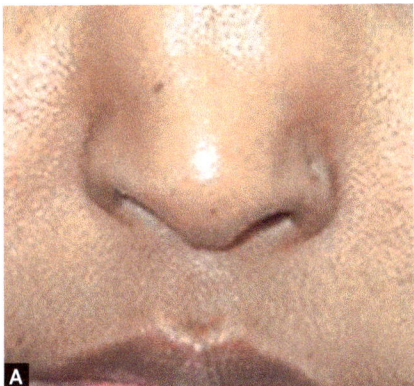 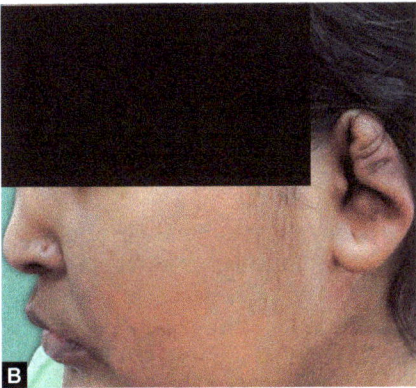

FIGURE 5: Recurrent attacks of cartilage inflammation resulted in significant destruction of auricular cartilage in a relapsing polychondritis patient.

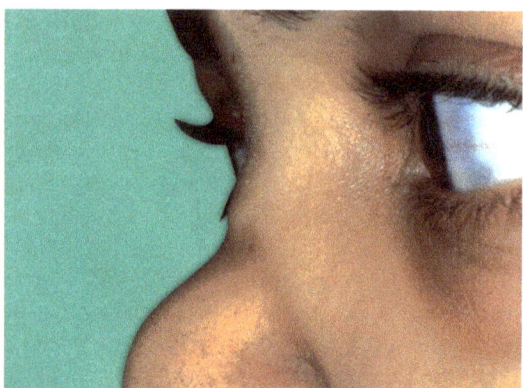

FIGURE 6: Relapsing polychondritis leading to saddle nose deformity.

during the course of relapsing polychondritis, probably as the cutaneous manifestation of the associated autoimmune disease. These include erythema nodosum, erythema multiforme, purpura, and livedo reticularis.[36] Mouth and genital ulcers, inflamed cartilage (MAGIC) syndrome has oral and genital aphthae as well, and may represent an overlap between relapsing polychondritis and Behçet's syndrome.[37] Systemic features can include valvular heart disease, renal dysfunction, and cranial nerve palsies and aseptic meningitis.[32-35]

Diagnosis

Diagnosis relies primarily on the clinical findings.[38] Biopsy of the affected cartilage may show breakdown of the normal lacunar structure of the cartilage, with neutrophilic (early stage) or lymphocytic (late stage) infiltration.[39] Autoantibodies against collagen-II may be found in about half of the patients.[40]

Treatment

Treatment options vary depending upon the severity of disease. Auricular or nasal chondritis and arthralgias may be treated with NSAIDs, colchicine or dapsone. More severe or visceral organ disease requires systemic steroids and other immunosuppressants, like azathioprine, methotrexate, cyclophosphamide, and biologics like TNF-α blockers.[32-34,41]

MULTICENTRIC RETICULOHISTIOCYTOSIS

Multicentric reticulohistiocytosis (MCRH) is a rare multisystemic non-langerhans cell histiocytosis, and is characterized by skin lesions and deforming arthritis (Box 7). Adults are usually affected, and there may be an increased risk of solid-organ malignancies in about one third of the patients.

Clinical Features

Skin lesions appear as skin-colored to red-brown firm papules present over the periarticular sites, usually over the hand joints (Fig. 7) and elbows. The lesions are arranged in a characteristic "coral bead" pattern on the proximal nail folds. Head and neck involvement is quite common, and may be severe enough to give rise to "leonine facies"

Box 7: Multicentric reticulohistiocytosis
- Self-limiting non-Langerhans cell histiocytosis
- Firm skin-colored to red-brown papules over the periarticular sites and head and neck region, characteristic "coral beading" on proximal nail folds
- Symmetric erosive arthritis affecting the small joints of hands, wrists, and knees
- Increased risk of solid-organ malignancies in about one third of the patients
- Skin biopsy shows dermal infiltrate of lymphocytes, histiocytes, and multinucleated giant cells having abundant eosinophilic homogenous "ground-glass" cytoplasm

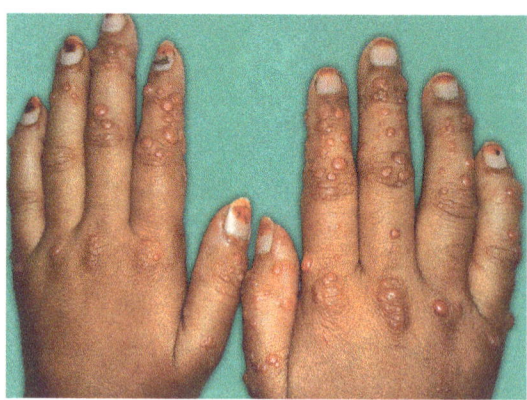

FIGURE 7: Multicentric reticulohistiocytosis lesions over hand.

Miscellaneous Rheumatological Disorders with Skin Manifestations

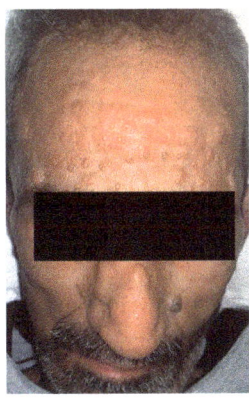

FIGURE 8: Multicentric reticulohistiocytosis lesions over face.

appearance (Fig. 8).[42] There is symmetric erosive arthritis affecting the small joints of hands, as well as the wrists and knees. "Arthritis mutilans" may be seen in about 45% cases.[43] Though joint disease is self-limited and usually "burns out" in 5–10 years, the patients are often left with significant residual disability.

Diagnosis

Skin biopsy shows characteristic changes, which include a dermal infiltrate of lymphocytes, histiocytes, and multinucleated giant cells having abundant eosinophilic homogenous "ground-glass" cytoplasm. Histiocytes stain positively for CD68 and are negative for S-100 and CD-1a.[44]

Treatment

Variable improvement has been seen with a variety of systemic agents including steroids, methotrexate, azathioprine, cyclophosphamide, chlorambucil, bisphosphonates, and TNF-α antagonists.

JUVENILE HYALINE FIBROMATOSIS AND INFANTILE SYSTEMIC HYALINOSIS

Juvenile hyaline fibromatosis and infantile systemic hyalinosis (ISH) (Box 8) are rare autosomal recessive genodermatosis which are characterized by deposition of hyaline material in the skin and internal organs. Juvenile hyaline fibromatosis and ISH share many overlapping features, and are considered to be in the same

> **Box 8: Juvenile hyaline fibromatosis or infantile systemic hyalinosis**
>
> - Autosomal recessive genodermatosis due to mutation in capillary morphogenesis protein-2
> - Onset in infancy or early childhood
> - Firm, pearly translucent papules and nodules on the head and neck, with a predilection for periorificial sites, and hands
> - Osteolytic bone lesions, flexion contractures of large joints
> - Infantile systemic hyalinosis has, in addition, diffusely thickened skin and systemic involvement

clinical continuum. The genetic mutation in both the disorders has been identified in the gene coding for capillary morphogenesis protein-2, a cell-surface receptor which binds to laminin and collagen IV, and plays a role in cell-cell and cell-matrix adhesions.[45]

Clinical Features

Onset is usually in infancy or early childhood. The cutaneous hallmark findings are the firm pearly, translucent papules, and subcutaneous nodules on the head and neck region, and the hands. The skin lesions have a predilection for periorificial sites, viz., around nose, mouth and ears. Gingival hyperplasia may also be seen. The osteoarticular manifestations include osteolytic bone lesions and disabling flexion contractures of the large joints.[46] Of the two diseases, ISH is more severe and is characterized by diffusely thickened skin, in addition to the hyaline papulonodular lesions, internal organ involvement, recurrent infections, intractable diarrhea, and reduced life-span.[47]

Diagnosis

Histological examination of the skin lesion shows an increased number of fibroblasts in a hyalinized periodic acid-Schiff positive connective tissue stroma occupying the dermis and subcutaneous tissue.[48]

Treatment

There is no effective therapy, and the treatment is directed towards improving the aesthetic appearance and minimizing the orthopedic

STIFF SKIN SYNDROME (CONGENITAL FASCIAL DYSTROPHY)

Stiff skin syndrome is a rare disorder characterized by stony-hard skin, mild hypertrichosis, and reduced joint mobility (Box 9). The genetic defect and mode of inheritance are not yet clearly established.

Clinical Features

The clinical manifestations appear during infancy or early childhood. Cutaneous features include rock-hard indurated skin on the buttocks and thighs, bound tightly down to the underlying tissue, with characteristic sparing of the inguinal folds. The overlying skin may show mild hyperpigmentation and hypertrichosis. There is flexion contracture of the large joints, especially the hip and knee joints. This leads to scoliosis, short stature, and narrow thorax. There is no internal organ involvement and life span is not adversely affected.[49]

Diagnosis

Histological examination of the affected skin shows fascial sclerosis without an inflammatory infiltrate. Giant "amianthoid-like" collagen fibrils in the fascia have been described as a characteristic finding. The overlying deep dermis may also show hyalinization of the collagen bundles, in some cases.[49]

Treatment

The treatment is largely supportive, and no definitive treatment exists.

> **Box 9: Stiff skin syndrome**
> - Onset in infancy and early childhood
> - Rock hard bound-down skin on buttocks and thighs with overlying hyperpigmentation and hypertrichosis, and characteristic sparing of inguinal folds
> - Flexion contracture of large joints, scoliosis

disability. The skin and gingival lesions can be surgically excised, but can recur. Release of contractures and physiotherapy may help in improving the joint deformities.

CONCLUSION

Apart from diseases which have characteristic pattern of skin lesions and arthritis (such as connective tissue diseases, Behcet's disease, psoriasis etc.), there are several other entities which can have variable cutaneous and joint involvement. Autoinflammatory syndromes are characterized by recurrent joint pains, fever and a variety of skin lesions. Certain skin lesions such as palisaded neutrophilic and granulomatous dermatitis and tophi may sometimes be the first manifestation of an underlying rheumatological disease. These miscellaneous conditions should be kept in mind while dealing with patients presenting with cutaneous and rheumatological manifestations not fitting in with the other more commonly encountered diseases.

REFERENCES

1. Nguyen TV, Cowen EW, Leslie KS. Autoinflammation: From monogenic syndromes to common skin diseases. J Am Acad Dermatol. 2013;68(5):834-53.
2. Tripathi SV, Leslie KS. Autoinflammatory diseases in dermatology: CAPS, TRAPS, HIDS, FMF, Blau, CANDLE. Dermatol Clin. 2013;31(3):387-404.
3. Cush JJ. Autoinflammatory syndromes. Dermatol Clin. 2013;31(3):471-80.
4. Krause K, Grattan CE, Bindslev-Jensen C, et al. How not to miss autoinflammatory diseases masquerading as urticaria. Allergy. 2012;67(12):1465-74.
5. Shohat M, Halpern GJ. Familial Mediterranean fever--a review. Genet Med. 2011;13:487-98.
6. Schmaltz R, Vogt T, Reichrath J. Skin manifestations in tumor necrosis factor receptor-associated periodic syndrome (TRAPS). Dermatoendocrinol. 2010;2(1):26-9.
7. Shoham NG, Centola M, Mansfield E, et al. Pyrin binds the PSTPIP1/CD2BP1 protein, defining familial Mediterranean fever and PAPA syndrome as disorders in the same pathway. Proc Natl Acad Sci U S A. 2003;100(23):13501-6.
8. Lindor NM, Arsenault TM, Solomon H, et al. A new autosomal dominant disorder of pyogenic sterile arthritis, pyoderma gangrenosum, and acne: PAPA syndrome. Mayo Clin Proc. 1997;72(7):611-5.
9. Naik HB, Cowen EW. Autoinflammatory pustular neutrophilic diseases. Dermatol Clin. 2013;31(3):405-25.
10. Ehrenfeld M, Samra Y, Kaplinsky N. Acne conglobata and arthritis: report of a case and review of the literature. Clin Rheumatol. 1986;5(3):407-9.
11. Kahn MF, Khan MA. The SAPHO syndrome. Baillières Clin Rheumatol. 1994;8(2):333-62.
12. Chamot AM, Benhamou CL, Kahn MF, et al. Acne-pustulosis-hyperostosis-osteitis syndrome. Results of a national survey. 85 cases. Rev Rhum Mal Ostéoartic. 1987;54(3):187-96.

13. Miceli-Richard C, Lesage S, Rybojad M, et al. CARD15 mutations in Blau syndrome. Nat Genet. 2001;29(1):19-20.
14. Alonso D, Elgart GW, Schachner LA. Blau syndrome: A new kindred. J Am Acad Dermatol. 2003;49(2):299-302.
15. Schaffer JV, Chandra P, Keegan BR, Heller P, Shin HT. Widespread granulomatous dermatitis of infancy: An early sign of Blau syndrome. Arch Dermatol. 2007;143(3):386-91.
16. Cush JJ. Adult-onset Still's disease. Bull Rheum Dis. 2000;49(6):1-4.
17. Prendiville JS, Tucker LB, Cabral DA, Crawford RI. A pruritic linear urticarial rash, fever, and systemic inflammatory disease in five adolescents: Adult-onset still disease or systemic juvenile idiopathic arthritis sine arthritis? Pediatr Dermatol. 2004;21(5):580-8.
18. Yamaguchi M, Ohta A, Tsunematsu T, et al. Preliminary criteria for classification of adult Still's disease. J Rheumatol. 1992;19(3):424-30.
19. Kadavath S, Efthimiou P. Adult-onset Still's disease-pathogenesis, clinical manifestations, and new treatment options. Ann Med. 2015;47(1):6-14.
20. Thissen CA, Frank J, Lucker GP. Tophi as first clinical sign of gout. Int J Dermatol. 2008;47 Suppl 1:49-51.
21. Shukla R, Vender RB, Alhabeeb A, et al. Miliarial gout (a new entity). J Cutan Med Surg. 2007;11(1):31-4.
22. Schlesinger N. Diagnosing and treating gout: A review to aid primary care physicians. Postgrad Med. 2010;122(2):157-61.
23. Terkeltaub R. Update on gout: New therapeutic strategies and options. Nat Rev Rheumatol. 2010;6(1):30-8.
24. Perez-Ruiz F, Calabozo M, Pijoan JI, et al. Effect of urate-lowering therapy on the velocity of size reduction of tophi in chronic gout. Arthritis Rheum. 2002;47(4):356-60.
25. Bremner R, Simpson E, White CR, et al. Palisaded neutrophilic and granulomatous dermatitis: An unusual cutaneous manifestation of immune-mediated disorders. Semin Arthritis Rheum. 2004;34(3):610-6.
26. Chu P, Connolly MK, LeBoit PE. The histopathologic spectrum of palisaded neutrophilic and granulomatous dermatitis in patients with collagen vascular disease. Arch Dermatol. 1994;130(10):1278-83.
27. Ackerman AB, Guo Y, Vitale P, et al. Clues to Diagnosis in Dermopathology. Chicago, IL: ASCP Press; 1993. pp. 309-12.
28. Antunes J, Pacheco D, Travassos AR, et al. Autoimmune thyroiditis presenting as interstitial granulomatous dermatitis. An Bras Dermatol. 2012;87(5):748-51.
29. Hu S, Cohen D, Murphy G, et al. Interstitial granulomatous dermatitis in a patient with rheumatoid arthritis on etanercept. Cutis. 2008;81(4):336-8.
30. García-Rabasco A, Esteve-Martínez A, Zaragoza-Ninet V, et al. Interstitial granulomatous dermatitis in a patient with lupus erythematosus. Am J Dermatopathol. 2011;33(8):871-2.
31. Crowson AN, Magro C. Interstitial granulomatous dermatitis with arthritis. Hum Pathol. 2004;35:779-80.
32. Sharma A, Gnanapandithan K, Sharma K, et al. Relapsing polychondritis: A review. Clin Rheumatol. 2013; 32(11):1575-83.
33. Trentham DE, Le CH. Relapsing polychondritis. Ann Intern Med. 1998;129(2):114-22.
34. Letko E, Zafirakis P, Baltatzis S, et al. Relapsing polychondritis: A clinical review. Semin Arthritis Rheum. 2002;31(6):384-95.
35. Zeuner M, Straub RH, Rauh G, et al. Relapsing polychondritis: clinical and immunogenetic analysis of 62 patients. J Rheumatol. 1997;24(1):96-101.
36. Francès C, el Rassi R, Laporte JL, et al. Dermatologic manifestations of relapsing polychondritis. A study of 200 cases at a single center. Medicine (Baltimore). 2001;80(3):173-9.
37. Orme RL, Nordlund JJ, Barich L, et al. The MAGIC syndrome (mouth and genital ulcers with inflamed cartilage). Arch Dermatol. 1990;126(7):940-4.
38. McAdam LP, O'Hanlan MA, Bluestone R, et al. Relapsing polychondritis: Prospective study of 23 patients and a review of the literature. Medicine (Baltimore). 1976; 55(3):193-215.
39. Riccieri V, Spadaro A, Taccari E, et al. A case of relapsing polychondritis: Pathogenetic considerations. Clin Exp Rheumatol. 1988;6(1):95-6.
40. Foidart JM, Abe S, Martin GR, et al. Antibodies to type II collagen in relapsing polychondritis. N Engl J Med. 1978;299(22):1203-7.
41. Kemta Lekpa F, Kraus VB, Chevalier X. Biologics in relapsing polychondritis: a literature review. Semin Arthritis Rheum. 2012;41(5):712-9.
42. Tajirian AL, Malik MK, Robinson-Bostom L, et al. Multicentric reticulohistiocytosis. Clin Dermatol. 2006;24(6):486-92.
43. Gorman JD, Danning C, Schumacher HR, et al. Multicentric reticulohistiocytosis: Case report with immunohistochemical analysis and literature review. Arthritis Rheum. 2000;43(4):930-8.
44. Barrow MV, Holubar K. Multicentric reticulohistiocytosis. A review of 33 patients. Medicine (Baltimore). 1969;48(4):287-305.
45. Dowling O, Difeo A, Ramirez MC, et al. Mutations in capillary morphogenesis gene-2 result in the allelic disorders juvenile hyaline fibromatosis and infantile systemic hyalinosis. Am J Hum Genet. 2003;73(4):957-66.
46. Malathi BG, Prabha CV, Padma SR, et al. Juvenile hyaline fibromatosis: A rare case report. Indian J Pathol Microbiol. 2006;49(2):257-9.
47. Giri PP, Raushan R, Ghosh A, et al. Infantile systemic hyalinosis. Indian Pediatr. 2012;49(1):62-4.
48. Gupta LK, Singhi MK, Bansal M, et al. Juvenile hyaline fibromatosis in siblings. Indian J Dermatol Venereol Leprol. 2005;71(2):115-8.
49. Liu T, McCalmont TH, Frieden IJ, et al. The stiff skin syndrome: Case series, differential diagnosis of the stiff skin phenotype, and review of the literature. Arch Dermatol. 2008;144(10):1351-9.

Appendix 1

6-minute walk test report of a systemic sclerosis patient presenting with dyspnea

DEPARTMENT OF MEDICINE
ALL INDIA INSTITUTE OF MEDICAL SCIENCES, NEW DELHI-110029
MEDICINE OPD, ROOM NO-30

Name: Age/Sex: 30 years/Female   UHID:

Date: Height (cm): 160 cm   Weight (kg): 58 kg

BMI (kg/m^2): 22.7 kg/m^2

6-MIN WALK TEST (6MWT)

	Baseline		3 months		6 months		12 months		18 months	
Total distance walked (m)	110 m		–	–	–	–	–	–	–	–
Time (min)	Walk	Rest	Walk	Rest	Walk	Rest	Walk	Rest	Walk	Rest
	2 min	4 min	–	–	–	–	–	–	–	–
	Pre	Post	Pre	Post	Pre	Post	Pre	Post	Pre	Post
Heart rate	117/min	155/min	–	–	–	–	–	–	–	–
Dyspnea (Borg scale)	1	2	–	–	–	–	–	–	–	–
Fatigue (Borg scale)	1	2	–	–	–	–	–	–	–	–
SatO$_2$ (%)	97	86	–	–	–	–	–	–	–	–

Borg Scale

0.	Nothing at all	6.	
0.5	Very, very slight (just noticeable)	7.	Very severe
1.	Very slight	8.	
2.	Slight (light)	9.	
3.	Moderate	10.	Very, very severe (maximal)
4.	Somewhat severe		
5.	Severe (heavy)		

Remarks: – Patient walked 110 meters
– Took rest for 4 minutes
– Significant tachycardia, desaturation, ↑ dyspnea and ↑ fatigue post exercise
– Repeat after 3 months

Resident, Medicine

INDEX

Page numbers followed by *b* refer to box, *f* refer to figure, *fc* refer to flowchart, and *t* refer to table.

A

Abatacept 228
Abscesses, neutrophilic 217*f*
Acanthosis, regular 217*f*
Achilles tendon 254*f*
Acidosis, renal tubular 21, 155
Ackerman's syndrome 318
Acne
  conglobate 240
  syndrome 240
Acquired immunodeficiency
  syndrome 245
Acral areas, involvement of 118
Acral desquamation 266*f*
Acral distribution, dystrophic
  calcification of 101
Acral purpura 4
Acrocyanosis 190*f*
Acrodermatitis chronica
  atrophicans 140*t*
Acrogeria 140
Acroosteolysis 98*f*
Acrosclerosis 135*t*, 136
Adalimumab 185*t*, 228*t*
Adamantiades 301
Airway disease, small 224
Alarcon-Segovia criteria 135*t*
Alcian blue 144
Alefacept 244
Alopecia areata 128*b*
Aluminum 166*t*
American College of
  Rheumatology 40, 56, 91, 92*t*,
  225, 225*t*, 275
  classification 264
  criteria 152, 153*b*
American European Consensus
  Group Criteria 152*b*
American Systemic Sclerosis
  Immune Suppression versus
  Transplant Trial 108

American Thoracic Society 165
Amyloidosis 224, 304
Amyopathic dermatomyositis,
  clinically 80
Anaphylactoid purpura 143
Anemia 56, 138, 224, 281
  aplastic 240*b*
  autoimmune hemolytic 57
  hemolytic 227*t*
  pernicious 125, 125*b*, 128*b*
Angina 103
Angioimmuno proliferative
  lesions 14
Angiomyxoma 141
Angiotensin converting enzyme
  166*t*, 179
  inhibitors 105, 114, 183
Angular cheilitis 155*f*, 156*f*, 157
Ankle joints, bilateral 105*f*
Annular sarcoidosis
  lesion 171*f*
  plaque 171*f*
Antibiotics 236*t*
Anticardiolipin antibodies 64, 64*b*
Anti-citrullinated peptide
  antibodies 21, 223
Antidepressants, tricyclic 162
Antiepileptics 236*t*
Antigen
  antibodies complexes 296
  presenting cell 168*f*
Antiglomerular basement
  membrane disease 292
Antihistamine 28, 87
Antihistone antibodies 118
Anti-inflammatory agents 218*t*
Antimalarials, oral 48
Antimicrobial agents 185*t*
Antineutrophil cytoplasmic
  antibody 4, 23, 23*f*, 24, 252,
  261*f*, 274, 281, 292

associated vasculitis 267, 267*f*,
  269*f*, 270*b*, 270*fc*, 271, 280*b*,
  282, 282*b*
  cutaneous arteritis of 269*f*
  prevalence of 24*t*
  related vasculitis, drug
    associated 298
Antinuclear antibody 5, 21, 22,
  22*f*, 22*t*, 37, 38, 60, 118
Antiphospholipid 66*fc*
  syndrome 57, 304
Antistreptolysin O titers 235*b*
Anti-thymocyte globulin 108
Antiviral therapies 192
Anxiety 205, 205*b*
Aortitis, granulomatous 224*t*
Apertognathia 100
Aphthous ulcer 303*f*, 304*f*
  oral 303*f*
Appendages, loss of 46*t*
Arteritis, subcutaneous 268
Arthralgia 154, 155, 157, 275
Arthritis 57, 105, 125, 134, 135*t*,
  136*b*, 137, 138, 155, 214, 216,
  245, 312*b*, 315*f*, 318, 318*b*
  asymmetric oligoarticular 214
  distal interphalangeal 197, 197*b*
  early 205
  inflammatory 21, 207
  juvenile idiopathic 21
  mild nonerosive symmetric 78
  mutilans 321
  onset of 214
  reactive 213, 214, 217, 218,
    218*fc*, 218*t*, 219, 220
  seronegative 240, 240*b*
  erosive 245*b*
Aspergillosis 178
Asteroid 177
Atrophic
  leukodermic patches 129

lichen sclerosus et atrophicus
    plaques 129f
  plaque, erythematous 32f
  stage 126
Atrophie blanche 250, 254, 265f
Atrophoderma
  of Pasini 123, 123f
  of Pierini 123, 123f
  vermiculata 35
Atrophy 42f, 171f
  progressive hemifacial 121
  subcutaneous tissue 35f
Autoantibody 20, 81, 91t
  myositis-associated 70t, 82
  tests 153
Autoimmune
  diseases 159, 189
  disorder 55, 125
Autoinflammatory syndromes
    312, 312b, 313, 313t
Autologous stem cell
    transplantation international
    scleroderma 108
Azathioprine 39, 48, 65fc, 86t,
    112, 112t, 162t, 163fc, 185t,
    270fc
Azotemia 56

B

Bacillus calmette-guérin 118
Balanitis xerotica obliterans 17,
    129
Barium swallow 105f
Basal cell
  carcinoma 141
    morpheaform 128, 131
  vacuolization 12f, 15f
Basal keratinocytes 46
Basement membrane 12, 46
Basilar pulmonary fibrosis 91, 92f
B-cell 55
  activating factor 152
  hyperactivity 154
Beau's line 199, 199f
Behçet's disease 38, 245, 301,
    301t, 303f, 304, 305f-308f, 309,
    322
  diagnosis of 304, 307b
  differential diagnosis of 304

etiopathogenesis of 302f
extracutaneous manifestations
    of 306t
Behçet's multiple symptom
    complex 301
Behçet's syndrome 236, 301, 320
Betamethasone 130
  dipropionate 126
Biopsy
  renal 281
  square outline of 16f
  subepithelial endobronchial
    178f
Birmingham vasculitis activity
    score 279
Bisphosphonates 114
Bladder 155
Blaschko's lines 35, 41
Blaschkoid morphea 121f
Blastomycosis 178
Blau syndrome 312, 314
  spectrum of 315f
Bleeding time 5
Bleomycin 118, 140
Blepharitis 160
Blood
  flow, reduction of 250
  vessel
    fibrinoid necrosis of 297f
    inflammation of 252
Bohan and Peter criteria 81b
Bone 224
Bony ankylosis 197, 200f
Borg scale 325
Borrelia afzelii 140
Borrelia burgdorferi 166
Boutonniere deformity 222f
Bowel disease, inflammatory
    143, 205, 236, 240, 304
Bowen's disease 37
Bowen's plaque 38f
Breast 169, 236
  lupus erythematosus
    profundus of 41
British Isles Lupus Assessment
    Group 66
Broken fishnet pattern 7
Bromocriptine 118, 140
Bronchiectasis 181f

Bronchoalveolar lavage 183
Bronchoscopy guided
    transbronchial lung biopsy
    178
Brucellosis 178
Buschke, scleredema of 140
Butterfly rash 11

C

Calcineurin inhibitors 47, 49, 65
  topical 130
Calcinosis 7, 77f, 87, 107
  cutis 9, 10f, 76, 80f, 85, 90, 114
    whitish plaques of 10f
  patchy cutaneous 10f
  severe cutaneous 76f
Calciphylaxis 256
Calcipotriene, topical 126
Calcium 87
  channel blockers 109, 163
Camouflage cream 127
Cancer 236
Capecitabine 28
Capillaroscopy 99f
  nail-fold 9
Caplan's syndrome 224
Carbamazepine 28
Carbidopa 140
Carbimazole 298
Carbon monoxide 10, 112, 183
  diffusion of 176
Carboplatin 140
Carcinoid syndrome 140
Carcinoma 178
  bronchogenic 277f
  en cuirasse 140
  low-grade 40
  ovary 70f
Cardiac magnetic resonance
    imaging 286f
Cardiac tamponade 57
Cardiomyopathy 224
Cardiovascular diseases 205
Cardiovascular system 308
Carpal tunnel syndrome 125
Cataract 182
Cat-scratch disease 178
Celiac disease 245
Cells, inflammatory 83f

Index

Central nervous system 56, 155, 158, 162, 278, 282, 296, 308
  involvement 176
  lupus, management of 66f
  pachymeningitis of 278
  vasculitis 224
Centromere proteins 22
Cerebrospinal fluid 156
Cerebrovascular accident 224
Certolizumab 228
Cervical
  necrotizing lymphadenitis, subacute 246
  spine involvement 223
Chapel Hill Consensus Conference, revised 274
Chemicals 140
Chemokine ligand 207
Chest
  computed tomography 286f
  contrast enhanced computed tomography scan 181f
  radiograph, abnormal 275
  X-ray 235
Chlamydia 213
  pneumoniae 213
  trachomatis 213, 214, 216, 219
Chloroquine 49, 185
Cholesterol embolization 256
Choroid 176
Churg-Strauss disease 18, 178
Churg-Strauss granuloma 245, 317
Churg-Strauss syndrome 24, 252, 282, 283
Cicatricial alopecia 32f, 61f
Cinnarizine 28
Circinate
  balanitis 214, 214f
  vulvitis 215f
Cirrhosis 191
  primary biliary 178, 240
Cisplatin 140
Citrullinated cyclic peptide 225
Clara cell 10 KD protein 166
Clinical disease activity index 230
Clobetasol 130
Clofazimine 244
Clostridium difficile 213, 214
Clotting time 5

Coccidioidomycosis 178
Colchicine 239, 246
Colitis, ulcerative 236, 240, 245
Complete blood count 5, 229
Complex musculoskeletal chronic inflammatory disorders 195
Computed tomography scan 181f, 277f, 278
Conjunctiva 176
Conjunctival injection 266f
Conjunctivitis 205
Connective tissue
  disease 245
  disorders 20
Contact dermatitis 59
Contusion 2
Corticosteroids 49, 64, 85, 208
  injectable 47
  intralesional 239
  systemic 48, 85, 88, 186, 239, 244, 295
  topical 47, 239
Cough 175
Coxsackie B virus 166
Cranial nerve 155, 177
C-reactive protein 20, 216, 225, 230, 278, 304, 312
Creatine phosphokinase, elevated level of 81
Cribriform scarring 241f
Crithidia lucillae 22
Crohn's disease 176, 178, 236, 240, 244
Cryoglobulinemia 21, 24
  idiopathic 188
Cryoglobulinemic vasculitis 188, 192, 193, 292
  classification criteria for 191
  infection-related 192
  pathogenesis of 189
  therapy of 192
Cryoglobulins 24, 191
  subtypes of 25t
Cryopyrin-associated periodic syndrome 313
Cryptococcosis 178
Cushing's syndrome 48
Cutaneous mucinoses, classification of 141b

Cutaneous sarcoidosis 168, 175t
  atrophic lesion of 171f
  psoriasiform
    lesion of 174f
    plaque of 174f
  umblicated lesion of 172f
Cutis marmorata 7
Cyclophosphamide 39, 48, 64, 65, 86, 108, 111, 112, 162, 163, 185, 192, 246, 270, 279
Cyclosporine 39, 48, 86, 207, 244, 246
  topical 160
Cyroglobulins 158
Cyst, mucinous 141
Cystic fibrosis transmembrane regulator 166
Cytarabine 48
Cytokines
  down regulates 127
  modulating drugs 185
Cytomegalovirus 27, 166, 178
Cytopenia 229
Cytotoxic T-lymphocyte-associated protein 4 302

D

Dactylitis 174f, 197, 201, 201f, 205, 216
Danazol 8, 257
Dapsone 48, 236
Darier-Roussy sarcoid 170, 175
Degos' disease 141
Dematomyositis 78t
Deoxyribonucleic acid 55
  antibodies, anti-single-stranded 118
  anti-double stranded 64, 64b
Depigmentation, postinflammatory 50f
Depression 120, 205
Dermatitis
  chronic discoid 37
  granulomatous 315f
  herpetiformis 14, 62
  neutrophilic granulomatous 245b, 317, 317b
  rheumatoid neutrophilic 18
  sclerotic 17
  seborrheic 263

Dermatofibrosarcoma
  protuberans 141
Dermatomyositis 7f, 9, 10f, 14,
  15, 15f, 19, 68, 69, 69f, 70t, 73f,
  75f, 76f, 77t, 81b, 82t-84t, 84,
  86t, 87, 141, 144, 233
  classification of 68, 68t
  complications of 81t
  differential diagnosis of 84t
  disease, cutaneous 85
  Gottron's rash of 59
  juvenile 69, 70, 71f, 74f, 79, 79f,
    80f, 80t
  malignancy-associated 80
  rash, background erythema
    of 70f
  severe 76f
  skin
    lesions of 71t
    severity index 85
    specific subcategories of 79
    worsening 87b
Dermatosis
  inflammatory 245
  neutrophilic 18
  pigmented purpuric 4f
Dermographism 19
Dermopathy, nephrogenic
  fibrosing 141
Dermoscopy 38
Dexamethasone
  cyclophosphamide pulse
    therapy 107
Diabetes mellitus 48, 66, 140,
  240, 245
Diarrhea 227
  bloody 245
Discoid lupus erythematosis 26,
  29, 29f, 31f, 36f-38f, 46, 46t,
  136
  lesions 30f, 31, 31f, 32f, 34f,
    39f, 60
  lichenoid hypertrophic plaque
    of 34f
  pathogenesis of 27fc
  plaque 29f, 34f, 37f
Disease activity score 230
Disease-modifying antirheumatic
  agents 213
  drugs 207, 218, 225, 227t, 314
  conventional 207

Distal extremity swelling 203
Diuretics 159
Diverticulitis 240
Diverticulosis
  esophageal 78
  intestinal 78
Dizziness 48
Docetaxel 28, 140
Donovanosis 178
Doppler echocardiography 177
D-penicillamine 110
Drugs 28, 140
  cytotoxic 185
  reactions 178
  topical 47
  toxicity, prevention of 66
Dyslipidemia 229
Dyspepsia 227
Dyspnea 175
Dystrophic nail, curved 99f

E

Ear lesions 4
Ecchymosis 2
Ecchymotic patches, multiple
  fresh 2f
Echocardiography 177
  two-dimensional 106
Ectropion 35
Eczema 263
Edema
  interstitial 83f
  pitting 203
  prominent periorbital 73f
Efalizumab 28
Ehlers–Danlos syndrome,
  ecchymoses of 5
Electrocardiogram 106, 177
Electromyography 83, 87
  myogenic pattern on 135
Elevated muscle enzymes
  creatine phosphokinase 135
Embolism 255
En coup de sabre 119, 121, 122f,
  125, 127
Endocarditis, subacute bacterial
  245
Endothelial cells 89
Endothelin receptor antagonists
  109

Enfuvirtide 131
Enthesitis 202, 216
Enzyme-linked immunosorbent
  assay 21, 24
Eosinophilia 224, 285
  myalgia syndrome 128, 140
Epidermis 12
Epidermolysis bullosa acquisita
  62
Epididymis 169
Episcleritis 205, 224
Epithelioid cell granuloma 178f
Epstein–Barr virus 166, 246
Erythema 29
  annular 157
  central 30f
  diffuse 147f
  elevatum diutinum 240
  mild 73f
  multiforme 45, 175f
  nail-fold 74f
  nodosum 174, 175f, 224, 233,
    234, 235b, 236, 263, 269f,
    306f
  chronic 235
  lesions, multiple 234f, 263f
  migrans 234
Erythematous macular discoid
  rash, pigmented 63f
Erythrocyte sedimentation rate
  20, 37, 216, 225, 230, 262, 304,
  312
Escherichia coli 213, 302
Esophageal dysfunction 90
Esophageal dysmotility 7, 125,
  135, 136
Esophageal screening 83
Esophagus 305f
  dilation of 135
Etanercept 28, 185, 228, 244
European Group for Blood
  and Bone Marrow
  Transplantation 108
European League Against
  Rheumatism 107, 110, 159,
  225, 295, 308
  Classification criteria for early
    diagnosis of rheumatoid
    arthritis 225t
  criteria 91

Criteria for systemic sclerosis 92*t*
Scleroderma Trials and Research Group 107
Sjögren's Syndrome Disease Activity Index 159, 163
European Vasculitis Study Group 279
Excimer laser 127
Eyelashes, loss of 35
Eyelid
  dermatitis 157
  margins 176
  mucinous carcinoma of 141
Eyes 169, 277
  dry 155*f*, 160
  medial canthus of 73*f*

F

Facial
  erythema 135
  expressions, loss of 94*f*
Fallopian tubes 169
Fanconi's anemia 240
Fascial dystrophy, congenital 322
Fasciitis, eosinophilic 17, 43, 128, 141
Fat lobules, periseptal areas of 235*f*
Fatigue 154
Fatty liver disease, nonalcoholic 205
Felty's syndrome 224
Fever 229, 252, 275
  familial mediterranean 313
  persistent 183
  rheumatic 18
F-fluorodeoxyglucose-positron emission tomography scan 182, 182*f*
Fibrinoid necrosis 177
Fibroblasts 89
Fibromatosis, juvenile hyaline 312, 321, 321*b*
Fibromyalgia syndrome 157, 163
Fibrosis 131, 179, 181*f*
  idiopathic pulmonary 112
  nephrogenic systemic 128
  perineural 269*f*
  pulmonary 135, 205

Fillers 127
Fingers edema 135, 136*f*
Flat epidermis 12*f*
Flexion contractures 99*f*, 100*f*
Fluid, hemorrhagic 237*f*
Fluorouracil 28
Focal granulomatous inflammation 269*f*
Focal mucinosis, cutaneous 141
Follicular
  ostia, dilated 32*f*
  plugging 29, 46
Folliculitis 304
Forced vital capacity 102, 112, 113, 162

G

Gangrene 107, 223*f*, 224
  digits 268*f*
  dry 101*f*
  fingers 95
  toes 95
Garland's sign 179
Gastrointestinal system 137
Gastrointestinal tract 91, 105, 107, 118, 236, 282
  disease of 240
Genetic testing 216
Genitourinary organs, carcinoma of 236
Genome-wide association study 196
Germinal blasts 152
Giant cell
  arteritis 261, 270
  myocarditis 178
Glans penis 129, 214
Glatiramer 131
Glaucoma 182
Glomerular filtration rate, reduced 205
Glomerulonephritis 190, 281
  cryoglobulinemic 190
  mesangioproliferative 191
  necrotizing 224, 280
  pauci-immune 23
Glucocorticoids 279
Glucose-6-phosphate dehydrogenase 229

Glutamic oxaloacetic transaminase 81
Glycosaminoglycans 140, 144
Golimumab 185, 228
Gottron's lesions, periungual lesions 85
Gottron's papules 15, 70, 71*f*, 72*f*, 82, 84, 136
  shiny atrophic 72*f*
Gottron's sign 71, 72*f*, 73*f*, 80*f*
Gout 312, 316, 316*b*
  arthritis of 316
Gouty tophi 317*f*
Graff classification 141
Graft versus host disease 15*f*, 128, 141, 159
Granulocyte colony stimulating factor 108, 236
Granulocytopenia 227
Granuloma
  actinic 178
  annulare 141, 178
  linear 245
  faciale 43
  formation 167
  necrobiotic 245
  palisading 245, 246*f*
  rheumatoid 245
    necrobiotic-palisaded 18
  sarcoidal 173*f*
Granulomatosis 24, 267, 269, 270, 274, 274*b*-277*f*, 278, 278*f*
  eosinophilic 24, 268*f*, 269, 270, 282, 282*b*, 284*f*-286*f*, 292
Granulomatous diseases
  infective 178
  noninfective 178
Granulomatous inflammation 275, 276, 280
Granulomatous reaction 178
Granulomatous rosacea 178
Grave's disease 150
Griseofulvin 28
Groove sign 120
Ground-glass
  appearance 103
  opacification 102
  opacities, multiple patchy 286*f*
Guttate lichen sclerosus et atrophicus 129*f*
Guttate morphea 119, 124

H

Hair
  depigmentation 227
  loss 60
Hallux valgus 222
Hamasaki-Wesenberg inclusion bodies 177
Hammer toes 222
Hand
  dorsum of 59
  X-ray of 172f
Headache 48, 228
Healing, superficial necrotic ulceration 253f
Heart
  disease, ischemic 224
  failure 229
Heat shock proteins 166, 302
Heel enthesopathy 202f
Heerfordt's-Waldenström syndrome 176t
Heliotrope rash 70f, 72, 73f, 79f, 84
  edema of 73f
Hematologic disease 240
Hematologic malignancy 224, 236
Hematologic system 138
Hematopoietic stem cell transplantation 108
Hematuria 5, 280
Hemoglobinemia 240
Hemoglobinuria, paroxysmal nocturnal 240
Hemogram, complete 235
Hemolytic uremic syndrome 245
Hemorrhage 23, 74f
  alveolar 280
  diffuse alveolar 277f
  subungual 199f
Henoch-Schönlein purpura 5, 292, 295, 296, 296f, 297, 297f
Hepatitis 125
  autoimmune 162
  B reactivation 229
  B virus 229, 264
  C 240
    antibodies 189
    virus 159, 166, 188, 229, 236
  chronic active 191, 240, 245

Herpes virus 166
Herpes zoster 59f
  varicella 280
Hidradenitis suppurativa 240
High-resolution computed tomography 102, 104f, 162, 179, 181, 181t
Hilar lymphadenopathy, bilateral 180f
Histocompatibility complex region 196
Histoplasmosis 178
Hodgkin's disease 178, 240
Hodgkin's lymphoma 245
Holster sign 75, 75f
Human herpesvirus-8 246
Human immunodeficiency virus 159, 166, 226, 240
Human leukocyte antigen 27, 135, 167, 167t, 196, 196t, 206, 216, 221, 306
  gene 167
  haplotypes 167t
Human leukocyte elastase 298
Humoral immune system 90
Huriez syndrome 140
Hutchinson Gilford syndrome 140t
Hyaluronidase 143
Hydrocarbons, chlorinated 128, 131
Hydroxychloroquine 49, 64, 86, 160, 163, 185, 227, 246, 257
Hypercalcemia 177
  persistent 183
Hypercalciuria 183
Hypergammaglobulinemic purpura 156f, 157
Hyperhidrosis 9
Hyperimmunoglobulin D syndrome 313
Hyperkeratosis 46
Hyperlipoproteinemias 159
Hyperoxaluria 256
Hyperparathyroidism 143
Hyperpigmentation 29, 39f, 95
  diffuse 95f
  localized 97f
  peripheral 30f
  postinflammatory 63, 63f, 265f
  severe 122f

Hyperplasia
  epidermal 13f
  psoriasiform 15f, 217f
Hypersplenism 176
Hypertension 56, 66, 227
  pulmonary 102, 103
    arterial 106, 107, 112, 134, 136
Hypocomplementemia 190
Hypomobility 105
Hypopigmentation 95
Hypothyroidism 140, 143, 150, 151

I

Imiquimod cream, topical 126
Immune
  complex vasculitis 274
    drug associated 298
  system, cells of 89, 90
Immunofluorescence 38, 46
Immunoglobulin G 188
  intravenous 49, 86, 162, 163, 263
Immunohistochemistry 87
Immunomodulators 28, 48
Immunomodulatory drugs 127
Immunoproliferative disorders 189
Immunosuppressants 48
Immunosuppressive
  agents 218
  therapy 160, 192
Indomethacin 183, 298
Infantile systemic hyalinosis 312, 321, 321b
Infections 236
  chronic 189
  risk of 228
  viral 228
Infectious diseases 253
Inflammation
  granulomatous 178
  markers of 20
  pattern of 11
Inflammatory
  diseases 159
  disorder 128
Infliximab 28, 185, 228, 246, 309

Infusion reaction 228, 229
Insomnia 48
Insulinomas, malignant 143
Interferon gamma 167
Interleukin 167, 207
International Chapel Hill
    Consensus Conference 260,
    260t, 292
International Study Group 303
Interphalangeal joint 98f, 100f,
    200f
Interstitial granulomatous
    dermatitis 18, 245, 312, 318,
    318b
    disease 245
Interstitial lung disease 21, 102,
    102t, 106, 107, 110, 112, 134,
    136, 156, 162, 224
    management of 113t
Iris 176
    synechiae 182
Iritis 205
Irritation 160
Ischemia
    critical digital 107
    visceral 224
Isolated dry eye syndrome 150
Isoniazid 298
Itching 160

J

Jessner's lymphocytic infiltration
    11, 43
Joint 199, 223
    aspiration 217
    assessment of 199
    contractures 105
    cricoarytenoid 223
    damage, biomarkers of 207t
    distal interphalangeal 198f,
        199, 200f
    manifestations 216
    metacarpophalangeal 91, 91f
    metatarsophalangeal 91, 222
    pain 105
    proximal interphalangeal 105f,
        200f, 222
    sacroiliac 201
    swelling 177

K

Kaposi-Irgang disease 41
Kartagener's syndrome 240
Kasukawa criteria 135
Kawasaki disease 265, 266, 266f,
    266fc, 267, 271
Kawasaki syndrome 266
Keratinocytes, necrotic 15f, 16f
Keratitis, stromal 35
Keratoconjunctivitis sicca 150, 224
Keratoderma blennorhagicum
    214, 214f
Keratopathy, superficial punctate
    35
Keratotic papules 215f
Kidney 91
    biopsy 64f
Kikuchi's disease 178
Kikuchi-Fujimoto disease 246
Koebner's phenomenon 30f, 32,
    59, 128
Kraurosis vulvae 129

L

Labia majora 214
Lacrimal functional unit 159
Lactation 227
Lambda and Panda patterns 180
Lansoprazole 28
Latent tuberculosis, reactivation
    of 228
Leeds enthesitis index 202
Leflunomide 28, 185, 207, 208,
    227
Leishmaniasis, cutaneous 178
Lennert's disease 178
Leonine facies 320
Leprosy lesions, all types of 178
Lesions 4
    biopsy of 249
Lethal midline granuloma 178
Leukemia 240
    acute myelogenous 236
    acute myeloid 242f
Leukocytes, polymorphonuclear
    305
Leukocytoclasis 294
Leukocytoclastic vasculitis 62f,
    136, 268, 269f, 292
    drug-induced 298

Leukonychia striata 33
Leukopenia 56, 57, 134, 138, 158
Lichen myxedematosus 141
Lichen planopilaris 263
Lichen planus 45, 128
    hypertrophic 37
    oral 37f
Lichen sclerosus 17, 17f
    et atrophicus 128, 128b, 129f,
        130f
    genital 129f, 130f
    plaques 128f
Lichenoid 175
    sarcoidosis 174
Light eruption, polymorphous
    43, 45
Limb length discrepancy 125
Lip dryness 156f
Lipodermatosclerosis 128, 130,
    131, 131f, 141
Livedo annularis 7
Livedo racemosa 7, 265f
Livedo reticularis 7, 136, 224,
    224f, 249, 249f, 251, 251f, 257
    causes of 251t
    treatment of 8, 257
    varieties of 8b
Livedoid vasculopathy 8f, 249,
    253, 254, 254f, 265f
    histopathology of 250f
Liver 154, 169
    function test 229
    involvement 183
Löfgren's syndrome 176t, 177, 183
Lower eyelid retraction 94f
L-tryptophan-induced
    eosinophilia-myalgia
    syndrome 141
Lung 154, 169
    cysts 240
    diffusing capacity of 106, 112
    disease, end-stage 179
    parenchyma, bilateral 277f
    sarcoidosis 179t
        parenchymal 183
    transplantation 112, 112t
Lupus anticoagulant assay 64
Lupus erythematosus 11, 12, 12f,
    13f, 14, 26, 35, 141, 233, 263
    acute 57, 59, 60f, 62
    cutaneous 26, 65

bullous 14
chilblain 14, 40, 40f, 61f
chronic cutaneous 26, 29, 30f, 39, 41f, 49f, 50, 57
classical discoid 29, 32f, 33f, 37f
cutaneous 11, 26, 27, 50
disease, subcutaneous 56
disseminated discoid 31
drug-induced 14, 63
erythematous chronic cutaneous 34f
extensive scalp discoid 33f
hemorrhagicus 35
lesion
   discoid chronic cutaneous 62f
   hypertrophic discoid 36f
hypertrophic discoid 36f
lichenoid discoid 40
linear discoid 32f
lip discoid 36f
lymphomatoid 14
mucosal discoid 37f
mucous membrane discoid 35
plaque
   hyperkeratotic chronic cutaneous 39f
   hyperkeratotic discoid 30f
   psoriasiform discoid 30f
profundus 35f, 41
rash
   generalized acute 58f, 59f
   maculopapular acute 59f
   psoriasiform subacute cutaneous 44f
   unilateral discoid 36f
scalp discoid 32f, 33f
specific skin diseases, classification of 26b
subacute 57
tumidus 29, 41, 43
ulcerated discoid 35f
uncommon cutaneous presentations of 14
vermiculatus 35f
verrucous chronic cutaneous 39f
Lupus hair 61f
Lupus nephritis 56
   management of 65fc

Lupus panniculitis 41
Lupus pernio 172f, 175
Lupus planus 40
Lupus pneumonitis, acute 57
Lupus profundus 13, 13f, 42f
   plaques 42f
Lupus tumidus 43f, 104f
Lupus vulgaris 37
Lymph nodes 168, 178
   extrathoracic 169
   intrathoracic 169
   para-aortic 181f
   peripheral 169
Lymphadenopathy 134, 135, 138, 154, 179
Lymphocytes 15f
   karyorrhexis of 12, 13f
Lymphocytic infiltrates, diffuse 13
Lymphoma 157, 158, 158b, 159, 178, 245
Lymphopenia 56, 57, 138
Lymphoproliferative disorders 189

M

Maastricht Ankylosing Spondylitis Enthesitis Score 202
Macrophage
   colony-stimulating factor 207
   inflammatory protein 1-alpha 167
   protein, natural resistance associated 166
Macular atrophic scarring 169
Macular erythema 74
Macular skin lesions, erythematous 284f
Macular violaceous erythema 75f, 76f, 79f
   confluent 74, 75f
Maculopapular pseudourticarial lesion 284f
Maculopapules 175
Magnetic resonance imaging 56, 66, 82, 126, 180, 200, 217, 225, 278, 308
Major histocompatibility complex 166, 168f

Malar rash 11, 12, 58, 58f, 134, 136, 137f
Mander enthesitis index 202
Mandibular condylosis, bilateral 100
Mannose-binding lectin 296
Measles, mumps, and rubella 118
Mechanics hand 74, 75f
Melanophages, dermal 15f
Melorheostosis, linear 128, 131
Metabolic syndrome 205
Metachromasia 143
Methadone 131
Methimazole 298
Methotrexate 86, 110, 127, 185, 207, 208, 226, 227, 230, 246, 270
   therapy 223
Methylenetetrahydrofolate reductase mutation 257
Methylprednisolone 65
   intravenous pulse of 85
Methysergide 140
Miescher's radial granulomas 236
Mikulicz's syndrome 176
Minocycline 114, 185, 298
Mixed connective tissue disease 22, 23, 134, 135, 135t, 136, 136b, 136f, 137f, 150
Mixed cryoglobulinemic vasculitis, noninfectious 193
Mohs micrographic surgery 131
Moll and Wright diagnostic criteria 204
Monoarthritis 177
Monoclonal gammopathy 145, 240
Mononeuritis multiplex 224, 280, 284
Mononucleosis, infectious 178
Morbidity 279
Morphea 16, 16f, 118, 128, 144
   associations of 125b
   bullous 119, 123
   clinical types of 118
   deep 119, 120
   en plaque 119, 120f
   extensive 122f

Index

frontoparietal 119
generalized 119, 123, 127
keloidal 119, 124
linear 119, 121, 121f, 124f
  limb 121, 127
mixed 119, 124
nodular 119, 124
over extremities 125
plaque 119
  multiple large 123f
prevalence of 124
profundus 119, 120
radiation-induced 128, 131
subcutaneous 119
superficial 119, 123, 123f
Morpheaform skin
  disorders 128
  lesions 128b
Moth-eaten appearance 74f
Mouth
  dryness of 21, 155, 155f, 160
  ulcer 320
Mucinoses 140
Mucinous nevus 141
Muckle-Wells syndrome 128, 313
Mucocutaneous disease 308
Mucocutaneous index 308
Mucocutaneous ocular syndrome 301
Multicentric reticulohistiocytosis 312, 320, 320b
  lesions 320f, 321f
Multisystem collagen vascular disorder 68
Multisystem disease, idiopathic 131
Muscle
  biopsy 82, 87
  enzymes 81
  fibers, degeneration of 83f
  histopathology of 83f
  imaging 83
  involvement 77
  testing, manual 78
  weakness 105, 125, 135
Myalgia 125
Myasthenia gravis 125
Mycobacteria
  atypical 166
  cell-wall deficient 166

Mycobacteriosis, atypical 178
Mycobacterium tuberculosis 165, 166
Mycophenolate 65, 270
  mofetil 48, 49, 86, 111, 127, 162, 163, 185
Mycoplasma 166, 178
Mycosis fungoides 45
  granulomatous 178
Myelofibrosis 240
Myeloma 240
Myeloperoxidase 24
Myeloproliferative disease 240
Myelosuppression 227
Myocarditis 57, 224
Myopathy 183
  idiopathic inflammatory 68, 73
Myositis 80, 135t, 136b, 137, 155, 183
Myxedema
  generalized 141
  pretibial 141
Myxomas 255
Myxosarcoma 141

N

Nail 60
  changes 216f
  dystrophy, psoriatic 205
Naproxen 28
Nasal
  cavity 172f
  inflammation 275
  mucosa 170
  philtrum 172f
  septum perforation 35
Nausea 227, 228
Necrobiosis lipoidica 173f, 178
Neodymium-doped yttrium aluminum garnet 162
Neoplasia 178
Nephritis, treatment for 65
Nephrocalcinosis 177
Nephrotic syndrome 56
Nervous system 56
  disorders of 106
Neuralgia, trigeminal 156
Neurofibroma 141
Neuromyotoxicity 227
Neuromyxoma 141

Neurosarcoidosis 183
Neutrophils 217f, 246f
New York Heart Association 226
Nodular episcleritis 307f
Nodular skin lesions 281f
Nodules 175
  multiple cavitating 276f
  pulmonary 23, 224, 227
  subcutaneous 18, 227
Non-Hodgkin's lymphoma 178t, 240b, 245b
Non-human leukocyte antigen 166
  candidate gene 166, 166t
Nonsteroidal anti-inflammatory drugs 28, 163, 207, 217, 218, 236, 308, 314, 316, 317
Nuclear antigens, extractable 22, 23

O

Obesity 66
Ocular disease, anterior 183
Olecranon 223
Oligoarthritis 177, 205
  asymmetric 201
Onycholysis, distal subungual 199f
Opioids 131
Optic nerve involvement 176
Orbit 176
  pseudotumor of 277f
Organ system 106, 224
Osler-Rendu-Weber disease 7
Osteoarthritis 240
Osteomyelitis, sterile chronic multifocal 240
Osteopenia 224
  periarticular 200f, 225f
Osteoporosis 48, 125, 224
Otitis media, chronic 23
Ovaries 169
Overlap diseases 158

P

Pachymeningitis 224
Paclitaxel 28
Pain 201
  abdominal 57
Painful oral lesions 303

Palisaded neutrophilic
   granulomatous dermatitis
   18, 245, 245f, 312, 317
Palmar erythema 224
Palmoplantar pustulosis 314
Palpable purpura 2, 2f, 190f
Pan sclerotic morphea 124f
Panda pattern 180
Panniculitis 13, 42f, 43
   eosinophilic 269f
   granulomatous 157
   lymphocytic 13
   subcutaneous 14
   traumatic 43
Papillary dermal melanophages 16f
Papular lesion 146f
Papular mucinosis 141
Papules 175
   purpuric 284f
Papulopustular lesions 304
Paraffin implant 131
Parakeratosis 13f, 15f, 217f
Paraneoplastic syndrome 304
Paraprotein, types of 147t
Paraproteinemia 142
Parenchymal nodules, bilateral 181f
Parotid enlargement, persistent 158
Parotid gland 169
   enlargement 161
   swelling 154
   tumors 159
Parry-Romberg syndrome 121, 123, 123f
Partial thromboplastin time 5
Parvovirus B19 246
Patient activity scale 230
Pawnbroker's sign 179
Peanut dust 166
Peau D'orange appearance 142
Pedal edema 103
   bilateral 168
Pediatric Rheumatology
   European Society Criteria 295
Pediatric Rheumatology
   International Trials
   Organisation 295

Pemphigoid, bullous 62
Pemphigus erythematosus 59
Pencil in cup deformity 200f
Penicillamine 110
Penile lichen sclerosis 129
Pentazocine 131
Pentoxifylline 185
Periadnexal lymphocytic
   infiltrate 12f
Periarteritis nodosa 245
Pericarditis 57, 78, 135, 138, 224
Periempolesis 14
Perinuclear antineutrophil
   cytoplasmic antibody 305
Periodic acid-Schiff stain 12, 12f
Periodic fever syndromes 312, 313
Periostitis 197
Peripheral nervous system 56, 155, 165, 278
Peripheral neuropathy 125, 191, 224
   therapy of 193
Peristomal pyoderma
   gangrenosum 242
Periungual calcinosis cutis,
   severe 76f
Petechia 2
Petechial spots 4f
Pheniramine 28
Phenylketonuria 140
Phenytoin 28
Phosphodiesterase inhibitors 110
Phospholipid syndrome 240
Photosensitivity 84, 136, 227
Phototherapy 126, 127, 219
Pine pollens 166
Pinkus follicular mucinoses 141
Piroxicam 28
Pityriasis
   rosea 45
   rubra pilaris 45
   versicolor 263
Plaques 175
   erythematous edematous 237f
   erythematous painful 33f
   psoriasis, severe chronic 197f
   psoriatic 199f
Plasma exchange 279
Plasmapheresis 86

Platelet
   dysfunction 5
   function, disorders of 5
Pleurisy 224
Pleuritis 57, 135
Pleuropericarditis 245
Pneumoconiosis 178
Pneumocystis jirovecii 178, 280
Pneumonia, chronic interstitial 178
Pneumonitis 227
   hypersensitivity 178
   lymphocytic interstitial 156, 162
   nonspecific interstitial 156, 162
Poikiloderma 76f
   atrophicans vasculare 74
Poikilodermatous patch 7f
Polyangiitis 24, 267, 268, 268f, 269, 270, 274, 274b, 275f-278f, 281f, 282, 282b, 284f-286f
   microscopic 24, 252, 267, 269, 270, 280, 280b, 282, 292
Polyarteritis nodosa 157, 252, 263, 264, 270, 304
   cutaneous 264, 265f
Polyarthralgias 21
Polyarthritis 135, 245
Polychondritis 319f, 320f
   relapsing 240, 312, 318, 318b
Polycyclic erythematous plaques 45f
Polycythemia vera 240
Polymyositis 68, 135
   classification of 68, 68t
Polyneuropathy, organomegaly,
   endocrinopathy, monoclonal
   gammopathy, and skin
   changes 140, 141, 147
Porphyria cutanea tarda 128, 131, 140
Potassium iodide 239
   oral 236
Pravastatin 28
Prazosin 9
Pregnancy 227, 236
Premature ageing syndromes 140
Prepuce 129

Proline-serine-threonine
    phosphatase interacting
    protein 1 313
Propionibacterium acnes 165,
    166
Propylthiouracil 298
Prostacyclins 109
Prostanoids 109
Prostate 169
    adenocarcinoma 245
Proteins 158
    major basic 123
Proteinuria 56
    nephritic 280
Proton pump inhibitors 114
Pseudofolliculitis 304
Pseudolymphoma 43
Pseudoscleroderma 144
    causes of 140*t*
Pseudoxanthoma elasticum 5
Psoralen 111, 207
Psoriasiform 175
    sarcoidosis 174
Psoriasis 37, 45, 125, 205, 207*t*,
    263
    and arthritis screening
        questionnaire 205
    assessment of 204
    epidemiology screening tool
        205
    evidence of 205
    scalp 198*f*
Psoriatic arthritis 195, 197, 197*b*,
    198, 198*f*, 200*f*, 203, 204,
    204*t*-207*t*, 209, 240
    associations of 205*b*
    classification of 204, 205*t*
    mutilans 202, 203*f*
    screening and evaluation tool
        205
Psychosis 48
Puffy fingers 134, 136*f*
Pulmonary function test 102,
    106, 112, 113, 162
Pulmonary sarcoidosis 172*f*,
    174*f*, 175*f*, 180*f*
    classic features of 181*t*
Pulse therapy 107
Pure red cell aplasia 224
Purkinje's system 177
Purpura 2, 4, 4*b*, 158, 224

clinical features of 4
extravascular causes of 3*t*
intravascular causes of 3*t*
vascular causes of 3, 3*t*
Purpuric lesions 2
Pustular lesion, recurrent 306*f*
Pustular pyoderma gangrenosum
    241
Pyoderma gangrenosum 18, 224,
    240, 240*b*, 241*f*, 242, 242*f*, 243,
    243*f*, 243*t*, 244, 262, 263*f*
    bullous 242
    extensive vegetative 242*f*
    hemorrhagic bullous 242*f*
    lesion 240*f*
    superficial
        granulomatous type of 263*f*
        vegetative 242*f*
    ulcer healing 241*f*
Pyogenic arthritis, 240
    pyoderma gangrenosum and
        acne syndrome 312, 313

R

Radiation 159
    dermatitis 6
Radio imaging studies 178
Radiodermatitis 141
Ranitidine 28
Rash 227, 229
    discoid 31*f*, 58*f*
    erythematosus 265
    facial 59*f*
    subactute cutaneous 136
    urticarial 157, 313
Raynaud's disease 136
Raynaud's phenomenon 7-9, 21,
    73, 90, 93, 101, 107, 109, 125,
    134-136, 138, 141, 146, 224,
    245
    causes of 9*b*
    management of 109
    presence of 118
    severe 98
Raynaud's syndrome 263
Red blood cells, extravasation
    of 294*f*
Reiter's disease 213
Renal disease 56, 64
    end-stage 56
Renal failure, chronic 56

Renal function tests 147
Reproductive organs 169
Respiratory tract infection, viral
    upper 295
Reticular dermis 46
Reticular erythematous
    mucinosis 141
Reticulate erythema 255*f*
Retiform purpura 253
Retina 176
Retinal damage, irreversible 227
Retinitis 78
Retinoids 236
    oral 49
    topical 47
Retrovirus 166
Rheumatism
    fibroblastic 141
    palindromic 21
Rheumatoid arthritis 18, 21, 134,
    143, 150, 195, 221, 233, 240,
    245, 251, 252, 317
    diagnosis of 20
    disease activity 230*t*
    extra-articular manifestations
        of 224*t*
Rheumatoid factor 20, 21, 135,
    223, 225, 278
    prevalence of 21*t*
Rheumatoid necrobiosis,
    superficial ulcerating 245
Rheumatoid nodules 18, 178,
    222*f*, 223, 224
    classical 18
Rheumatoid papules 245, 317
Rheumatoid vasculitis 18
Rheumatologic disease 240
    dermatopathology of 11
Rheumatologic disorders 1, 2, 11,
    20, 233, 312, 312*b*
Rhinorrhea 239
Ribonucleic acid, cytoplasmic
    158
Ribonucleoproteins 22, 23, 158
Rickettsia helvetica 166
Rifampicin 298
Rituximab 49, 112, 185, 229, 270,
    279
Rocker-bottom foot 223
Rodnan skin scoring, modified
    93

Rope sign 318
Rowell syndrome 60, 62f
Rupioid keratotic plaques 215f

S

Saddle nose deformity 276, 320f
Salivary gland ultrasound 159
Salt and pepper
  depigmentation 97f
  pigmentary anomaly 95f, 96f
Sarcoidosis 37, 131, 165, 166t, 167b, 167t, 168, 169t, 171, 173f, 177, 178t, 179t, 181f, 183b, 184fc, 186, 240, 245, 304
  acute 169, 169t, 177
  angiolupoid 173f
  cardiac 183
  case control etiologic study of 165
  causes of 165
  chronic 169, 169t
  clinicopathological differential diagnosis of 178t
  cutaneous 168, 175, 175t
  hypopigmented 174
  ichthyosiform cutaneous 173f
  immunopathophysiology of 168f
  lesion
    papular 170f
    papulomacular 170f
    polymorphous 171f
    subcutaneous 172f
  maculopapular 169
  morpheaform 128, 131
  ocular 176t
  pattern of 167t
  plaque 171f
  psoriasiform 174
  subcutaneous 43, 172f, 175
  symptomatic pulmonary 183
  syndromes of 176
  systemic 175
  treatment of 185t
  tumoral 171
Scars
  digital pitted 91, 92f
  extensive hypertrophic 243f
  ischemic 92f
  pitted 98f
  post-traumatic 173f
  sarcoidosis 173f, 175
Schaumann's inclusion bodies 177
Schistosomiasis 178
Schulman's syndrome 17
Scleredema 140, 141, 142f, 143f, 144
  differential diagnosis of 144t
  rule out 147
Scleritis 205, 224
  necrotizing 277f
Sclerodactyly 7, 21, 90, 91, 92f, 118, 134, 135, 136
Scleroderma 9, 16, 17f, 78, 89, 108, 135, 136, 138
  linear 124
  localized 16, 124
  proximal 91
  renal crisis 105, 107
Sclerodermatomyositis 79, 80f
Scleroedema 143
Sclerokeratitis, necrotizing 240
Scleromalacia 224
  perforans 277
Scleromyxedema 140, 141, 144–146, 146f, 147f, 148
  classification of 146b
Sclerosing panniculitis 130
Sclerosis 17, 128, 131, 140
  causes of 144
  central 120f
  multiple 125, 245
Sclerotic septal panniculitis 16
Secondary calcinosis cutis 101f
Sectoral episcleritis 307f
Seizures 48
Selective serotonin reuptake inhibitor 163
Sensory neuropathy 106
Serologic tests 5, 135
Shawl sign 74, 75f
Shuster's sign 32f
Sialoadenitis, focal lymphocytic 152
Sicca syndrome 136
Sickle cell anemia 255
Sildenafil 9, 110
Silica dust 140
Silicone 131

Simplified disease activity index 230t
Simvastatin 28
Sinus computed tomography 285f
Sinusitis 285f
  chronic 23, 275
Six-minute walk test 325
Sjögren's syndrome 19, 21, 22, 106, 136, 143, 144, 150, 156f, 157, 162, 189, 233, 234, 245
  extraglandular versus exocrine predominant 150
  primary 150, 151f, 154t, 157, 157b
  secondary 150
Skin 91, 93, 119t, 136, 154, 157, 169, 223, 233, 262, 277, 303
  binding 107
  down of 110
  biopsy 5, 11, 82, 107, 216, 235, 235f, 238, 239f, 246f, 259, 285, 318, 321
  dry 157
  induration 118
  involvement 168
  lesions 157b, 182, 190, 303, 316
    basic 2
    diagnosis of 178
    erythematous edematous 313
    lupus specific 11
    nonvasculitic 269, 270, 270b
    ulcerative 281f
  manifestations 267, 312
  over face, tightening of 94f
  pigmentation 227
  rash 136
  small vessel vasculitis of 292, 293f, 294f
  ulcer, vasculopathic 80f
Slender fibrocytes 46
Sneddon syndrome 253
Soft tissue swelling 225f
Sonography 106
Spinal cord 155
Spine 223
Spleen 169
Spondylitis 201, 240
  clinical features of 201

Index

Spondyloarthritides 197
Spondyloarthropathy 213
Squamous cell carcinoma 17, 38, 39, 39f, 40, 125
  transformation 130f
Stanozolol 8, 257
Stem cell
  therapy 185
  transplantation 107, 108
Steroid 57
  injection, intralesional 126
  myopathy 87b
  pulse therapy 107
  sparing immunosuppressive agents 239
  drugs 244
  systemic 127, 236
  topical 126, 130, 160, 183
Stevens-Johnson syndrome 45
Stiff skin syndrome 140, 312, 322, 322b
Still's disease 19, 312, 315, 316
  adult-onset 19, 316
Stomach 105
Stratum corneum 217f
Streptococcal infection 245b
Streptococcal pharyngitis 295
Subacute cutaneous lupus erythematosus 12f, 26, 41f, 43, 45f, 46, 46t, 49fc
  pathogenesis of 27fc
Subepidermal clefts 12f
Submandibular gland swelling 154
Sudeck's dystrophy 141
Sulfa drugs 244
Sulfasalazine 207, 208, 227, 244
Superficial dermal
  dense neutrophilic infiltrate 263f
  small vessels, prominent fibrinoid necrosis of 269f
Swan neck deformity 222f
Sweet's syndrome 18, 236, 237f, 238, 238t, 304, 314
  classical 236-238
  drug-induced 236, 238
  etiology of 236t
  histiocytoid 238
  solitary lesion of 237f
  subcutaneous 238

Swollen
  fingers 135, 136
  hands 135
  joint count 230
Symblepharon 35
Symmetrical additive inflammatory small joint polyarthritis 275
Sympathectomy 110
Syncope, exertional near 103
Synovial fluid 305
  analysis of 206
Synovitis, acne, pustulosis, hyperostosis and osteitis syndrome 312, 314
Systemic amyloidosis, primary 140
Systemic lupus erythematosus 10, 21, 22, 23, 26, 41f, 55-57, 59f, 60f, 64b, 125, 128, 134, 135, 240, 245, 251, 253, 304, 317
  bullous 62f
  classification criteria 55
  diagnosis of 64
  disease activity index 66
  lesion 63f
  neuropsychiatric 56
  vasculitis of 252
Systemic sclerosis 6, 8f, 10, 10f, 16, 23, 89, 92f, 94f, 95f, 97f, 98, 98f, 99f-101f, 103t-107f, 111t-113t, 114, 118, 128, 144, 233, 245
  diffuse cutaneous 91, 91t
  fingers of 100f
  localized cutaneous 91
  management of 106
  pathogenesis of 89
  prevalence of 89
  pulmonary manifestations of 102
  treatment of 107
Systemic therapy 47, 85, 244

T

Tacrolimus ointment, topical 126
Tadalafil 9
Takayasu's aortitis 245, 262, 263f, 270

Takayasu's arteritis, dermatologic manifestations of 263t
Takayasu's syndrome 240
Tamoxifen 28
Tattooing 178
T-cell 55
  activation 166t
  expression, normal 167
  lymphoma 14, 43
    cutaneous 141
Tears, artificial 160
Telangiectasia 6, 7, 7f, 74f, 90, 136
  causes of 6b
  dermal 12f
  hereditary hemorrhagic 6
  matt-like 6f, 97f
  nail-fold 6
  periungual 73, 74f
  primary 6
  secondary 6
  spider 7
Telmisartan 9
Tendon
  bombe-shaped aspect of 202
  sheaths, synovial proliferation of 222
Tendonitis 105
Tenosynovitis 177
Terbinafine 28
Testis 169
Tetanus 118
Texier's disease 131
Thalidomide 185, 244
Throat culture 235
Thrombocytopenia 5, 135, 183, 227
  essential 240
  mild 56
Thrombocytosis 5, 224, 281
Thrombosis 253
Thrombotic thrombocytopenic purpura 245
Thyroid 155
Thyroiditis 125
  autoimmune 159, 245
Tinea incognito 37
Tocilizumab 229
Toluidine blue 144
Tongue, severe 156f

Tophi 316
Topical therapy 47, 85, 243
Toronto psoriatic arthritis screen 205
Total lung capacity 113
Toxic epidermal necrolysis 45, 59f
Toxic oil syndrome 128, 140, 141
Toxoplasmosis 178
Transbronchial lung biopsy, bronchoscopy guided 178
Transforming growth factor 90, 167
Transmural inflammation 269f
Triaditis, mild 191
Trichinosis 144
Tuberculin skin test 229, 235
Tuberculosis 178, 236
  infections like 159
Tumor 141
  mesenchymal 141
  necrosis factor 206, 207, 218
    alpha 69, 166, 167, 197, 213, 244, 309, 312
    receptor associated periodic syndrome 313
  neural 141
  solid 236

U

Ulcer 59f, 250
  cutaneous 101f, 190f
  digital 109
  genital 303, 320
  healing 254f
  ischemic 100f, 125f
  mucosal 276f
  oral 227
  over lower leg 214f
  recurrent painful nonhealing 259
  superficial 4f
    retiform necrotic 8f
Ulcerative nodular cutaneous polyarteritis nodosa lesions 259f

Ultrasound 106
Ultraviolet
  A 207
  B 28
  light 28
Upper respiratory tract 236
Urethritis, inflammatory noninfective 205
Urinary abnormalities 56
Urticaria 43, 141, 313, 313t
Ustekinumab 185
Uterus 169
Uveitis 205, 224, 315f

V

Valsartan 9
van Bijsterveld's scoring system 152
Vaquez disease 240
Vascular endothelial growth factor 166
Vasculitic disorder 260
  classification of 261f
Vasculitic lesion 190f
Vasculitic purpura 157
Vasculitides
  classification of 260
  systemic 274
Vasculitis 106, 155, 157, 224, 245, 252, 269, 292
  cryoglobulinemic 189
  cutaneous 224, 268, 268f
    leukocytoclastic 292
    small vessel 2f, 4f
  drug-induced 292, 298
  renal 191
  small vessel 292, 293f, 294f
  systemic 157, 245
  urticarial 43
Vasculopathy, digital 109
Venereal Disease Research Laboratories 5
Vesicle, biopsy of 14
Vessel
  vasculitides 259
  wall disorders 256

Vibration disease 141
Vinca alkaloids 140
Vinyl chloride 140
Violaceous erythematous granulomatous swelling 172
Violaceous papular sarcoidosis lesions 172
Viscera, abdominal 176
Vitamin
  B12 118
  D
    analogue 126
    receptor 166
    supplementation 87
  K injections 118
  K1, oil-soluble 131
Vitiligo 125
Vulvitis 214

W

Waldenstrom's macroglobulinemia 143
Warts, viral 263
Watermelon stomach 105
Wegener's granulomatosis 24, 38, 178, 240, 245, 252, 274, 292, 304, 317
Weight loss 183, 227, 275
Werner's syndrome 140
Wheezing 175
Wickham's striae 37f
Winchester syndrome 128, 140
Wrinkles, loss of 147f
Wrists joint 222

X

Xeroderma 157
Xerostomia 154

Z

Zirconium 166, 178
Zosteriform morphea 119, 124

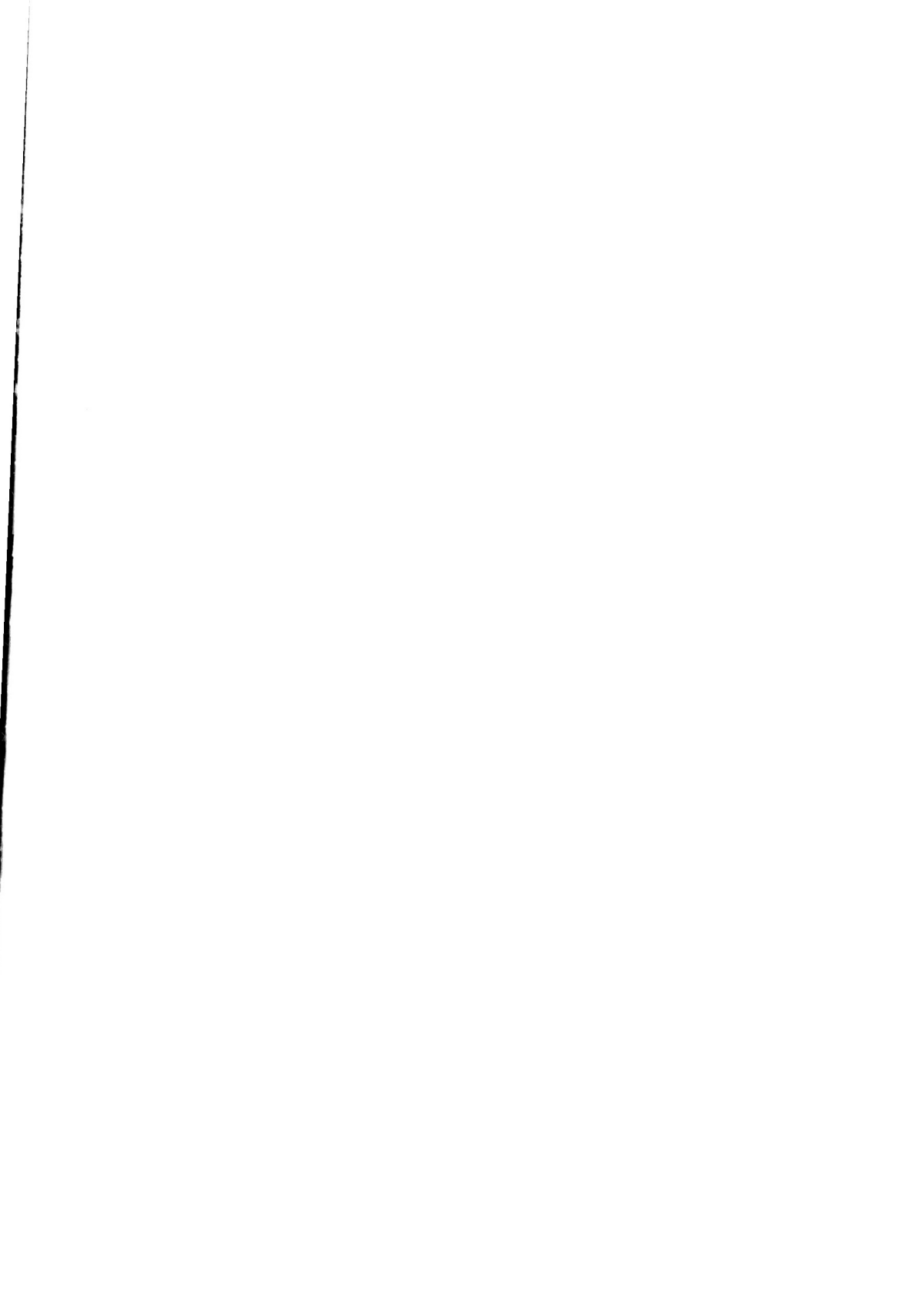

EU GSPR Authorised Reprsentative
Logos Europe, 9 rue Nicolas Poussin
1700, La Rochelle, France
Phone: +33 (0) 6 67 93 73 78
E-mail: contact@logoseurope.eu

www.ingramcontent.com/pod-product-compliance
Ingram Content Group UK Ltd.
Pitfield, Milton Keynes, MK11 3LW, UK
UKHW061147270326
469420UK00003B/13